MCGRAW-HILL
ONLINE RESOURCES

IMPORTANT:

HERE IS YOUR REGISTRATION CODE TO ACCESS
YOUR PREMIUM McGRAW-HILL ONLINE RESOURCES.

For key premium online resources you need THIS CODE to gain access. Once the code is entered, you will be able to use the Web resources for the length of your course.

If your course is using **WebCT** or **Blackboard**, you'll be able to use this code to access the McGraw-Hill content within your instructor's online course.

Access is provided if you have purchased a new book. If the registration code is missing from this book, the registration screen on our Website, and within your WebCT or Blackboard course, will tell you how to obtain your new code.

Registering for McGraw-Hill Online Resources

TO gain access to your MCGRaw-Hill web resources simply follow the steps below:

1. USE YOUR WEB BROWSER TO GO TO: **http://www.mhhe.com/hahn7e**

2. CLICK ON **FIRST TIME USER**.

3. ENTER THE REGISTRATION CODE* PRINTED ON THE TEAR-OFF BOOKMARK ON THE RIGHT.

4. AFTER YOU HAVE ENTERED YOUR REGISTRATION CODE, CLICK **REGISTER**.

5. FOLLOW THE INSTRUCTIONS TO SET-UP YOUR PERSONAL UserID AND PASSWORD.

6. WRITE YOUR UserID AND PASSWORD DOWN FOR FUTURE REFERENCE.
KEEP IT IN A SAFE PLACE.

TO GAIN ACCESS to the McGraw-Hill content in your instructor's **WebCT** or **Blackboard** course simply log in to the course with the UserID and Password provided by your instructor. Enter the registration code exactly as it appears in the box to the right when prompted by the system. You will only need to use the code the first time you click on McGraw-Hill content.

Thank you, and welcome to your MCGRaw-Hill online Resources!

* YOUR REGISTRATION CODE CAN BE USED ONLY ONCE TO ESTABLISH ACCESS. IT IS NOT TRANSFERABLE.
0-07-297387-0 T/A HAHN: FOCUS ON HEALTH, 7E

REGISTRATION CODE

TJF6-35EJ-RPN6-7NQ6-W8SE

Learning to Go:HEALTH

Welcome to Learning to Go: Health!

Learning to Go: Health is an Internet-based learning reinforcement system that delivers fun, interactive lessons to help you retain and practice what you learn in your Personal Health course.

Each lesson includes 3 action steps that will help you boost your retention of one core skill – reinforced through quizzes, exercises, tips, and web links. Each lesson takes 10 to 15 minutes.

YOU choose when you want your lessons to arrive, and they are pushed to your browser at that time each day or week. Each bite-sized lesson puts the skills to work for you – and helps you build the habits of success.

STUDY TODAY'S PRINCIPLE IN-DEPTH

Learning to Go: Health is provided in addition to the premium content resources located on your text's Online Learning Center.

To register:

- Go to the Online Learning Center that accompanies this book (the URL is listed on the back cover or inside cover of the text).

- Select the Register Link.

- Follow the registration instructions, which indicate where you'll need to enter your password/ registration code.

- Once you're registered, you'll receive instructions for how to download and install Learning to Go: Health to your PC.

- Access is provided if you have purchased a new book. This code may be used only once. If you have purchased a used book, select the Register Link and then click on the link for used book owners.

P/N 292078-5

Your Learning To Go: Health password/registration code is:

8gs4t-s2wdb-573pa

focus on health

focus on health

Seventh Edition

Dale B. Hahn, Ph.D.

Wayne A. Payne, Ed.D.

Ellen B. Mauer, Ph.D.

All of Ball State University
Muncie, Indiana

Boston   Burr Ridge, IL   Dubuque, IA   Madison, WI   New York   San Francisco   St. Louis
Bangkok   Bogotá   Caracas   Kuala Lumpur   Lisbon   London   Madrid   Mexico City
Milan   Montreal   New Delhi   Santiago   Seoul   Singapore   Sydney   Taipei   Toronto

To all of our students, with the hope that the decisions they make will be healthy ones.

The McGraw-Hill Companies

 Higher Education

FOCUS ON HEALTH
Published by McGraw-Hill, a business unit of The McGraw-Hill Companies, Inc., 1221 Avenue of the Americas, New York, NY 10020. Copyright © 2005, 2003, 2001, 1999, 1997, 1994, 1991, by The McGraw-Hill Companies, Inc. All rights reserved. No part of this publication may be reproduced or distributed in any form or by any means, or stored in a database or retrieval system, without the prior written consent of The McGraw-Hill Companies, Inc., including, but not limited to, in any network or other electronic storage or transmission, or broadcast for distance learning.
Some ancillaries, including electronic and print components, may not be available to customers outside the United States.

This book is printed on acid-free paper.

1 2 3 4 5 6 7 8 9 0 DOW/DOW 0 9 8 7 6 5 4

ISBN 0-07-284415-9

Vice president and editor-in-chief: *Emily Barrosse*
Publisher: *William Glass*
Sponsoring editor: *Nicholas Barrett*
Director of development: *Kate Engelberg*
Developmental editor: *Ann Kirby-Payne*
Senior marketing manager: *Pamela S. Cooper*
Media producer: *Lance Gerhart*
Project manager: *Jill Moline-Eccher*
Production supervisor: *Janean A. Utley*
Senior designer: *Kim Menning*
Lead media project manager: *Marc Mattson*
Photo research coordinator: *Alexandra Ambrose*
Art editor: *Emma C. Ghiselli*
Manager, photo researcher: *Brian Pecko*
Art director: *Jeanne Schreiber*
Cover design: *Yvo Riezebos*
Interior design: *Jeanne Calabrese*
Typeface: *10.5/12 Minion*
Compositor: *The GTS Companies, Inc.*
Printer: *R.R. Donnelley and Sons Inc.*
Cover image: © *David Madison*

The credits section for this book begins on page C-1 and is considered an extensive of the copyright page.

Library of Congress Cataloging-in-Publication Data
Hahn, Dale B.
    Focus on health / Dale B. Hahn, Wayne A. Payne, Ellen B. Mauer.—7th ed.
        p. cm.
    Includes index.
    ISBN 0-07-284415-9 (softcover : alk. paper)
    1. Health. I. Payne, Wayne A. II. Mauer, Ellen B. III. Title.
RA776.H142 2005
613—dc22
                                                2004045697

www.mhhe.com

learning to go: health

Your online coach for health behavior change

HERE'S HOW IT WORKS

Learning to Go: Health is designed to complement your new McGraw-Hill Personal Health textbook. It uses the Internet and "push technology" to bring lessons that relate to this book directly to your computer. You choose the time of day, and the lessons will automatically appear on your screen. You'll spend 15 minutes a day on one lesson that focuses on a single topic.

This feature is based on the following 4-step system:

1 Core Principle—Focus on one topic per lesson.

2 Lesson Overview—Review more information about that principle to help yourself learn it.

3 Action Steps—Three action steps per lesson help you learn by doing and taking action. Knowledge isn't powerful until you put it into action.

4 Reinforcements—Interact and learn through various means: Quotations, Reality Checks, Health Tips, True or False, Tic-Tac-Toe, and Learn More.

HERE'S HOW TO GET STARTED

- Go to the Online Learning Center for this book at:
  www.mhhe.com/hahn7e
- Click on *Learning to Go: Health*.
- Follow the steps for registration.
- Once you're registered, set your preferences.
- Then you'll be ready for your first lesson!

contents in brief

contents

part one: the mind

part three: preventing drug abuse and addition

part four: preventing diseases

part five: sexuality and reproduction

part six: Consumer and safety issues

preface

As a health educator, you already know that personal health is one of the most exciting courses a college student will take. Today's media-oriented college students are aware of the critical health issues of the new millennium. They hear about environmental issues, substance abuse, sexually transmitted diseases, fitness, and nutrition virtually every day. The value of the personal health course is its potential to expand students' knowledge of these and other health topics. Students will then be able to examine their attitudes toward health issues and modify their behavior to improve their health and perhaps even prevent or delay the onset of certain health conditions.

Focus on Health accomplishes this task with a carefully composed, well-documented text that addresses the health issues most important to both instructors and students. As health educators, we understand the teaching issues you face daily in the classroom and have written this text with your concerns in mind.

We are pleased that this seventh edition of *Focus on Health* has been infused with an exciting new perspective through the major contributions of a third author. Ellen B. Mauer, Ph.D., serves as the Associate Director of the Ball State University Counseling Center. Each academic year she connects with thousands of Ball State students through classroom presentations on her specialty areas of emotional health, stress management, eating disorders, and positive body image. As a licensed psychologist, Dr. Mauer regularly counsels students and also maintains a private clinical practice. For this seventh edition, Dr. Mauer wrote significant revisions for Chapters 2 (Achieving Psychological Health), 3 (Managing Stress), 5 (Understanding Nutrition and Your Diet), and 6 (Maintaining a Healthy Weight). Because of her additions to Chapter 2, we felt it was no longer necessary to include an appendix on mental health, so that element has been taken out of this edition. We are proud to have Dr. Mauer join our team.

Hallmarks of the Text

Several unique themes and features set *Focus on Health* apart from other personal health texts. These successful features continue to define *Focus on Health* in its seventh edition.

A Text for All Students

This book is written for college students in a wide variety of settings, from community colleges to large four-year universities. The content is carefully constructed to be meaningful to both traditional- and nontraditional-age students. We have paid special attention to the increasing numbers of nontraditional-age students (those over age 25) who have decided to pursue a college education. The topics covered in the text often address the particular needs of these nontraditional-age students. *Focus on Health* continues to encourage students of all ages and backgrounds to achieve their goals.

Two Central Themes

Two central themes—the multiple dimensions of health and the developmental tasks—are presented in Chapter 1. Together, these two themes offer students a foundation for understanding their own health and achieving positive behavior change. A helpful illustration (Figure 1-2 on page 13) depicts the role of multidimensional health in the completion of developmental tasks.

Flexible Organization

The seventh edition of *Focus on Health* has seventeen chapters. The first stands alone as an introductory chapter that explains the focus of the book. The arrangement of the remaining chapters follows the recommendations of both the users of previous editions of the book and reviewers for this edition. Of course, professors can choose to cover the chapters in any sequence that suits the needs of their courses.

Wellness and Disease Prevention

Throughout this new edition, students are continually urged to be proactive in shaping their future health. Even the chapter titles invite students to take control of their own health behavior.

Integrated Presentation of Aging

Topics of interest to midlife and older adults are integrated into appropriate chapters according to subject. This organization allows both traditional-age and nontraditional-age students to learn about the physical and emotional changes that take place as we age. Similarly, issues related to death and dying—from considering organ donation to preparing a living will—have been incorporated into relevant chapters.

Timely Coverage of Cancer and Chronic Conditions

Rapid developments in cancer prevention, diagnosis, and treatment warrant a comprehensive chapter on cancer, in which we present the latest research and information. The chapter also includes information on some of the most common chronic conditions.

Technology: The Key to Teaching and Learning

Just a quick glance through the pages of *Focus on Health* shows that technology is woven throughout every chapter, both in the content and in the chapter pedagogy. Similarly, the package of supplements that accompanies the text emphasizes technology while acknowledging that printed materials also have merit. Together, the text and its supplements offer the ideal approach to teaching and learning—one that integrates the best tools that technology has to offer, challenging both instructors and students to reach higher.

Updated Coverage

As experienced health educators and authors, we know how important it is to provide students with the most current information available. The seventh edition of *Focus on Health* has been thoroughly updated with the latest information, statistics, and findings. Throughout each chapter, we have incorporated new examples and discussions, from information on newly available prescription drugs and medications (Chapters 2, 3, 11, and 15), to the latest information on dieting and supplements (Chapters 5, 6, and 15), to recent findings on air quality and health (Chapter 17).

Another exciting change in this edition of *Focus on Health* is the addition of a new Chapter 17, The Environment and Your Health. Prepared by David LeBlanc, Ph.D., Professor of Biology at Ball State University, this chapter presents pertinent information on a variety of environmental factors—ranging from naturally occurring hazards like radon and ultraviolet radiation to human-made problems like water and air pollution—that can adversely affect personal health. Even more importantly, the chapter includes practical advice for protecting oneself from harmful environmental factors and proactive measures for working toward environmental change.

In addition to these topics, we have once again included chapter-ending "As We Go To Press" boxes in relevant chapters. These unique boxes allow us to comment on breaking news right up to press time, ensuring that the most current issues in health are addressed. For example, we discuss changes to fast food menus in response to consumer and government concerns over obesity in Chapter 5, and the controversy over gay marriages in Chapter 13.

New or Expanded Topics

Following is a sampling of topics that are either completely new to this edition or are covered in greater depth than in the previous edition:

Chapter 1: Shaping Your Health

- Chapter introduction revised to more clearly emphasize the costs of failing health
- Prochaska's six stages of change
- Keys to living longer
- Episodic health care

Chapter 2: Achieving Psychological Health

- The Internet and psychological health
- Taking positive steps toward psychological health
- Nonverbal communication
- Self-esteem, self-concept, emotional intelligence, and personality
- Laughter and enhancing psychological health
- Managing conflict
- Learned helplessness and learned optimism
- Treatments and drug therapies for specific disorders
- Mood disorders
- Anxiety disorders

Chapter 3: Managing Stress

- Stress management techniques
- Technology and stress
- Three stages of stress
- Costs and benefits of stress

- Yerkes-Dodson law
- Student stress
- Perfectionism
- Type A and Type B personalities
- Stress in the aftermath of 9/11

Chapter 4: Becoming Physically Fit

- New definitions for exercise, physical activity, and physical fitness
- Health-related physical fitness
- Performance-related physical fitness
- High-intensity aerobic activity
- Benefits of physical activity/aerobic fitness in reducing some health risks
- Muscular fitness and muscular endurance
- Isotonic resistance exercise
- Developing a cardiorespiratory fitness program
- Calculating your target heart rate
- Stretching and flexibility
- Childhood obesity

Chapter 5: Understanding Nutrition and Your Diet

- Artificial sweeteners
- Religious food restrictions
- The importance of fats in satisfying appetite
- Trans fats
- Benefits of fiber
- New figures on current USDA food guidelines vs. the average American diet
- Healthy eating pyramid
- Fast food restaurant choices
- Probiotic products
- Food allergies and food intolerance
- Food safety
- Vegetarianism

Chapter 6: Maintaining a Healthy Weight

- Food and emotions
- The weight loss industry
- Obesity and underweight
- Body dysmorphic disorder
- Lifestyle change for weight management
- Supplements and appetite suppressants, including Phenylpropanolamine (PPA), and dietary supplements, including Ephedrine, Aristolochia Fangchi, Meridia, Orlistat
- Gastric band surgery
- Eating disorders

Chapter 7: Making Decisions About Drug Use

- Gamma-hydroxybutyrate (GHB), also known as liquid ecstasy or Georgia Home Boy
- Ephedra
- Crystal meth
- Ritalin abuse
- Date rape depressants
- Long- and short-term effects of marijuana
- Oxycontin

Chapter 8: Taking Control of Alcohol Use

- Moderate drinking
- Low-carbohydrate beer
- Effects of alcohol by number of drinks
- Hangovers

Chapter 9: Rejecting Tobacco Use

- Tobacco settlement results
- Chippers and part-time smokers
- Genetic influences on nicotine addiction
- Toxic and carcinogenic components of cigarette smoke
- New tobacco/nicotine products: "safe" cigarettes and nontobacco sources of nicotine (nico water, patches, etc.)
- Smoking cessation programs and aids

Chapter 10: Reducing Your Risk of Cardiovascular Disease

- New statistics on hypertension, smoking, diabetes, and overweight/obesity as risk factors for heart disease
- New information on link between estrogen replacement therapy and heart attacks and strokes
- C-reactive protein
- Cholesterol screening and treatments for high cholesterol
- New information on defibrillators and CPR
- Echocardiography
- Diagnostic techniques such as positron emission tomography (PET), electron beam computed tomography (EBCT), and magnetic resonance imaging (MRI)
- Hypertension and pre-hypertension

Chapter 11: Living with Cancer and Chronic Conditions

- Survivability
- Staging cancer and naming conventions for cancers
- Risk factors and treatments

- Hormone replacement therapy and cancer
- Genetic links to cancer
- Tamoxifen
- Thinprep pap test
- Uterine cancer among African American women
- Prostate cancer and overtreatment
- Alternative screening tests for colorectal cancer
- Progress in the "War On Cancer"
- Multiple sclerosis
- Diabetes and obesity
- Reactive and functional hypoglycemia

Chapter 12: Preventing Infectious Diseases

- SARS
- Stem cell research and treatments
- Childhood and adult immunizations
- Pneumococcal infections and vaccine
- Influenza and flu shots
- Passive vs. active immunity
- Hepatitis B infections and immunizations
- New AIDS medications, information on AIDS vaccines
- T cells and B cells
- West Nile virus and Lyme disease
- Sexually transmitted diseases (STDs)

Chapter 13: Understanding Sexuality

- Effects of aging on the male reproductive system
- Female genital mutilation
- Endometriosis
- New Star box on alternatives to hormone replacement therapy
- Link between cancer and hormone replacement therapy discussed
- Roots/causes of hetero/homosexuality
- Gay and lesbian partnerships and the battle over gay marriage
- The challenges bisexuals face
- The mainstreaming of gay culture
- 2003 U.S. Supreme Court ruling striking down Texas sodomy laws
- Cohabitation arrangements vs. marriage

Chapter 14: Managing Your Fertility

- Updated coverage of several forms of birth control, including the contraceptive ring and contraceptive patch, vaginal spermicides, cervical cap, triphasic pills, and IUDs
- Emergency contraception

- Update on abortion laws
- Human cloning
- Intracytoplasmic sperm injection

Chapter 15: Becoming an Informed Health Care Consumer

- Health interests of American youth
- Communicating with physicians
- Primary health care providers
- Acupuncture
- Reflexology
- Herbal supplements and recent FDA efforts to tighten control over their sale and use
- Nursing shortage
- Self-care and when to see a physician
- Medicare and Medicaid
- Prescription drug issues, including prescription vs. over-the-counter drugs, purchasing medications from Canada, costs of research and development, and insurance
- Advance medical directives and living wills
- Organ donation
- Prepaying a funeral

Chapter 16: Protecting Your Safety

- The aftermath of 9/11 terror attacks and subsequent War on Terror
- Domestic/child abuse
- Gun violence
- Guns on campus
- Identity theft
- Watch dogs
- Recreational safety
- Firearm safety
- Motor vehicle safety

Chapter 17: The Environment and Your Health

Topics in this new chapter include:

- Indoor air quality
- Drinking water
- Noise
- Radio frequency radiation
- Air pollution
- Water pollution
- Land pollution
- Loss of green space
- Radiation
- Human population explosion
- Global climate change

- Stratospheric ozone depletion
- Loss of natural habitats and species extinction
- Ecoterrorism
- The high-tech revolution and e-waste

Student-Friendly Chapter Pedagogy

Each chapter of *Focus on Health* is rich with pedagogical features that offer a variety of ways to address new and emerging health issues and to pique student interest in particular topics.

Chapter Objectives

Each chapter begins with a set of clear objectives that help students distill the most important concepts in the pages that follow.

Taking Charge of Your Health

Located at the end of each chapter, these bulleted lists invite students to put the knowledge and information they've gleaned from the chapter to work in their everyday lives. Cross-referencing the text with Internet links and real-world situations allows students to see how what they've learned can be applied in their own lives.

Online Learning Center Resources

Online Learning Center boxes, found on the opening page of each chapter, direct students toward the useful resources available on the Online Learning Center that accompanies this text. These resources include chapter key terms and definitions, student interactive question-and-answer sites, and self-scoring chapter quizzes.

Talking It Over (NEW)

This feature focuses on communication and health issues. It encourages students to begin each chapter by thinking about how they would discuss a specific health topic with their friends, their doctor, or their family. It also prompts them to think about controversial health issues from different viewpoints. Topics vary from how to communicate your sexual needs to your partner to the pros and cons of legalization of marijuana. CommunicationLinks suggest websites that students can explore to learn more about each topic.

Eye on the Media

Face it—a student's world revolves around media of all types, especially the web. Students get most of their health information not from instructors and textbooks, but from television, self-help books, popular news magazines, the web, and the radio. To meet students on this familiar ground, we've included Eye on the Media boxes (see the inside front cover for a list of these boxes), which take a critical look at these media sources of health information.

Discovering Your Spirituality

Spirituality has become an important focus in health courses. Discovering Your Spirituality boxes (see the inside front cover for a list of these boxes) highlight the spiritual dimension of health and its effect on overall wellness. The boxes cover topics such as body image, living well with cancer or a chronic infectious disease, making decisions about sex, and having an enjoyable social life without abusing alcohol or other drugs.

Talking Points

Interspersed throughout each chapter, Talking Points offer students opportunities to explore how they might start a dialogue about specific health-related issues and situations.

Changing for the Better

These unique question-and-answer boxes show students how to put health concepts into practice. Each box begins with a real-life question, followed by helpful tips and practical advice for initiating behavior change and staying motivated to follow a healthy lifestyle.

Health on the Web Behavior Change Activities

Today's computer-savvy students can find reliable health information at their fingertips when they search the world wide web. New activities direct students to important health websites related to the material in each chapter. For each activity, students explore a website and then complete a quiz or self-assessment offered at the site. These activities help students think critically about valuable health information.

HealthQuest Activities

Many chapters contain an activities box to complement the HealthQuest CD-ROM that accompanies the text. These activities allow students to assess their health behavior in each of nine different areas. HealthQuest's exciting graphics and interactive approach will encourage students to learn about topics such as condom use, cancer prevention, and healthy eating behavior as they complete the activities.

Learning from Our Diversity

These boxes expose students to alternative viewpoints and highlight what we can learn from the differences that make us unique. Topics include the Mediterranean Food Pyramid, the male contraceptive pill, and special issues related to infectious disease among older adults.

Focus On . . . Articles

The Focus On articles examine current issues that students are hearing about in today's news, such as genetically modified food, drinking and violence, extreme sports, and job-related illness. These often controversial health-related topics are a perfect starting point for class or group discussions. Because these essays are placed at the end of each chapter, they can be covered or not at the instructor's option.

InfoLinks

InfoLinks boxes placed at the end of many of the Changing for the Better boxes and Focus On . . . articles give students a starting point for exploring health information on the Internet. Log onto the MADD website to learn how to host a party responsibly. Get tips on the most healthful menu choices at ethnic restaurants. Check out helpful advice for preparing for exams and coping with test anxiety. InfoLinks will get students plugged in to the possibilities for learning about health online.

Star Boxes

In each chapter, special material in Star boxes encourages students to delve into a particular topic or closely examine an important health issue.

Personal Assessments

Each chapter contains at least one Personal Assessment inventory. These self-assessment exercises serve three important functions: to capture students' attention, to serve as a basis for introspection and behavior change, and to provide suggestions for carrying the applications further.

Definition Boxes

Key terms are set in boldface type and defined in corresponding boxes. Pronunciation guides are provided where appropriate. Other important terms in the text are set in italics for emphasis. Both approaches facilitate student vocabulary comprehension.

Chapter Summaries

Each chapter concludes with a bulleted summary of key concepts and their significance or application. The student can then return to any topic in the chapter for clarification or study.

Review Questions

A set of questions appears at the end of each chapter to aid the student in review and analysis of chapter content.

Comprehensive Health Assessment

The Comprehensive Health Assessment at the beginning of the book allows students to take a close look at their current state of health, typical health behavior, and risk factors. Using this assessment, students can pinpoint trouble spots in their own health behavior and find out what they can do to reduce their risk of disease or other health conditions. At the end of the semester, they can take a look at their previous answers to see how their behavior changed as they learned more about health and wellness issues.

Health Reference Guide

The updated Health Reference Guide at the back of the book lists many commonly used health resources. Internet addresses, phone numbers, and mailing addresses of various organizations and government agencies are provided as available. The guide is perforated and laminated, making it durable enough for students to keep for later use.

Vegetarian Food Pyramid

Many students now follow or are considering a vegetarian diet. To help them understand how such a diet meets nutrient needs, we have printed a vegetarian food pyramid along with the USDA Food Guide Pyramid in Chapter 5.

Comprehensive Glossary

At the end of the text, all terms defined in boxes, as well as pertinent italicized terms, are merged into a comprehensive glossary.

Supplements

An extensive supplements package is available to qualified adopters to enhance the teaching-learning process. We have made a concerted effort to produce supplements of extraordinary utility and quality. This package has been carefully planned and developed to help instructors derive the greatest benefit from the text. We encourage instructors to examine them carefully. Many of the products can be packaged with the text at a discounted price. Beyond the following brief descriptions, additional information about these supplements is available from your McGraw-Hill sales representative.

Integrated Instructor's Resource CD

Organized by chapter, the Instructor's Resource CD includes resources to help you teach your course. The CD will work in both Windows and Macintosh environments and includes the following elements:

- **Course Integrator Guide** This guide includes all the useful features of an instructor's manual, such as learning objectives, suggested lecture outlines, suggested activities, media resources, and web links. It also integrates the text with all the related resources McGraw-Hill offers, such as the Online Learning Center, the HealthQuest CD-ROM, and the Health and Human Performance Discipline Page. The guide also includes references to relevant print and broadcast media.
- **Test Bank** This file includes more than 1,000 questions, including multiple-choice, true/false, and short essay. It has been rewritten to enhance clarity, and it now includes critical thinking questions and more applications questions.
- **Computerized Test Bank** McGraw-Hill's Computerized Testing is the most flexible and easy-to-use electronic testing program available in higher education. The program allows instructors to create tests from book-specific test banks and to add their own questions. It accommodates a wide range of question types, and multiple versions of the test can be created. The program is available for Windows, Macintosh, and Linux environments.
- **PowerPoint** A complete set of PowerPoint lecture slides for the course is included on the Instructor's Resource CD, as well as on the instructor's portion of the Online Learning Center. This presentation, ready to use in class, was prepared by a professional in the field of health and fitness. It corresponds to the content in each chapter of *Focus on Health*, making it easier for you to teach and ensuring that your students can follow your lectures point by point. You can modify the presentation as much as you like to meet the needs of your course.

Online Learning Center

The Online Learning Center to accompany this text offers a number of additional resources for both students and instructors. Many study tools are open to all students. Premium content such as assessments and PowerWeb require student registration using the passcode that comes free with new books. Visit this website to find useful materials such as the following:

For the instructor:

- Downloadable PowerPoint presentations
- Course Integrator Guide

For the student:

- Self-scoring chapter quizzes and online study guides
- Flash cards and crossword puzzles for learning key terms and their definitions
- Learning objectives
- Interactive activities
- Web links for study and exploration of topics in the text
- Online labs
- Wellness worksheets
- PowerWeb
- Newsfeeds
- Internet guide

HealthQuest CD-ROM, by Bob Gold and Nancy Atkinson

The HealthQuest CD-ROM helps students explore their wellness behavior using state-of-the-art interactive technology. Students can assess their current health status, determine their risks, and explore options for positive lifestyle change. Tailored feedback gives students a meaningful and individualized learning experience without using valuable classroom time. Modules include the Wellboard (a health self-assessment); Stress Management and Mental Health; Fitness; Nutrition and Weight Control; Communicable Diseases; Cardiovascular Health; Cancer; Tobacco, Alcohol, and Other Drugs. An online Instructor's Manual presents ideas for incorporating HealthQuest into your course.

Fitness and Nutrition Log

This logbook helps students track their diet and exercise programs. It serves as a diary to help students monitor their behaviors. It can be packaged with any McGraw-Hill textbook for a small additional fee.

PowerWeb

www.dushkin.com/online

The PowerWeb website is a reservoir of course-specific articles and current events. Students can visit Power-Web to take a self-scoring quiz, complete an interactive exercise, click through an interactive glossary, or check the daily news. An expert in each discipline analyzes the day's news to show students how it relates to their field of study.

PowerWeb is part of the Online Learning Center. Students are also granted full access to Dushkin/McGraw-Hill's Student Site, where they can read study tips, conduct web research, learn about different career paths, and follow links on the web.

Wellness Worksheets

This collection of activities and assessments helps students become more involved in their own wellness and better prepared to implement behavior change programs. It includes 120 assessments under the topics of General Wellness and Behavior Change; Stress Management; Psychological and Spiritual Wellness; Intimate Relationships and Communication; Sexuality; Addictive Behaviors and Drug Dependence; Nutrition; Physical Activity and Exercise; Weight Management; Chronic Diseases: Cardiovascular Disease and Cancer; Infectious Diseases; Aging, Dying and Death; Consumer Health; Personal Safety; and Environmental Health. They are available online in the premium content or may be packaged with the text at minimal cost.

NutritionCalc Plus

http://nutritioncalc.mhhe.com

NutritionCalc Plus (ISBN 0-07-292084-X) is a dietary analysis program with an easy-to-use interface that allows users to track their nutrient and food group intakes, energy expenditures, and weight control goals. It generates a variety of reports and graphs for analysis, including comparisons with the Food Guide Pyramid and the latest Dietary Reference Intakes (DRIs). The database includes thousands of ethnic foods, supplements, fast foods, and convenience foods, and users can add their own foods to the food list. NutritionCalc Plus is available on CD-ROM or in an online version.

Video Library

The McGraw-Hill Video Library contains many quality videotapes, including selected videos from the *Films for Humanities* series and all the videos from the award-winning *Healthy Living: Road to Wellness* series. Digitized video clips are also available (see Healthy Living Video Clips CD-ROM). The library also features *Students on Health,* a unique video filmed on college campuses across the country that includes eight brief segments, 8 to 10 minutes long, featuring students involved in discussion and role play on health issues. Finally, an additional video—*McGraw-Hill Health Video*—is available. This video features brief clips on a wide range of topics of interest in personal health courses. Contact your McGraw-Hill sales representative to discuss eligibility to receive videos.

PageOut: The Course Website Development Center

www.pageout.net

PageOut, free to instructors who use a McGraw-Hill textbook, is an online program you can use to create your own course website. PageOut offers the following features:

- A course home page
- An instructor home page
- A syllabus (interactive and customizable, including quizzing, instructor notes, and links to the text's Online Learning Center)
- Web links
- Discussions (multiple discussion areas per class)
- An online gradebook
- Links to student web pages

Contact your McGraw-Hill sales representative to obtain a password.

Course Management Systems

www.mhhe.com/solutions

Now instructors can combine their McGraw-Hill Online Learning Center with today's most popular course management systems. Our Instructor Advantage program offers customers access to a complete online teaching website called the Knowledge Gateway, prepaid, toll-free phone support, and unlimited e-mail support directly from WebCT and Blackboard. Instructors who use 500 or more copies of a McGraw-Hill textbook can enroll in our Instructor Advantage Plus program, which provides on-campus, hands-on training from a certified platform specialist. Consult your McGraw-Hill sales representative to learn what other course management systems are easily used with McGraw-Hill online materials.

Classroom Performance System

Classroom Performance System (CPS) brings interactivity into the classroom/lecture hall. It is a wireless response system that gives instructors and students immediate feedback from the entire class. The wireless response pads are essentially remotes that are easy to use and that engage students. CPS is available for both IBM and Mac computers.

The Wellness Workbook from Quia

The Wellness Workbook, developed in collaboration with Quia™, offers an electronic version of assessments and quizzes compiled from the text and its main supplements. This new online supplement offers students such benefits as interactive assessments, self-scoring quizzes, and instant feedback. Instructors benefit from a grade book that automatically scores, tracks, and records students' results and provides the opportunity to review individual and class performance. Instructors also have the ability to customize activities and features for their course by using Quia's™ activity templates. To find out more about this new online supplement and how you can package it with your textbook, contact your McGraw-Hill sales representative.

Primis Online

www.mhhe.com/primis/online

Primis Online is a database-driven publishing system that allows instructors to create content-rich textbooks, lab manuals, or readers for their courses directly from the Primis website. The customized text can be delivered in print or electronic (eBook) form. A Primis eBook is a digital version of the customized text (sold directly to students as a file downloadable to their computer or accessed online by a password). *Focus on Health*, seventh edition, is included in the database.

You Can Make a Difference: Be Environmentally Responsible, Second Edition, by Judith Getis

This handy text is organized around the three parts of the biosphere: land, water, and air. Each section contains descriptions of the environmental problems associated with that part of the biosphere. Immediately following the problems, or challenges, are suggested ways in which individuals and communities can help solve or alleviate them.

Annual Editions

Annual Editions is an ever-enlarging series of more than seventy volumes, each designed to provide convenient, low-cost access to a wide range of current, carefully selected articles from some of the most important magazines, newspapers, and journals published today. The articles, drawn from more than 400 periodical sources, are written by prominent scholars, researchers, and commentators. All *Annual Editions* have common organizational features, such as annotated tables of contents, topic guides, unit overviews, and indexes. In addition, a list of annotated websites is included. An Instructor's Resource Guide with testing suggestions for each volume is available to qualified instructors.

Taking Sides

www.dushkin.com/takingsides

McGraw-Hill/Dushkin's *Taking Sides* series currently consists of twenty-two volumes, with an instructor's guide with testing material available for each volume. The *Taking Sides* approach brings together the arguments of leading social and behavioral scientists, educators, and contemporary commentators, forming eighteen to twenty debates, or issues, that present the pros and cons of current controversies in an area of study. An Issue Introduction that precedes the two opposing viewpoints gives students the proper context and historical background for each debate. After reading the debate, students are given other viewpoints to consider in the Issue Postscript, which also offers recommendations for further reading. *Taking Sides* fosters critical thinking in students and encourages them to develop a concern for serious social dialogue.

Acknowledgments

The publisher's reviewers made excellent comments and suggestions that were very useful to us in writing and revising this book. Their contributions are present in every chapter. We would like to express our sincere appreciation for both their critical and comparative readings.

For the Seventh Edition

Kari Barnumon
Moorpark College

Carol Biddington
California University of Pennsylvania

Susie Cousar
Lane Community College

William Ebomoyi
University of Northern Colorado

Caroline Crowther Fuller
Clemson University

Holly Henry
Chemeketa Community College

Marshall J. Meyer
Portland Community College–Sylvania

Lorette Oden
Western Illinois University

Todd Russell
University of Great Falls

Scott Wolf
Southeastern Illinois College

For the Sixth Edition

M. Betsy Bergen
Kansas State University

Sandra Bonneau
Golden West College

Sandra DiNatale
Keene State College

Lisa Everett
Las Positas College

Albert J. Figone
Humboldt State University

Neil E. Gallagher
Towson University

Amy Goff
Scottsdale Community College

Sharrie A. Herbold-Sheley
Lane Community College

Katie Herrington
Jones Junior College

Cathy Kennedy
Colorado State University

Mary Mock
University of South Dakota

Leonid Polyakov
Essex County College

Debra Tavasso
East Carolina University

Jennifer Thomas
Emporia State University

Martin Turnauer
Radford University

Dale Wagoner
Chabot College

Mary A. Wyandt
University of Arkansas

Beverly Zeakes
Radford University

For the Fifth Edition

John Batacan
Idaho State University

Steve Bordi
West Valley Community College

Judy Drolet
Southern Illinois University–Carbondale

Don Haynes
University of Minnesota–Duluth

Mary Iten
University of Nebraska at Kearney

Emogene Johnson Vaughn
Norfolk State University

Patricia Lawson
Arkansas State University

Rosalie Marinelli
University of Nevada

Marilyn Morton
SUNY-Plattsburgh

Trish Root
North Seattle Community College

Walt Rehm
Cuesta College

Betty Shepherd
Virginia Western Community College

Ladona Tournabene
University of South Dakota

Glenda Warren
Cumberland College

Katie Wiedman
University of St. Francis

For the Fourth Edition

S. Eugene Barnes
University of Southern Alabama

Anne K. Black
Austin Peay State University

Susan Ceriale
University of California–Santa Barbara

Bridget M. Finn
William Paterson University

Marianne Frauenknecht
Western Michigan University

Edna Gillis
Valdosta State University

Joe Goldfarb
University of Missouri–Columbia

Phil Huntsinger
University of Kansas

Gordon B. James
Weber State University

Sylvia M. Kubsch
University of Wisconsin–Green Bay

Frederick M. Randolph
Western Illinois University

Dell Smith
University of Central Arkansas

B. McKinley Thomas
Augusta State University

Chuck Ulrich
Western Illinois University

For the Third Edition

Dayna S. Brown
Morehead State University

Diane M. Hamilton
Georgia Southern University

Joe Herzstein
Trenton State College

Rebecca Rutt Leas
Clarion University

Dorinda Maynard
Eastern Kentucky University

Steven Navarro
Cerritos College

Mary Beth Tighe
The Ohio State University

For the Second Edition

James D. Aguiar
Ithaca College

Carolyn M. Allred
Central Piedmont Community College

Joan Benson
University of Utah

Daniel E. Berney
California State University–Dominguez Hills

Ronnie Carda
Emporia State University

Barbara Funke
Georgia College

William C. Gross
Western Michigan University

Richard Hurley
Brigham Young University

L. Clark McCammon
Western Illinois University

Dan Neal
Southwestern Oregon Community College

David Quadagno
Florida State University

Leslie Rurey
Community Colleges of Spokane

Scott E. Scobell
West Virginia State College

Raeann Koerner Smith
Ventura College

Karen T. Sullivan
Marymount University

Joan Tudor
Chapman University

Stuart L. Whitney
University of Vermont

For the First Edition

Sandra L. Bonneau
Golden West College

Richard A. Kaye
Kingsborough Community College

Donald Haynes
University of Minnesota–Duluth

J. Dale Wagoner
Chabot College

Special Acknowledgments

Authors do not exist in isolation. To publish successful textbooks, an entire team of professionals must work together for a significant time. During the past three decades, we have worked with many talented people to publish seventeen successful textbooks.

For this edition of *Focus on Health*, we used the professional expertise and writing talents of a team of four contributing authors. Leonard Kaminsky, Ph.D., Professor and Coordinator of Ball State University's Adult Fitness and Cardiac Rehabilitation Programs, took on the task of revising and updating Chapter 4 (Becoming Physically Fit) and Chapter 10 (Reducing Your Risk of Cardiovascular Disease). Chapter 7 (Making Decisions About Drug Use) and Chapter 8 (Taking Control of Alcohol Use) were revised by Alison Cockerill, M.S., Health Educator in the Ball State Student Health Center. Robert Pinger, Ph.D., Professor and Chairperson of the Department of Physiology and Health Science at Ball State, revised Chapter 16 (Protecting Your Safety). And our new Chapter 19, The Environment and Your Health, was written by David LeBlanc, Ph.D., Professor of Biology at Ball State University. We thank these contributors for their professional dedication to this book and their personal commitment to the health of college students with whom they work on a daily basis.

There are many others whom we would like to thank for their contributions to this book. Ann Kirby-Payne did an exceptional job as our developmental editor. She took over the project at a rather challenging point but "rallied the troops" and always maintained her excitement and positive outlook. Ann found engaging ways to incorporate the revisions and perspectives of our new author, Ellen B. Mauer, and the four contributing authors. We believe that this seventh edition is a major reflection of Ann's insight, vision, and determination.

We remain grateful to Vicki Malinee, who saw us through nine book projects. This latest edition of *Focus on Health* also bears the imprint of Nick Barrett, Executive Editor, Health and Human Performance. Although Nick joined this project in its final stages, his infectious enthusiasm for *Focus on Health* and his positive vision for the future of our personal health texts make us especially proud to be McGraw-Hill authors. We look forward to working with Nick on upcoming projects.

Special recognition goes to Pam Cooper, Executive Marketing Manager, who is as energetic a person as we have seen in college publishing. We are confident that her experience, expertise, and talent will allow this book to reach many of our teaching colleagues.

We are also grateful to those who worked behind the scenes at McGraw-Hill on the production of this book. Lynda Huenefeld made a major contribution to the development of both the book and its supplements package. Project Manager Jill Moline-Eccher juggled this book and its larger version simultaneously with remarkable grace and good humor, all the while keeping watch over every detail and deadline. Senior Designer Kim Menning created an exciting, dynamic new look for the seventh edition. And Photo Research Coordinator Alexandra Ambrose culled a fine selection of colorful, thought-provoking images.

Finally, we would like to thank our families for their continued support and love. More than anyone else, they know the energy and dedication it takes to write and revise textbooks. To them we continue to offer our sincere admiration and loving appreciation.

Dale B. Hahn
Wayne A. Payne
Ellen B. Mauer

a visual guide to focus on health

Whether you're trying to get in shape, looking for sound health advice, trying to interpret the health information you see in the media, or just working toward a good grade, *Focus on Health* is designed to help you succeed. Here's a brief guide to some of the useful and eye-opening features you'll find inside.

Chapter Objectives
Each chapter opens with a set of clear learning goals; check them out before you begin reading the chapter, and use them for review once you've completed it.

Online Learning Center Resources
A wealth of study aids and other resources to help you prepare for exams and improve your grade are available at **www.mhhe.com/hahn7e.**

Talking It Over
How would you approach a doctor, family member, friend, or partner about a specific health problem? Where do you stand on today's controversial health issues? Are you honest with yourself about your own health? Use these boxes to role play and sharpen your communication skills.

Eye on the Media
Curious about all those ads you see for various drugs? Wondering about the reliability of the health information you find on the Internet? This feature investigates the way that written, broadcast, and electronic media shape our perceptions about health, health care, and wellness.

Health on the Web Behavior Change Activities
Surfing the web can be good for your health! These activities guide you to interactive self-assessments on the web. How much stress are you under? What form of contraception is best for you? Log on and find out!

HealthQuest Activities
You received a free HealthQuest CD-ROM with your new copy of *Focus on Health.* This feature provides activities to help you explore HealthQuest and assess your health behavior in areas like cancer prevention, fitness, and nutrition.

---

chapter seventeen

the environment and your health

Chapter Objectives

After reading this chapter, you should be able to:

- identify several environmental factors that can impact your personal health in either positive or adverse ways.
- explain how your personal health is influenced by different environmental factors on several scales, including personal environment, the community and regional environment, and the global environment.
- describe specific actions that you can take to minimize health risks associated with your personal environment—your home, your automobile, your workplace.
- describe the distinction between a "point source" versus a "nonpoint source" of community/regional air or water pollution.
- detail several specific actions that you can take to minimize environmental health risks at the community and regional level.
- describe several global environmental health issues, and offer several actions that you might take to foster change.

Online Learning Center Resources

www.mhhe.com/hahn7e

Log on to our Online Learning Center (OLC) for access to theses additional resources:

- Chapter key terms and definitions
- Learning objectives
- Student interactive question-and-answer sites
- Self-scoring chapter quiz
- Online assessments
- Key term flash cards

Talking It Over

Talking—and Acting—Like an Environmentalist

One of your classmates claims to be an avid environmentalist who loves hiking, camping, and other outdoor activities. He is involved with several organizations that lobby the government for environmental reform. So, when you see him drive a large, gas-guzzling SUV up to the recycling center, where he deposits neatly sorted paper, bottles, and cans for recycling, does this image strike you as contradictory? Do you think he recycles to ease a guilty conscience about driving an SUV? Would it matter more if you were standing in the middle of New York City (far from any dirt roads), or in Salt Lake City (surrounded by vast wildlands)? If his love of the great outdoors requires a larger vehicle (to haul camping gear, kayak, etc.), might he have made a more environmentally sound choice?

CommunicationLinks:
www.thedetroitproject.com
http://www.ecocenter.org/auto.shtml

Eye on the Media

Does Eco-Terrorism Really Work to Protect Our Environment?

On August 23, 2003, several automobile dealerships were attacked by arsonists who left graffiti claiming that they destroyed or damaged gas-guzzling SUVs to protect the environment. The unknown perpetrators claimed to be acting in accordance with the Earth Liberation Front, or ELF. According to their Internet website, ELF is an internet ... underground organi.... over $100 million in damages to entities who profit from the destruction of life and the planet.

Many people are angered by the degradation of our shared natural environment, but is direct action/eco-terr.... ... justified in a democratic soci....

Health on the Web

Behavior Change Activities

Following a Healthy Lifestyle

Students who take a personal health course usually want to improve their health behavior. *Prevention* magazine offers an excellent general health website that addresses subjects such as health, weight loss and fitness, food, and community. The content varies, but it's always useful and worthwhile. Click on **www.healthyideas.com**, and choose a path that interests you.

Exploring Lifestyle Links

If you're seeking information on a multitude of lifestyle choices, this is the site for you. Topics include fitness, weight, exercise, food, nutrition, ... , material arts, an.... .....lubs. Click on **w.....ess.com,**

HealthQuest Activities

- Use the Wellboard to report your life score (number of years out of 114) and the score percentages for each of the eight health areas.
- Fill out the Wellboard using data from a fictional college student. On the first assessment screen, change the demographics to show how gender, ethnicity, age, marital status, and community affect average life expectancy.

Changing for the Better

Eating on the Run

I am always in a hurry and don't have time to cook, and so a lot of my meals end up being fast food. Are there better choices I can make when eating on the run?

The typical American eats about three hamburgers and four orders of French fries each week so you aren't alone. With over 300,000 fast-food restaurants in the United States, fast food is definitely part of the American lifestyle. Here are some things to consider when eating at fast food restaurants:

- Don't supersize! Go for the "small" or "regular" size.
- Don't wait until you are starving because that leads to overeating and supersizing!
- Decide what you w̶ ̶ ̶ ̶ ̶ ahead of time and d̶ ̶ ̶ ̶ ̶ ̶ued

- Order grilled instead of fried chicken or fish.
- Look for the "light" choices.
- Limit your condiments. Mustard, catsup, salsa, or low-fat or fat-free condiments and dressing are preferable to regular mayonnaise or high-fat dressings.
- For breakfast, choose cereal and milk or pancakes rather than a breakfast sandwich (which can have about 475 calories, 30 grams of fat, and 1,260 mg of sodium).
- Bring fast food from home! Buy portable foods at the grocery store to take with you that can be eaten quickly and easily such as portable yogurt, a banana or apple, low-fat granola bar, or breakfast bar.
- Order̶ ̶ ̶ ̶ ̶ skim milk or water i̶ ̶ ̶ ̶ ̶ ̶ soda. ̶ ̶ ̶ ̶to se̶
  ̶ ̶ ̶ ̶nt k̶ ̶ ̶ ̶

Discovering Your Spirituality

Yoga: Creating Peaceful Time

In a typical college day that includes academic, social, and financial pressures, you can lose the sense of who you really are. Do you ever find yourself wondering why you're making certain choices and what's really important to you? Meditative practices such as yoga offer you the chance to slow down and recapture a sense of yourself.

The word *yoga* comes from a Sanskrit root meaning "union" or "joining," referring to the integration of body, mind, and spirit. Yoga has evolved from ancient beginnings in the Himalayan mountains of India. Accounts of its origin differ, and some suggest that it reaches back 6,000 years. Yoga is practiced by people of all social, economic, ̶nd religious backgr̶ ̶ ̶ ̶ ̶Many past yoga master̶ ̶ ̶

but th̶ ̶ ̶ ̶ ̶brace or e̶ ̶ ̶ ̶ ̶ ̶m

Each exercise, called an *asan* or *ansana*, has specific effects. The "diamond pose," for example, limbers the lower back, hips, and groin muscles. Specialized workouts—to address pregnancy, sports, weight-loss programs, and other needs—can be created by including carefully selected exercises.

Yoga requires no special equipment and can be practiced in a small space such as a bedroom. Instructors in the United States have worked to make yoga accessible to the American lifestyle by developing special routines that can be pursued during travel, business, or the acade̶ ̶ ̶ ̶Classes are frequently offe̶ ̶ ̶ ̶college campuses or̶ ̶ ̶ ̶but any lar̶ ̶ ̶ ̶ ̶ ̶ ̶ ̶ ̶oks tha̶

Learning from Our Diversity

Understanding Kosher Laws

Food has been part of many religious practices and customs for centuries. Some foods have symbolic meanings related to major life experiences, and ceremonies and religious rites involving food are associated with certain events. Understanding the dietary restrictions of your friends, classmates, and colleagues can help you to be more sensitive to their needs when dining out, or when you entertain at home.

While many religions have specific dietary restrictions, perhaps the most familiar are those that govern the diets of many Jews. Foods selected and prepared according to the "Rules of Kashruth" are referred to as kosher, meaning "fit or proper." These laws dictate that no pork or shellfish shall be consumed, and all other types of meat must be ̶eticulously clea̶ ̶ ̶ ̶all blood. Animal̶ ̶ ̶ ̶ ̶ ̶ ̶he eaten must be

For many Jews, following a kosher diet is a not merely a matter of following tradition or of being aware of what they eat. The laws governing the kosher diet are an important part of Jewish law, spelled out in the Torah. Many of these laws are in essence guidelines for safe and sanitary food; indeed, the laws governing the butchering of animals are so humane and sanitary that the federal government exempts kosher butchers and slaughterhouses from many USDA regulations.[1] For this reason, many non-Jews choose to eat only kosher meat, noting that it is not only very safe to eat, but also tastes better.[2] In the wake of the first reported cases of Mad Cow Disease in the United States at the end of 2003, many more consumers began to seek kosher beef, noting that the kosher law prohibits the slaughter of cows that cannot walk, and does ̶ ̶ ̶ ̶animals to be killed by h̶ ̶ ̶ ̶ ̶or shot in the head. w̶ ̶ ̶ad bra̶ ̶ ̶ ̶ ̶ ̶ ̶ ̶ke o̶ ̶ ̶ ̶ ̶ ̶ ̶blood̶

personal assessment

how stressed are you?

A widely used life stress scale called the Social Readjustment Rating Scale by Holmes and Rahe has been used to determine the degree of stress that you are experiencing due to life events over the past year. It also projects your chances of developing an illness- or stress-related health condition. Stress can lead to some serious health problems, and the more stress you have in your life, the more vulnerable you are to being susceptible to illness. Let's see how you score.

Trouble with in-laws	29	___
Outstanding personal achievement	28	___
Begin or end school	26	___
Partner begins/stops working	26	___
Change in living conditions	25	___
Change in personal habits	24	___
Trouble with supervisor	23	___
Change in work ho̶ ̶ ̶	20	___
̶ ̶ ̶ ̶ ̶		

focus on

the changing picture of infectious disease

Just a generation ago, many scientists believed we were wiping out infectious disease. Armed with improved sanitation, better hygiene practices, antibiotics, and pesticides, humankind had malaria, cholera, and tuberculosis (TB) on the run and smallpox and polio well on the way to ̶tion. I̶ ̶ ̶ ̶ ̶disea̶

(SIV), but don't become sick. Of course, HIV/AIDS is a dangerous virus, but Ebola is more infective and runs a shorter disease course. As one author put it, "Ebola does in ten days what it takes AIDS ten years to accomplish."[1] This is terrible for the nine out of ten people infected with ̶hola v̶ ̶ ̶ ̶ ̶ ̶ ̶r of days̶

the rodent population exploded in the Four Corners area of New Mexico, Arizona, Colorado, and Utah. The rodent population spread hantavirus to sixteen states. This virus killed half of the ninety-four people it infected.[3] More recently, the first case of hantavirus transmission be-̶ ̶ ̶n hum̶ ̶ ̶ ̶ ̶ ̶rgenti̶

Changing for the Better
Learn to put health concepts into practice by following these useful tips. This feature provides practical advice for making positive changes and staying motivated to follow a healthy lifestyle.

Discovering Your Spirituality
A healthy body and a healthy mind go hand in hand. This feature will help you tap into your spiritual side to improve your self-esteem, foster good relationships with others, and jump-start your physical health.

Talking Points
Throughout each chapter, you'll find these tips for starting a dialogue about sensitive health topics.

TALKING POINTS How would you show support for a friend who is struggling with the dietary requirements of diabetes?

Learning from Our Diversity
These unique boxes invite you to explore the rich diversity of your own campus, and to gain perspective on the way such characteristics as age, racial/ethnic background, physical abilities, and sexual orientation can shape individuals' lives and well-being.

Personal Assessment
Do you eat too much fat? What's the best method of birth control for you if you are sexually active? Are you a perfectionist? Each chapter in *Focus on Health* includes an assessment to help you learn the answers to these and many other questions.

Focus On...
Every day you hear the buzz about hot health topics ranging from extreme sports to emerging diseases. Read these articles and decide where you stand on these controversial issues.

comprehensive health assessment

Social and Occupational Health

	Not true/ rarely	Somewhat true/ sometimes	Mostly true/ usually	Very true/ always
1. I feel loved and supported by my family.	1	2	3	4
2. I establish friendships with ease and enjoyment.	1	2	3	4
3. I establish friendships with people of both genders and all ages.	1	2	3	4
4. I sustain relationships by communicating with and caring about my family and friends.	1	2	3	4
5. I feel comfortable and confident when meeting people for the first time.	1	2	3	4
6. I practice social skills to facilitate the process of forming new relationships.	1	2	3	4
7. I seek opportunities to meet and interact with new people.	1	2	3	4
8. I talk with, rather than at, people.	1	2	3	4
9. I am open to developing or sustaining intimate relationships.	1	2	3	4
10. I appreciate the importance of parenting the next generation and am committed to supporting it in ways that reflect my own resources.	1	2	3	4
11. I recognize the strengths and weaknesses of my parents' childrearing skills and feel comfortable modifying them if I choose to become a parent.	1	2	3	4
12. I attempt to be tolerant of others whether or not I approve of their behavior or beliefs.	1	2	3	4
13. I understand and appreciate the contribution that cultural diversity makes to the quality of living.	1	2	3	4
14. I understand and appreciate the difference between being educated and being trained.	1	2	3	4
15. My work gives me a sense of self-sufficiency and an opportunity to contribute.	1	2	3	4
16. I have equal respect for the roles of leader and subordinate within the workplace.	1	2	3	4
17. I have chosen an occupation that suits my interests and temperament.	1	2	3	4
18. I have chosen an occupation that does not compromise my physical or psychological health.	1	2	3	4
19. I get along well with my coworkers most of the time.	1	2	3	4
20. When I have a disagreement with a coworker, I try to resolve it directly and constructively.	1	2	3	4

Points _____

Spiritual and Psychological Health

	Not true/ rarely	Somewhat true/ sometimes	Mostly true/ usually	Very true/ always
1. I have a deeply held belief system or personal theology.	1	2	3	4
2. I recognize the contribution that membership in a community of faith can make to a person's overall quality of life.	1	2	3	4

3. I seek experiences with nature and reflect on nature's contribution to my quality of life.	1	2	3	4
4. My spirituality is a resource that helps me remain calm and strong during times of stress.	1	2	3	4
5. I have found appropriate ways to express my spirituality.	1	2	3	4
6. I respect the diversity of spiritual expression and am tolerant of those whose beliefs differ from my own.	1	2	3	4
7. I take adequate time to reflect on my own life and my relationships with others and the institutions of society.	1	2	3	4
8. I routinely undertake new experiences.	1	2	3	4
9. I receive adequate support from others.	1	2	3	4
10. I look for opportunities to support others, even occasionally at the expense of my own goals and aspirations.	1	2	3	4
11. I recognize that emotional and psychological health are as important as physical health.	1	2	3	4
12. I express my feelings and opinions comfortably, yet am capable of keeping them to myself when appropriate.	1	2	3	4
13. I see myself as a person of worth and feel comfortable with my own strengths and limitations.	1	2	3	4
14. I establish realistic goals and work to achieve them.	1	2	3	4
15. I understand the differences between the normal range of emotions and the signs of clinical depression.	1	2	3	4
16. I know how to recognize signs of suicidal thoughts and am willing to intervene.	1	2	3	4
17. I regularly assess my own behavior patterns and beliefs and would seek professional assistance for any emotional dysfunction.	1	2	3	4
18. I accept the reality of aging and view it as an opportunity for positive change.	1	2	3	4
19. I accept the reality of death and view it as a normal and inevitable part of life.	1	2	3	4
20. I have made decisions about my own death to ensure that I die with dignity when the time comes.	1	2	3	4

Points _____

Stress Management

	Not true/ rarely	Somewhat true/ sometimes	Mostly true/ usually	Very true/ always
1. I accept the reality of change while maintaining the necessary stability in my daily activities.	1	2	3	4
2. I seek change when it is necessary or desirable to do so.	1	2	3	4
3. I know what stress-management services are offered on campus, through my employer, or in my community.	1	2	3	4
4. When necessary, I use the stress-management services to which I have access.	1	2	3	4
5. I employ stress-reduction practices in anticipation of stressful events, such as job interviews and final examinations.	1	2	3	4
6. I reevaluate the way in which I handled stressful events so that I can better cope with similar events in the future.	1	2	3	4
7. I turn to relatives and friends during periods of disruption in my life.	1	2	3	4
8. I avoid using alcohol or other drugs during periods of stress.	1	2	3	4
9. I refrain from behaving aggressively or abusively during periods of stress.	1	2	3	4

	Not true/rarely	Somewhat true/sometimes	Mostly true/usually	Very true/always
10. I sleep enough to maintain a high level of health and cope successfully with daily challenges.	1	2	3	4
11. I avoid sleeping excessively as a response to stressful change.	1	2	3	4
12. My diet is conducive to good health and stress management.	1	2	3	4
13. I participate in physical activity to relieve stress.	1	2	3	4
14. I practice stress-management skills, such as diaphragmatic breathing and yoga.	1	2	3	4
15. I manage my time effectively.	1	2	3	4

Points _____

Fitness

	Not true/rarely	Somewhat true/sometimes	Mostly true/usually	Very true/always
1. I participate in recreational and fitness activities both to minimize stress and to improve or maintain my level of physical fitness.	1	2	3	4
2. I select some recreational activities that are strenuous rather than sedentary in nature.	1	2	3	4
3. I include various types of aerobic conditioning activities among the wider array of recreational and fitness activities in which I engage.	1	2	3	4
4. I engage in aerobic activities with appropriate frequency, intensity, and duration to provide a training effect for my heart and lungs.	1	2	3	4
5. I routinely include strength-training activities among the wider array of fitness activities in which I engage.	1	2	3	4
6. I routinely vary the types of strength-training activities in which I participate in order to minimize injury and strengthen all of the important muscle groups.	1	2	3	4
7. I do exercises specifically designed to maintain joint range of motion.	1	2	3	4
8. I believe that recreational and fitness activities can help me improve my physical health and my emotional and social well-being.	1	2	3	4
9. I include a variety of fitness activities in my overall plan for physical fitness.	1	2	3	4
10. I take appropriate steps to avoid injuries when participating in recreational and fitness activities.	1	2	3	4
11. I seek appropriate treatment for all injuries that result from fitness activities.	1	2	3	4
12. I believe that older adults should undertake appropriately chosen fitness activities.	1	2	3	4
13. My body composition is consistent with a high level of health.	1	2	3	4
14. I warm up before beginning vigorous activity, and I cool down afterward.	1	2	3	4
15. I select properly designed and well-maintained equipment and clothing for each activity.	1	2	3	4
16. I avoid using performance-enhancing substances that are known to be dangerous and those whose influence on the body is not fully understood.	1	2	3	4
17. I sleep seven to eight hours daily.	1	2	3	4
18. I refrain from using over-the-counter sleep-inducing aids.	1	2	3	4
19. I follow sound dietary practices as an important adjunct to a health-enhancing physical activity program.	1	2	3	4
20. My current level of fitness allows me to participate fully and effortlessly in my daily activities.	1	2	3	4

Points _____

Nutrition and Weight Management

	Not true/ rarely	Somewhat true/ sometimes	Mostly true/ usually	Very true/ always
1. I balance my caloric intake with my caloric expenditure.	1	2	3	4
2. I obtain the recommended number of servings from each of the food groups.	1	2	3	4
3. I select a wide variety of foods chosen from each of the food groups.	1	2	3	4
4. I understand the amount of a particular food that constitutes a single serving.	1	2	3	4
5. I often try new foods, particularly when I know them to be healthful.	1	2	3	4
6. I select breads, cereals, fresh fruits, and vegetables in preference to pastries, candies, sodas, and fruits canned in heavy syrup.	1	2	3	4
7. I limit the amount of sugar that I add to foods during preparation and at the table.	1	2	3	4
8. I consume an appropriate percentage of my total daily calories from carbohydrates.	1	2	3	4
9. I select primarily nonmeat sources of protein, such as peas, beans, and peanut butter, while limiting my consumption of red meat and high-fat dairy products.	1	2	3	4
10. I consume an appropriate percentage of my total daily calories from protein.	1	2	3	4
11. I select foods prepared with unsaturated vegetable oils while reducing my consumption of red meat, high-fat dairy products, and foods prepared with lard (animal fat) or butter.	1	2	3	4
12. I carefully limit the amount of fast food that I consume during a typical week.	1	2	3	4
13. I consume an appropriate percentage of my total daily calories from fat.	1	2	3	4
14. I select nutritious foods when I snack.	1	2	3	4
15. I limit my use of salt during food preparation and at the table.	1	2	3	4
16. I consume adequate amounts of fiber.	1	2	3	4
17. I routinely consider the nutrient density of individual food items when choosing foods.	1	2	3	4
18. I maintain my weight without reliance on over-the-counter or prescription diet pills.	1	2	3	4
19. I maintain my weight without reliance on fad diets or liquid weight loss beverages.	1	2	3	4
20. I exercise regularly to help maintain my weight.	1	2	3	4

Points _____

Alcohol, Tobacco, and Other Drug Use

	Not true/ rarely	Somewhat true/ sometimes	Mostly true/ usually	Very true/ always
1. I abstain or drink in moderation when offered alcoholic beverages.	1	2	3	4
2. I abstain from using illegal psychoactive (mind-altering) drugs.	1	2	3	4
3. I do not consume alcoholic beverages or psychoactive drugs rapidly or in large quantities.	1	2	3	4
4. I do not use alcohol or psychoactive drugs in a way that causes me to behave inappropriately.	1	2	3	4
5. My use of alcohol or other drugs does not compromise my academic performance.	1	2	3	4

	Not true/ rarely	Somewhat true/ sometimes	Mostly true/ usually	Very true/ always
6. I refrain from drinking alcoholic beverages or using psychoactive drugs when engaging in recreational activities that require strength, speed, or coordination.	1	2	3	4
7. I refrain from drinking alcoholic beverages while participating in occupational activities, regardless of the nature of those activities.	1	2	3	4
8. My use of alcohol or other drugs does not generate financial concerns for myself or for others.	1	2	3	4
9. I refrain from drinking alcohol or using psychoactive drugs when driving a motor vehicle or operating heavy equipment.	1	2	3	4
10. I do not drink alcohol or use psychoactive drugs when I am alone.	1	2	3	4
11. I avoid riding with people who have been drinking alcohol or using psychoactive drugs.	1	2	3	4
12. My use of alcohol or other drugs does not cause family dysfunction.	1	2	3	4
13. I do not use marijuana.	1	2	3	4
14. I do not use hallucinogens.	1	2	3	4
15. I do not use heroin or other illegal intravenous drugs.	1	2	3	4
16. I do not experience blackouts when I drink alcohol.	1	2	3	4
17. I do not become abusive or violent when I drink alcohol or use psychoactive drugs.	1	2	3	4
18. I use potentially addictive prescription medication in complete compliance with my physician's directions.	1	2	3	4
19. I do not smoke cigarettes.	1	2	3	4
20. I do not use tobacco products in any other form.	1	2	3	4
21. I minimize my exposure to secondhand smoke.	1	2	3	4
22. I am concerned about the effect that alcohol, tobacco, and other drug use is known to have on developing fetuses.	1	2	3	4
23. I am concerned about the effect that alcohol, tobacco, and other drug use is known to have on the health of other people.	1	2	3	4
24. I seek natural, health-enhancing highs rather than relying on alcohol, tobacco, and illegal drugs.	1	2	3	4
25. I take prescription medication only as instructed, and I use over-the-counter medication in accordance with directions.	1	2	3	4

Points _____

Disease Prevention

	Not true/ rarely	Somewhat true/ sometimes	Mostly true/ usually	Very true/ always
1. My diet includes foods rich in phytochemicals.	1	2	3	4
2. My diet includes foods rich in folic acid.	1	2	3	4
3. My diet includes foods that are good sources of dietary fiber.	1	2	3	4
4. My diet is low in dietary cholesterol.	1	2	3	4
5. I follow food preparation practices that minimize the risk of food-borne illness.	1	2	3	4
6. I engage in regular physical activity and am able to control my weight effectively.	1	2	3	4
7. I do not use tobacco products.	1	2	3	4
8. I abstain from alcohol or drink only in moderation.	1	2	3	4
9. I do not use intravenously administered illegal drugs.	1	2	3	4
10. I use safer sex practices intended to minimize my risk of exposure to sexually transmitted diseases, including HIV and HPV.	1	2	3	4

	Not true/rarely	Somewhat true/sometimes	Mostly true/usually	Very true/always
11. I take steps to limit my risk of exposure to the bacterium that causes Lyme disease and to the virus that causes hantavirus pulmonary syndrome.	1	2	3	4
12. I control my blood pressure with weight management and physical fitness activities.	1	2	3	4
13. I minimize my exposure to allergens, including those that trigger asthma attacks.	1	2	3	4
14. I wash my hands frequently and thoroughly.	1	2	3	4
15. I use preventive medical care services appropriately.	1	2	3	4
16. I use appropriate cancer self-screening practices, such as breast self-examination and testicular self-examination.	1	2	3	4
17. I know which chronic illnesses and diseases are part of my family history.	1	2	3	4
18. I know which inherited conditions are part of my family history and will seek preconceptional counseling regarding these conditions.	1	2	3	4
19. I am fully immunized against infectious diseases.	1	2	3	4
20. I take prescribed medications, particularly antibiotics, exactly as instructed by my physician.	1	2	3	4

Points _____

Sexual Health

	Not true/rarely	Somewhat true/sometimes	Mostly true/usually	Very true/always
1. I know how sexually transmitted diseases are spread.	1	2	3	4
2. I can recognize the symptoms of sexually transmitted diseases.	1	2	3	4
3. I know how sexually transmitted disease transmission can be prevented.	1	2	3	4
4. I know how safer sex practices reduce the risk of contracting sexually transmitted diseases.	1	2	3	4
5. I follow safer sex practices.	1	2	3	4
6. I recognize the symptoms of premenstrual syndrome and understand how it is prevented and treated.	1	2	3	4
7. I recognize the symptoms of endometriosis and understand the relationship of its symptoms to hormonal cycles.	1	2	3	4
8. I understand the physiological basis of menopause and recognize that it is a normal part of the aging process in women.	1	2	3	4
9. I understand and accept the range of human sexual orientations.	1	2	3	4
10. I encourage the development of flexible sex roles (androgyny) in children.	1	2	3	4
11. I take a mature approach to dating and mate selection.	1	2	3	4
12. I recognize that marriage and other types of long-term relationships can be satisfying.	1	2	3	4
13. I recognize that a celibate lifestyle is appropriate and satisfying for some people.	1	2	3	4
14. I affirm the sexuality of older adults and am comfortable with its expression.	1	2	3	4
15. I am familiar with the advantages and disadvantages of a wide range of birth control methods.	1	2	3	4
16. I understand how each birth control method works and how effective it is.	1	2	3	4
17. I use my birth control method consistently and appropriately.	1	2	3	4
18. I am familiar with the wide range of procedures now available to treat infertility.	1	2	3	4

	Not true/ rarely	Somewhat true/ sometimes	Mostly true/ usually	Very true/ always
19. I accept that others may disagree with my feelings about pregnancy termination.	1	2	3	4
20. I am familiar with alternatives available to infertile couples, including adoption.	1	2	3	4

Points _____

Safety Practices and Violence Prevention

	Not true/ rarely	Somewhat true/ sometimes	Mostly true/ usually	Very true/ always
1. I attempt to identify sources of risk or danger in each new setting or activity.	1	2	3	4
2. I learn proper procedures and precautions before undertaking new recreational or occupational activities.	1	2	3	4
3. I select appropriate clothing and equipment for all activities and maintain equipment in good working order.	1	2	3	4
4. I curtail my participation in activities when I am not feeling well or am distracted by other demands.	1	2	3	4
5. I repair dangerous conditions or report them to those responsible for maintenance.	1	2	3	4
6. I use common sense and observe the laws governing non-motorized vehicles when I ride a bicycle.	1	2	3	4
7. I operate all motor vehicles as safely as possible, including using seat belts and other safety equipment.	1	2	3	4
8. I refrain from driving an automobile or boat when I have been drinking alcohol or taking drugs or medications.	1	2	3	4
9. I try to anticipate the risk of falling and maintain my environment to minimize this risk.	1	2	3	4
10. I maintain my environment to minimize the risk of fire, and I have a well-rehearsed plan to exit my residence in case of fire.	1	2	3	4
11. I am a competent swimmer and could save myself or rescue someone who was drowning.	1	2	3	4
12. I refrain from sexually aggressive behavior toward my partner or others.	1	2	3	4
13. I would report an incident of sexual harassment or date rape whether or not I was the victim.	1	2	3	4
14. I would seek help from others if I were the victim or perpetrator of domestic violence.	1	2	3	4
15. I practice gun safety and encourage other gun owners to do so.	1	2	3	4
16. I drive at all times in a way that will minimize my risk of being carjacked.	1	2	3	4
17. I have taken steps to protect my home from intruders.	1	2	3	4
18. I use campus security services as much as possible when they are available.	1	2	3	4
19. I know what to do if I am being stalked.	1	2	3	4
20. I have a well-rehearsed plan to protect myself from the aggressive behavior of other people in my place of residence.	1	2	3	4

Points _____

Health Care Consumerism

	Not true/ rarely	Somewhat true/ sometimes	Mostly true/ usually	Very true/ always
1. I know how to obtain valid health information.	1	2	3	4
2. I accept health information that has been deemed valid by the established scientific community.	1	2	3	4

	Not true/ rarely	Somewhat true/ sometimes	Mostly true/ usually	Very true/ always
3. I am skeptical of claims that guarantee the effectiveness of a particular health-care service or product.	1	2	3	4
4. I am skeptical of practitioners or clinics who advertise or offer services at rates substantially lower than those charged by reputable providers.	1	2	3	4
5. I am not swayed by advertisements that present unhealthy behavior in an attractive manner.	1	2	3	4
6. I can afford proper medical care, including hospitalization.	1	2	3	4
7. I can afford adequate health insurance.	1	2	3	4
8. I understand the role of government health care plans in providing health care to people who qualify for coverage.	1	2	3	4
9. I know how to select health care providers who are highly qualified and appropriate for my current health care needs.	1	2	3	4
10. I seek a second or third opinion when surgery or other costly therapies are recommended.	1	2	3	4
11. I have told my physician which hospital I would prefer to use should the need arise.	1	2	3	4
12. I understand my rights and responsibilities as a patient when admitted to a hospital.	1	2	3	4
13. I practice adequate self-care to reduce my health care expenditures and my reliance on health care providers.	1	2	3	4
14. I am open-minded about alternative health care practices and support current efforts to determine their appropriate role in effective health care.	1	2	3	4
15. I have a well-established relationship with a pharmacist and have transmitted all necessary information regarding medication and use.	1	2	3	4
16. I carefully follow labels and directions when using health care products, such as over-the-counter medications.	1	2	3	4
17. I finish all prescription medications as directed, rather than stopping use when symptoms subside.	1	2	3	4
18. I report to the appropriate agencies any providers of health care services, information, or products that use deceptive advertising or fraudulent methods of operation.	1	2	3	4
19. I pursue my rights as fully as possible in matters of misrepresentation or consumer dissatisfaction.	1	2	3	4
20. I follow current health care issues in the news and voice my opinion to my elected representatives.	1	2	3	4

Points _____

Environmental Health

	Not true/ rarely	Somewhat true/ sometimes	Mostly true/ usually	Very true/ always
1. I avoid use of and exposure to pesticides as much as possible.	1	2	3	4
2. I avoid use of and exposure to herbicides as much as possible.	1	2	3	4
3. I am willing to spend the extra money and time required to obtain organically grown produce.	1	2	3	4
4. I reduce environmental pollutants by minimizing my use of the automobile.	1	2	3	4
5. I avoid the use of products that contribute to indoor air pollution.	1	2	3	4
6. I limit my exposure to ultraviolet radiation by avoiding excessive sun exposure.	1	2	3	4
7. I limit my exposure to radon gas by using a radon gas detector.	1	2	3	4

8. I limit my exposure to radiation by promptly eliminating radon gas within my home.	1	2	3	4
9. I limit my exposure to radiation by agreeing to undergo medical radiation procedures only when absolutely necessary for the diagnosis and treatment of an illness or disease.	1	2	3	4
10. I avoid the use of potentially unsafe water, particularly when traveling in a foreign country or when a municipal water supply or bottled water is unavailable.	1	2	3	4
11. I avoid noise pollution by limiting my exposure to loud noise or by using ear protection.	1	2	3	4
12. I avoid air pollution by carefully selecting the environments in which I live, work, and recreate.	1	2	3	4
13. I do not knowingly use or improperly dispose of personal care products that can harm the environment.	1	2	3	4
14. I reuse as many products as possible so that they can avoid the recycling bins for as long as possible.	1	2	3	4
15. I participate fully in my community's recycling efforts.	1	2	3	4
16. I encourage the increased use of recycled materials in the design and manufacturing of new products.	1	2	3	4
17. I dispose of residential toxic substances safely and properly.	1	2	3	4
18. I follow environmental issues in the news and voice my opinion to my elected representatives.	1	2	3	4
19. I am aware of and involved in environmental issues in my local area.	1	2	3	4
20. I perceive myself as a steward of the environment for the generations to come, rather than as a person with a right to use (and misuse) the environment to meet my immediate needs.	1	2	3	4

Points _____
YOUR TOTAL POINTS _____

Interpretation

770–880 points

Congratulations! Your health behavior is very supportive of high-level health. Continue to practice your positive health habits, and look for areas in which you can become even stronger. Encourage others to follow your example, and support their efforts in any way you can.

550–769 points

Good job! Your health behavior is relatively supportive of high-level health. You scored well in several areas; however, you can improve in some ways. Identify your weak areas and chart a plan for behavior change, as explained at the end of Chapter 1. Then pay close attention as you learn more about health in the weeks ahead.

330–549 points

Caution! Your relatively low score indicates that your behavior may be compromising your health. Review your responses to this assessment carefully, noting the areas in which you scored poorly. Then chart a detailed plan for behavior change, as outlined at the end of Chapter 1. Be sure to set realistic goals that you can work toward steadily as you complete this course.

Below 330 points

Red flag! Your low score suggests that your health behavior is destructive. Immediate changes in your behavior are needed to put you back on track. Review your responses to this assessment carefully. Then begin to make changes in the most critical areas, such as harmful alcohol or other drug use patterns. Seek help promptly for any difficulties that you are not prepared to deal with alone, such as domestic violence or suicidal thoughts. The information you read in this textbook and learn in this course could have a significant effect on your future health. Remember, it's not too late to improve your health!

To Carry This Further . . .

Most of us can improve our health behavior in a number of ways. We hope this assessment will help you identify areas in which you can make positive changes and serve as a motivator as you implement your plan for behavior change (see Chapter 1). If you scored well, give yourself a pat on the back. If your score was not as high as you would have liked, take heart. This textbook and your instructor can help you get started on the road to wellness. Good luck!

focus on health

chapter one

shaping your health

Chapter Objectives

Upon completing this chapter, you should be able to:

▌ understand how your health affects your lifestyle.

▌ recognize how the delivery of health care influences definitions of health.

▌ detail some of the health concerns outlined by the Institute of Medicine and Healthy People 2010.

▌ suggest additional reasons why health behavior change is difficult, beyond those outlined in your textbook.

▌ speculate on strategies for encouraging health behavior change, and offer reasons why health behavior change is difficult.

▌ list Prochaska's six stages of change.

▌ describe and compare the range of traditional and nontraditional students on your campus.

▌ describe the developmental tasks of adulthood, and assess your current level of progress in mastering them.

▌ monitor your own activities, and list the dimensions of health from which resources were drawn.

▌ compare wellness and health promotion, noting both the differences and the similarities between the two concepts.

▌ describe your textbook's new definition of health, and compare it with definitions of episodic health care and health promotion.

Online Learning Center Resources

www.mhhe.com/hahn7e

Log on to our Online Learning Center (OLC) for access to these additional resources:

- Chapter key terms and definitions
- Learning objectives
- Student interactive question-and-answer sites

- Self-scoring chapter quiz
- Online assessments
- Key term flash cards

Talking It Over

Getting in Shape Together: That's What Friends Are For

Shaping up can be a lonely business—unless you use the buddy system. But convincing a friend to get out and walk, run, or play volleyball can be tricky. Even a good friend might think you're saying he's flabby or lazy.

Try this approach: Say that *you* need to get in shape and want your friend's help and support. Make it clear to your friend that you don't want to become a marathon runner, just improve your cardiovascular fitness.

Tell your friend that it won't be punishment—it might even be fun! Check out the websites below for ideas on getting started.

CommunicationLinks
www.healthfinder.gov
www.healthworld.com

Eye on the Media

Where Does Our Health Information Come From?

Today our health information comes from a variety of media—some more reliable than others. Eye on the Media will appear in each chapter of this text, highlighting the important issue of which ones are good (in other words, valid and reliable) sources for learning about health.

Radio and Television

When you think of radio, the first thing that may come to mind is your favorite music. But two areas of radio are especially important for news and information: talk radio and public radio networks such as National Public Radio (NPR) and Public Radio International (PRI).

Talk radio raises the question of validity of information. For example, if you're listening to a talk show about HIV exposure, the perceptions and opinions of the host (which may be strong or even extreme) are an important part of the show. When this point of view is combined with the opinions of callers, whose "facts" may come from unauthoritative sources, what you're hearing is probably not solid information. It's certainly not a good basis for making your health decisions.

NPR and PRI, on the other hand, take a scholarly approach to news, featuring experts who do not always agree on an issue. In general, the news reports on NPR and PRI are long enough to present an in-depth, balanced treatment of health-related topics.

Television, too, is often an important source of health information. Coverage ranges from brief health-related segments on national or local news programs to entire cable programs devoted to health topics, such as those seen on the Learning and Discovery channels. While these programs can be timely and accurate, television also provides an array of "Infomercials" promoting health products that should be evaluated more critically.

Newspapers and Magazines

Let's assume that most people read only one or two newspapers a day—their local paper and perhaps a national newspaper such as *The New York Times* or *USA Today.* If so, the health information they are receiving is typically from wire services like the Associated Press; it is condensed and simplified but accurate within these limitations. When health-related information in newspapers is accompanied by illustrations and identification of the original source of information (such as a professional journal), it is more helpful to the reader.

Unlike newspapers, magazines are so diverse in terms of ownership, intended audience, and standards of validity that it is difficult to determine the reliability of their health-related content. In general, the national news magazines, such as *Time* and *Newsweek,* are very careful about the accuracy of their reporting, often including primary (original) sources. Their content is considered "state of the art." In contrast, the checkout-lane tabloids, such as *The Globe* and *The National Enquirer,* are known for printing stories with "health" content that few readers take seriously. Between these two extremes is a wide array of general content magazines, such as *The Saturday Evening Post,* and health-oriented magazines, such as *Prevention,* that vary greatly in validity and reliability.

Professional Journals

Your college library probably offers a broad selection of professional journals. Through these publications, the members of an academic discipline share the latest developments and issues in their field with their colleagues and other readers. Because the study of health is so multifaceted, drawing on different disciplines for information, health-related journals are plentiful. The vast majority of articles that appear in publications such as *The New England Journal of Medicine* and *The Journal of the American Dietetic Association* are peer-reviewed. This means that professionals in the particular field review and judge the content of a submitted article to determine whether or not it should be published. Then, if a study being reported was not carefully controlled, or if its underlying theory seems to be flawed, the article is returned to the author(s) for refinement. This process greatly reduces the risk of publishing invalid information. Currently, journals are beginning to appear in fields such as complementary (alternative) health care. When reading such publications, you need to consider whether they are backed by a peer-review process.

Government Documents

Each year various departments of the federal government, particularly the Department of Health and Human Services (DHHS), release the results of research being done under the oversight of its many divisions and agencies. These documents, such as the annual *Surgeon General's Report on Smoking and Health,* become the source of much of the health-related news reported by other media sources, including textbooks and professional journals. These publications generally can be purchased through the U.S. Government Printing Office. They are also available through urban public libraries and large university libraries. With few exceptions, the information in these publications is reviewed by the most respected authorities in each field.

Books

Books continue to be a vast source of information on health-related topics. Today's health books, in addition to academic health textbooks such as **Focus On Health** fall into three categories: reference books, medical encyclopedias, and single-topic trade (retail) books.

Included in the category of reference books are important professional publications such as *The Merck Manual* and the *Physi-*

cians' Desk Reference. These books, intended for professionals in various health fields, contain the most current information on specific aspects of health. Although these books can be purchased by the general public, their content is technical and complex, and their language is often difficult for non-professional readers to follow.

More valuable to the typical American household are the various medical (health) encyclopedias, such as *The Johns Hopkins Home Medical Handbook* and *The Mayo Clinic Family Health Book.* Such books usually include a wide array of medical conditions and offer valuable information about health promotion and disease prevention. Their clear writing styles and highly valid information make these books excellent home references.

Single-topic health-related trade books, such as those about diets and health problems, are readily available from retail outlets like bookstores and the Internet. Like magazines, these books are difficult to assess because of their quantity and the varying backgrounds of the authors. Some are very sound in terms of content and philosophy. Others may be misleading and may contain advice that could be dangerous to your health. Included in this group are self-help books, the best-selling health books of all.

The Internet

Today, at least 60% of all U.S. households can access the Internet directly, with 72% of those headed by college graduates having direct Internet access. Internet access is also available through libraries, educational institutions, and the workplace. With just a few clicks, you can reach many health-related websites that offer a wide range of health information. Chat rooms provide a forum for individuals to share their personal health experiences. Because the Internet is such an important source of health information for both professionals and the general public, this textbook highlights helpful websites in all chapters. To learn about criteria for assessing the validity and reliability of Internet information, see Chapter 15.

Source: Percentage of Internet-connected Households Soars to 60% in 2000; In-Stat Reveals Results in Buying and Internet Usage Trends. *In-Stat MDR Press Release.* March 28, 2000. http://www.in-stat.com

"Take care of your health, because you'll miss it when it's gone," younger people hear often from their elders. This simple and heartfelt advice is given in the belief that young people take their health for granted and assume that they will always maintain the state of health and wellness they now enjoy. Observation and experience should, however, remind all of us that youth is relatively brief, and health is always changing—often in a downward direction. In fact, as health deteriorates, our ability to participate in meaningful life activities can be compromised or even lost. Consider, for example, how failing health might affect the following activities:

- Your ability to pursue an education or career
- Your opportunity to socialize with friends and family
- The chance to travel—for business, relaxation, or adventure
- The opportunity to meet and connect with a spouse or partner
- The ability to conceive children or the opportunity to raise a family
- Participation in hobbies or physical activities, from skydiving to stamp collecting
- Your enjoyment of a wide range of foods
- The opportunity to enjoy a high-level of physical activity

It is quality of life issues such as these that your parents and grandparents are thinking about when they advise you to take care of your health. As you will learn in this chapter, health is intertwined with activities such as these—indeed, your authors will present a new definition of health specifically related to accomplishing these important life tasks. But first, a few familiar perceptions of health, each of which is concerned primarily with illness and death, will be reviewed, and strategies for changing health behaviors will be discussed.

Definitions of Health

By the time they reach college age, most Americans are familiar with the many ways in which health care is provided. Here are some easily recognizable examples, all of which serve to reinforce our traditional definitions of health. As you will learn, these definitions are centered in the cure or management of illness and the extension of life. Note the concerns over **morbidity** and **mortality** present in the descriptions that follow.

Episodic Health Care

The vast majority of Americans use the services of professional health care providers during periods (episodes) of

Keys to Longer Living

Experts generally agree on basic lifestyle characteristics that support greater longevity and, hopefully, a higher quality of life. Small adjustments that promote this improvement include:

- Testing your cholesterol level regularly and taking a 30-minute brisk walk every day.
- Wearing a seat belt in the car and a helmet while riding a bicycle, motorcycle, or while skating.
- Substituting olive oil instead of butter.
- Quitting smoking or at least reducing the amount of tobacco used daily. Lung cancer is the most frequent cause of cancer-related death in the United States.
- Avoiding sun exposure from 11 A.M. until 2 P.M. when UV radiation is most dangerous. Stay inside during those peak hours and always wear sunscreen outdoors.
- Asking questions of your doctor or pharmacist about concerns, test results, diagnosis, or treatments. It is often helpful to take someone with you to important appointments.
- Don't worry! Even if everyone was overly cautious, we would still not live in a risk free world—unnecessary worry can stress the mind and body.

illness and injury, that is, when we are "unhealthy." We consult providers seeking a diagnosis that will explain why we are not feeling well. Once a problem is identified, we expect to receive effective treatment from the practitioner that will lead to our recovery (the absence of illness) and a return to health. If we are willing to be compliant with the care strategies prescribed by our practitioner, we should soon be able to define ourselves as "healthy" once again.

The familiarity of episodic health care is evident in the 823.5 million times that Americans visited physicians during 2000. Although some of these visits were for preventive health care (see discussion on page 5), the vast majority were in conjunction with illness. When viewed by racial groups, Whites averaged 3.2 visits, Asians 2.9, Blacks 2.1 and Native Americans 0.8 visits during that year.[1]

TALKING POINTS Would you be hesitant to talk to your doctor about health advice you found on the Internet? How would you approach the subject?

Key Terms

morbidity pertaining to illness and disease.

mortality pertaining to death.

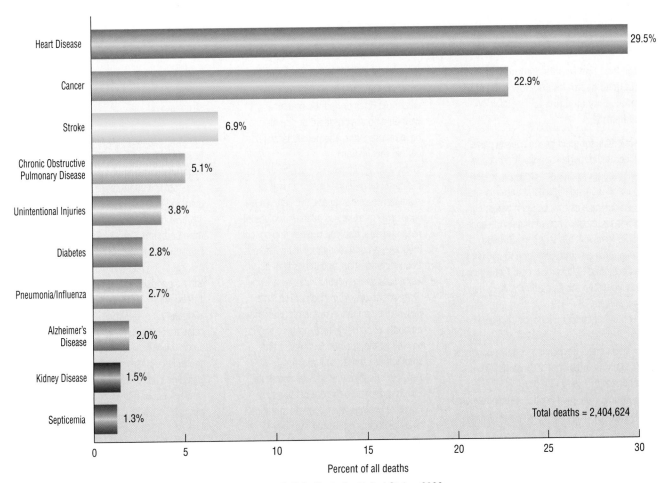

Figure 1-1 The 10 leading causes of death as a percentage of all deaths in the United States, 2000.

Source: *Deaths and death rates by leading causes of death and ages: 2000.* U.S. National Center for Health Statistics. Vital Statistics of the United States, Annual: National Vital Statistics Report (NVSR). 2002.

Preventive or Prospective Medicine

Simple logic suggests that it makes more sense to prevent illness than to deal with it through episodic health (medical) care. This philosophy characterizes **preventive** or **prospective medicine.** Unfortunately, however, many physicians say they have little time to practice preventive medicine because of the large number of episodically sick people who fill their offices every day.

When physicians do practice preventive or prospective medicine, they first attempt to determine their patient's level of risk for developing particular conditions. They make this assessment by identifying **risk factors** (and **high-risk health behaviors**) with a variety of observational techniques and screening tests, some of which may be invasive (taking tissues from the body such as a biopsy or blood draw). Additionally, an important tool in assessing risk is an accurate family health history, something that over one-third of all adults cannot adequately provide to their health care providers.[2] However, when you

are certain that any of the conditions shown in Figure 1-1 have occurred in your family, this information should be shared with your health care provider.

At age 34, I find that I'm getting lazy about good health habits. How can I start to refocus my thoughts and actions on good health?

Prescriptions for good health usually place considerable importance on *risk reduction.* Health care professionals stress the importance of identifying behavioral patterns and biomedical indexes that suggest the potential for illness or death. Each of us has the opportunity to receive information, counseling, behavior change strategies, and medical therapies designed to lower our risk. The extent to which we act on this opportunity is our degree of *compliance.*

Some risk factors cannot be reduced. For example, gender, race, age, and genetic predisposition make developing certain conditions more likely. Being aware of these risk factors is important.

To refocus on good health, concentrate on these actions, which can reduce risk factors:

- *Refrain from using tobacco in any form.* This rule is so critically important that the surgeon general of the United States has identified smoking as the single most important reversible factor contributing to illness and early death.

- *If you drink alcohol, do so in moderation.* This is particularly important for people who must drive or operate machinery, women who are pregnant or planning to become pregnant, and people taking certain medications.

- *Engage in regular exercise designed to train the cardiorespiratory system as well as maintain muscle strength.* You can use a wide array of exercises as the basis of a fitness program, and you can develop specific programs around recommendations about frequency, duration, and intensity of activity.

- *Eat a balanced diet that includes a wide array of choices from each of the food groups.* Pay attention to the recommended amounts of carbohydrate, protein, and fat, as well as the specific food items that supply these three nutrients.

- *Develop effective coping techniques for use in moderating the effects of stress.* Effective coping can reduce the duration of physiological challenge the body faces during periods of unexpected change. Remember, however, that some forms of coping can themselves be sources of additional stress.

- *Maintain normal body weight.* Persons who are excessively overweight or underweight may experience abnormal structural or functional changes, predispose themselves to chronic illnesses, and unnecessarily shorten their lives. Lifelong weight management is preferable to intermittent periods of weight gain and loss.

- *Receive regular preventive health care from competent professionals.* This care should include routine screening and risk-reducing lifestyle management, early diagnosis, and effective treatment if needed.

- *Maintain an optimistic outlook.* Anger, cynicism, and a pessimistic outlook on life can erode the holistic basis on which high-level health is built. Several chronic conditions, including cardiovascular diseases and cancers, occur more frequently in persons who lack a positive outlook on their own lives and life in general.

- *Establish a personally meaningful belief system.* Over the course of long life the presence of such a system and the supportive faith community usually associated with it may prove to be the most beneficial health resource we will possess.

Once they have identified levels of risk in patients, health practitioners try to lower those risk levels through patient education, lifestyle modification, and, when necessary, medical intervention. Continued compliance on the part of the patients will result in a lower level of risk that will continue over the years. Note that preventive medicine is guided by practitioners, and patients are expected to be compliant with the direction they are given.

Although preventive medical care appears to be a much more sensible approach than episodic care in reducing morbidity and mortality, third-party payers (insurance plans) traditionally have not provided coverage for these services. Managed health care plans that earn a profit by preventing sickness, such as health maintenance organizations, or HMOs (see Chapter 15), should be much more receptive to the concept and practice of preventive medicine.

Health Promotion

Throughout the United States, YMCA/YWCA-sponsored wellness programs, commercial fitness clubs, and corporate fitness centers offer risk-reduction programs under the direction of qualified instructors, many of whom are university graduates in disciplines such as exercise science, wellness management, and **health promotion.** Using

> **Key Terms**
>
> **health promotion** movement in which knowledge, practices, and values are transmitted to people for use in lengthening their lives, reducing the incidence of illness, and feeling better.

approaches similar to those employed in preventive medicine, these nonphysician health professionals attempt to guide their clients toward activities and behaviors that will lower their risk of chronic illness. Unlike preventive medicine, with its sometimes invasive assessment procedures and medication-based therapies, health promotion programs are not legally defined as medical practices and thus do not require the involvement of physicians. In addition, the fitness focus, social interaction, and healthy lifestyle orientation these programs provide tend to mask the emphasis on preventing chronic illness that would be the selling point of such efforts if they were undertaken as preventive medicine. In fact, it is likely that people receiving health promotion in these settings do not recognize it as such. Rather, they are only submitting to assessments and listening to health-related information as incidental parts of personal goals, such as losing weight, preparing for their first marathon, or simply meeting friends for lunch hour basketball.

Community Health Promotion

In addition to the practices just described, a group-oriented form of health promotion is offered in many communities. This approach to improving health through risk reduction is directed at empowering community groups, such as church congregations or a neighborhood association, so they can develop, operate, and financially sustain their own programs with little direct involvement of health promotion specialists.[3,4]

The key to successful community-based health promotion is **empowerment.**[5,6] In the context of health, empowerment refers to a process in which individuals or groups of people gain increasing control over their health. To take control over health matters, individuals and groups must learn to "liberate" themselves from a variety of barriers that tend to restrict health enhancement.

Empowerment programs have produced positive health consequences for individuals and groups that traditionally have been underserved by the health care system, such as minority populations. Once such people are given needed information, inroads into the political process, and skills for accessing funding sources, they become better able to plan, implement, and operate programs tailored to their unique health needs. In many communities, empowered people have organized grassroots campaigns to prevent neighborhood violence, improve childhood nutrition, promote healthy lifestyles, or prevent drug use among youth. When successful, these programs stand as excellent examples of the reality that people can make a difference when they become empowered.

Healthy People 2000 and Healthy People 2010

To identify all of the health-related concerns identified by members of the health community would be a monumental undertaking far beyond the scope of this book. However, in 2003, the Institutes of Medicine released a list of priority health concerns that they believe need particular attention. Among these priority concerns are:[7]

- treatment of asthma
- coordination of care for the 60 million persons with chronic health conditions
- reduction in the development of diabetes
- development of evidence-based cancer screening
- enhanced rates of immunization, particularly for flu and pneumonia
- improved detection of depression, which is now inadequately diagnosed and treated
- aggressively promoted prevention of cardiovascular disease, presently the leading killer of American adults
- concerted efforts to reduce the rate of nosocomial infections (infections that occur as a result of medical care) that kill an estimated 100,000 Americans annually
- reduction of tobacco dependence through cessation and prevention of smoking
- widened availability of prenatal care

While improvements in these areas are greatly needed, the Institutes of Medicine have no specific programs in place at this time to address them. In comparison, a well-established and ongoing program, Healthy People 2000, has established specific goals and objectives to improve the health of Americans in many of these areas. A brief description of this ongoing program follows.

In 1991 a U.S. government document titled *Healthy People 2000: National Health Promotion and Disease Prevention Objectives*[8] outlined a strategic plan for promoting the health of the American public. The plan included 300 health objectives in twenty-two priority areas.

Key Terms

empowerment the nurturing of an individual's or group's ability to be responsible for their own health and well-being.

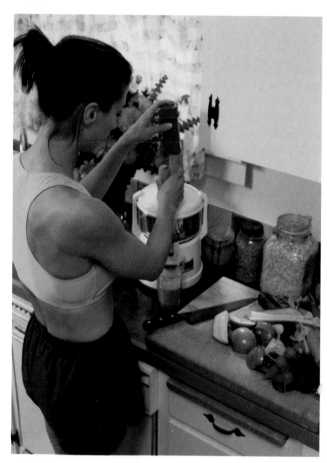

Many students have been able to change a specific health-related behavior, such as replacing poor eating habits with nutritious food choices.

Forty-seven of the 300 objectives were defined as "sentinel" ones, that is, particularly significant goals that could be used to measure the progress of the 1990s health promotion objectives.

Progress toward achieving the objectives was assessed near the middle of the decade and reported in a document titled *Healthy People 2000: Midcourse Review and 1995 Revisions.*[9] Although progress was reported in some areas, little or no progress was reported in many. Subsequently, a new plan, called *Healthy People 2010: Understanding and Improving Health,*[10] was formulated, refined, and is now being implemented.[11]

Healthy People 2010: Understanding and Improving Health is a health promotion program intended to be implemented at all levels, ranging from individual involvement through multinational cooperative efforts, including *Health for All in the 21ˢᵗ Century,*[12] a World Health Organization health promotion initiative. Al-

though the goals of *Healthy People 2000: National Health Promotion and Disease Prevention Objectives* and *Healthy People 2010: Understanding and Improving Health* are similar, the latter focuses on the projected needs of the United States during the first decade of the new century. Newly emerging demographics, such as the increasing number of older adults, and technologies, including new vaccines and HIV antiviral drugs, are better addressed in *Healthy People 2010: Understanding and Improving Health.*

Central to the design of *Healthy People 2010: Understanding and Improving Health* are two paramount goals: (1) increasing quality and years of life, and (2) eliminating health disparities in areas such as gender, race, and ethnicity, as well as income and education level. These goals in turn provide twenty-eight more focused objectives. Progress in accomplishing these objectives is anticipated through the manipulation of the behavioral, biological, and environmental determinants of health as they relate to ten of the leading health indicators: (1) physical activity, (2) weight management, (3) tobacco use, (4) substance abuse, (5) responsible sexual behavior, (6) mental health, (7) injury and violence, (8) environmental quality, (9) immunization, and (10) access to health care.

The success of *Healthy People 2010: Understanding and Improving Health* will not be known until nearer the end of the decade. However, if its goals are ultimately reached, Americans can anticipate an improved quantity and quality of life.

Changing Health-Related Behavior

Although some health concerns can be successfully addressed collectively though local, state, national, or international efforts such as those just outlined, most are ultimately based on the willingness and ability of persons to change aspects of their own behavior.

Why Behavior Change Is Often Difficult

Several factors can strongly influence a person's desire to change high health-risk behaviors, including those listed below.

1. A person must know that a particular behavioral pattern is clearly associated with (or even causes) a particular health problem. For example: Cigarette smoking is the primary cause of lung cancer.
2. A person must believe (accept) that their behavioral pattern will make (or has made) them susceptible to this particular health problem. For example: My

cigarette smoking will significantly increase my risk of developing lung cancer.

3. A person must recognize that risk-reduction intervention strategies exist and that should they adopt these in a compliant manner they too will reduce their risk for a particular health condition. For example: Smoking cessation programs exist, and following such a program could help me quit smoking.

4. A person must believe that benefits of newly adopted health-enhancing behaviors will be more reinforcing than the behaviors being given up. For example: The improved health, lowered risk, and freedom from dependence resulting from no longer smoking are better than the temporary pleasures provided by smoking.

5. A person must feel that significant others in their lives truly want them to alter their high-risk health behaviors and will support their efforts. For example: My friends who are cigarette smokers will make a concerted effort to not smoke in my presence and will help me avoid being around people who smoke.

When one or more of the conditions listed above is not in place, the likelihood that persons will be successful in reducing health-risk behaviors will be greatly diminished.

Stages of Change

The process of behavioral change unfolds over time and progresses through defined stages.[13,14] James Prochaska, John Norcross, and Carol DiClemente outlined six predictable stages of change. They studied thousands of individuals who were changing long-standing problems such as alcohol abuse, smoking, and gambling. While these people used different strategies to change their behavior, they all proceeded through six consistent stages of change in the process referred to as **Prochaska's Stages of Change.**[15]

Precontemplation Stage

The first stage of change is called *precontemplation,* during which a person might think about making a change, but ultimately finds it too difficult and avoids doing it. For example, during this phase a smoker might tell friends, "Eventually I will quit," but have no real intention of stopping within the next 6 months.

Contemplation Stage

For many, however, progress toward change begins as they move into a *contemplation* stage, during which they might develop the desire to change but have little understanding of how to go about it. Typically, they see themselves taking action within the next 6 months.

Preparation Stage

Following the contemplation stage, a *preparation* begins, during which change begins to appear to be not only desirable but possible as well. A smoker might begin making plans to quit during this stage, setting a quit date for the very near future (a few days to a month), and perhaps enrolling in a smoking cessation program.

Action Stage

Plans for change are implemented during the *action* stage, during which changes are made and sustained for a period of about 6 months.

Maintenance Stage

The fifth stage is the *maintenance* stage, during which new habits are consolidated and practiced for an additional 6 months.

Termination Stage

The sixth and final stage is called *termination,* which refers to the point at which new habits are well established and so efforts to change are complete.

Today's Health Concerns

To this point in the chapter your textbook has identified some health concerns and addressed the desirability of health-related behavior change. Earlier in the chapter, your textbook looked at those illnesses that are the major causes of death that afflict the American public. Beyond those mentioned, it is evident that, in spite of astonishing progress on many fronts, we continue to face a number of serious health challenges. Heart disease, cancer, accidents, drug use, and mental illness all are important concerns for each of us, even if we are not directly affected by them. Also becoming increasingly troublesome are the complex problems of environmental pollution, violence, health

---

Key Terms

Prochaska's Stages of Change the six predictable stages— precontemplation, contemplation, preparation, action, maintenance, and termination—people go through in establishing new habits and patterns of behavior.

Table 1.1 Leading Causes of Death in the United States by Age Group, 2000

1–4 Years	Number of Deaths
Unintentional injuries	1,780
Birth defects	471
Cancer	393
5–14 Years	
Unintentional injuries	2,878
Cancer	1,017
Homicide	364
15–24 Years	
Unintentional injuries	13,616
Homicide	4,796
Suicide	3,877
25–44 Years	
Unintentional injuries	24,817
Cancer	20,200
Heart disease	15,267
45–64 Years	
Cancer	136,363
Heart disease	97,334
Unintentional injuries	18,252
65 Years and Older	
Heart disease	545,440
Cancer	392,052
Stroke	146,725

Source: Deaths and death rates by leading causes of death and ages: 2000. U.S. National Center for Health Statistics. *Vital Statistics of the United States, Annual: National Vital Statistics Report* (NVSR). 2002.

Health: More than the Absence of Illness?

What exactly is health? Is it simply the absence of disease and illness, as Western medicine has held for centuries—or does health embrace other elements we ought to consider now that the twenty-first century has begun?

Rather routinely national news magazines (and other media) feature articles describing advances in modern medicine.[16,17] These articles describe vividly in words and images the impressive progress being made in fields such as cancer treatment, gene manipulation, computer-aided surgery, and complementary medical care. Because of articles like this that relate health to medical care, most of us continue to hold to our traditional perception of health as (1) the virtual absence of disease and illness (low levels of morbidity) and (2) the ability to live a long life (reduced risk of mortality). However, in striving to be fully "health educated" in the new century, perhaps we need to consider a broader definition that more accurately reflects the demands associated with becoming functional and satisfied persons as we transition through each adult stage of life—*young adulthood, middle adulthood,* and, finally, *older adulthood.* With this in mind, look forward to another definition of health—one that recognizes the importance of the more familiar definitions of health, but is focused on the demands of our own growth and development. However, before looking at this newer perception of health and its relationship to young adulthood let's meet the reader of this book, today's college students, each of whom are or once were young adults.

Today's College Students

Readers of this textbook are college students, but they are also young adults, middle age adults, or even older adults. In some cases their decision to be a student has placed

care costs, and the international scope of the HIV/AIDS epidemic, as well as other sexually transmitted diseases. Figure 1-1 on page 4 lists the ten leading causes of death in the United States expressed as a percentage of all deaths. Table 1.1 depicts the leading causes of death at various age levels. World hunger, over-population, and the threat of domestic and international terrorism are other health-related issues that will affect us, as well as the generations that follow.

The health concerns just mentioned are by no means unmanageable. Fortunately, we as individuals can reduce the likelihood of encountering many of these conditions by making choices in the way we live our lives. On a personal level, we can decide to pursue a plan of healthful living to minimize the incidence of illness and disease and to extend life.

OnSITE/InSIGHT

Learning to Go: Health

Getting tired of your study routine? Click on Learning to Go: Health on the Online Learning Center at **www.mhhe.com/hahn7e** for a different slant on studying. Check out these lessons, which make a good match for this chapter:

Lesson 1: Chart a plan for behavior change.

Lesson 2: Strive for multidimensional health.

them in settings far different from those being experienced by other people their age. For many students, college classes are sandwiched in between other obligations—for example a full-time job, parenting, community involvement, even the care of older parents. Some might be the first members of their families to pursue higher education. Many students come from economic, racial, or ethnic backgrounds quite different from that of the majority of their classmates. Thus, today there is no one type of college student, but nevertheless, all of them are progressing through life in predictable, yet unique ways.

Traditional-Age Undergraduate College Students

Statistics indicate that more than 13.4 million students were enrolled in degree-granting U.S. colleges and universities in 2001. Nearly 60% of these students are women. Minority students make up approximately 28% of American college students and foreign students total 10.1%.[18]

Because two-thirds (66%) of all undergraduates are traditional-age students[19], this book is directed first at these students. However, because of significant growth in the proportion of older students, we will also address a variety of life experiences appropriate to these students. Unquestionably, the nontraditional-age students in our classes help our traditional-age students understand the wide and varied role that health plays throughout the life cycle.

TALKING POINTS You are in charge of a campus event for students of various ages from several cultural groups. How would you go about finding out what would make the event attractive to students with backgrounds different from your own?

Nontraditional-Age Undergraduate College Students

In 1999, nearly 33% of American undergraduate college students were classified as **nontraditional-age students.**[18] Included in this vast overlapping group are part-time students, military veterans, students returning to college, single parents, older adults, and evening students. These students enter the classroom with a wide assortment of life experiences and observations. Most of these students are twenty-five to forty years old. Read the Learning from Our Diversity box for a closer look at nontraditional-age students.

Many nontraditional-age students are trying to juggle an extremely demanding schedule. The responsibilities of managing a job, a schedule of classes, and perhaps a fam-

Ages of Undergraduate College Students (Full- and Part-time), Projected for 2001

Age	Number	Percentage of Total
14–17	170,000	1.1
18–19	3,543,000	23.1
20–21	3,101,000	20.2
22–24	2,457,000	16.1
25–29	1,863,000	12.2
30–34	1,223,000	8.0
35+	2,943,000	18.8
		99.5%

Source: *Total fall enrollment in degree-granting institutions, by attendance status, sex, and age: 1970 to 2001.* U.S. Census Bureau. Statistical Abstract of the United States: 2002 (122nd Edition)

ily present formidable challenges. Performing these tasks on a limited budget compounds the difficulty. For undergraduate students, concerns over paying next month's rent, caring for aging parents, or finding affordable child care are as common as the challenges that confront students of traditional age.

For these reasons, we want to make this textbook meaningful for both traditional-age and nontraditional-age students. Much of the information we present applies to both categories of students. We ask nontraditional-age students to do two things as you read this book: (1) reflect on your own young adult years, and (2) examine your current lifestyle to see how the decisions you made as a younger adult are affecting the quality of your life now. As a nontraditional-age student, you may have young adult children whose lives you can observe in light of the information you will find in this book.

Minority Students

Although enrollment patterns at colleges and universities vary, the overall number of minority students is increasing.

> **Key Terms**
>
> **nontraditional-age students** administrative term used by colleges and universities for students who, for whatever reason, are pursuing undergraduate work at an age other than that associated with the traditional college years (18–24).

To anyone who's visited an American college campus in the last ten years, it's abundantly clear that the once typical college student—white, middle class, between the ages of eighteen and twenty-four—is not always a majority on campus. In most institutions of higher learning, today's student body is a rich tapestry of color, culture, language, ability, and age. Wheelchair-accessible campuses roll out the welcome mat for students with disabilities; the air is filled with the music of a dozen or more languages spoken by students from virtually every part of the world; students in their 60s chat animatedly with classmates young enough to be their grandchildren.

Of all the trends that are changing the face of college enrollment in the United States, perhaps the most significant is the increasing diversity in the age of students now on campus. Older students today are both a common and welcome sight in colleges and universities across the country. Many women cut short their undergraduate education—or defer graduate school—to marry and raise children. Divorcees, widows, and women whose children are grown often return to college, or enroll for the first time, to prepare for professional careers. And increasingly, both men and women are finding it desirable, if not essential, to further their education as a means of either keeping their current job or qualifying for a higher position.

Just as children are enriched by the knowledge and experience of their grandparents and other older relatives, so too is today's college classroom a richer place when many of the seats are filled by students of nontraditional age. Without being didactic or preachy, older students can provide valuable guidance and direction to younger classmates who may be uncertain of their career path, or who may be wrestling with decisions about marriage and parenthood. In doing so, nontraditional-age students can gain helpful insights about young people's feelings, attitudes, challenges, and aspirations.

Among the many important benefits of today's increasingly diverse college campus, surely one of the most significant is the enhanced opportunity for intergenerational communication and understanding made possible by the growing numbers of students of nontraditional age.

In your classes, how would you characterize the interactions between traditional-age students and those of nontraditional age? In what ways are they enriching each other's college experience?

In 1999, slightly over 26% of all college students were minority students, with African Americans, Hispanic Americans, Asian Americans, and Native Americans representing the largest groups of minority students.[20] These students bring a rich variety of cultural influences and traditions to today's college environment.

Students with Disabilities

People with reported disabilities are another rapidly growing student population, currently comprising 9.3% of all undergraduates.[21] Improved diagnostic, medical, and rehabilitation procedures coupled with improved educational accommodations have opened up opportunities for these students at an increasing rate. In addition to students who have visible disabilities, such as blindness, deafness, or a physical disability requiring use of a wheelchair, a greater number of students with "hidden" disabilities are appearing on campuses. Examples are students with learning disabilities (including attention deficit disorders), those with managed psychiatric and emotional problems, and those recovering from alcohol and substance abuse. Interestingly, many students with reported "hidden disabilities" often do not consider themselves to be disabled.[21]

TALKING POINTS When controversial subjects are discussed in class, do you think that your opinions (or how you present them) are affected by the fact that students of different cultural backgrounds are involved in the discussion?

Developmental Tasks of Young Adulthood

Because most of today's undergraduate college students range between the ages of eighteen and perhaps forty, we will address several areas of growth and development (defined as *developmental tasks*) that characterize the lives of people in this age group (Figure 1-2). When people sense that they are making progress in some or all of these areas, they are likely to report a sense of life satisfaction or, as we describe it, a sense of well-being.

Forming an Initial Adult Identity

For most of childhood and adolescence, most young people are seen by adults in their neighborhood or community as someone's son or daughter. With the onset of young adulthood, that stage has almost passed; both young people and society are beginning to look at each other in new ways.

Why Men Die Young

The extra longevity of women in our society is well established. In fact, the difference in life expectancy for male and female infants born today is projected to be 80 years for females, but only 75 for males. This five-year difference has commonly been attributed to genetic factors. However, new evidence demonstrates that this discrepancy may be affected more by male behavior rather than genetic traits.

Men outrank women in all of the top fifteen causes of death except for Alzheimer's disease. Men's death rates are twice as high for suicide, homicide, and cirrhosis of the liver. In every age group, American males have poorer health and higher risk of mortality than do females. Common increased risks include:

- More men smoke than women.
- Men are twice as likely to be heavy drinkers, or to engage in other risky behaviors such as abusing drugs and driving without a seatbelt.
- More men work in dangerous settings than women, and men account for 90% of on-the-job fatalities.
- More men drive SUVs that are rollover prone, and suffer fatalities in motorcycle accidents.

Perhaps some of these increased risks are associated with deep-seated cultural beliefs about men's bravery and machismo, which reward them for taking risks and facing danger head-on. This "macho" attitude seems to extend to the care that men take of their own physical and mental health. Women are twice as likely to visit their doctor on an annual basis and explore preventative medical treatments than are men. Men are more likely to ignore symptoms and less likely to schedule checkups or seek follow-up treatment. Psychologically, men tend to internalize their feelings or stressors, or even self-medicate to deal with stress, while women tend to seek psychological help. Almost all stress-related diseases are more common in men.

In the final analysis, men and women alike must be responsible for their own health and well-being. By making sound choices regarding diet, exercise, medical care, and high-risk behaviors, both genders can attempt to maximize the full potential of their life expectancy.

As emerging adults, most young people want to present a unique identity to society. Internally they are constructing perceptions of themselves as the adults they wish to be; externally they are formulating the behavioral patterns that will project this identity to others.

Completion of this first developmental task is necessary for young adults to establish a foundation on which to nurture identity during later stages of adulthood. As a result of their experiences in achieving an initial adult identity, they will become capable of answering the

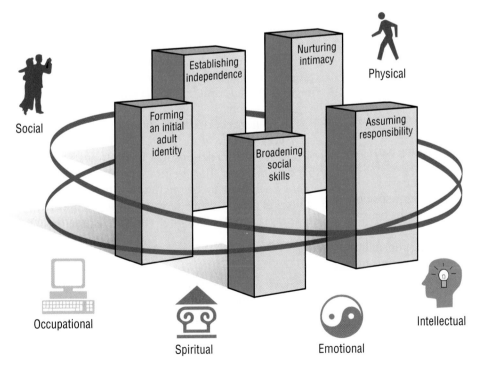

Figure 1-2 Mastery of the developmental tasks through a balanced involvement of the six dimensions of health will lead to your enjoying a more productive and satisfying life.

central question of young adulthood: "Who am I?" Most likely, many nontraditional-age students are also asking themselves this question as they progress through college and anticipate the changes that will result from completing a high level of formal education.

Establishing Independence

In contemporary society the primary responsibility for socialization during childhood and adolescence is assigned to the family. For nearly two decades the family is the primary contributor to a young person's knowledge, values, and behaviors. By young adulthood, however, students of traditional college age should be demonstrating the desire to move away from the dependent relationship that has existed between themselves and their families.

 TALKING POINTS What does being an adult mean to you at this point? How would you explain this to your best friend?

Travel, peer relationships, marriage, military service, and, of course, college have been traditional avenues for disengagement from the family, although most undergraduates return home during summers.[22] Generally the ability and willingness to follow one or more of these paths will help a young adult establish independence. Success in these endeavors will depend on the willingness to use a variety of resources we will explore later.

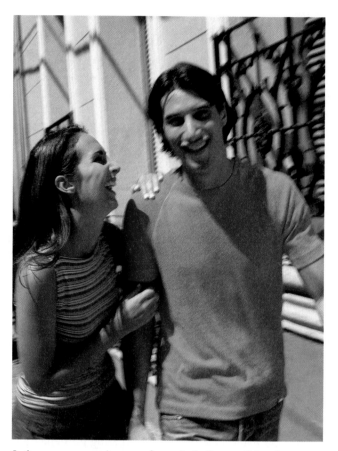

Intimacy can occur in many forms, including traditional dating relationships.

Assuming Responsibility

The third developmental task in which traditional-age college students are expected to progress is the assumption of increasing levels of responsibility. Young adults have a variety of opportunities to assume responsibility. College-age young adults may accept responsibility voluntarily, such as when they join a campus organization or establish a new friendship. Other responsibilities are placed on them when professors assign term papers, when dating partners exert pressure on them to conform to their expectations, or when employers require consistently productive work. In other situations they may accept responsibility for doing a particular task not for themselves but for the benefit of others. As important and demanding as these areas of responsibility are, a more fundamental responsibility awaits young adults: the responsibility of maintaining and improving their health and the health of others.

Broadening Social Skills

The fourth developmental task of the young adult years is broadening the range of appropriate and dependable so-

cial skills. Adulthood ordinarily involves "membership" in a variety of groups that range in size from a marital pair to a national political party or international corporation. These memberships will require the ability to function in many different social settings and with a wide variety of people.

The college experience traditionally has prepared students very effectively in this regard, but interactions in friendships, work relationships, or parenting may require that they make an effort to grow and develop beyond levels they achieved by belonging to a peer group. Young adults will need to refine a variety of social skills, including communication, listening, and conflict management.

Nurturing Intimacy

The task of nurturing intimacy usually begins in young adulthood and continues through midlife. During this time it is developmentally important to establish one or more intimate relationships. Most people in this age group are viewing intimacy in its broadest sense as a deeply close, sharing relationship. Intimacy may unfold in the context of dating relationships, close friendships, and certainly mentoring relationships.

Involvement in intimate relationships varies, with some people having many relationships and others having only one or two. The number does not matter. From a developmental standpoint, what matters is that we have others with whom to share our most deeply held thoughts and feelings as we attempt to validate our own unique approach to living.

Related Developmental Tasks of Young Adulthood

In addition to the five developmental tasks of young adulthood just described, two additional areas of growth and development seem applicable to 18- to 24-year-olds. These include obtaining *entry-level employment and the developing of parenting skills.*

For at least the last sixty years, students in increasing numbers have pursued a college education in large part to gain entry into many occupations and professions. Students of today certainly anticipate that a college degree will open doors for their first substantial employment or entry-level employment.

In many respects employment needs go beyond those associated purely with money. Employment provides the opportunity to assume new responsibilities in which the skills learned in college can be applied and expanded. Employment also involves taking on new roles (such as colleague, mentor, mentee, or partner) that may play an important part in the way we define ourselves for the remainder of our lives. In addition, employment provides a new, more independent arena in which friendships (intimacy) can be pursued. By no means least important, entry-level employment provides the financial foundation on which we can establish independence.

For many people, young adulthood marks the entry to parenthood, one of the most important responsibilities anyone can choose to assume. The multitude of decisions associated with this commitment will, naturally, shape the remainder of one's life. Examples of these decisions are whether to parent or not, and, if so, when to begin, how many children to have, what interval between children, and what role parenting will play in the context of overall adulthood. The ability to make sound decisions and to develop the skills and insights necessary to parent effectively may be the most challenging aspect of growth and development that confronts young adults.

The Multiple Dimensions of Health

In an earlier section of the chapter your authors promised a new definition of health that would be less focused on morbidity (illness) and mortality (death) than most others. Before we do this, however, let us introduce a multidimensional concept of health (or **holistic health** —a requirement for any definition of health that moves beyond the cure/prevention of illness and the postponement of death.

> **Key Terms**
>
> **holistic health** a view of health in terms of its physical, emotional, social, intellectual, and spiritual makeup.

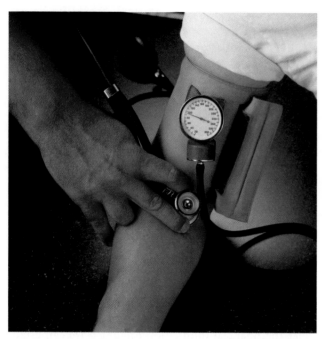

Although not interested in illness or premature death, wellness practitioners find it critically important that they inform their clients about the role of elevated blood pressure in the development of cardiovascular disease.

Although our modern health care community too frequently acts as if the structure and function of the physical body is the sole basis of health, common experience supports the validity of a *holistic* nature to health. In this section we will examine six component parts, or dimensions, of health, all interacting in a synergistic manner allowing us to engage in the wide array of life experiences.

Physical Dimension

Most of us have a number of physiological and structural characteristics we can call on to aid us in accomplishing the wide array of activities that characterize a typical day, and, on occasion, a not so typical day. Among these physical characteristics are our body weight, visual ability, strength, coordination, level of endurance, level of susceptibility to disease, and powers of recuperation. In certain situations the physical dimension of health may be the most important. This almost certainly is why traditional medicine for centuries has equated health with the design and operation of the body.

Emotional Dimension

We also possess certain emotional characteristics that can help us through the demands of daily living. The emo-

tional dimension of health encompasses our ability to cope with stress, remain flexible, and compromise to resolve conflict.

For young adults, growth and development often give rise to emotional vulnerability, which may lead to feelings of rejection and failure that can reduce productivity and satisfaction. To some extent we are all affected by feeling states, such as anger, happiness, fear, empathy, guilt, love, and hate. People who consistently try to improve their emotional health appear to enjoy life to a much greater extent than do those who let feelings of vulnerability overwhelm them or block their creativity.

Social Dimension

A third dimension of health encompasses social skills and insights. Initially, family interactions, school experiences, and peer group interactions foster social skill development, but future social interactions will demand additional skill development and refinement of already existing skills and insights. In adulthood, including young adulthood, the composition of the social world changes, principally because of our exposure to a wider array of people and the expanded roles associated with employment, parenting, and community involvement.

The social abilities of many nontraditional-age students may already be firmly established. Entering college may encourage them to develop new social skills that help them socialize with their traditional-age student colleagues. After being on campus for a while, nontraditional-age students are often able to interact comfortably with traditional-age students in such diverse places as the library, the student center, and the bookstore. This interaction enhances the social dimension of health for both types of students.

Intellectual Dimension

The ability to process and act on information, clarify values and beliefs, and exercise decision-making capacity ranks among the most important aspects of total health. In fact, for many college-educated persons, this dimension of health may prove to be the most important and satisfying of the six. In fact, for all of us, at least on certain occasions, this will hold true. Our ability to analyze, synthesize, hypothesize, and then act upon new information enhances the quality of our lives in multiple ways.

Spiritual Dimension

The fifth dimension of health is the spiritual dimension. Although certainly it includes religious beliefs and practices, many young adults would expand it to encompass more diverse belief systems, including relationships with other living things, the nature of human behavior, and the need and willingness to serve others. All are important components of spiritual health.

Through nurturing the spiritual dimension of our health, we may develop an expanded perception of the universe and better define our relationship to all that it contains, including other people. To achieve growth in the spiritual dimension of health, many people undertake a serious study of doctrine associated with established religious groups and will assume membership in a community of faith. For others, however, spiritual growth is believed to occur, in the absence of a theist-based belief system, as they open themselves to new experiences that involve nature, art, body movement, or stewarding of the environment.

Interestingly, the role of the spiritual dimension of health was given an increased measure of credence when studies published in the scientific literature, including a statistical review of forty-two earlier studies, demonstrated a consistently longer life for persons who regularly participated in religious practices, particularly for women.[23,24] This was true even when factors such as smoking, alcohol use, and income were statistically eliminated. Contradictory to these findings, however, was a report suggesting that the ability of prescriptive prayer (prayers of intercession) to enhance healing and extend life could not be supported by current research due to design flaws in the studies made to date.[25]

Occupational Dimension

A significant contribution made by the currently popular wellness movement is that it defines for many people the importance of the workplace to their sense of well-being. In today's world, employment and productive efforts play an increasingly important role in how we perceive ourselves and how we see the "goodness" of the world in which we live. In addition, the workplace serves as both a testing ground for and a source of life-enhancing skills. In our place of employment we gain not only the financial resources to meet our demands for both necessities and luxuries, but also an array of useful skills like conflict resolution, experiences in shared responsibility, and intellectual growth that can be used to facilitate a wide range of nonemployment-related interactions. In turn, the workplace is enhanced by the healthfulness of the individuals who contribute to its endeavors.

Wellness

Expanded perceptions of health are the basis for **wellness.** Recall that episodic health care, preventive medicine, and community health promotion are directly aligned with concerns over morbidity and mortality, while health promotion at the individual level is focused on aspects of appearance, weight management, body composition, and physical performance capabilities. Wellness differs from these kinds of health care because it virtually has no interest in morbidity and mortality.

Practitioners describe wellness as a process of extending information, counseling, assessment, and lifestyle modification strategies, leading to a desirable change in the recipients' overall lifestyle, or the adoption of a wellness lifestyle. Once adopted, the wellness lifestyle produces a sense of well-being (also called wellness) that in turn enables recipients to unlock their full potential.

Key Terms

wellness the promotion and achievement of optimal health, including physical, emotional, social, spiritual, intellectual, and occupational well-being.

This explanation of how wellness differs from episodic health care, preventive medicine, and health promotion does, on first hearing, seem progressive and clearly devoid of interest in morbidity and mortality concerns. But in practice, wellness programs are not all that different from other kinds of health care. Your authors have consistently noted that wellness programs, as carried out on college campuses, in local hospital wellness centers, and in corporate settings, routinely transmit familiar health-related information and engage in the same risk-reduction activities that characterize preventive medicine and health promotion. It is in the final aspect of wellness, the "unlocking of full potential," that wellness differs from other concepts of health. More than the absence of chronic illness, it involves achieving optimal health across all six of the dimensions of health discussed in the previous section.

A New Definition of Health

At the beginning of the chapter we asked you to consider a new way to view health—a view that would be far less centered in morbidity and mortality concerns than traditional concepts of health and even of wellness. The definition that we propose takes into account the differences between *what health is for* (its role) and *what health is* (its composition).

The Role of Health

The role of health in our lives is very similar to the role of a car. Much as a car (or other vehicle) takes us to places we need or want to be, health enables us to accomplish the activities that collectively transition us into and through developmental tasks associated with young adulthood (see pages 12 through 15). Recall that the process of moving through each stage of adulthood does not occur simply because of the passage of time, but rather because we actively participate, on a day-to-day basis, in demands of life appropriate to our life stage.

The Composition of Health

Now that you know what the role of health is, its composition can be seen as being more than simply having a body free of illness and apparently destined for a long life. Rather, the composition of health is that of a collection of resources, from each dimension of health (see pages 15 through 17), determined to be necessary for the successful accomplishment of activities that you need or want to do. Some of these needed resources will already be within you (intrinsic), while others will need to come from outside (extrinsic). However, regardless of their origin, once they are accessed and applied to activities, small forward growth steps will occur. Obviously, to recognize what resources are needed, you must be a student of society's expectations for persons of your age, as well as your own highly personalized developmental aspirations.

Our Definition of Health

By combining the role of health with the composition of health, we offer a new definition of health that we believe is unique to this textbook.

> Health is a reflection of your ability to use the **intrinsic** and **extrinsic** resources related to each dimension of health to participate fully in the activities that contribute to your growth and development, with the goal of feeling a sense of well-being as you evaluate your progress through life.

In light of this definition, do not be surprised when your textbook asks whether you are resourceful (healthy) enough for the goals you wish to reach, or whether you are healthy enough to sustain a particular behavioral pattern that you have adopted, or whether you are experiencing the sense of well-being to which you aspire.

Taking Charge of Your Health

- Complete the Comprehensive Health Assessment on p. xxxi. Develop a plan to modify your behavior in the areas in which you need improvement.
- Take part in a new spiritual activity, such as meditating, creating art or music, or appreciating nature.
- To promote the social dimension of your health, try to meet one new person each week during the semester.

- Choose one developmental task you would like to focus on, such as assuming responsibility, and plan the steps you can follow to progress in this area.
- Volunteer to be an assistant in a community service program, such as a literacy project or a preschool program.

Summary

- When used to define health, morbidity and mortality relate to the prevalence of particular diseases and illnesses and to death resulting from those diseases and illnesses.
- When we seek the services of health care practitioners because of symptoms of illness or disease, we are said to be seeking episodic health care.
- Preventive medical care attempts to minimize the incidence of illness and disease by identifying early indicators of risk to bring them under control.
- Individual health promotion involves risk-reduction activities similar to those used in preventive medical care, except that the techniques cannot be invasive, and are directed by professionals who are not physicians.
- Community health promotion involves the empowerment of individuals so that they can organize and participate in their own health promotion activities.
- Healthy People 2010 is a federally funded program to improve the nation's health, increase life expectancy, and expand access to comprehensive health care.
- A decision to change a health behavior is often difficult to make because of a multiplicity of factors underlying the behavior, making the behavior one that results in immediate gratification.
- Health behavior change requires movement through a multistaged process, including precontemplation, contemplation, preparation, action, and maintenance.
- A wide array of health problems (for example, cancer, cardiovascular disease, HIV/AIDS) persist despite today's highly sophisticated health care technology.
- Today's college campus is a dynamic blend of students of both traditional and nontraditional ages and of diverse background, cultures, and attributes.
- Young adulthood is characterized by five key developmental tasks: forming an initial adult identity, establishing independence, assuming responsibility, broadening social skills, and nurturing intimacy.
- Personal development during young adulthood involves a set of developmental tasks that are common to all, yet may be undertaken differently by each individual.
- Multidimensional definitions of health, including holistic health, have existed for decades—although the primary emphasis has always been on the physical dimension.
- Current multidimensions of health may include many or all of the following dimensions: physical, emotional, social, intellectual, spiritual, and occupational.
- Wellness contends a disinterest in morbidity and mortality, rather emphasizing living a wellness lifestyle that leads to a sense of well-being.
- The role of health, as seen by your textbook, is to enable individuals to participate in the activities that collectively constitute growth and development.
- The composition of health, as seen by your textbook, is the intrinsic and extrinsic resources on which individuals can draw to participate fully in their own growth and development.

Review Questions

1. What are morbidity and mortality, and how are they involved in the more traditional definitions of health?
2. When and from whom do people seek episodic health care?
3. In preventive medical care, who determines a person's level of risk and decides what risk-reduction techniques should be implemented?
4. In terms of professional personnel and the type of risk reduction techniques used, how does health promotion at the individual level differ from preventive medical care?
5. What does the term *empowerment* mean and how would it appear as a component of a community-based health promotion program?
6. What are the two primary goals of *Healthy People 2010,* the federally funded program to improve the health of the American population?
7. What are the six stages that persons pass through as they consider and then attempt to change their health behavior?
8. What are several of the more pressing health problems that confront the American people?
9. In what ways is the current American college student population more diverse that any coming before?
10. What are the developmental tasks of young adulthood and how can the accomplishing of one influence the accomplishing of any of the remaining four?
11. How does the term *multidimensional* apply to the concept of holistic health?
12. What are the most frequently included dimensions within a holistically centered definition of health?
13. What is the underlying reason that proponents of wellness give for being disinterested in morbidity and mortality?

14. How does your textbook's definition of health differ from traditional definitions?
15. How does your textbook define the role of health?
16. How is composition of health defined by your textbook? What would be examples of resources from each of the five dimensions of health?

17. Why is it necessary to understand developmental expectations before we can answer the question, "Are you healthy enough to . . . ?"

References

1. Centers for Disease Control and Prevention: *National Ambulatory Medical Care Survey: 2000.* July, 2002.
2. Roper Center for Public Opinion Research (for Pfizer Women's Health), University of Connecticut: *Adults know their family history.* USA Today. May 30, 2000. p.5D.
3. Cottrell RR, Girvan JT, McKenzie JF. *Principles and foundations of health promotion and education.* Benjamin Cummings, 2002.
4. Kreuter MW, Lezin NA, Kreuter MW, Green LW. *Community health promotion ideas that work: a field-book for practitioners.* Jones and Bartlett Publishers, 2003.
5. McKenzie, JF, Smeltzer JL. *Planning, implementing and evaluating health promotion programs,* 3rd ed. Allyn and Bacon, 2001.
6. Bensley RJ, Brookins-Fisher J (Editors). *Community health education methods: a practitioner's guide.* Jones and Bartlett Publishers, 2003.
7. *Priority areas for national action: transforming healthcare quality (2003).* The National Academies Press, 2003.
8. *Healthy people 2000: national health promotion and disease prevention objectives* (full report with commentary). U.S. Department of Health and Human Services. Public Health Service, 1991.
9. *Healthy people 2000: midcourse review and 1995 revisions.* 1995. Department of Health and Human Services. Public Health Service.
10. *Healthy people 2010: understanding and improving health.* Department of Health and Human Services. Public Health Service, 2000.
11. *Healthy people 2010: understanding and improving health,* 2nd ed. Department of Health and Human Services. Public Health Services, 2000.
12. Health for all in the 21st century. World Health Organization, 1979. **www.who/int/archives/hfa/policy.htm**
13. Prochaska JO, Velicer WF. The transtheoretical model of health behavior change. 1994. *Am J of Health Promotion.* 12:38–48.
14. Norcross JC, Prochaska JO. Using the stages of change. 2002. *Harv Ment Health Lett.* 18(11):507.
15. Prochaska JO, Norcross JC, Clemente CC. *Changing for good.* William Morrow and Company, 1994.
16. *Drugs of the future.* (Special issue.) *Time* 157:02, January 15, 2001.
17. The science of alternative medicine. *Newsweek.* December 02, 2002.
18. U.S. Census Bureau: *Statistical Abstract of the United States: 2002* (122nd Edition)
19. U.S. Department of Education. National Center for Education Statistics, Integrated Postsecondary Education Data System, "Fall Enrollment, 1999" Survey. 2001.
20. U.S. Department of Education. National Center for Education Statistics, Integrated Postsecondary Data System (IPEDS). *Fall enrollment in institutions of higher education: projections of education statistics to 2009,* July 1999. **http://nces.ed.gov/[ibs2000/digest99/**
21. U.S. National Center for Education Statistics: *Profile of undergraduates in U.S. postsecondary education institutions, 1999–2000.* July 2000.
22. Most college student living with the folks. *USA Today.* August 27, 2002. p.5D. Source: *Collegeclub.com* online survey of 3,188 self-selected respondents. June 7, 2002.
23. Hummer RA et al. Religious involvement and U.S. adult mortality. *Demography* 1999; 36(2): 272–285.
24. McCullough ME et al. Religious involvement and mortality: a meta-analytic review. *Health Psychology* 2000; 19(2): 211–222.
25. Sloan RP et al. Should physicians prescribe religious activities? *N Engl J Med* 2000; 342(25): 1913–1916.

At the heart of preventive medical care is the need on the part of physicians to identify areas of risk that foretell chronic illnesses for their patients. The taking of detailed family medical histories, combined with the results of an array of screening procedures assessing biomedical indices, augment physicians' observational skills in identifying areas of concern and the high-risk behaviors associated with each. From the information gleaned, physicians should counsel their patients toward risk reduction. But how frequently does this important patient education occur?

In a recent assessment of patient education efforts made by physicians practicing in Derby, Connecticut, and reported in *Preventive Medicine,* the results were not encouraging. For example, about one half of the physicians failed to discuss with their patients two important areas of behavior related to the potential for chronic illness: dietary practices and exercise. Even more discouraging, only three-fourths of physicians reported talking to their patients about the importance of discontinuing cigarette smoking—the single most powerful high-risk health behavior relating to the development of cancer and cardiovascular disease. Researchers concluded that competing priorities for physicians' time, the lack of physician self-efficacy, and financial restraints might be the underlying factors reducing the likelihood of physicians' engaging in important patient education.

In spite of the less than ideal level of patient education reported above, it is encouraging to note that when physicians did counsel (educate) their patients regarding exercise and dietary practices, patients were encouragingly compliant. In contrast, however, patient education regarding the importance of stopping cigarette smoking was largely ignored. Thus, the authors concluded that patient education was a moderately motivating factor in changing patients' high-risk health behaviors.

the diversity of today's college students

It's the fall of 1950, and you're about to meet Joe College, a student in a freshman health class at State University. Joe is an 18-year-old white man who graduated from City High School last summer in the top half of his class. He lives in State U's dormitory. Because his tuition is being paid by his parents, he can devote himself to his studies and college life on a full-time basis. When Joe looks around his health class, he sees some women and a few minorities and older students, but most of the students are much like himself. Joe College is a typical college student.

Flash forward to today. When you look around your health classroom, what kinds of students do you see? Students like Joe College are probably still there, but they don't make up the overwhelming majority of the student body. The many changes in American society that have taken place over the last 50 years are reflected in today's colleges and universities. Currently, slightly more women than men are graduating from college. As more older people find that they need better skills, more training, or a college degree to keep their present jobs or find new ones, the average age of college students has risen. Also, schools are increasing their efforts in actively recruiting minority students. Finally, recent laws affirming the rights of Americans with disabilities to have access to most public facilities are giving individuals with disabilities the opportunity to attend college.

Causes Behind the Changes

Why are these changes occurring? Several factors seem to be affecting enrollment figures in the United States. Clearly, the changing climate of the economy has influenced enrollment. Corporate trends toward a more streamlined workforce and the gradual shift to a service-oriented marketplace have caused many workers to seek training for new careers or additional training for their current jobs. As a result, people who never thought they would see the inside of a classroom again are drawn back to school.

In response to the economic changes just described, colleges have become more accessible in recent years. The trend toward open admissions, especially at community colleges, has opened the doors of higher education to those who otherwise might be held back by low high school grades or low test scores. Colleges are attempting to meet the needs of these new students with remedial courses and special programs designed to prepare them to meet strong academic standards.

Social changes have also played an important role in the changing demographics on college campuses. The Civil Rights movement of the 1950s and 1960s was instrumental in making a college education available to minorities, and minority enrollment has increased as overall awareness of civil rights becomes more entrenched in society. Students with various physical disabilities are also finding it easier to obtain a college education. The Americans with Disabilities Act, signed into law in 1990, guarantees that people with disabilities will have access to employment, education, and public services. As a result, people with disabilities can pursue careers that were previously inaccessible to them, and many are heading to college to receive training for those careers.

As higher education has become more accessible, an attitude change about going to college has occurred. The feeling that everyone should go to college after high school is now more prevalent.

Unfortunately, this emphasis on college has produced a cost to many important skilled trades, such as tool- and dye-making and construction. Students who might have once entered apprentice programs in these areas now feel compelled to seek a college degree. The military services have also experienced a similar effect as more and more high school graduates are moving on to college campuses.

Practical Implications of Diversity on Campus

With the rise of new populations on campuses, many practical changes have taken place to reflect the needs and interests of those students. For example, most college and universities now offer developmental education programs for students who need skill enhancement in reading, writing, and mathematics. Flexibility in the timing of course offerings is designed to accommodate the employment and parenting demands of nontraditional-age students. Many institutions also provide preschool centers for the children of parents who would otherwise find college attendance more difficult or even impossible.

The college student population is also changing in terms of increased numbers of individuals of different racial backgrounds, ethnic groups, and national origin. In response to these developments, a wider range of courses in areas such as history, literature, fine arts, music, drama, and political science is reflected in course catalogs. Faculty composition is also diversifying; however, in some cases, the pool of qualified applicants is small in relation to demand. Campus libraries have expanded the diversity of their collections to accommodate the changing campus population. Likewise, college bookstores offer a wider range of reading and musical selections. The increasing diversity of today's student bodies has also influenced the number and types of extracurricular offerings. Culturally diverse student associations, student political organizations, honor societies, and interest-based groups such as dance troupes are evident on many college campuses. Greater accessibility to the Internet has brought even the most isolated college campuses into the growing diversity that characterizes population as a whole.

Changing Campuses and the Study of Health

Why mention the many changes taking place on college campuses in a health text? Because of increasing diversity, students who are studying health (and most other disciplines) need to be aware of issues that affect students of different backgrounds. For example, many people are unaware of the fact that most pharmaceutical research is performed on men and then generalized to apply to women. This is a potentially dangerous practice because women are at a greater risk for adverse drug reactions. Another example is the use of complementary (alternative) medical practitioners. Native Americans view health care as a holistic, rather than a symptom-based, process. They are more likely to respond to a healer who looks at both the physical and spiritual person, than to a physician, who focuses only on the body. Similarly, some Mexican Americans will either rely on (or supplement traditional health care with) *curanderismo,* a medical system that combines Western health care practices with folklore, magic, herbalism, and religion. Knowledge of these and other related cultural health care issues will help college students understand all members of our culturally diverse society.

Bringing cultural awareness into the health classroom introduces students to concepts they might not otherwise be exposed to. During your college career, you will encounter students from a variety of backgrounds. They may be young or old, rich or poor, from a rural or urban environment, or from an ethnic group different from yours. Just as your culture has its own unique health concerns, every other culture also has its own set of health concerns, and you need to be aware of them.

chapter two

achieving psychological health

Chapter Objectives

Upon completing this chapter, you will be able to:

▌ define the terms *self-esteem* and *self-concept* and describe how they apply to you.

▌ describe the characteristics of psychologically healthy people.

▌ define the term *emotional intelligence* and explain how it relates to psychological health.

▌ define the term *learned optimism* and its components, and explain how it relates to psychological health.

▌ describe how humor can improve psychological health.

▌ explain Maslow's Hierarchy of Needs and how it can apply to your daily activities.

▌ describe strategies to enhance communication skills.

▌ describe mood disorders, including the difference between having "the blues" and clinical depression.

▌ describe anxiety disorders.

▌ explain the treatment modalities for psychological disorders.

Online Learning Center Resources

www.mhhe.com/hahn7e

Log on to our Online Learning Center (OLC) for access to these additional resources:

- Chapter key terms and definitions
- Learning objectives
- Student interactive question-and-answer sites
- Online assessments
- Key term flash cards
- Self-scoring chapter quiz

Talking It Over

Becoming More Assertive

While visiting your home, which has a "smoke-free" policy, your friend lights up a cigarette. How would you handle this situation? If you're an assertive person, you would firmly but courteously ask your friend to smoke outside. If you tend to be passive, you might remain silent but feel angry. If you're an aggressive person, you might yell.

Regardless of the communication style you grew up with, you can learn to become more assertive, asking for what you need or want while respecting other people. When you become an assertive person, your psychological health and self-esteem will soar.

CommunicationLinks

www.lifeclinic.com/focus/stress/
　communicating.asp
www.wellsource.com

Eye on the Media

**Self-Help via the Internet—
Guidance to Wellness or Path to Destruction?**

According to a recent poll conducted by Harris Interactive, about 98 million American adults use the Internet to find health-related information.[1] However, much of the time this information is not accurate and may cause harm if the reader accepts the information without question.

Some people feel more comfortable accessing psychological information and asking questions regarding their mental health via the Internet. There are also self-help and support groups, counseling, and assessments available through the Web. However,

this is where the Internet can potentially be a dangerous tool as people can diagnosis themselves through taking online surveys, which may lack validity or reliability. In fact, a study conducted by the UCLA Internet project[2] reported that half of the information they accessed on the Internet was reliable and accurate. A person reading about bulimia may self-diagnose and decide that he or she does not meet the criteria when in fact s/he may be developing this disorder. You may

Eye on the Media *continued*
purchase an herbal medicine that claims to alleviate depression when there is no research to support this and it may actually cause harm. There are also websites that instruct people on how to commit suicide or become better anorexics, again causing greater distress rather than offering assistance to better psychological health.

The number of resources on the Internet is growing by leaps and bounds, doubling in size about every year. In addition, anyone can publish on the Internet, and since there are over 800 million Internet sites, the accuracy of what is out on the Net is difficult if not impossible to regulate. Unfortunately, many people believe that if it is on the Internet, it must be true, which is not necessarily the case.

How can you be reasonably sure that the information you are reading is correct? Here are some important questions to consider:

- What are the author's qualifications and credentials? Is the resource from an expert or scholar in the field or from an individual's own opinion and experience?
- Is there any evidence of quality control? This would be more likely if the informa-tion is part of an official organizational website, such as an affiliation with a college or university or recognized professional organization such as the American Psychological Association.
- What is the reliability of the information presented? Does it seem consistent with other things you have read? Is it error free? Are the sources listed?
- What is the motivation of the author? Does the author stand to gain financially from the way the information is presented? Is there evidence of bias, was some information omitted, or was the material presented in a one-sided way?
- How current is the information? What was the last date the information was revised? Are there up-to-date links listed?

There are of course many positive reasons for accessing the Internet for information, support, and help. Technology has become more innovative in the way that assistance can be provided to people via the Internet including providing mental and medical advice. For example, Ball State University has started a new program in which students can ask health-related questions using their computers. They can receive medical care without leaving their residence hall room! The students can see the nurse but the nurse cannot see them. The nurse can also present pictures, video clips, or documents to the student via Web browser to help discuss and diagnose the student's condition.[3]

There have been some efforts from American Accreditation HealthCare Commission towards organizing an advisory committee from a variety of groups such as the Internet Healthcare Coalition, Hi-Ethics, and the American Medical Association to begin developing a standard for accrediting health websites. Until this group or some other agency is formed to regulate the credibility or the information on the Internet, it is advisable to be a critical consumer of Internet information.

[1] International Food Information Council Foundation: *Navigating for Health: Finding Accurate Information on the Internet.* Nov/Dec. 2000.
[2] The UCLA Internet Report Surveying the Digital Future: *Internet Access and Use: 2000, 2001 and 2002.*
[3] *The Chronicle of Higher Education.* April 11, 2003. Ball State Tests System for Answering Students' Health Questions Online.

The terms *emotional wellness* and *psychological health* have been used interchangeably to describe how people function in the affective and cognitive realms of their lives. **Psychological health** relates to how people express their emotions, cope with stress, adversity, and success, and adapt to changes in themselves and their environment, as well as to cognitive functioning—the way people think and behave in conjunction with their emotions. There is some debate about whether thoughts influence feelings or feelings cause us to think and behave a certain way. However, the most accepted view is that the way we think can directly change how we feel about an event or situation. Thus, you can change your feelings about something by changing your perspective about a situation. This has implications for how we can increase our self-esteem and confidence level and improve interactions with others. You will learn more about psychological health as you study this chapter.

Psychological Health

How do you feel about yourself? When you apply the resources from the multiple dimensions of health (see Chapter 1) in ways that allow you to direct your growth, assess deeply held values, deal effectively with change, and have satisfying relationships with others, you are

> ### Key Terms
>
> **psychological health** a broadly based concept pertaining to cognitive functioning in conjunction with the way people express their emotions, cope with stress, adversity, and success, and adapt to changes in themselves and their environment.

psychologically healthy. Research in the area of health psychology has shown that there is a mind–body connection in which biological, psychological, and social factors interact to influence health or illness. This is referred to as the **biopsychological model.**[1] We know that your psychological state has a significant effect on physical health: stress, depression, and anxiety have been associated with how your immune system responds and can impair physical health. Studies have shown that terminally ill cancer patients who had better psychological health lived longer lives and reported having a higher quality of life.[2] Psychological health does not just refer to your emotional state but also to your cognitive and social functioning as well.

Psychological health has also been associated with developing and maintaining a positive **self-esteem,** positive **self-concept,** and a high level of **emotional intelligence.** Each of these concepts will be explained further. However, as you will see, psychological health is much more than just the absence of mental illness.

Characteristics of Psychologically Healthy People

Psychologically healthy people are not perfect. They have their share of problems, flaws, and mistakes. However, it is how they perceive themselves and how they cope with their stress and failures that separates them from unhealthy individuals.

Psychologically healthy people have the following characteristics:

- Accept themselves and others
- Like themselves
- Appropriately express the full range of human emotions, both positive and negative
- Give and receive care, love, and support
- Accept life's disappointments
- Accept their mistakes
- Express empathy and concern for others
- Take care of themselves
- Trust others as well as themselves
- Establish goals, both short and long term
- Can function both independently and interdependently
- Lead a health enhancing lifestyle that includes regular exercise, good nutrition, and adequate sleep

Normal Range of Emotions

Do you know people who seem to be "up" all the time? These people appear to be confident, happy, and full of good feelings 24 seven. Although some people are like

that, they are truly the exceptions. For most people, emotions are more like a roller coaster ride. Sometimes they feel good about themselves and others, but other times nothing seems to go right. This is normal and healthy. Life has its ups and downs, and the concept of the "normal range of emotions" reflects these changes.

Self-Esteem

What is self-esteem? How do you know when someone is lacking in self-esteem? Most people answer this question by saying that they define positive self-esteem as:

- Having pride in yourself
- Treating yourself with respect
- Considering yourself valuable, important, worthy
- Feeling good about yourself
- Having self-confidence, being self-assured
- Accepting yourself

People with lower levels of self-esteem tend to allow others to mistreat them, don't take care of themselves, and have difficulty being by themselves. In addition, they have little self-confidence and so avoid taking risks and have trouble believing that other people care about them. People with low self-esteem tend to take things personally, are sometimes seen as "overly sensitive" and perfectionistic, criticize themselves and others, and believe that they can't do anything right. These individuals tend to have a pessimistic outlook on life, and see themselves as undeserving of good fortune. Some strategies for enhancing self-esteem are outlined in the Changing for the Better box on page 28. We will explore the concepts of optimism and pessimism as they relate to psychological health in a later section of this chapter.

Key Terms

biopsychological model a model that addresses how biological, psychological, and social factors interact and affect psychological health.

self-esteem an individual's sense of pride, self-respect, value, and worth.

self-concept an individual's internal picture of him or herself; the way one sees oneself.

emotional intelligence the ability to understand others and act wisely in human relations and measure how well you know your emotions, manage your emotions, motivate yourself, recognize emotions in others, and handle relationships.

TALKING POINTS You've noticed that one of your friends always seems to be critical of herself and allows others to take advantage of her. What might you say to help her to increase her self-esteem?

Self-Concept

People with low self-esteem also have a poor self-concept, meaning that their internal picture of themselves, how they see themselves, is very negative. Because of this poor self-concept, people with low self-esteem are more vulnerable to allowing others to mistreat or abuse them, and fail to be assertive. Many psychological problems have their underpinnings in low self-esteem, including eating disorders, substance abuse problems, depression, and anxiety disorders.

Where do we get our self-esteem? Most people would say from their parents, teachers, peers, siblings, religious institutions, and the media. While these factors certainly can positively or negatively affect our self-esteem, they are all external factors. Self-esteem relates to our *internal* self-perception. If self-esteem truly came from outside ourselves, then we would need to change our environment and the people around us. This is the reason that people tend to tell themselves, "If I just made more money, had a nicer car, were married, or had a more prestigious job, I would feel better about myself." This can become a vicious cycle, leaving the person always seeking more, and perpetually unsatisfied with him- or herself. This can also lead to perfectionism and not accepting yourself.

It is generally accepted that self-esteem comes from within ourselves and is ultimately within each individual's control. Moreover, self-esteem in not an all-or-none commodity, as most people have varying degrees of self-esteem, depending upon their stage of development, events in their lives, and their environment.[3]

Emotional Intelligence

A third aspect of psychological health is the degree of emotional intelligence you possess. Emotional intelligence refers to "the ability to understand others and act wisely in human relations."[4] Furthermore, emotional intelligence can be broken down into 5 main domains:

- **Knowing your emotions.** This is considered to be the cornerstone of emotional intelligence and relates to how much self-awareness and insight you have. How quickly you are able to recognize and label your feelings as you feel them determines the level of your emotional intelligence.

- **Managing your emotions.** How well can you express your feelings appropriately and cope with your emotions? People who have trouble coping with anxiety,

OnSITE/InSIGHT

Learning to Go: Health

Did you know that psychological health is just as important as physical health? Click on Learning to Go: Health on the Online Learning Center at **www.mhhe.com/hahn7e** to explore these lessons, which are ideal for this chapter:

Lesson 3: Boost your psychological health.

Lesson 4: Expand your communication skills.

Lesson 5: Approach your life proactively.

Lesson 6: Get a handle on mood disorders.

Lesson 7: Battle against depression.

Lesson 8: Seek both emotional and psychological health.

distress, and failures tend to have lower levels of emotional intelligence.

- **Motivating yourself.** People who can motivate themselves tend to be more highly productive and independent than those who rely on external sources for motivation. The more you can self-motivate and engage in goal-directed activities, the higher your emotional intelligence.

- **Recognizing emotions in others.** Another aspect of emotional intelligence is the degree of empathy you have or how sensitive you are to the feelings of others and how you come across to other people.

- **Handling relationships.** This refers to your level of social skills. The more interpersonally effective you are and able to negotiate conflict and build a social support network, the more emotional intelligence you possess.

Of course, people have differing levels of emotional intelligence and may have higher levels in one domain than in another. People with overall high levels of emotional intelligence tend to take on leadership roles, are confident, assertive, express their feelings directly and appropriately, feel good about themselves, are outgoing, and adapt well to stress.[4]

Enhancing Psychological Health

Most people have the opportunity to function at an enhanced level of psychological well-being. This state is often achieved by improving certain skills and abilities, including improving verbal and nonverbal communication, learning to use humor effectively, developing better conflict resolution skills, and taking

I keep getting into unhealthy romantic relationships and have come to expect that the person I am dating will eventually find something wrong with me and leave me. What can I do to feel better about myself and change my attitude toward my chances of having a successful relationship?

As the saying goes, it is hard to allow others to love you when you don't love yourself. So the first step is to start accepting and liking yourself and develop a more positive self-concept. The activities listed below can help you to start the process of enhancing your self-esteem:

Write down 3 things you like about yourself every day. Ask yourself what you did well today—not what you did wrong. Pay attention to your successes and accomplishments, not to your mistakes.

Share this list with a friend. It is generally more accepted to share your flaws and problems rather than your successes or positive qualities. We often hear people say "That was a stupid thing for me to say" rather than "I was proud of how I was able to answer a question in class today."

Accept compliments. Frequently we deflect or laugh away compliments rather than accept them. One of the ways to test yourself to see if you really took in the compliment is to see if you remember what that person said about you an hour later. Another way to check if you are accepting of compliments is to focus on how you are feeling—do you feel more positive, confident, happier with yourself?

Give compliments. Sometimes people with low self-esteem criticize others in order to feel better about themselves. To get out of this pattern, look for positives in other people and share your feedback, without belittling yourself. Instead of saying, "You do that so much better than I do," just say, "You are really good at that."

Watch your body posture. Making eye contact with others, keeping your head up, shoulders back, and not folding your arms in front of you, but keeping an open body posture helps to build self-esteem and confidence and projects this image to others.

Take a risk, do something different. People with lower levels of self-esteem tend to tell themselves, "I can't do that," and so don't even try. Don't be afraid of making a mistake or looking foolish. Take a risk and do something new and different—you might surprise yourself and be more successful than you anticipated.

Disarm the critic. Don't listen to the critical voice in your head that tells you that you are stupid, lazy, or not good enough. Sometimes this critical voice is the voice of our parents, teachers, or someone else in our lives who told us these negative messages. Replace the negative statements with positive ones and tell the critic to ease up a bit.

Reward yourself and be good to yourself. We frequently do nice things for other people or wait for others to reward us. Do something fun or nice for yourself everyday.

Signs and symbols of self-worth. Keep your list of positive qualities where you will see it, perhaps in your room or in your car. Have things around you that remind you that people care about you and that you are a worthwhile person, such as notes from friends, pictures of enjoyable times with others, or an item that is special to you in some way.

Set realistic goals and expectations for yourself. Changing patterns takes time and practice. You didn't develop your self-concept overnight and it will take some time to change the way you talk to yourself and see yourself. Notice how much progress you have made rather than how much more you have to go.

InfoLinks

www.self-esteem-nase.org

---

an optimistic approach to life. This section explores each of these facets of psychological health.

Improving Verbal Communication

Communication can be viewed in terms of your role as sender or receiver. In sending messages, you can enhance the effectiveness of your *verbal* communication in several ways. First, take time before speaking to understand what needs to be said. For example, does the audience/listener need information, encouragement, humor, or something else? Focus on the most important thoughts and ideas. Talk *with,* rather than at, listeners to encourage productive exchanges. Begin verbal exchanges on a positive note, and maintain a positive environment. Use "minimal encouragers," such as short questions, to gain feedback. Avoid using sarcasm, which can be destructive to communication. Recognize when other forms of communication, such as e-mail messages or handwritten notes, would be better for transmitting information or ideas.

You also need to be a skilled listener. First, listen attentively in order to hear everything that is being said. In a polite way, stop the speaker at certain points and ask him or her to repeat or rephrase the information. This technique helps you to understand what the speaker really means rather than focusing on your own responses. Ask for clarification and summarize what you think you heard the speaker saying to ensure you have received the message accurately. Also try to focus on one main topic and don't go off on tangents.

Nonverbal Communication

Strengthening your nonverbal communication skills may also enhance your psychological health. Nonverbal communication is what is communicated by your facial expressions, body posture, tone of voice, movements, and even the way you breathe—such as when you sigh or yawn. Nonverbal communication is a very powerful and sometimes more important aspect of the message than what is verbally communicated. In fact, people use information from facial cues more than any other source.[5] Facial cues, particularly from the eyes, are attended to more than any other type of nonverbal communication, even when information from other sources—such as from hand and body movements—may provide a more accurate picture of what the person is feeling. The following suggestions can enhance your nonverbal communication skills:

- *Facial expressions.* Facial expressions have been cited as one of the most important sources of nonverbal communication in terms of a person's emotional state.[5] When people speak with their eyebrows raised, they tend to be seen as more animated, excited, and happier. Flushing of one's face can indicate embarrassment, and crinkling one's nose can mean that you don't like something. Every part of your face can communicate some type of emotional reaction.

- *Eye contact.* Maintaining eye contact is an important component of positive nonverbal communication, while looking away or shifting your eyes can be read as seeming dishonest. But don't stare—5 to 7 seconds seems to be the maximum amount of time to look at someone's eyes before they begin to feel scrutinized.

- *Personal space.* There are cultural differences in how much personal space or distance is comfortable and acceptable when sitting or standing next to another person. For example, Americans' personal space— about 3 to 4 feet for a casual conversation—tends to be much greater than that of Arabs or Italians but less than Japanese or Britons. Gender and age and degree of familiarity are other factors that can determine the amount of personal space you are comfortable having between you and another person.

- *Body posture.* Assertiveness is equated with people who carry themselves with their heads up, shoulders back, and maintaining eye contact. Folded arms, crossed legs, and turning your body away from the speaker can indicate defensiveness and rejection.

Enhancing Conflict Management Skills

Communication can be especially challenging when there is a conflict or disagreement. Emotions such as anger, hurt, and fear might alter your ability to communicate as effectively as you would like. Some techniques for managing angry or upset people or conflictual situations are:

- *Listen and acknowledge the other person's point of view, even if it differs from your own.* Sometimes people are

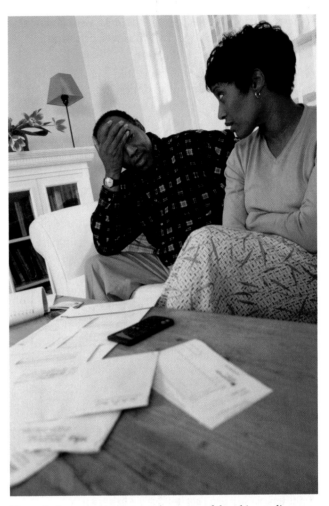

Nonverbal communication can be a powerful tool in sending messages to others through body language and posture as well as facial expressions.

so busy thinking of the next thing they want to say that they don't pay attention to what the other person is saying. To ensure that you have heard the person accurately and to let that person know you are listening to them, repeat back or summarize what you heard and ask if you misunderstood something that was said.

- *Use assertive communication.* Using "I" statements rather than "You" helps to avoid putting people on the defensive and is especially helpful when negotiating conflict or disagreements. Rather than saying, "You are inconsiderate," you can say, "I feel upset when you're late and haven't called to let me know."

- *Focus not just on what you say but how you say it.* Pay attention to your tone of voice and speak in a conversational tone. People tend to talk louder because they erroneously think they will be heard if they speak louder. This can result in a shouting match in which neither person hears the other.

- *Acknowledge the other person's feelings.* Use statements like "I can understand why this is so frustrating for you."

- *Watch your body posture.* Don't fold your arms in a closed, defensive posture, maintain eye contact, be aware of your facial expression so that you are not conveying hostility nonverbally. Make sure your nonverbal communication matches your verbal communication.

- *Accept valid criticism.* If you made a mistake, admit to it and apologize for whatever you think you did to contribute to the misunderstanding or conflict. This will open the door for the other person to take responsibility for their part in the conflict as well.

- *Focus on the problem at hand.* Don't bring up past hurts and problems. If you try to resolve every disagreement you have ever had with this person, you'll just wind up feeling frustrated and overwhelmed, and won't accomplish much. Stay on track by talking about the present situation.

- *Take a team approach.* Engage in mutual problem solving. This alleviates the winner-versus-loser paradigm. Look for areas of compromise and find a middle ground you can both agree to and live with.

- *Agree to disagree.* There is probably more than one right answer and you can agree that you will not persuade the other to change his or her point of view.

- *Agree to discuss this at a later time.* Sometimes the conversation becomes too volatile and heated. Some time and distance from the problem can be beneficial.

Enhancing Psychological Health Through Humor

Having a sense of humor is another important component of psychological health. Humor helps to put things in their proper perspective, alleviating tension and pain by releasing more endorphins in our bodies. In addition, laughter reduces stress,[6] boosts the immune system,[7] alleviates pain[8] stabilizes mood,[9] decreases anxiety,[10] enhances communication,[11] and inspires creativity.[12] The research suggests that we need to laugh 30 minutes total per 24-hour period to attain these benefits. This is an easy task for children who on average laugh 250 times a day but more challenging for adults who tend to only laugh 15 times a day.[13] Employers have been putting the benefits of laughter to good use to increase productivity in factories. Factories in India have created "laughing clubs" in which workers laugh together for 20 minutes a day, resulting in less absenteeism and better performance.[14]

Recognizing the humor in everyday situations and being able to laugh at yourself will make you feel better about yourself. People who build humor into their daily lives generally feel more positive, and others enjoy being around them. Some people will say that if they don't laugh about a particular situation, they will cry, and laughing seems the better choice. In fact, humor is viewed as one of the higher-level defense mechanisms, compared to denying the problem, rationalizing or minimizing the problem, or blaming others. Some researchers have suggested that recovery from an injury or illness is enhanced when patients maintain a sense of humor.[15]

Taking an Optimistic Approach to Life

Another key to psychological health is your ability to manage and express your thoughts, feelings, and behavior in a positive manner. Do you believe that your happiness is within your control? Are people born naturally happy or sad? One important key to psychological health is the way that you think about and interpret events in your life. For example, if you say "hello" to someone and you don't get a response, do you begin to wonder if that person is

Changing for the Better

Communication Counts in a Close Relationship

My partner and I have been living together for 2 years. We get along well most of the time, but when we try to talk about problems, we just can't connect. How do we learn to communicate better?

- Schedule the conversation so that you and the other person will be prepared for it.
- Choose a neutral setting to lessen the possibility of hostility.
- Set aside any preoccupations before starting the discussion.
- State your position clearly and nonaggressively.
- Keep your tone, manner of speaking, and body language respectful.
- Focus on the topic at hand.
- Be specific when you praise or criticize.
- Listen to what the other person is saying—not just the words but the feelings behind them.
- Avoid using trigger words that might turn a discussion into an argument.
- Suggest and ask for ideas about a course of action that will help resolve the problem.

If you follow these suggestions, you'll be taking into account the psychological health of the other person and yourself. This creates a sense of equality within the intimate relationship. Since both of you will be aware of acknowledging and respecting the other person, you'll begin on a positive note.

angry with you? Or do you surmise that he or she didn't hear you or perhaps was distracted? Research shows that having a positive interpretation of life's events, particularly how you cope with adversity, can make a significant difference in terms of your health and academic and work performance as well as how long you will live.[16] Do you see the glass half empty, as pessimists do, or half full, like optimists? Does it matter? Again studies overwhelmingly contend that your perspective makes a tremendous difference in your psychological health. Compared to pessimists, optimists tend to:

- Contract fewer infectious diseases
- Have better health habits
- Possess stronger immune systems
- Be more successful in their careers
- Perform better in sports, music, and academics

We do know that people can learn to be helpless and ultimately become depressed and even suicidal. Pavlov demonstrated the concept of "learned helplessness" in his classic study in which he administered an electric shock to dogs that were harnessed and couldn't escape the shocks. When he moved the dogs to another room, the dogs lay down and whimpered and didn't try to avoid the shocks. This time the dogs were not harnessed and could have easily escaped the shocks by moving to another side of the room. This reaction has been referred to as **learned helplessness,** as the dogs learned that there was nothing they could do to affect their lives and they lost hope and felt trapped and powerless.[17] We have seen this same phenomenon with humans. College students volunteered for an experiment in which they were subjected to an ear-splitting noise and their efforts to stop the noise were unsuccessful. Later, when they were placed in another situation where they could have easily pulled a control lever to turn off the noise, they made no effort to do so and just suffered with the noise until the experimenter stopped it.[18] Battered women have demonstrated this same sense of powerlessness and helplessness in their ability to escape the abuse they are subjected to by their partners.

If people can learn to be helpless and pessimistic, can they also learn to feel more optimistic, powerful, and in control? Martin Seligman conducted studies to prove that this is possible and called this concept **learned optimism.** He identified three key factors that contribute to having an optimistic or pessimistic perspective. Learned optimism refers to your explanatory style, in other words, if you describe the glass as being half full or half empty.

The first dimension of learned optimism is **permanence.** Pessimists tend to give up easily because they believe the causes of bad events are *permanent.* They say things like "Things never work out for me," "That won't ever work," or "He's always in a bad mood." Such permanent language—words like *never, always,* and *forever*—imply that these negative situations are not temporary but will continue on indefinitely. Optimists tend to use temporary language—words like *sometimes, frequently,* and *often*—and they blame bad events on transient conditions. Examples of optimistic language are "It didn't work out this time," "Doing it that way didn't work," or "He's in a bad mood today." Optimists see failure as a small, transitory setback and are able to pick themselves up, brush themselves off, and persevere towards their goals.

The second aspect of learned optimism is **pervasiveness.** This refers to whether you perceive negative events as universal and generalize them to everything in your life, or if you can compartmentalize and keep them defined to the specific situation. Pessimists tend to make universal explanations for their problems, and, when something goes wrong in one part of their lives, they give up on everything. While a pessimist would say that they are not good at math, an optimist would say that they didn't perform well in that particular class with that type of math. "I'm good at algebra but not as good with geometry."

The last aspect of learned optimism is determined by whether you blame bad things on yourself or on other people or circumstances. Pessimism and low self-esteem tend to come from **personalization**—blaming oneself and having an internal explanatory style for negative events. An optimist might say, "The professor wrote a very poor exam and that is the reason I received a lower score," while the pessimist would say, "I am stupid" or "I didn't study enough." This is different from not taking responsibility for

---

| **Key Terms** |

learned helplessness a theory of motivation explaining how individuals can learn to feel powerless, trapped, and defeated.

learned optimism how people explain both positive and negative events in their lives, accounting for success and failure.

permanence the first dimension of an individual's attribution style, related to whether certain events are perceived as temporary or long-lasting.

pervasiveness the second dimension of an individual's attribution style, related to whether they perceive events as specific or general.

personalization the final dimension of attribution style, related to whether an individual takes things personally or is more balanced in accepting responsibility for positive and negative events.

one's actions and blaming other people for your problems or mistakes. The idea is to have a balanced perspective and outlook on life. Pessimists tend to give credit to other people or circumstances when good things happen and blame themselves when bad events occur. For example, a pessimist would say, "That was just dumb luck," rather than taking credit for a success. However, if pessimists fail, they readily blame themselves, saying, "I messed up." On the other hand, optimists tend to give themselves credit for their accomplishments, saying, "I worked hard and did a good job," and don't belittle themselves when things go wrong.

Seligman conducted many studies to test how an optimistic explanatory style might be useful in daily living. For example, he worked with a swimming team from the University of California, Berkeley, to see how optimism or pessimism might affect their performance. He had their coaches tell the athletes that their times were slower than they actually were. The swimmers were then asked to swim the event again as fast as they could. The performance of the pessimists deteriorated in their hundred-yard event by two seconds, the difference between winning the event and finishing dead last. The optimists got faster by two to five seconds, again enough to be the difference between losing and winning the race.[16] So how you interpret events, your attribution style, can make a tremendous difference in the eventual success or failure in your endeavors.

So how can you learn to be more optimistic? Albert Ellis developed a cognitive framework to become more positive in how you think and feel about things that happen in your life called the ABC method. When you encounter adversity, the "A" part of the formula, you try to make sense out of it and explain what has happened. For example, if you receive a notice from the bank that you have over-drawn your checking account, you start to think, "How did this happen?" These thoughts are associated with our beliefs, the "B" in ABC. You might think, "I'm irresponsible for letting this happen. I can't manage my money." Then you begin to feel badly about yourself, worthless and upset. Your beliefs affect your feelings, and so you can control your emotions by changing your beliefs and thoughts.[19] If you said, "The bank probably made a mistake" or "I might have added something incorrectly," you will most likely feel much better about yourself and the situation. The "C" aspect is the consequence of the event, how you end up feeling about the situation. When someone feels depressed, he or she feels hopeless, trapped, and powerless. By adopting a more positive way of reframing or thinking about events, you create options, hope, and a strategy for solving problems rather than staying stuck, like the whimpering dogs laying down and putting up with being shocked. In the previously described scenario with the overdraft, you can generate ideas such as "I need to check with the bank, go over my bank statement, be more careful in recording and calculating my balances, and request overdraft protection to prevent this from becoming a problem again."

Everyone encounters adversity sometime in his or her life. You can become discouraged by these events, blame yourself, and feel hopeless, worthless, and cynical about the world. Or you can be persistent and become stronger by overcoming these obstacles by having positive beliefs, and seeing these problems as short-lived, specific, and not as a flaw in your character. When you embrace an optimistic perspective, you will feel more hopeful, stronger, and confident. You will be able to accept new challenges and take more risks in your life.

 TALKING POINTS Think about something bad that has happened in your life recently. What were your beliefs about this event? How did you feel? Using the concepts of permanence, pervasiveness, and personalization, how can you change your beliefs about this situation? How do you feel differently about the event?

Taking a Proactive Approach to Life

In addition to the approaches already discussed, the plan that follows is intended to give you other strategies for enhancing your psychological health. The following is a four-step process that continues throughout life: constructing perceptions of yourself, accepting these perceptions, undertaking new experiences, and reframing your perceptions based on new information.

Constructing Mental Pictures

Actively taking charge of your psychological health begins with constructing a mental picture of what you're like. Use the most recent and accurate information you have about yourself—what is important to you, your values, and your abilities. To construct this mental picture, set aside a period of uninterrupted quiet time for reflection.

Before proceeding to the second step, you also need to construct mental pictures about yourself in relation to *other people and material objects*; including your residence and college or work environment, to clarify these relationships.

For example, after graduating from college with a degree in fine arts, Allison moved to a large city to become a jewelry designer. Two years later, her small business was thriving and she was living in a spacious loft apartment with room for her studio. Still, Allison felt that something was missing. She constructed a mental picture in which she saw herself as a resourceful, creative, independent person who was comfortable in her new surroundings. However, Allison realized that she wanted a partner to share her success and her life.

Accepting Mental Pictures

The second step of the plan involves an *acceptance* of these perceptions. This implies a willingness to honor the truthfulness of the perceptions you have formed about yourself and other people. For example, Allison acknowledges her professional success and her artistic ability, and she also accepts that she has been unable to establish a satisfying long-term romantic relationship.

Emotional development is rarely a passive process. You must be willing to be *introspective* (inwardly reflective) about yourself and the world around you.

Undertaking New Experiences

The next step of the plan is to test your newly formed perceptions. This *testing* is accomplished by *undertaking a new experience* or by reexperiencing something in a different way.

New experiences do not necessarily require high levels of risk, foreign travel, or money (see Learning from Our Diversity, on page 34). They may be no more "new" than deciding to move from the dorm into an apartment, to change from one shift at work to another, or to pursue new friendships. The experience itself is not the goal; rather, it's a means of collecting information about yourself, others, and the objects that form your material world.

For instance, Allison volunteered to teach art therapy classes to chronically ill patients at a local hospital. This work was enjoyable and fulfilling for her, and she formed friendships with a few of the other hospital volunteers. Allison also met and began dating Mark, a staff physical therapist.

Reframing Mental Pictures

When you have completed the first three steps in the plan, the new information about yourself, others, and objects becomes the most current source of information. Regardless of the type of new experience you have undertaken and its outcome, you are now in a position to modify the initial perceptions constructed during the first step. Then you will have new insights, knowledge, and perspectives.

Allison reframed her mental pictures in light of the changes that had taken place in her life. Her volunteer work gave her a renewed appreciation for art. Also, she now saw herself as part of a circle of friends and as a partner

in a long-term relationship with Mark. With her proactive approach to life, Allison had created challenges for herself that allowed her to change and grow.

Challenges to Psychological Health

In spite of their best efforts to be positive and resilient, many people have a less than optimal level of psychological health. There is some debate about how much control people actually do have over their psychological health. A general consensus is that two factors, **nature** and **nurture**,

Key Terms

nature the innate factors that genetically determine personality traits.

nurture the effect that the environment, people, and external factors have on personality.

influence psychological health, but there are differing views on how much each contributes to our psychological makeup. Nature refers to the innate factors we are born with that genetically determine our degree of psychological health. Nurture is the effect that the environment, people, and external factors have on our psychological health.[20] We all know some people who are high strung or anxious by nature, and others who are cheerful and naturally outgoing. We seem to be born with a predisposition towards a certain psychological health, which is often similar to our parents. "She is serious like her father" or "He is funny like his mother" are remarks people may make alluding to this genetic link. Environmental factors such as social relationships, family harmony, financial resources, job and academic concerns, stressful situations or events and even the weather can influence your degree of psychological health.

Psychological Disorders

In the course of one year, an estimated 22% of Americans, about one in five, suffer from a diagnosable mental disorder.[21] In addition, four of the ten leading causes of disability in the United States and other developed countries are mental disorders such as depression, bipolar disorder, schizophrenia, and obsessive-compulsive disorder.[22] However two-thirds of those suffering from psychological disorders will not receive treatment due to the stigma and cost associated with mental health treatment.[23] Overall, minorities share the same prevalence rate of mental disorders as Caucasians; however, there are great disparities in the rate of mental health care for minorities as compared to the non-minority population.

While there are over 300 different types of mental illness that can be diagnosed, we will cover three major

categories of mental disorders: mood disorders, including depression and bipolar disorder; anxiety disorders; and schizophrenia.[24] Over 450 million people worldwide are affected by mental disorders at any given time, and these numbers are expected to increase in the future.[25]

Mood Disorders

Mood disorders, such as depression, seasonal affective disorder, and bipolar disorder, refer to psychological problems in which the primary symptom is a disturbance in mood.[24] You might see someone as moody, unable to predict if the person will be in a good or bad mood from one day to the next.

People who suffer from depression tend to feel hopeless and unmotivated, and withdraw from others, which then increases their feelings of being trapped and stuck.

Depression

About one in ten Americans suffer some form of depression, with women experiencing **clinical depression** twice as often as men.[26] The incidence of depression starting in childhood and adolescence has dramatically increased over the past ten years. We have already begun to see this trend, as the number of college students with depression has doubled over the last 13 years.[27] While depression can develop at any age, the average age of onset is the mid-twenties.

How can you tell the difference between having the blues and clinical depression? The symptoms of depression are:

- Depressed mood most of the day, nearly every day
- Frequent crying
- Withdrawing, isolating oneself from others
- Lack of interest in activities that are typically enjoyable
- Increase or decrease in appetite resulting in significant weight loss or weight gain
- Insomnia, disturbed or restless sleep, or sleeping more than usual
- Feeling tired most of the time, regardless of how much sleep you have had
- Low self-esteem, feelings of hopelessness and worthlessness
- Difficulty concentrating, remembering things, and focusing on a task, and indecisiveness
- Frequent thoughts of suicide

Many people have experienced some of these symptoms at one point or another in their lives; however, clinically depressed individuals experience most of these symptoms every day and have felt this way for at least two weeks. Most people can find ways of pulling themselves out of feeling down, but when you have clinical depression, the normal methods you have used in the past to cope with the blues don't work. Clinical depression can range from mild to severe depression and can result in significant impairment in functioning, such as not being able to get out of bed to attend classes or go to work or have the energy or motivation to take care of your basic needs for food, hygiene, and rest. Some depressed people tend to become irritable, negative, and uncommunicative, which can cause greater stress and conflict in their relationships. Depression has been described as constantly having a black cloud over your head, and not being able to get out from underneath it no matter what you do.

There are several causes or triggers for depression to develop. Research suggests that if you have a family history of depression or any type of mood disorder, you are more prone to developing a depressive disorder. In fact, rates of depression for a child with a depressed parent are two to four times greater than for children without this type of heredity.[28] While there is no single gene that causes depression, your genetic makeup can make you more vulnerable to depression. Neurotransmitters and hormone levels play a major role in the way your brain regulates your mood and emotions. Two neurotransmitters, serotonin and norepinephrine, are often found to be deficient in people with depression.

However, biological processes are not the only explanation for depression. You may have a family history of depression and never develop depressive symptoms as this only puts you in a higher risk category for this disorder. Other life events, stressors, and losses can activate this predisposition, causing depression. In addition, you may have no genetic predisposition and still become clinically depressed. Depression can be caused by many factors such as:

- loss of a significant relationship
- death of a family member or friend
- physical or sexual abuse or assault
- serious illness or health problems
- experiencing numerous setbacks and problems simultaneously

Having a support system, effective coping strategies, and a positive attributional style can make the difference between succumbing to depression or being protected during stressful and adverse times in our lives.

There are many ways to treat depression, but the most efficacious treatment approach is a combination of counseling and medication. Counseling can help people develop effective and healthy coping skills, learn stress management strategies, focus on developing an optimistic explanatory style, and improve relationships and social skills. Medication, such as antidepressants, have been found to be very helpful in the treatment of depression, as they act to increase the serotonin or norepinephrine levels to a normal and functional range. Some of the newer antidepressants are Prozac, Paxil, Zoloft, Serzone, Remeron, Effexor, and Lexapro. It takes 4 to 6 weeks for an antidepressant to be fully effective, and there may be side effects such as dry mouth, decreased sexual drive, drowsiness, constipation, or diarrhea. Most of these will disappear after 2 weeks of taking the medication.

> ### Key Terms
>
> **clinical depression** a psychological disorder in which individuals experience a lack of motivation, decreased energy level, fatigue, social withdrawal, sleep disturbance, disturbance in appetite, diminished sex drive, feelings of worthlessness and despair.

Most people take an antidepressant for 6 months to a year and then are able to taper off of the medication without a reoccurrence of symptoms. If you have had three separate episodes of depression, recovering from each episode and then relapsing, this can be a sign that your depression is chemically caused and an indication that you may need to continue taking an antidepressant medication long-term.

Herbal supplements, such as St. John's Wort, have also been touted as a treatment for depression, although there is some debate as to how effective they truly are. Most health care providers agree that St. John's Wort can be somewhat effective in alleviating mild depression, but not for more moderate or severe types of depression. As is the case with all herbal supplements, St. John's Wort is not subject to FDA approval nor has it been put through the clinical trials prescription medication has undergone to establish its therapeutic dose and efficacy. However, the National Institute of Mental Health, the National Center for Complementary and Alternative Medicine, and the Office of Dietary Supplements are currently conducting a $4 million collaborative four-year study to investigate the safety and effectiveness of St. John's Wort, and so more definitive information will be available in the near future.

Exercise and activity level also play a significant role in alleviating and insulating people from depression. Again it seems that the endorphin levels and effects on brain chemistry and hormonal levels are part of the explanation for why this is a powerful antidote for depression.[29]

 TALKING POINTS Have you ever felt depressed? If so, what did you do to cope with these feelings? What did you do that worked and/or didn't help you to feel better?

Suicide

Suicide is the third leading cause of death for young adults 15 to 24 years old and the eleventh leading cause of all deaths in the United States. Men commit suicide four times more often than women do, and 72% of all suicides are committed by white men. Suicide occurs most often among Americans age 65 and older.[30] However, women are three times more likely than men to attempt suicide. Men tend to employ more lethal methods such as using firearms, hanging, or jumping from high places, while women tend to use slower methods such as overdosing with pills or cutting their wrists, which allow more time for medical attention. Twice as many Whites complete suicide as African Americans, with Asian Americans being one of the lowest risk groups

Electroconvulsive Therapy (ECT) as Another Treatment for Depression

Electroconvulsive therapy (ECT) is another form of treatment for depression, with 100,000 Americans receiving this treatment each year. While ECT had fallen out of favor in the past 25 years (due in part to depictions of it in the film *One Flew Over the Cuckoo's Nest*), it has recently regained popularity. The procedure involves delivering a 90-volt burst of electricity, equal to the electricity in a 40-watt light bulb, to the brain for about a minute, causing a grand mal seizure. The patient is under anesthesia and receives muscle relaxants prior to administering the shock, and the heart rate and oxygen level are constantly monitored during the treatment. Most patients receive three ECT treatments each week, for a total of six to twelve sessions. Proponents of ECT claim that shock treatments produce positive treatment effects for depression when no other antidepressant or treatment regime has worked. Critics of ECT say that it causes brain damage and memory loss, and that the decrease in depressive symptoms are only temporary.[31] Although ECT has been used for the past 60 years, no one knows exactly how it works or why it alleviates depression.

in terms of ethnicity. The suicide rate for the Hispanic population is lower than for Whites but higher than for African Americans.

Why do people attempt or commit suicide? The majority of suicidal people have depressive disorders and feel helpless and powerless over their lives. They say things like "I just want the pain to stop" and don't see any other options available to them. There are some risk factors associated with suicidal behavior such as having:

- little to no support system
- made previous suicide attempts
- a family history of mental illness, including substance abuse
- a family history of suicide
- problems with drugs or alcohol

- possession of a firearm
- exposure to suicidal behavior of others, including through the media

It is estimated that there are 300,000 suicide attempts made each year in the United States, or more than one every 2 minutes. Some people say that suicidal gestures or threats are merely a cry for attention and ignore them. But left ignored, the person may go ahead and take the next step to attempt suicide because no one seems to care. It is always best to take any threats or talk about suicide seriously and act accordingly. What should you do if a friend or family member talks to you about thoughts of suicide? See the Star box for the Do's and Don'ts of Suicide Intervention.

The Do's and Don'ts of Suicide Intervention

Don't . . .

1. **Avoid talking about suicide or dance around the topic.** Talking about suicide doesn't upset people more. In fact, often people who are thinking about killing themselves say it is a relief to talk about it and it helps them to let go of this idea, not pursue it further.

2. **Be judgmental or argumentative.** Now is not the time to debate the morality of suicide—you will lose the debate and possibly the person.

3. **Assume that the person is not serious.** Saying "You're not serious" or "You don't mean that" may inadvertently encourage the person to show you how serious she or he truly is.

4. **Argue.** Telling a suicidal person that things aren't that bad, or that other people have it worse, can make them feel worse about themselves and guilty about their feelings of unhappiness.

5. **Promise not to tell anyone.** If you keep this promise and something happens to this person, how will you feel?

Do . . .

1. **Remain calm.** Talk about the person's feelings of sadness and helplessness.

2. **Offer support and assistance.** Tell the person he or she is not alone.

3. **Encourage problem solving** and taking positive steps.

4. **Emphasize the temporary nature of the problem.** Suicide is a permanent solution to a temporary problem.

5. **Seek help and don't try to handle this problem on your own.** This might involve the person's family, religious advisor, friends, or teachers, or calling a mental health agency for consultation.

6. **Make a no-suicide contract.** Ask the person to promise not to hurt or kill him/herself.

7. **If possible, stay with the person** until you can get further assistance.

Bipolar Disorder

Another important mood disorder is **bipolar disorder,** a condition that was previously known as manic depression. Bipolar refers to the extreme mood swings individuals with this disorder experience, from feeling euphoric, energetic, and reckless to feeling depressed, powerless, and listless. It is the least common of the mood disorders. Men and women are equally likely to develop this condition, and the average age of onset for the first manic episode typically occurs in the early twenties. This change in mood or "mood swing" can last for hours, days, weeks, or months, and it is found among all ages, races, ethnic groups, and social classes. The illness tends to run in families and appears to have a genetic link, as it is more likely to affect the children of parents who have the disorder.[24] When one parent has bipolar disorder, the risk to each child is estimated to be 15 percent to 30 percent. When both parents have bipolar disorder, the risk increases to 50 percent to 75 percent.

We have already described depression in great detail in the previous section. Bipolar disorder involves both having depressive periods and manic episodes. **Mania** is characterized by the following:

- Excessive energy, needing little sleep
- Racing thoughts, feeling as though your mind is going 50 mph
- Rapid speech, changing from topic to topic quickly in conversation
- Irritability

- Impulsive and reckless behavior, for example, going on spending sprees, increased involvement in sexual activity, and drug and alcohol use
- Trying to do too much, feeling as though you can accomplish a great deal
- Being easily distracted
- Exciteability

Many people with bipolar disorder will tell you that they enjoy the "highs" but dread the lows. However, manic behavior can become very destructive because when people are in a manic phase they can create enormous credit card debt, abuse drugs and alcohol, drive recklessly, and often feel invincible. They stay up all night and feel very little need for rest or food and eventually their bodies can't function and they collapse. Mood stabilizers such as Lithium and Lithobid and anticonvulsant medications such as Depakote, Neurontin, Topomax, and Lamictal have been used to treat bipolar disorder, along with psychotherapy.

Key Terms

bipolar disorder a mood disorder characterized by alternating episodes of depression and mania.

mania an extremely excitable state characterized by excessive energy, racing thoughts, impulsive and/or reckless behavior, irritability, and being prone to distraction.

Anxiety Disorders

Bill, a very talented and bright twenty-six-year old, has a very promising career as an executive in a large accounting firm. However, he is in jeopardy of losing his job because of his absenteeism and tardiness. He has missed several important meetings with clients and not been able to get his work done on time as a result. It can take him hours to get to work even though he lives 15 minutes away, and sometimes he doesn't go to work even though he is in the car and ready to go. Bill has a routine in the morning that involves checking the windows, doors, iron, stove, and garage door five times to ensure that things are secure and safe. Sometimes he drives away and then returns to the house to check again. He feels a need to turn the handles on doors five times, and if he loses track, he starts all over again.

Susan has been having such severe panic attacks in the car while driving to work that she has needed to pull over. Her heart races, her breathing is labored, and she sometimes feels as though she is having a heart attack and might die. She is frightened of being in the car alone and having an attack and being unable to get help, or of having a car accident. She is beginning to be afraid to leave her house and feels safer at home. She has declined invitations to go out with her friends and only goes out when absolutely necessary. She feels as though she is losing control of her life.

John worries constantly about what other people think of him. When he hears people laughing, he assumes that they are laughing at him. He has trouble having conversations with people because he believes whatever he says will sound stupid and that people will not like him. He also plays conversations over and over in his head when he is trying to go to sleep, thinking about what he should have said and worrying about how people are judging him.

Bill, Susan, and John are all suffering from *anxiety disorders*. While everyone tends to feel nervous or worry about something at some point in their lives, people with anxiety disorders feel anxious most, if not all, of the time. They also feel out of control and powerless to alleviate their anxiety, and tend to worry about becoming anxious, so their anxiety causes them even greater anxiety. Anxiety is related to fear and is part of daily life. Some anxiety can even be helpful and motivating at times. Anxiety is a physiological, adaptive response to danger or potential threat and can enhance performance and keep us out of harm's way. In Chapter 3, Managing Stress, we will discuss the flight or fight response and how the stress response is related to anxiety. Anxiety disorders are differentiated from daily stress as characterized by:

- intense, often debilitating, in which people sometimes think they are going to die

- long lasting, persisting after the danger or stressful event has passed
- dysfunctional, causing significant interference in your life

Anxiety disorders include **generalized anxiety disorder (GAD), obsessive-compulsive disorder (OCD)** such as Bill's problem, post traumatic stress disorder, **panic disorder** which describes Susan's symptoms, and phobias such as the **social phobia** John suffered from in the example above.[32] Approximately 19 million Americans have an anxiety disorder, and women are twice as likely as men to suffer from panic disorder, post-traumatic stress disorder, generalized anxiety disorder, agoraphobia, and other specific phobias. There are no gender differences with obsessive-compulsive disorder or social phobia.[33] There is a genetic component associated with developing an anxiety disorder as studies suggest that you are more likely to develop one if your parents have one. Certainly environmental stressors and events can be instrumental in whether this predisposition is activated or not.

The treatment for anxiety disorders usually involves a combination of medication and counseling. There is some evidence that a deficiency in the neurotransmitter serotonin or a disturbance in metabolizing serotonin is associated with this condition and taking an antidepressant increases the serotonin levels in the brain. Individuals

---

Key Terms

generalized anxiety disorder (GAD) an anxiety disorder that involves experiencing intense and nonspecific anxiety for at least 6 months, in which the intensity and frequency of worry is excessive and out of proportion to the situation.

obsessive-compulsive disorder (OCD) an anxiety disorder characterized by obsessions—intrusive thoughts, images, or impulses causing a great deal of distress—and compulsions—repetitive behaviors aimed at reducing anxiety or stress that is associated with the obsessive thoughts.

panic disorder an anxiety disorder characterized by panic attacks, in which individuals experience severe physical symptoms. These episodes can seemingly occur "out of the blue" or because of some trigger, and can last for a few minutes or for hours.

social phobia a phobia characterized by feelings of extreme dread and embarrassment in situations in which public speaking or social interaction is involved.

suffering from anxiety disorders can also benefit from learning stress management, relaxation, and ways of coping with the stress.[32] Exercise, good nutrition, and avoidance of stimulants such as caffeine can also be helpful in alleviating anxiety.

Schizophrenia

Schizophrenia is one of the most severe mental disorders as it is characterized by profound distortions in one's thought processes, emotions, perceptions, and behavior. People with schizophrenia experience hallucinations (seeing things that are not there, hearing voices), delusions (believing that you are Jesus, the CIA is after you, or that radio waves are controlling your mind), and disorganized thinking (wearing multiple coats, scarves, and gloves on a warm day, shouting and swearing at passersby, maintaining a rigid posture and not moving for hours). The movie *A Beautiful Mind* gives a glimpse into the life of one schizophrenic, John Nash, and his recovery.

There are several types of schizophrenia: paranoid, disorganized, catatonic, and undifferentiated. This disabling illness affects 1 percent of the U.S. population, and symptoms typically surface in people in their late teens and early twenties. Men and women are equally likely to develop schizophrenia, and it seems to run in families. Schizophrenia is often confused with multiple personality disorder, which is an entirely separate and distinct mental illness. While people with multiple personality disorder display two or more distinct identities or personalities that take control of the person's life, people with schizophrenia do not have multiple, separate, enduring personalities.

There are many theories to explain what causes schizophrenia. Some research suggests that heredity accounts for about 80 percent of the cause of schizophrenia and the other 20 percent is due to environmental stressors or situations. Researchers have also identified a number of abnormalities in the brains of diagnosed schizophrenics, including smaller temporal lobes, enlargement of the ventricles, and cerebral atrophy in the frontal lobes. There is further investigation looking at how the variations in chromosome-22 genes may be linked to schizophrenia. Individuals with schizophrenia also seem to have nearly double the number of dopamine receptors in their brains, leading to the theory that too much dopamine is being released into the brain pathways and causing schizophrenia symptoms. The antipsychotic medications act to block the receptors and prevent the transmission of dopamine, reducing the amount of dopamine in the system that is creating this chemical imbalance.[1]

While there is no cure for schizophrenia, there are antipsychotic medications, such as Seroquel, Risperidone,

Zyprexa, Geodon, and Abilify that can effectively treat this illness and enable people to live functional, satisfying lives. Psychotherapy can be helpful in developing problem-solving approaches, in addition to identifying stressors and triggers, and early detection of a psychotic episode. Unfortunately some people with schizophrenia are unable to recognize that they are delusional or irrational, and so do not get treatment or take their medications on a regular basis.

Reflections of Psychological Health

What characterizes people who have developed their psychological health to their highest potential? The following discussion suggests three areas in which psychological health is evident. These include (1) movement toward fulfilling the highest level of need (as defined by Maslow), (2) development of a mature level of spirituality, and (3) expression of creativity.

Maslow's Hierarchy of Needs

Abraham Maslow has been among the significant contributors to the understanding of personality and psychological health. Central to Maslow's contribution to twentieth-century American psychological thought is his view of psychological health in terms of the individual's attempt to meet inner needs, what he called *the hierarchy of needs* (Figure 2-1).[20]

Maslow's theory is a positive, optimistic theory of human behavior. He believed that people are motivated to grow and fulfill their potential, referring to this phenomenon as **self-actualization.** He described self-actualization as "the need to become more and more what one is, to

---

> ### Key Terms
>
> **schizophrenia** one of the most severe mental disorders, characterized by profound distortions in one's thought processes, emotions, perceptions, and behavior; symptoms may include hallucinations, delusions, disorganized thinking, and/or maintaining a rigid posture and not moving for hours.
>
> **self-actualization** the highest level of psychological health at which one reaches his or her highest potential and values truth, beauty, goodness, faith, love, humor, and ingenuity.

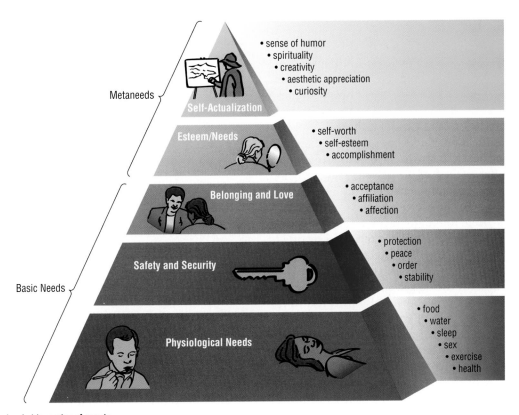

Figure 2-1 Maslow's hierarchy of needs.

become everything that one is capable of becoming."[34] Maslow differentiated between two different categories of needs: **basic needs** and **metaneeds.** Basic needs, physiological needs, belonging and love, and esteem needs are the deficiency needs and are essential and urgent. Metaneeds come into play once the basic needs are met and include spirituality, creativity, curiosity, beauty, philosophy, and justice. Maslow's hierarchy of needs is arranged with the basic needs on the bottom, as they are the most fundamental and powerful needs. Lower level needs must be met before the next level of needs can be satisfied. Maslow believed that the fulfillment of metaneeds is needed to be-

come a completely developed human being. Left unfulfilled, people can become cynical, apathetic and lonely.[35]

Maslow arrived at this model by examining what he considered to be exceptionally healthy people, people he defined as having developed to their fullest potentials. Self-actualized people that Maslow identified included Albert Einstein, Albert Schweitzer, Eleanor Roosevelt, and Abraham Lincoln. He perceived these people to share similar personality characteristics such as being comfortable with themselves, having a strong ethical and moral code of conduct, innovative, compassionate, altruistic, goal oriented, and internally motivated.[36]

HealthQuest Activities

Mental wellness is more than the absence of mental health problems. It means having balanced perspective, effective coping skills, and an ability to enjoy and accept one's life. Go to the Stress Management and Mental Health module of HealthQuest and complete the Wellness Activity called "How is Your Mental Wellness?"

Key Terms

basic needs deficiency needs that are viewed as essential and fundamental, including physiological needs, belonging and love, and esteem needs.

metaneeds secondary concerns, such as spirituality, creativity, curiosity, beauty, philosophy, and justice, that can be addressed only after the basic needs are met.

Spiritual Health

Having a sense of purpose, direction, and awareness are some of the dimensions of spiritual health. This aspect of psychological health also refers to how well we integrate our beliefs and values with our behavior. People with spiritual health seek meaning and purpose in their lives and have a deep appreciation for a sense of unity and community. Spiritual health also includes one's morals, ethics, intrinsic values, and beliefs. It also refers to an awareness and appreciation of the vastness of the universe, and recognition of a dimension beyond the natural and rational, involving perhaps a belief in a force greater than oneself.[37] Spirituality has been found to increase psychological health as people that incorporate it into their lives reported better psychological coping, increased well-being, increased satisfaction with life, lower anxiety and depressive symptoms, less hostility and anger, and greater happiness in general.[38] Similarly, spirituality has also been related to better physical health. Studies have shown that no matter how spirituality was defined or measured, it has a positive effect on reducing coronary heart disease, high blood pressure, stroke, cancer, and increasing life expectancy.[39]

As a resource for the spiritual dimension of health, spirituality provides a basis on which a belief system can mature and an expanding awareness of life's meaning can be fostered. Spirituality also gives meaning to your career and helps you better understand the consequences of your vocational efforts. In addition, spirituality influences many of the experiences that you will seek throughout life and tempers your emotional response to these experiences.

In nearly all cultures, spirituality provides individuals and groups with rituals and practices that foster a sense of community—"a community of faith." In turn, the community nurtures the emotional stability, confidence, and sense of competence needed for living life fully.[39]

Creative Expression

Another characteristic of people who have developed their psychological health is creativity. Allowing yourself to express your thoughts, feelings, and individuality in a creative manner entails having self-confidence, self-esteem, and flexibility. Confidence and self-esteem are essential so that you don't feel embarrassed by your creativity and feel free to share your creative side with others. Children can easily do this when they draw a picture or make up a dance and say, "Look at me. Look at what I made." However, as we age, some of us become inhibited and don't allow ourselves to be creative or to share this part of ourselves. Like muscles, if you don't exercise your creative side, it can begin to atrophy.

What are some resources that you might need to develop in order to foster your creativity?

- *Nonconformity.* Creative individuals aren't terribly concerned about what other people think of them. They are willing to risk looking foolish or proposing ideas that are divergent from others or traditional ways of thinking.

- *Independence.* Highly creative people tend to work well alone and sometimes prefer this to working in a group. As children, they often were encouraged to

Discovering Your Spirituality

Solitude: Time to Reflect, Regroup, Renew

Have you taken a moment today to be quiet and just be with yourself? Time alone can help you step away from a busy, fragmented world and draw inward for renewal. It provides an opportunity to reflect and to have new and deeper observations. Having strengthened awareness of yourself in both mind and body allows you to experience the fullness of the moment, even to feel in sync with the universe.

Solitude can also help you establish your identity, clarify what's important to you, and strengthen your independence. Because most of our time is spent living with, caring for, or responding to others, it is only when we are alone that we have the opportunity to fully emerge and become ourselves.

Any time you take for this meditation will be restorative. You may start with just five minutes every morning. You will need a place where you feel comfortable to be alone with your own thoughts, whether it be at the kitchen table, in bed, in the bath, at a coffee shop, in the library, or in the garden. Go for a walk, listen to music, weed the garden, write a letter to a friend, paint, read a poem, or just be still and concentrate on your breathing. All of these are solitary actions that, in the end, reconnect you to a life force and to others. Pretty soon you may feel that your time of solitude is more energizing than sleep! When you are faced with a difficult project, a household disaster, or something more serious, such as sickness or death, these reflective moments will give you mental and spiritual renewal.

It's not selfish to carve out whatever time you need alone to refresh yourself. By claiming solitude regularly, you're reconnecting to your inner self. This nourished spirit is what you can share with others, whether family, friends, coworkers, or strangers. Through your appreciation of a deep, rich, inner reality, you will feel rapture in the mystery and gift of just *being* here.

A New Problem . . . Internet Addiction

The Internet has changed the way we work, socialize, and educate ourselves. While the Internet has provided connections that otherwise could not be made very easily with people all around the world, it has also created unique psychological problems for some individuals. There is some question about the psychological implications the Internet may be having on our society as we are moving from a world in which we used to know our neighbors and interact with people face to face to developing serious and deep relationships with people from a distance. Marriages have broken up, affairs have taken place, and teenagers have been kidnapped by people they met over the Internet. In fact, one teenager was encouraged to overdose on drugs by his Internet friends and died while communicating over the Net to this group.

There is a feeling of anonymity that is created by talking on the Web. You can be who you want to be, reveal as much or as little as you want, and not be judged by your appearance. Of course this also means people can be deceitful and dishonest about who they are and what they want from you. In addition, there is a blending of home and work and increased solitary. Studies show that greater use of the Internet is associated with less communication among family members, decreased socializing with local friends, and increased depression and loneliness.[1] One study showed that using the Internet more than 5 hours a week resulted in less time with friends, family, and social activities.[2]

In fact, there is such concern about the potential adverse effects of spending too much time on the Internet that there are mental health professionals that propose adding "Internet addiction" as a diagnosable mental disorder. How can you tell if you are addicted? Here are some warning signs:

1. Preoccupation with the Internet—planning and thinking about the next time you can get online.
2. Increased use of the Internet over time.
3. Repeatedly making unsuccessful attempts to curtail your use of the Internet.
4. Feeling irritable, restless, and moody when you attempt to cut down your use of the Internet or are prevented from getting online when you would like.
5. Unaware of how much time you are spending on the Internet, staying online more than you originally intended.
6. Lying to family members and friends about your use of the Internet.
7. Jeopardizing your job or risking losing a relationship because of the time you are spending on the Web.
8. Using the Internet as a way of escaping from problems, coping with depression.
9. Declining invitations to spend time with family and friends because you would rather be online.

Of course, answering "yes" to one of these questions does not indicate a concern. However, if you can answer "yes" to more than half of these questions, then you may want to

examine your use of the Internet. Here are some ways you can avoid being an Internet addict:

- Decide how much time you want to spend on the Internet before you get online and set an alarm for that time. Stick to that time allotment and don't say "5 more minutes" which can then become an hour.
- Take frequent breaks. Spend at least 5 minutes out of every hour or 15 to 20 minutes of every 3 hours on unwired activity. Take a walk, stretch your body, eat a snack, or listen to music.
- Visit the Net with a purpose and a strategy. Surfing the Web aimlessly can lead to being online for longer than you anticipated.
- Interact with people in a nonwired world. Make a commitment to socially interact at least once a day with someone who is not online.
- Don't let the Internet be the center of your existence or the most important, enjoyable part of your day. Remind yourself of your life goals, values, and interests. What are other ways to achieve these goals besides via the Web?[3]

1 Kraut R., Patterson M., Lundmark V., Kiesler S., Mukopadyay T. & Scherlis W., Internet Paradox: A social technology that reduces social involvement and psychological well-being? *American Psychologist,* 53(9), 1998.
2 Streitfeld D., Study finds heavy Internet users are isolated. *Washington Post,* February 16, 2000.
3 Goldstein D. & Flory J., Best of the Net: *Online Guide Book Series.* New York: McGraw-Hill Irwin Professional Publishing Inc. 1996.

solve problems on their own rather than having someone else to do so for them.

- *Motivation.* Creative people are motivated by intrinsic rather than external rewards, meaning they like to be creative for their own pleasure, not to please others or because it is expected of them. They don't fear failure and success is not the main goal. They enjoy creativity for creativity's sake alone and not to reap rewards or praise from others.
- *Curiosity.* Creative people have a wide range of interests and a broad base of knowledge. They are open to new experiences and question things that other people ignore or take for granted.

- *Persistence.* This is seen as one of the most important traits of a creative person. As Thomas Edison said, "Genius is one-tenth inspiration and nine-tenths perspiration." Persistence requires not giving up when your first efforts are not successful and continually to think of new ways of doing something, problem solving, or thinking "outside of the box."[40]

Some people reviewing the preceding list may recognize many of these characteristics as being already well developed in their own personalities. Others may not have demonstrated some of the traits listed, and they may appear far beyond their reach. Nevertheless, most people can increase their creativity by giving themselves permission to be creative. Some people state, "I'm not a creative person" and yet they haven't explored that part of their personality, perhaps since childhood. There are many avenues of creativity and the first step is to experiment, to be open and spontaneous. In this way, you can gain greater psychological health from accessing your inner strengths and resources.

Psychological Health: A Final Thought

As you can see, psychological health involves how your emotions, thoughts, and behavior interplay with each other and with the world around you. There is an important mind–body connection in terms of your psychological health having a significant impact on your physical health and vice versa. Psychological health is not just the absence of mental illness, and there is a range or continuum of psychological health. Possessing a positive self-concept, developing high self-esteem, and cultivating an optimistic attitude towards life can promote psychological health and enhance relationships with others. While heredity plays a role in the development of personality and psychological health, environmental factors and stressors seem to have an equally important role. As people age and come across developmental milestones, they encounter new challenges, obstacles, and resources in continuing to maintain their psychological health.

Taking Charge of Your Health

Assess how effective and healthy your style of communication is by considering the following questions:

- Do you know the difference between passive, aggressive, and assertive behavior?
- Do you use assertive language such as "I" statements rather than "you" statements?
- Do you have assertive body language such as making eye contact and keeping an open body posture without crossing your arms in front of you?
- Are you aware of your nonverbal communication?
- Are you aware of the volume and tone of your voice and the message you might be conveying?

- Do you acknowledge the other person's feelings and point of view before stating your own?
- Do you feel comfortable saying "no" to requests?
- Do you feel comfortable asking for someone's help, disagreeing with someone, or giving your opinion about something?

Having a positive and effective communication style is an important aspect of psychological health and can have a significant impact on your relationships, success at work, and your self-worth. Learn to be more optimistic in your attitude and communication by considering the characteristics of an optimist on page 31.

Summary

- There is a mind–body connection in which biological, psychological, and social factors interact to influence health or illness. This is referred to as the biopsychological model.
- Psychological health has also been associated with developing and maintaining a positive self-concept, positive self-esteem, and emotional intelligence.
- Psychologically healthy people display a wide range of emotions.
- There is a continuum for self-esteem, and people can enhance their self-esteem through the use of several effective techniques.
- People with overall high levels of emotional intelligence tend to take on leadership roles, are confident and assertive, express their feelings directly and appropriately, feel good about themselves, are outgoing, and adapt well to stress.

- Two factors, nature and nurture, influence the shaping of personality. Nature refers to the innate factors we are born with that genetically determine our personality traits while nurture is the effect that the environment, people, and external factors have on our personality.
- Maintaining a sense of humor is a key to psychological health and well-being.
- Nonverbal communication is what is communicated by your facial expression, body posture, tone of voice, and movements.
- Maslow's theory is a positive, optimistic theory of human behavior. He believed that people are motivated to grow and fulfill their potential, referring to this phenomenon as self-actualization.
- People with spiritual health seek meaning and purpose in their lives and have a deep appreciation for a sense of unity and community.

- Having a positive interpretation of life's events, particularly how you cope with adversity, can make a significant difference in terms of your health and academic and work performance, as well as how long you will live.
- Clinical depression can range from mild to severe and can result in significant impairment in functioning.

- The majority of suicidal people have depressive disorders and feel helpless and powerless over their lives. It is always best to take any threats or talk about suicide seriously and act accordingly.
- Schizophrenia is one of the most severe mental disorders as it is characterized by profound distortions in one's thought processes, emotions, perceptions, and behavior.

Review Questions

1. What is the name of the model that talks about a mind–body connection in which biological, psychological, and social factors interact to influence health or illness?
2. What are three factors that have been associated with psychological health?
3. What are the characteristics commonly demonstrated by psychologically healthy people?
4. What is the definition of self-esteem and how can self-esteem be enhanced?
5. What characterizes people with overall high levels of emotional intelligence?
6. What are the main two factors thought to influence the shaping of personality?
7. What relationship is there between humor and psychological health?
8. What is nonverbal communication?
9. Describe Maslow's theory of the hierarchy of needs.
10. What traits are associated with people with spiritual health?
11. How can having a positive interpretation of life's events make a significant difference in people's health?
12. How is clinical depression different from having the "blues"?
13. How should you respond to someone threatening or talking about committing suicide?
14. What disorder is considered one of the most severe mental disorders?

References

1. Papalia D and Olds S. *Psychology,* 2nd edition. New York: McGraw-Hill, 1988.
2. Seligman M. *Learned Optimism.* New York: Simon & Schuster Inc., 1990.
3. McKay M and Fanning P. *Self-Esteem,* 3rd edition. Oakland, CA: New Harbinger Publications. 1992.
4. Goleman D. *Emotional Intelligence.* New York: Bantam Books, 1997.
5. Collier G. *Emotional Expression.* Hillsdale, N.J. Lawrence Erlbaum Associates, 1985.
6. Castro B, Eshleman J, Shearer R. Using humor to reduce stress and improve relationships. *Seminar Nurse Management* 7(2), 90–92, 1999.
7. Berk LS, et al. Immune System Changes During Humor Associated Laughter. *Clinical Research* 39, 124a, 1991.
8. Cogan R, et al. Effects of Laughter and Relaxation on Discomfort Thresholds. *Journal of Behavioral Medicine,* 139–144, 1987.
9. Martin RA and Lefcourt HM. Sense of Humor as a Moderator Between Stressors and Moods. *Journal of Personality and Social Psychology,* 45, 1313–1324, 1983.
10. Nezu A, Nezu C, and Blissett S. Sense of humor as a moderator of the relationship between stressful events and psychological distress. *Journal of Personality and Social Psychology* 54, 520–525, 1988.
11. Miller J. Jokes and joking: A serious laughing matter, in Durant J and Miller J, Eds: *Laughing Matters: A Serious Look at Humor.* Longman Scientific and Technical, Essex England, 1988.
12. Lefcourt HM and Martin RA. *Humor and Life Stress: Antidote to Adversity,* Springer-Verlag, New York, 1986.
13. Kuhn C. *Humor Techniques for Health Care Professionals.* Presentation at Ball Memorial Hospital, April 22, 1998.
14. Nair M. A Documentary: *"The Laughing Clubs of India,"* 2001.
15. Berk L, et al. Modulation of neuroimmune parameters during the eustress of humor associated mirthful laughter. *Altern There Health Med* 7(2), 67–72, 2001.
16. Seligman M. *Learned Optimism.* New York: Pocket Books, 1990.
17. Pavlov IP. *Conditioned reflexes.* New York: Oxford University Press, 1927.
18. Hiroto D. Locus of control and learned helplessness. *Journal of Experiential Psychology* 102, 187–93, 1974.
19. Ellis A. *Reason and emotion in psychotherapy.* New York: Lyle Stuart, 1962.

20. Spear P, Penrod S, and Baker T. *Psychology: Perspective on Behavior.* New York: John Wiley & Sons, 1988.

21. Regier DA, Narrow WE, Rae DS, et al: The de facto mental and addictive disorders service system. Epidemiologic Catchment Area prospective 1-year prevalence rates of disorders and services. *Archives of General Psychiatry* 50(2), 85–94, 1993.

22. Murray CJL, Lopez AD, eds. *Summary: The global burden of disease: a comprehensive assessment of mortality and disability from diseases, injuries, and risk factors in 1990 and projected to 2020.* Cambridge, MA: Published by the Harvard School of Public Health on behalf of the World Health Organization and the World Bank, Harvard University, 2003.

23. Lehrer J. Transcript from On Line News Hour. Living with Mental Illness, December 13, 1999.

24. American Psychiatric Association. *Diagnostic and Statistical Manual on Mental Disorders,* fourth edition (DSM-IV-TR). Washington, DC: American Psychiatric Press, 2000.

25. World Health Organization. *Mental Health,* 2003.

26. National Institute of Mental Health, 2003.

27. Dramatic Increases Seen in College Students' Mental Health Problems over the Last 13 Years. *Journal of Professional Psychology: Research and Practice,* February 2003. Maslow, AH: *The farthest reaches of human nature.* Peter Smith, 1983.

28. Peterson K. Resilience, talking can help kids beat depression. *USA Today,* June 4, 2002.

29. Exercise Better than Drugs for Depression. *British Journal of Sports Medicine* 35, 114–117, April 2001.

30. Robins L, Regier D, eds. *Psychiatric disorders in America: the Epidemiologic Catchment Area Study.* New York: *The Free Press,* 1991.

31. Study puts spotlight on electroshock therapy. *USA Today,* March 13, 2001.

32. Bourne E. *The Anxiety and Phobia Workbook.* Oakland: CA. New Harbinger Publications Inc., 1995.

33. Narrow W, Rae D, and Regier D. NIMH epidemiology note: prevalence of anxiety disorder. *One year prevalence best estimates calculated from ECA and NCS data.* Population estimates based on U.S. Census estimated residential population age 18 to 54 on July 1, 1998.

34. Maslow AH. *Motivation and personality,* 2nd ed. New York: Van Nostrand, 1970.

35. Maslow AH. *The farthest reaches of human nature.* Peter Smith, 1983.

36. Lindzey G, Thompson R, and Spring B. *Psychology,* 3rd ed. New York: Worth Publishers, Inc. 1988.

37. Hemenway JE, et al. *Assessing Spiritual Needs: A Guide for Caregivers.* Augsburg Press, 1993.

38. Ayele H, Muligan T, Gheorghiu S, and Reyes-Oritiz C. Religious activity improves life satisfaction for some physicians and older patients. *Journal of the American Geriatrics Society,* 43, 453–455, 1999.

39. Levin JS. Religion and health: Is there an association, is it valid and is it causal? *Social Science Medicine* 38(11), 1475–1482, 1994.

40. Wade C and Tavris C. *Psychology.* New York: Harper & Row Publishers, 1987.

As We Go to Press

When teenagers seem irritable, sullen, or complain of unhappiness, it is often dismissed as a "passing phase" or a normal stage of development, such as the "rebellious teenage years." However, this may be a sign of something much more serious and potentially lethal. Having trouble sleeping, eating more or less than usual, moodiness, being critical of oneself, and losing interest in things you normally like to do may be a sign of clinical depression. With suicide being the third leading cause of death for ten to twenty-year-olds, this is certainly a group that is at risk for depression. It is no wonder that the use of anti-depressants has dramatically increased for this age group, along with the FDA's nod of approval for use of Prozac to treat depression for children and adolescents. There is some debate as to whether kids are more depressed today, as 8% of adolescents and 2% of children are clinically depressed, or if there is just a greater recognition of this problem. With the increased divorce rate, violence, and rising social and academic pressures facing adolescents, it is no wonder that we are seeing more teenagers succumb to what was once thought of as an "adult disease."

The NIMH recently launched a major 12-city initiative called the "Treatment for Adolescents with Depression Study" to further investigate the reasons behind teenage depression and effective treatment interventions. While there is evidence supporting the idea that short-term behavioral therapy can be helpful in treating depression, along with anti-depressants, this seems to work for only 60% of the cases. In addition, half of those who improved, relapsed within a year of stopping treatment. The NIMH research study is hoping to find which treatment is best for particular individuals with specific types of symptoms, as not all people exhibit depressive symptoms in the same way. There is also a continuum in terms of severity of the symptoms and so they are examining what type of treatment might work best for different levels of depression. Hopefully we will soon find ways to detect who might be at risk and how to intervene before we lose more victims to this illness.

Sources: "Young and Depressed," *Newsweek,* October 7, 2002. "FDA Approves Prozac for Children, *USA Today,* January 3, 2003.

lending a helping hand: becoming a volunteer

From now on in America, any definition of a successful life must include serving others.

—Former President George H. W. Bush

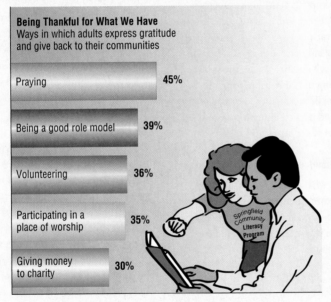

Being Thankful for What We Have
Ways in which adults express gratitude and give back to their communities

Praying — 45%

Being a good role model — 39%

Volunteering — 36%

Participating in a place of worship — 35%

Giving money to charity — 30%

Springfield Community Literacy Program

Many of us have been fortunate enough not to experience poverty, serious illness, or lack of education. Do you think it's important to express gratitude by giving something back to your community?

For nearly 40 years, two federally funded voluntary agencies, Peace Corps and VISTA (Volunteers in Service to America), have provided American adults of all ages an opportunity to put their idealism into action by using their skills in service to others. More recently, a third avenue for extending services to others, AmeriCorps, was established. This agency is a paid service initiative that lowers the cost of college for participants. Today, thousands of programs at the local, state, national, and international levels provide a similar opportunity.

Americans traditionally have expended their time, talents, and energy in support of others more freely than have the citizens of many other highly industrialized nations. Recent examples of this admirable American response were the clean-up efforts following devastating tornadoes in Oklahoma, assistance to those affected by the massive earthquake damage in Turkey, and victims of flooding in North Carolina following Hurricane Floyd. Less visible are the thousands of American volunteers who serve on committees, babysit, coach, and lead scout

troops. Various international programs also provide opportunities for Americans to volunteer in other countries. Two such programs are Amigos de las Americas (a program for teens to live and volunteer in Latin America) and World Teach (a program for college graduates to teach English in a foreign country). The monetary value of this free (or nearly free) service given by Americans is difficult to determine accurately, but most recently it was estimated to be worth at least $200 billion per year.[1]

Helping Others and Improving Yourself

Although volunteer service benefits those in need, volunteering is also good for the volunteer. It provides companionship, friendship, and fellowship in working toward a common goal. Volunteer service allows us to use skills and talents that we normally don't use at our daily jobs. It encourages us to branch out, learn new things, and become more well-rounded. The decision to become a volunteer fosters decision making and expands the scope of the volunteer's self-directed behavior. Most important, volunteering brings people of diverse backgrounds together, makes those being served feel a greater sense of self-worth, and raises the aspirations of all involved.

Today, the importance of volunteering, referred to as *service learning,* is reflected in the fact that many colleges and high schools are requiring its inclusion in their curricula.[2,3] Students who have participated in volunteering programs appear to profit in terms of their academic performance, perhaps because of the time management skills and discipline involved. They also report an increased sense of concern for the well-being of others and a greater ability to respond empathetically, as well as sympathetically, to people in need.

Employers are beginning to notice—and value—the inclusion of volunteering on the transcripts of recent graduates. Some members of the academic community question the appropriateness of *requiring* students to volunteer. Perhaps offering opportunities for students to volunteer (for credit) and to develop job-related skills is a good reason to include it in the curricula. Volunteering broadens the volunteer's world and sharpens his or her focus, combining to enhance both occupational performance and psychological well-being.

Diversity Among Volunteers

Volunteers are a very diverse group. Examples of recent American Institute of Public Service's Jacqueline Kennedy Onassis Awards for outstanding local community service include: Isaac Pope who overcame a segregated boyhood in Tennessee to earn a medical degree. After being diagnosed with cancer 10 years ago, he sold his medical practice to open a clinic for severely disabled children.

John Beal of Seattle restored environmentally crippled streams in the Duwamish River watershed in South Seattle. In 23 years of tireless work, he's brought teeming life back to Hamm Creek.

Another Onassis Award recipient is Lenny Larson who has helped people with AIDS to cope with the deadly disease, providing support through the Northwest AIDS Foundation, the Chicken Soup Brigade, and the Seattle AIDS Support Group, three organizations he co-founded.

Elizabeth Thomas, another award recipient, provided care and comfort to children in need as a dedicated pediatric nurse practitioner at the Odessa Brown Children's Clinic in Seattle.

Peter Truong of Burien, a war refugee who fled his native Vietnam in 1975, volunteers his time to assist Asian immigrants in dealing with an unfamiliar culture and country—when he's not working as a community service officer for the King County Sheriff's Office.

The many volunteers who do not receive official recognition for their efforts are just as important. Millions of Americans volunteer their expertise, time, and energy in various ways. Many "silent" volunteers are lobbying for the preservation of free speech and privacy on the Internet, participating in Habitat for Humanity, working on behalf of abused or neglected animals, and participating in countless other types of service.

Ways to Volunteer

No matter what your interests, abilities, or time commitments, there is much that you can do. Just a few of the volunteer opportunities you might consider include the following:

AIDS
Arts/cultural enrichment
Business assistance
Citizenship
Civic affairs
Consumer services/legal rights
Day care/Head Start
Disaster response/emergency
  preparedness
Drug abuse/alcoholism
Education
Employment
Health issues
Law enforcement/crime prevention
Literacy
Mental health
Nutrition

Physical environment
Psychosocial support services
Recreation and sports
Teen pregnancy prevention
Parenting
Transportation and safety
Animal welfare
Women's crisis centers

You can make a difference alone, with a few friends, or as part of an established organization. The Student Environmental Action Coalition (with chapters at 2,300 high schools and colleges), VISTA, Peace Corps, United Way, the Salvation Army, and the American Red Cross are just a few of the national organizations that need volunteers. To volunteer, contact one of these agencies or your local church, hospital, nursing home, city recreation department, or scout council directly.

For Discussion . . .

Do you currently volunteer? Why or why not? If you decided to become a volunteer, what areas of work would interest you most? Can you think of a way that a volunteer has touched your life? How do you feel about compulsory service as a component in college and high school curricula? Should time spent volunteering be counted as a contribution for income tax purposes (as is a monetary contribution to a nonprofit agency would)?

References

1. Wofford H, Waldlman S, Bandow D: AmeriCorps the beautiful? *Policy Review* 79:28–36, 1996.
2. Sax L, Justin A: The benefits of service: evidence from undergraduates, *EducationalRecord*, Summer/Fall: 25–33, 1997.
3. Calderon J: Making a difference: service-learning as an activism catalyst and community builder, *American Association for Higher Education Bulletin* 52(1):7–9, 1999.

personal assessment

how does my self—concept compare with my idealized self?

Below is a list of fifteen personal attributes, each portrayed on a 9-point continuum. Mark with an X where you think you rank on each attribute. Try to be candid and accurate; these marks will collectively describe a portion of your sense of self-concept. When you are finished with the task, go back and circle where you wish you could be on each dimension. These marks describe your idealized self. Finally, in the spaces on the right, indicate the difference between your self-concept and your idealized self for each attribute.

Decisive							Indecisive	____
9	8	7	6	5	4	3	2	1

Anxious							Relaxed	____
9	8	7	6	5	4	3	2	1

Easily influenced							Independent thinker	____
9	8	7	6	5	4	3	2	1

Very intelligent							Less intelligent	____
9	8	7	6	5	4	3	2	1

In good physical shape							In poor physical shape	____
9	8	7	6	5	4	3	2	1

Undependable							Dependable	____
9	8	7	6	5	4	3	2	1

Deceitful							Honest	____
9	8	7	6	5	4	3	2	1

A leader							A follower	____
9	8	7	6	5	4	3	2	1

Unambitious							Ambitious	____
9	8	7	6	5	4	3	2	1

Self-confident							Insecure	____
9	8	7	6	5	4	3	2	1

Conservative							Adventurous	____
9	8	7	6	5	4	3	2	1

Extroverted							Introverted	____
9	8	7	6	5	4	3	2	1

Physically attractive							Physically unattractive	____
9	8	7	6	5	4	3	2	1

Lazy							Hardworking	____
9	8	7	6	5	4	3	2	1

Funny							Little sense of humor	____
9	8	7	6	5	4	3	2	1

To Carry This Further . . .

1. Overall, how would you describe the difference between your self-concept and your self-ideal (large, moderate, small, large on a few dimensions)?

2. How do these differences for any of your attributes affect your sense of self-esteem?

3. How do you think someone who knows you well would rate you? Would they rate you in a similar way to how you see yourself? If not, why not?

4. Identify several attributes that you realistically believe can be changed to narrow the difference between your self-concept and your self-ideal and, thus, foster a well-developed sense of self-esteem.

chapter three

managing stress

Talking It Over

Communication and Stress

You just found out that your sister has been diagnosed with cancer, and you're feeling very stressed. You need to talk to someone, but who? First, figure out what you want. Is it emotional support, advice, affection, or help with errands? The answer will lead you to the best person. Second, explain what you're going through as clearly as you can. Tell the person what you need—whether it's a sympathetic ear or someone to drive you to the hospital. Third, talk to your sister as normally as possible. She needs you to talk—and listen—to her now more than ever.

CommunicationLinks

www.wellsource.com
www.webmd.com
www.cancer.org

Eye on the Media

New Technology, New Stresses

The Internet has connected an estimated 13 million computers in 195 countries on every continent, even Antarctica. The way we work, shop, access information, take classes, and socialize with others has all changed thanks to the Internet. While the Internet has connected the world in ways once unimaginable, along with the convenience and easy access to information have come new risks, and subsequently, new stress. Vulnerability to hackers, identity thieves, and viruses—not to mention endless piles of junk e-mail—can make the Internet a scary place. Your private journal or letter to someone might be read by someone you didn't intend to read it, your credit card information might fall into the wrong hands, or information about your medical records might be disbursed to people you didn't authorize to have this information.

Information can be corrupted when it is available on an insecure network. This means that unauthorized changes are made to information, whether by human error or intentional tampering. If you pay your bills online, or use the Internet for activities such as electronic funds transfers and financial accounting, this could cause you considerable stress should the information become

51

What Is Stress?

How do you know when you are stressed? You might experience headaches, stomach aches, or back and neck aches, or you might feel irritable, tired, anxious, and depressed. Some people eat more, while others find eating difficult when they are stressed. **Stress** refers to physiological and emotional responses to a significant or unexpected change or disruption in one's life. It can be brought on by real or imagined factors or events.

Stress was first described in the 1930s by Hans Selye, who observed that patients suffering from a variety of illnesses all showed common symptoms, such as fatigue, appetite disturbance, sleep problems, mood swings, gastrointestinal problems, and diminished concentration and recall. He called this collection of symptoms—this separate stress disease—stress syndrome, or the **general adaptation syndrome (GAS).** He also described this as "the syndrome of being ill."[1] We'll discuss Selye's discovery further later in the chapter.

Selye defines stress as "the nonspecific response of the body to any demand whether it is caused by or results in pleasant or unpleasant conditions."[1] Stress can be both positive or negative: again it is our response to stress—how we manage stress—that makes a difference in terms of how it affects us. Stress resulting from unpleasant events or conditions is called **distress** (from the Latin *dis*, meaning bad, as in displeasure). Stress resulting from pleasant events or conditions is called **eustress** (from

> ### Key Terms
>
> **stress** the physiological and psychological state of disruption caused by the presence of an unanticipated, disruptive, or stimulating event.
>
> **general adaptation syndrome (GAS)** sequenced physiological responses to the presence of a stressor, involving the alarm, resistance, and exhaustion stages of the stress response.
>
> **distress** stress that diminishes the quality of life; commonly associated with disease, illness, and maladaptation.
>
> **eustress** stress that enhances the quality of life.

the Latin *eu,* meaning good, as in euphoria). Both eustress and distress elicit the same physiological responses in the body, as noted in Selye's General Adaptation Syndrome model.

While stress may not always be negative, our responses to it can be negative, problematic, or unhealthy. Both positive and negative stressful situations place extra demands on the body—your body is reacting to an unexpected change or a highly emotional experience, regardless of whether this change is good or bad. If the duration of your stress is relatively short, the overall effect is minimal and your body will rest, renew itself, and everything returns to normal. But as you will learn in this chapter, long-lasting stress, experiencing multiple stressors simultaneously, and not managing your stress effectively, can take a toll on your body.

How We Respond to Stress

When we are stressed, we react in specific ways. The **stress response** is the result of learned and conditioned habits adopted early in life as a way of coping with problems, conflict and disruptive events. But many of our responses to stress are innate, basic human survival mechanisms left over from our primordial roots. In prehistoric times, the best response to perceived danger, such as seeing a saber-tooth-tiger coming your way, might be to either fight the animal or to run away. Stress in modern times remains the same except that we are responding to 21st century threats and dangers

rather than to saber-tooth tigers. Again it is not the events that determine how stressed we will feel but our response to these stressors. We will discuss the way that this innate stress response affects our modern lives in the section that follows.

Fight or Flight Response

Our response to stress involves many physiological changes that are collectively called the **fight or flight response.** In situations in which you must react immediately to danger, it is advisable to either fight off the danger or flee. For example, you are walking back from class at night, thinking about all the studying you need to do and you begin to cross the street. Suddenly, out of nowhere, you see a car with its headlights coming right at you. Since your best response is probably not to fight the car, you run as fast as you can to the other side of the road. In that split second,

Key Terms

stress response the physiological and psychological responses to positive or negative events that are disruptive, unexpected, or stimulating.

fight or flight response the physiological response to a stressor that prepares the body for confrontation or avoidance.

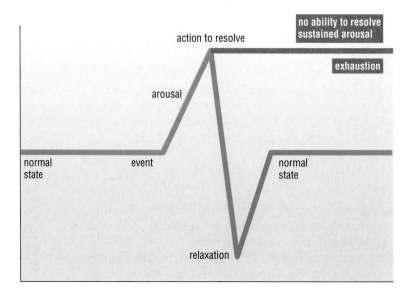

Figure 3-1 Resolving Stress There is a tremendous difference in how long your body remains at a high level of physiological arousal depending upon how quickly and effectively you act to resolve the stress.

Source: Selye "The Stress of Life."

when you see the car careening quickly towards you, your muscles tense, your heart beats faster, your adrenaline is pumping faster and being released at higher levels into your blood stream, your breathing becomes more shallow and rapid, and your pupils dilate to see the car better.

This is the fight or flight response. Again, all of these changes are very adaptive and helpful to your survival in getting out of harm's way. In the above example, when you get to the other side of the road and realize that you are okay, your body begins to relax and return to its normal state. You take a large, deep breath, expressing a big sigh of relief. Your muscles may feel even weaker than usual, your breathing may become deeper and heavier than is typical, and you may feel shaky as your body goes from extreme arousal to relaxing very quickly. Figure 3-1 depicts these changes from your normal state to an arousal state to a very relaxed state then back to normal.

Chronic Stress

Now let's consider a different situation. You have a test in a week that you are very concerned about. It seems to be preoccupying your every waking thought and you have trouble sleeping as well. You are worried that you won't perform well on the test and you really need to do better than you did on your last test. Your parents have been putting a great deal of pressure on you to do better in school in general. Because our bodies respond similarly to perceived or anticipated threat, you can have the same response to something that hasn't yet occurred. In other words, your heart races, breathing becomes labored, muscles are tense, body sweats, and blood flow is con-

stricted to the extremities and digestive organs and increases to the major muscles and brain. Your body is becoming ready to fight or flee the danger. However, you cannot take any action and make a fight or flight response, because nothing has really happened. You haven't taken the test yet and even once you do, you don't know your grade. So your body remains at this high level of arousal.

Remaining in a continued state of physiological arousal for an extended period of time is called **chronic stress.** This high level of arousal is similar to putting your foot on the accelerator of your car while it is in park and not letting up on the gas pedal. Since the fight or flight response is meant to be a very quick, short acting response, your body begins to wear down if kept at this physiological state of arousal for too long; eventually, you will begin to experience the physical and psychological symptoms of chronic stress. This is also the reason that people cope better with anxiety by taking some action, doing something about whatever they are worried about rather than stewing about their problems. Thus the fight or flight response

---

Key Terms

chronic stress refers to remaining at a high level of physiological arousal for an extended period of time; it can also occur when an individual is not able to immediately react to a real or perceived threat.

can be triggered inappropriately in response to phobias, irrational beliefs, an overactive imagination, or hallucinations or delusions.

The Three Stages of Stress

Once under the influence of a stressor, people's bodies respond in remarkably similar, predictable ways. For example, when asked to give a speech for a class, your heart rate may increase, your throat becomes dry, palms sweat, and you may feel lightheaded, dizzy, and nauseous. If an individual lost her or his job or discovered that her or his partner wanted to terminate their relationship, s/he might experience similar sensations. It is clear that different stressors are able to evoke these common physical reactions.

Selye described the typical physical response to a stressor in his general adaptation syndrome model[1] discussed earlier in the chapter. Selye stated that the human body moves through three stages when confronted by stressors as follows.

Alarm Stage

Once exposed to any event that is perceived as threatening or dangerous, the body immediately prepares for difficulty, entering what Selye called the **alarm stage.** These involuntary changes described in Figure 3-2, are controlled by the hormonal and nervous system, and trigger the fight or flight response. For example, you realize that the final exam you thought was today was actually scheduled for yesterday. You may begin to experience: fear, panic, anxiety, anger, depression, and restlessness.[2]

Resistance Stage

The second stage of a response to a stressor is the **resistance stage,** during which the body attempts to reestablish its equilibrium or internal balance. The body is geared for survival and because staying in the alarm stage for a prolonged amount of time is not conducive for the body's optimal functioning; it will resist or attempt to resolve the problem and reduce the intensity of the response to a more manageable level. Specific organ systems, such as the cardiovascular and digestive systems, become the focus of the body's response.[2] During this phase, you might take steps to calm yourself down and relieve the stress on your body: You might deny the situation, withdraw and isolate yourself from others, and shut down your emotions. Thus, in the example above, you may not tell anyone about missing the exam, may tell yourself that you don't care about that class anyway and go back to bed.

Exhaustion Stage

Your ability to move from the alarm stage to a less damaging resistance stage will determine the impact that the stressor has on your physical and psychological health. As you gain more control and balance is reestablished, you can begin to recover from the stress.

The length of time, energy and effort demanded in accomplishing this will decide how exhausted your body becomes as a result of the stressor. Of course, the longer your body is under stress and out of balance, the more negative the impact. Long-term exposure to a stressor or coping with multiple stressors at the same time often results in overloading your system. Specific organs and body systems that were called upon during the resistance stage may not be able to resist a stressor indefinitely. When all the psychological and physical resources we rely on to deal with stress are used up, an **exhaustion stage** results, and the stress producing hormones such as adrenaline rise again.[2] This is when chronic and serious illnesses can begin to develop. In the above example, the individual may develop clinical depression.

Sources of Stress

There are other causes of stress besides experiencing positive or negative events in your life. What events or situations trigger stress for you? For some it is financial worries, for others it might be relationship conflict, and for others it is work-related stress. Even positive events, such as getting married, starting a new job, moving to a new place can be **stressors.** Going on vacation can be stressful as you get things done ahead of time to prepare for being away, pack your belongings, spend money on

---

> **Key Terms**
>
> **alarm stage** the first stage of the stress response involving physiological, involuntary changes which are controlled by the hormonal and nervous system; the fight or flight response is activated in this stage.
>
> **resistance stage** the second stage of the stress response during which the body attempts to reestablish its equilibrium or internal balance.
>
> **exhaustion stage** the third stage of the stress response and the point at which the physical and psychological resources used to deal with stress have been depleted.
>
> **stressors** factors or events, real or imagined, that elicit a state of stress.

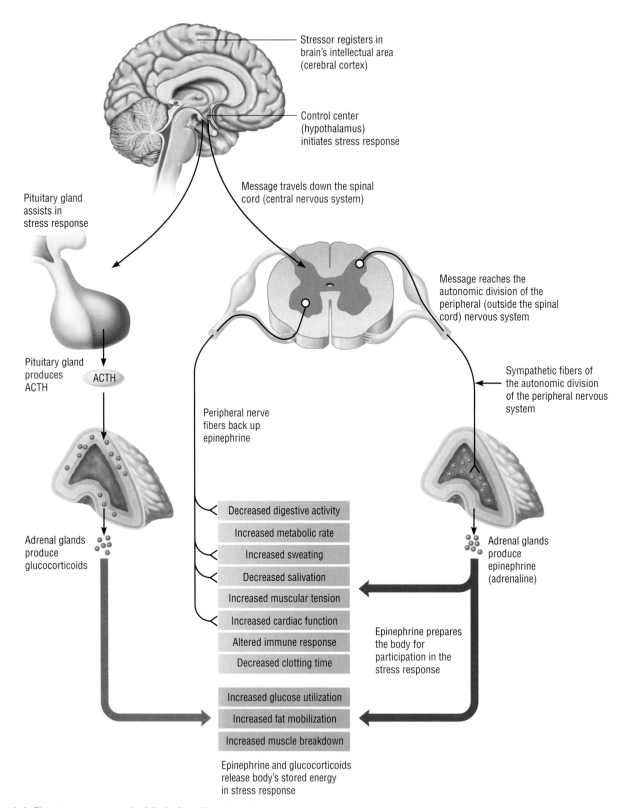

Stressor registers in brain's intellectual area (cerebral cortex)

Control center (hypothalamus) initiates stress response

Message travels down the spinal cord (central nervous system)

Pituitary gland assists in stress response

Pituitary gland produces ACTH

ACTH

Adrenal glands produce glucocorticoids

Message reaches the autonomic division of the peripheral (outside the spinal cord) nervous system

Sympathetic fibers of the autonomic division of the peripheral nervous system

Peripheral nerve fibers back up epinephrine

Adrenal glands produce epinephrine (adrenaline)

Decreased digestive activity

Increased metabolic rate

Increased sweating

Decreased salivation

Increased muscular tension

Increased cardiac function

Altered immune response

Decreased clotting time

Epinephrine prepares the body for participation in the stress response

Increased glucose utilization

Increased fat mobilization

Increased muscle breakdown

Epinephrine and glucocorticoids release body's stored energy in stress response

Figure 3-2 The stress response: physiological reactions to a stressor.

the trip and completely change your routine. Any type of change in your life has the potential to trigger a stressful response.

Because stress involves a physiological response, it has a direct link to your physical and psychological health. The work of Thomas Holmes and Richard Rahe have found direct connections between changes in people's lives and physical illness. They developed a widely used inventory, called the Social Readjustment Rating Scale, to assess the degree of stress people experience in connection with particular life events. While one of these events alone might be tolerable, a combination of too many life changes within a short period of time is more likely to lead to illness.[3] To assess your level of stress and potential vulnerability to illness, complete the personal assessment inventory at the end of this chapter.

The Costs and Benefits of Stress

Stress can be costly, taking a toll on our physical and mental health as well as our finances.

Constant arousal and increased levels of adrenaline in your system will eventually wear down your body's immunological system. As this occurs, you will be less able to cope with stress, and so it takes less and less to cause a stress reaction. When you are chronically stressed, it takes very little to frustrate you and you feel easily irritated and stressed at the littlest thing. Your body is both psychologically as well as physically less able to cope with stress. This can cause your immune system to become compromised, and you may become ill more easily. It may also take longer for you to recover from illness. There are a variety of medical problems that have been associated with stress, such as cardiovascular problems, gastrointestinal problems, sleep disorders, sexual dysfunction, infertility, and allergies.[4]

While too much stress can have a negative impact and cause some serious health problems, a moderate level of stress is positive and beneficial. Stress can be very motivating and energizing. Without some stress, many of us may not get much accomplished in our day or even get out of bed! Look at the diagram in Figure 3-3 on this page, what do you notice? Too little and too much stress is not helpful. When you are not stressed at all, you can be apathetic and lethargic. When you are too stressed, you are paralyzed with fear, like deer in the headlights. This is referred to as the **Yerkes-Dodson Law** that shows a bell shaped curve demonstrating that there is an optimal level of stress for peak performance (see Figure 3-3). This holds true for any type of performance from academic or work activities to music or athletics.[5] Recognizing your appropriate level of stress for your ideal performance level is important in reaching your potential.

Figure 3-3 The Yerkes-Dodson Law Too little or too much stress is not helpful, but a moderate level of stress encourages peak performance.

Source: Hebb DO. Drive and the CNS (central nervous system). *Psychological Review* 62(4) 243–254, 1955.

Student Stress

Going to college has been likened to "crossing into a new culture," and there are unique challenges and stressors that students face.[6] Similar to going to live in another country, students must learn new customs and traditions, new ways of doing things, a new language, and must leave comfortable and familiar surroundings. This can cause a high level of stress for students, many of whom have left their support system behind to live in a place where they know few people. In the sections that follow, we will cover some of the specific stressors college students face and offer ways to manage these situations.

Coping with Homesickness

Homesickness is one of the most common problems facing college students—which is understandable given that

---

Key Terms

Yerkes-Dodson Law a bell-shaped curve demonstrating that there is an optimal level of stress for peak performance; this law states that too little and too much stress is not helpful, while a moderate level of stress is positive and beneficial.

Journaling: Self-Help for Stress

Feeling anxious about your college experience? Trying to put past events in perspective? Want to record your experiences? Focused, regular writing—journaling—is growing in popularity as a way to approach these issues.

Writing in a journal each day slows down your pace. You sit and reflect. You connect with an experience by recalling details you may have forgotten, then write them down. For 15 to 30 minutes a day, you pause to make sense of your life.

Journaling generally gets easier the more you do it, so start by writing about nonthreatening topics. Try this: Each day, ask yourself a simple question, and then write the answer in your journal. As you gain experience, you may want to tackle more difficult issues.

Here are some journaling tips. Use an easy-to-carry spiral-bound notebook with a thick cover, so you can write anywhere. Or you may want to set aside a regular time and place so you won't be disturbed. Once you start writing, keep your pen moving continuously. Don't go back to correct spelling or punctuation. That will only slow you down and distract you from your thoughts, which are more important than perfect writing. Give yourself permission not to have to share your journal with others as this may inhibit your writing, making it less honest and open.

One powerful form of journaling is therapeutic, or healing journaling, in which the individual writes about a traumatic event for 15 to 30 min-utes a day, on three or four consecutive days. Studies by James W. Pennebaker, M.D. and colleagues noted lowered blood pressure and heart rates in healthy people who wrote about their innermost feelings for 20 minutes on three consecutive days.

Therapeutic writing can be very difficult and should be approached with caution. In particular, if you have been under medical treatment, check with your health-care professional before you begin a therapeutic journaling program. If you write about private events, you can shred or burn your pages. Be aware of not just writing about negative events or emotions. Don't allow this to be a journal about "how I messed up today."

Want to know more about journaling? *Personal Journaling Magazine* (*www.journalingmagazine.com*) is a good place to start. You'll find that journaling takes many forms, including memoirs, dream journals, chronicles of daily life, and "blogging" on the Internet.

In college, most of the things you write, such as papers and reports, are assigned and judged by an instructor. But when you write in a journal, it's for yourself—no judgments, no grades.

Tired of being stressed out all the time? Want to clear out the cobwebs in your head? Take out paper and pen and embark on one of the most exciting trips you'll ever take—the journey into yourself.

---

you are separated from your friends and family and learning to live in an entirely new environment.[6] When undergoing a great deal of change in your life, it is helpful to have the comfort and security of your home base remaining stable and consistent. Moving from home to college can disrupt this sense of safety. While this can be an exciting and challenging time in your life, you may be missing your friends and family at home with whom you normally

---

Changing for the Better

I just started college and my family and friends are 5 hours away from me. I tend to be on the shy side and don't know anyone at my college. I miss my friends and family and don't feel like I belong here. I am thinking about withdrawing from school and going home. What should I do?

The following are some strategies to combat these feelings:

- Get involved! Become active in noncurricular, social activities such as special interest clubs, student government, religious clubs, fraternities and sororities. Clubs associated with your major are a great way to meet people, further your academic and career interests, and keep you from feeling homesick.

- Call, e-mail, or write your family and friends regularly and let them know you would like to hear from them.

- Be open to meeting new people. Introduce yourself to people in your classes and exchange e-mail addresses and phone numbers. This is also an excellent way to get a study partner or study group together. Keep your door open when you are in your room, and spend time in public, common areas—not just hiding away in your room when you have spare time. Strike up a conversation while doing your laundry in the common laundry room area.

- Don't eat alone. Ask someone to join you to eat, or ask people at a table if you can eat with them.

- Don't go home on the weekends. Even though it may be tempting to visit your family and friends, the weekends are the best time to meet people and participate in the activities going on around campus.

- Be patient with yourself. Accept that loneliness and longing for home is normal and it will take some time for you to adjust to all of the changes you are experiencing. Don't decide to throw in the towel after the first few days! It may take a month before you begin to feel more comfortable in your new home. Give yourself some time to face this new challenge.

Figure 3-4 Percentages of college students who also work at paying jobs.

Source: Data from the U.S. Department of Labor.

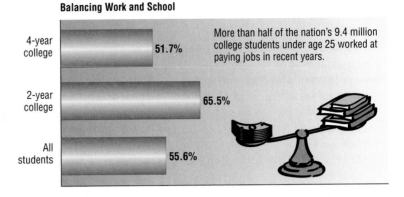

Balancing Work and School

4-year college 51.7%

2-year college 65.5%

All students 55.6%

More than half of the nation's 9.4 million college students under age 25 worked at paying jobs in recent years.

share these events. You may have also lost your sense of belonging while you struggle with finding a way to fit in with and navigate your new surroundings.

Often homesickness doesn't hit until a few weeks or maybe a month after you have moved, as the first few weeks are filled with meeting new people, social activities, and unpacking. After the dust settles, some people begin to feel lonely and alone. See Changing for the Better on page 58 for advice on how to deal with homesickness.

Relationship Problems

Along with homesickness, another very common stressor for students is relationship problems. Often students are separated by long distances from their best friends and romantic partners. While it can be difficult to maintain long distance relationships, it is not impossible. Studies show that the key to effective long distance relationships is communication.[7] The quality of a long distance relationship is increased if you both are committed to each other, you can talk openly about your concerns, feelings, and fears, and you can agree on the rules of the relationship such as dating other people. In addition, there needs to be a strong level of trust between the couple, as this is often tested in long distance relationships. Both of you will change and it is important that you share these changes so that you can grow together, not apart. Communicate how often you will see each other, call or e-mail, and focus on spending quality time together.

It can be beneficial to have your friends visit you at college (rather than you going home) so that they can interact with you in your new environment and meet your new friends. Often students feel as though they live in two worlds, home and school, and it can be stressful to negotiate going from one to the other. The more you can connect these two worlds, the less stress you will experience. So it can be helpful to share what you are doing in your day—activities around campus, details of your classes, even who you ate lunch with—with your friends and family back home, and ask the same about them.

Balancing Work, Home, and School

It is estimated that about three-quarters of students work along with going to college and more students are working full-time to pay for the costs of tuition (see Figure 3-4). In addition it is estimated that between 5 to 10 percent of college students also have children. This, of course, adds more stress to a student's life in balancing time for school, children, work, and household responsibilities. This is partly as a result of a nationwide trend of more women in their mid twenties or older who are starting or returning to college. In fact, a national study by the University of Michigan showed that the number of full-time female students over 25 years old grew by 500% over the past 30 years.[8]

While some campuses offer child care, many do not and this leaves students having to coordinate schedules and juggle responsibilities even more, causing potentially more stress. Also the cost of child care can be exorbitant for some and can certainly add to financial worries. Managing your time well and having a strong support system is essential for students with children, particularly single parents. Often there is little to no time available for relaxation, socializing, or exercising, and so employing these stress relief strategies can be challenging.

Test Anxiety

You have studied for the test you are about to take and are well prepared. You look at the first test question and suddenly your mind goes blank. The harder you try to think, the more nervous and distressed you feel. You just can't think clearly and feel like you have some type of mental block—what is happening? One-fifth of students

Do You Suffer from Test Anxiety?

Test anxiety is a commonly experienced problem and can significantly impair your academic performance. Similar to managing other types of stress and anxiety, test anxiety can be coped with by using the following suggestions:

- Prepare well in advance. Don't cram at the last minute for the test. Rehearsal and repetition are the best ways of remembering information.
- Improve your odds by getting a good night's sleep before the test and eating a nutritious meal to give your brain needed energy.

- Have a positive attitude and watch your test talk. Don't talk about the test beforehand with friends as this tends to increase anxiety. Go into the test with a confident attitude, reminding yourself that you are well prepared and have taken many tests and performed satisfactorily in the past.
- Activity reduces anxiety. If you stumble on a question, don't linger over it; go onto the next question and return to that one later.
- Ask for clarification if you don't understand a question or something on the test.

- Don't pay attention to the people around you. Focus on the test and don't allow yourself to get distracted.
- Take deep breaths, allow your breathing to help you to relax and bring more oxygen to the brain so you can think more clearly.
- Pace yourself and be aware of your time. Know when you need to be half way through the test according to the time allotted for the exam.

Source: Newman E. *No More Test Anxiety.* Los Angeles, CA: Learning Skills Publications, 1996.

---

experience these feelings, referred to as **test anxiety.** Exams are one of the greatest sources of stress for college students. The physical sensations associated with test anxiety are similar to those of general anxiety, such as fidgeting, having the feeling of butterflies in your stomach, rapid heart rate, difficulty breathing, nausea, tension in your neck, back, jaw and shoulders, headaches, sweaty palms, and feeling shaky. People suffering from test anxiety make more mistakes on their tests, don't read the test accurately, and tend to make simple mistakes, such as spelling errors or adding something incorrectly. Many don't pace themselves well, and have a hard time finishing exams. Test anxiety is a form of performance anxiety, as people anticipate that they will perform poorly on the test.[9] In order to assess your test anxiety level, complete the inventory at the end of this chapter.

TALKING POINTS What are some problems with stress described in this chapter that you have experienced?

Speech Anxiety

As was mentioned in the previous chapter, speech anxiety, or fear of public speaking, is one of the most common anxiety disorders. Since students are frequently required to give oral presentations, expected to engage in class discussion, and graded on class participation points, this can present a problem for some.

In addition to the basic stress management techniques outlined in this chapter, it is also advised to do the following in coping with speech anxiety:

- Volunteer to go first. It is advisable to go first since anxiety is dealt with best by taking action. The pressure and expectations tend to mount with each person that takes a turn. Another advantage is that your performance is judged on its own merit without being compared to anyone else.
- Practice in front of a mirror and for your friends. Solicit feedback: do you need to slow down or speak louder? This will also help you to remember your talk so that you aren't reading it word for word which can seem less interesting to your audience.
- Engage in positive visualization. Taking deep, comfortable breaths, imagine yourself giving your speech with confidence and receiving positive feedback and compliments regarding your performance.
- Vary your presentation style and format. Use visuals such as slides, illustrations or photographs and engage your audience in discussion so that they are an active not a passive part of your presentation.

Math Anxiety

Another common stressor for college students is math anxiety. Math anxiety is an intense emotional feeling of

---

Key Terms

test anxiety a form of performance anxiety that generates extreme feelings of distress in exam situations.

anxiety that some people have about their ability to understand mathematics. People who suffer from math anxiety feel that they are incapable of performing well in activities and classes that involve math. The incidence of math anxiety among college students has risen significantly over the last decade. Many students have even chosen their college major on the basis of how little math is required for the degree. Math anxiety has become so prevalent on college campuses that many schools have designed classes and special counseling programs to help math-anxious students. Typically, people with math anxiety have the potential to perform well in math and it is more of a psychological, rather than intellectual, problem.

Students who fear math often avoid asking questions to save embarrassment, sit in the back of the classroom, fail to seek help from the professor, and usually put off studying math until the last moment. All of these negative behaviors are intended to reduce the student's anxiety but actually result in more intense anxiety. However, you can take a number of positive steps to facilitate learning and performance in math classes. A student can use a number of the following strategies to overcome math anxiety.

1. Be sure to have developed a solid arithmetic foundation. As complex concepts build cumulatively on more simplistic ones, a remedial course or short course in arithmetic is often a significant first step in reducing the anxiety response to math.
2. If you have a choice, take an easier, slower math course as opposed to a faster paced, more challenging one. It is better to stack the odds in your favor than to risk reinforcing your negative experiences with math.
3. Be aware of thoughts, feelings, and actions as they are related to math. Cultivate positive math talk rather than self-defeating, negative statements.
4. There is safety in numbers! Math anxiety is learned and reinforced over a long period of time and may take time to eliminate. You can reduce your anxiety with the help of a tutor, studying with a friend, or talking with your instructor.

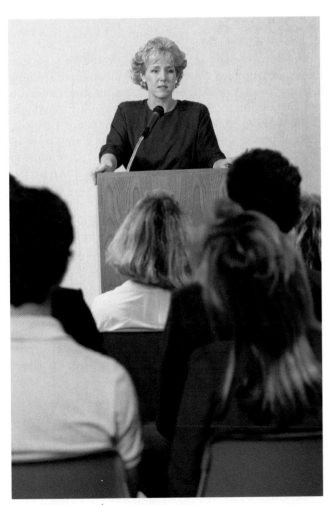

Speech anxiety or fear of public speaking is one of the most common anxiety disorders.

5. Sit near the front of the class where you will experience fewer distractions and feel more a part of what is being discussed.

6. If you have questions or can't keep up with the instructor ask for clarification and to repeat something you missed.[10]

7. Review the material. As with most things, skill in math comes from practice and repetition. Make sure you review the material covered in that class, and identify questions you need to ask the instructor as soon as possible after the class. Research shows that you will remember 50 percent of what you heard in class if you review it immediately after class, but only 20 percent is retained 24 hours later if you don't review it right away.[11]

Stress and Learning

How does stress affect learning? Research suggests that people that are highly anxious tend to perform better than others at simple learning tasks but less well than others at difficult tasks, particularly with reasoning activities and time-limited tests. An interesting study was conducted that showed college students with average scholastic ability earned significantly better grades when they had low levels of anxiety as compared to highly anxious average students.[12] When you are more stressed or anxious, you have a diminished ability to concentrate, to recall information, and to engage in problem-solving activities. You may find yourself reading the same page in your textbook over and over again and not knowing what you read.[9]

Using Time Effectively

An overwhelming number of students identify time management as the reason for their academic success or failure. Setting priorities and goals, balancing academic life with your social life, and finding time for sleeping, eating, exercising, and working along with studying is an essential aspect of managing your stress effectively.

Time Management

Managing your time effectively can help you cope with your stress by feeling more in control, having a sense of accomplishment, and having a sense of purpose in your life. Establishing good time management habits can take 2 to 3 weeks. By using specific systems, even the most disorganized person can make their lives less chaotic and stressful.

Assess Your Habits

The first step is to analyze how you are spending your time. When is your more productive and least productive time of day or night? Do you tend to underestimate how long

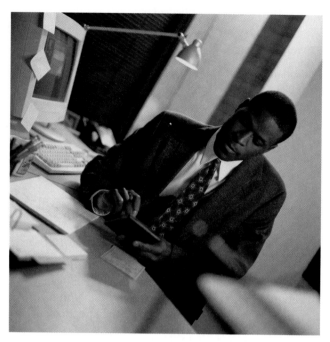

Managing your time well can greatly reduce your stress level.

something will take you to complete? Do you waste time or allow interruptions to take you off the task? Carrying a notebook with you for a week and writing down how you spend your time might provide you with some insight into the answers to these questions and how you spend your time. You might find that you've been devoting most of your time to less important tasks. Perhaps it is tempting to do your laundry rather than to start writing that term paper, but this is probably not the best use of your time.

Use a Planner

Keeping a daily planner to schedule your time is the next step in managing your time more effectively. First block off all of the activities that are consistent, regular, weekly activities such as attending classes, eating meals, sleeping, going to meetings, exercising, and working. Then look at the open, available time remaining. Schedule regular study time, relaxation time, and free time. Remember to schedule your study time during the more productive part of your waking hours. When you have a 1-hour block of

HealthQuest Activities

Each day brings its own challenges and frustrations. How do you react to situations throughout a typical day? Complete the CyberStress Exploration in the Stress Management and Mental Health Module to see how well you currently handle stress.

time, what can you realistically get done in that time? This may be a good time to review your notes from class, pay bills, or get some reading done.

Set Goals and Prioritize

It is advisable to set goals for the week as well as for each day. If something unexpected interferes with your time schedule, modify your plans but don't throw out the entire schedule.

Making a to-do list can be helpful, but it is only the first step. Breaking the larger tasks into smaller, more manageable pieces and then prioritizing them is the key to effective time management. When you prioritize your tasks, it is beneficial to use the "ABC" method of task management. The A tasks are those items that are most urgent and must be done today. Then the B tasks are those things that are important but, if need be, could wait 24 hours. The C tasks are activities that can easily wait a few days to a week. Don't fall into the C trap which is when you do the less important tasks because they are quick and can be checked off your list with ease. This can lead to procrastinating the more important A activities, leaving them until you feel stressed and overwhelmed.[13] We will discuss more about procrastination in the next section.

Procrastination

Procrastination means postponing something that is necessary to do to reach your goal.[14] Putting things off is a common problem that plagues students and can cause stress. A survey of college students found that approximately 23% of students said they procrastinated about half of the time and 27% of students said they procrastinated most of the time.[15] Procrastination has been seen as a time management problem but it is really more than that, and so time management strategies tend to be ineffective in resolving this problem. Procrastination is also different from indecision, as people can make a decision but have trouble implementing their decisions.

Typically there is a psychological aspect to procrastination as we tend to delay doing things we don't want to do. Emotions such as anxiety, guilt, and dread often accompany thinking about the task. By putting the dreaded activity off, you can temporarily alleviate your anxiety and discomfort, and this is a reinforcing aspect of procrastination. In the short term, procrastination seems like a good solution and helps you to feel better. However, in the long run, procrastinating activities usually leads to bigger problems and more work. For example putting off paying your bills may feel good in the moment, but when your electricity is turned off and you have to pay late fees, and your roommates are upset with you because they thought you had paid the bill, your pleasurable feelings soon turn sour.

Many people who procrastinate report feeling overwhelmed and highly anxious. They have difficulty tuning out external stimulation and concentrating on the task at hand. They also worry about how their performance will be judged by others and have perfectionistic standards for themselves. Students who procrastinate tend to perform less well and retain less than students who do not.[16] We will discuss perfectionism in the next section of this chapter.

Some techniques for combating procrastination involve time management, stress management, assertiveness training, and increasing self-esteem and self-acceptance. Procrastinators tend to both over- and underestimate how much time a task will take. When they underestimate the time, they feel justified in procrastinating because they erroneously believe they have plenty of time to complete the task. When they overestimate the time needed, they feel intimidated by the magnitude of the job, feel anxious, and so have trouble getting started. Most students explain that their anxiety stems from a fear of failure or being evaluated. Sometimes their anxiety manifests itself because they don't understand the material or what the instructor is wanting but are afraid to ask for clarification.

People also report procrastinating when they feel forced or pressured to do something they don't want to do. Rather than communicating assertively, they rebel by agreeing to do something but constantly put it off, which can be a passive-aggressive way of behaving. They fear the consequences of saying no or not fulfilling their obligations, but are also angry about what they perceive as unfair expectations and demands on them. This is where some assertiveness training may be helpful. Finally, increasing self-esteem can solve problems with procrastination as feeling better about yourself relieves you of worrying about what others think of you and having to prove yourself to them constantly. Some procrastinate because they think they need to do everything perfectly or not at all. With increased self-esteem, you are more accepting of mistakes and don't expect yourself to perform perfectly.

Perfectionism

Perfectionism leads to undue stress, because perfection is an unattainable goal. By setting the standard at perfect, you will set yourself up to fail. Perfectionists tend to be

---

Key Terms

procrastination a tendency to put off completing tasks until some later time, sometimes resulting in increased stress.

perfectionism a tendency to expect perfection in everything one does, with little tolerance for mistakes.

their own worst critic; they are harder on themselves than anyone else is on them, and they are also critical of others. These individuals are described as neat and organized, seeming to "have it all together" and to be able to do more than most people and do it exceptionally well. Often people envy perfectionistic people because they seem very confident and competent; however, individuals who are perfectionist never feel good enough and often feel out of control in their lives.[17] People who are perfectionists focus on what they haven't accomplished or haven't done right rather than on what they have completed or have done well. Making mistakes feels especially humiliating to persons who are perfectionistic, and they tend to feel a strong sense of shame and low self-esteem when someone catches them in error. They have difficulty with criticism or any negative feedback as much of their self-esteem is based upon being accurate, competent, and being the best. While striving to do your best is an admirable quality, expecting to be perfect in everything you do and never making a mistake places a great deal of stress and pressure on yourself.

In alleviating the stress of perfectionism, it is helpful to develop your self-esteem from who you are rather than what you do. This involves accepting yourself and others unconditionally, including the imperfections. Lowering your expectations of yourself and others and aiming for 80% rather than 100% is another strategy in battling perfectionism. Notice what you are doing well and have accomplished rather than what is still left to do. Time management strategies such as those outlined above can be useful in managing your expectations of yourself. Push yourself to take risks and allow yourself to make mistakes. It can be useful to make mistakes on purpose in order to get accustomed to this experience and realize that people still like and accept you and nothing bad will happen. Relaxation and stress management techniques such as the ones described at the end of this chapter can also help alleviate the stress that comes with perfectionism. You might want to take the survey at the end of this chapter to assess your level of perfectionism.

Managing Stress: Effective Coping Strategies

The research on how people cope with crisis and stress in their lives has shown that people tend to resolve problems within 2 weeks of experiencing a crisis. Because stress involves a disruption in your equilibrium, and the body does not function well in a chronic state of disequilibrium, it is human nature to seek a way to alleviate the stress your body is experiencing and return to a steady state. As discussed previously, our bodies cannot function for very long in the fight or flight response without serious damage, and so you will naturally strive to

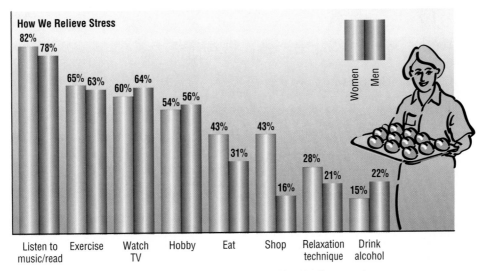

Figure 3-5 People have different ways of relaxing and relieving stress, such as cooking, reading a mystery novel, or swimming: How do you cope with stress?

make changes to resolve the stress for survival. However, it is important to note that the way that you resolve your problems and alleviate your stress may be positive or negative.

There are a number of negative ways of dealing with stress that are quite common and often quite harmful. As indicated in Figure 3-5, some turn to alcohol and drugs to avoid their problems and numb their feelings, and cigarettes are also cited as a way of relieving stress. Many people use food to comfort themselves. Procrastinating distasteful tasks and avoiding stressful situations is another negative way of coping with stress. Some people use sleep as a way of escaping their problems and certainly depression has been associated with not having the ability to effectively manage stress. In the next section, we will discuss ways of effectively managing stress.

What are some positive, effective methods to cope with stress? There are different strategies and methods for stress management involving the physical, social, environmental, and psychological aspects of your stress. We will review techniques and strategies within each of these dimensions, and you will need to practice and experiment to find the stress management techniques that are right for you.

The Physical Aspects of Stress Management

The physical aspects of stress management involve meeting your basic needs of nutrition, sleep and exercise as was discussed in Chapter two under Maslow's hierarchy of needs.[18]

Nutrition

In Chapter 5 you will learn that nutrients provide the necessary fuel the body needs to function. When people are stressed, they often skip meals or eat on the run. Since the fight or flight response requires more energy than is normally needed, it is even more essential that you eat a balanced, nutritious diet during stressful times. Without proper nutrition, the body will begin the breakdown of its own tissues in an effort to obtain the energy required to survive. The immune system can then become compromised and the body is more susceptible to disease. It is not a coincidence that many people who are under a great deal of stress for prolonged periods of time become ill and regaining their health takes longer than for those who are managing their stress well.

As was previously mentioned, people often use food to cope with stress and can overeat, typically eating high sugar and high fat foods such as chips, candy, and cookies, when under stress. Eating too much or too little is not an effective way to manage stress and can eventually lead to more serious health problems such as obesity, eating disorders, diabetes and hypertension.

Sleep

As with eating, too much sleep or too little is also an ineffective way of managing stress. Most adults require 7 to 8 hours of sleep a night.[19] Sometimes people get very little sleep during the week and they try to "catch up" over the weekend, sleeping 14 hours at a time or taking naps during the day. Sleep is not like a bank account in which you can make deposits and withdrawals, and so

Exercising is one of the best ways to manage your stress.

getting an average of 7 to 8 hours a night over a week's time is not the same thing as sleeping this amount each night.

It is also important that you experience uninterrupted sleep. Normal **circadian rhythms,** the biological process related to the 24-hour light/dark cycle, are necessary for normal sleep and optimal daytime functioning. Our sleep patterns relate to these biological cycles which also impact our patterns of hunger and eating, body temperature, and hormone release. It is important that these cycles be in harmony to have a sense of well-being during our waking hours.[20] Research also shows that sleeping too much can result in increased depression and decreased energy levels. Sleep deprivation has been found to cause losses in higher cognitive processing tasks, decline in the performance of simple tasks, memory loss, and, with prolonged sleep deprivation, temporary psychosis such as hallucinations and delirium.[21] So getting adequate rest is an essential aspect of stress management.

Exercise

Exercise is another physical aspect of stress management. Exercising aerobically at least three times a week for 20 to 30 minutes has been found to manage stress effectively for several reasons. First, exercising requires you to focus on your breathing and to breath deeply, the key to stress management. By tensing and releasing the muscles through exercise, you are allowing your body to relax and unwind. Secondly, exercise can alleviate stress through the release of endorphins, naturally occurring chemicals in the brain. Endorphins help to counter stress, subdue pain, and increase pleasure, which is the reason people talk about the runner's high. Hitting a racquet ball against the wall or playing basketball can be a great way to release the frustrations of the day and let go of tension and stress. Aerobic exercise includes walking briskly, running, bicycling, skating, and dancing. The benefits of exercise will be further discussed in Chapter 4.

The Social Aspects of Stress Management

It is also important in managing your stress effectively for you to make time to have fun and play. Like exercise, laughter increases the release of endorphins and requires you to breath deeply, and so having humor in your life is an essential part of stress management.[22] Research has

---

Key Terms

circadian rhythms the internal, biological clock that helps coordinate physiological processes related to the 24-hour light/dark cycle.

shown that stress can be related to having inadequate social interactions.[23] Hugging and human contact has also been demonstrated as having a significant effect in reducing the harmful physical effects of stress.[24] Participating in social activities such as social organizations, sports or just talking with friends can give you the break you need to rest your mind and focus on something other than work.

Actually you don't even have to have human contact to reduce stress—as just owning a pet can make the difference. Studies have shown that just petting an animal produces calming effects such as lowered blood pressure and decreased heart rate. Cardiac patients who own pets tend to live much longer than those who have no pets.[25]

The Environmental Aspects of Stress Management

To effectively manage your stress, you need to take into consideration environmental stressors such as the noise level, amount of light, and aesthetic quality of the space you inhabit. Stress has been linked to being exposed to prolonged, daily noise such as in a factory.[26] We know that depression can be related to the amount of light to which you are exposed, and this can also affect your circadian rhythms.[27] Natural light tends to elevate your mood while prolonged exposure to artificial lighting can increase your stress level. There is also research to suggest that different colors can raise or lower your stress and energy level. Some people associate the color red with feelings of anger or hostility and blue with feeling more depressed. Having plants or photos of friends and family around your living and workspace can also alleviate stress.

Smell can also play a significant role in managing stress. As the saying goes, "Stop and smell the roses." Studies have shown that aromatherapy, using different aromas or odors therapeutically, can lower stress levels. When you breathe in these oils, they send a direct message to your brain via your olfactory nerves, where they can then affect the endocrine and hormonal systems via the hypothala-

mus. Odors have an amazing effect on our emotional states because they hook into the emotional or primitive parts of our brains such as the limbic system. Aromatherapy has been used to relieve pain, enhance relaxation and stress relief, unknot tense muscles, soften dry skin, and enhance immunity. So it is wise to pay attention to your aromatic surroundings, as they may affect you much more than you may realize.

While social interaction has been shown to have positive results on lessening the effects of stress, it does make a difference as to the type of friends with whom you surround yourself. Spending time with negative, pessimistic people can increase your stress level rather than decrease it. It is obviously more advantageous to surround yourself with positive, optimistic friends to better manage your stress.[28] Feeling crowded in a room and not having enough personal space can also lead to an increase in stress.[29] Interestingly, it is not being in crowds itself but how familiar you are with the people, the activity that is taking place, and how much control you feel over your personal space that makes the difference. In other words, being in a crowded room filled with your friends during a party feels subjectively different than feeling trapped in a crowded restaurant filled with strangers.

Other important aspects of managing stress in your environment include having meaningful work and challenging and interesting classes. Having work that is stimulating but not beyond your abilities helps to keep your stress response at a moderate, optimal level for performance.

The Psychological Aspects of Stress Management

Lastly, you can effectively cope with stress by using a variety of cognitive and psychological strategies. There are several different techniques, but as you will see, many are focused on deep breathing, which is the key to managing stress.

Relaxation and Deep Breathing

The relaxation response is a powerful weapon in ensuring you do not remain in the stress response for too long. It is effective because it entails the opposite of the stress response. Rather than taking shallow breaths, you are required to breathe deeply, inhaling to a count of four and exhaling to a count of four while sitting in a comfortable position. As you breathe deeply, your muscles unwind and relax, again the opposite of the stress response. It is generally advised not to cross your legs or arms so that your muscles can relax easily. Blood flows to the extremities and your heart rate slows. In fact, experienced users of this technique can temporarily lower their breathing rate from a typical rate of fourteen to eighteen breaths per minute to as few as four breaths per minute. Body temperature decreases and blood pressure is lowered as well. The entire nervous system is slowed, in direct opposition to its role in the stress response. You are instructed to focus on your breathing and inner experience and become less aware of your external environment. To help to tune out the outside world, you are instructed to close your eyes and let go of the worries and concerns of the day.[31]

To try this technique, take a moment to focus on your breathing and breathe in for a count of four and out for four. After doing so a few times, tighten your body, clench your hands, teeth, and jaw, close your eyes tightly, and pull your shoulders up while you are still breathing deeply. Are you able to do so? It is virtually impossible to tense your body and breathe deeply, as they are mutually exclusive activities. Thus, the relaxation response is the foundation of most of the stress management techniques that will be described in this chapter. Deep breathing is the fundamental aspect of stress management.

Progressive Muscle Relaxation (PMR)

Progressive Muscle Relaxation involves learning to recognize the difference between contracted and relaxed muscles, in order to gain a sense of control over your body and the stress response. Progressive muscle relaxation enables you to intentionally put certain muscles into a controlled state of relaxation and reduce your overall stress level.

PMR is based on the use of positioning your body in a comfortable position, sitting or lying down, and concentrating on certain muscle groups. As you inhale, breathing in for a count of four, you contract your muscles starting with your forehead and counting for four as you exhale and relax your muscles. Continue to clench and relax the muscles, using your breathing to help you to tighten and release, working your way down your body all the way to your feet and toes. Concentrate on the sensations of relaxation and how different this feels from feeling tense and stressed. Fifteen minutes, twice a day, is the recommended schedule. In 1 to 2 weeks, you will have mastered the basics and will be aware of which muscles need more attention in order to relax. You will also be more sensitive to the buildup of tension in your body so that you will be able to decrease your stress level before it becomes overwhelming.[31]

Guided Imagery and Visualization

Guided imagery involves having someone describe a beautiful, relaxing scene while focusing on taking deep, comfortable breaths. While in a comfortable position, in an environment free from interruptions and distractions, you breathe deeply, relaxing your muscles and imagining a pleasant scene. The imagery includes all of the senses,

not just what you see, but pleasant smells, sounds, touch, and even taste. Guided imagery can be self-taught or you can listen to recordings of narrated scripts.

Visualization is similar to guided imagery with the scene being more specifically focused on something you are about to do, want to accomplish, or some performance or activity that may be causing you distress. Guided imagery and visualization techniques help you to consciously program change through positive mental images. For example, you might imagine yourself auditioning for a part in a play, seeing yourself go through your lines effortlessly and flawlessly, and feeling confident and proud of yourself. You are probably already skilled at visualization. Unfortunately we frequently engage in negative visualization and are unaware of doing so: we imagine ourselves making fools of ourselves or making mistakes.

Athletes are trained in using positive visualization to improve their performance and visualize their goals.[32] Positive visualization has also been used in managing pain, especially chronic pain management. This technique has also been effective in weight management, smoking cessation, insomnia, and for almost any type of behavior change.

Meditation and Hypnosis

Meditation allows the mind to transcend thought effortlessly when the person concentrates on a focal point. In Transcendental Meditation, a widely recognized approach to meditation, people repeat a mantra, or a personal word, while using deep breathing and relaxation techniques. In other meditation approaches, alternative focal points are used to establish the depth of concentration needed to free the mind from conscious thought. Physical objects, music, relaxing environmental sounds or breathing can be used as focal points.

Hypnosis is an artificially induced state, resembling, but physiologically distinct from, sleep. It involves a heightened state of suggestibility that creates flexible and intensified attention and receptiveness, and an increased responsiveness to an idea or to a set of ideas. The focus is on the unconscious rather than on the conscious state of mind, using deep breathing and relaxation techniques. Hypnosis is perhaps the oldest and most misunderstood type of relaxation technique. It has been given a bad reputation by stage entertainers who use hypnosis to have unsuspecting audience members engage in embarrassing behavior.

Hypnosis is a natural state of mind that occurs spontaneously in nearly every person. It is a trancelike state, similar to those that you experience upon awakening, prior to falling asleep, or when you are engrossed in thought while performing other tasks—such as driving down a highway—on autopilot. It is possible to learn self-hypnosis from a trained professional or participate in hypnosis sessions with a qualified hypnotherapist.

Similar to the other techniques described, meditation and hypnosis are best when you are in a comfortable, quiet environment and are practiced at least once a day, every day, for 15 to 20 minutes.

Biofeedback

Biofeedback is a training technique in which people are taught to improve their health and performance by using signals from their own bodies. It operates on the premise that individuals can alter their involuntary responses by being "fed back" information either visually or audibly about what was occurring in their bodies. In addition, studies have shown that we have more control over so-called involuntary bodily functions than we once thought possible.

One commonly used device, for example, picks up electrical signals from the muscles and translates the signals into a form that people can detect. This device triggers a flashing light or activates a beeper every time muscles become more tense. If one wants to relax tense muscles, one must try to slow down the flashing or beeping. People learn to associate sensations from the muscle with actual levels of tension and develop a new, healthy habit of keeping muscles only as tense as is necessary for as long as necessary. After treatment, individuals are then able to repeat this response at will without being attached to the sensors. Other biological functions that are commonly measured and used in a similar way to help people learn to control their physical functioning are skin temperature, heart rate, sweat gland activity, and brainwave activity. In this way, you can manage your stress by decreasing the physiological components of the stress response.

Stress Inoculation

Similar to being protected from influenza by injecting some of the flu strain into your system, stress inoculation involves exposing an individual to specific stressful situations, a little at a time, under controlled, safe conditions. Stress inoculation teaches individuals to relax using deep breathing and progressive muscle relaxation while exposing them to stressful situations rather than avoiding them.

The first step is to construct your personal list of stressful situations and arrange the list from the least to the most stressful items, and learn how to evoke each of these situations in your mind while at the same time focusing on your breathing and relaxing your muscles. The second step is to create an arsenal of stress-coping thoughts, such as "I'm going to be all right," "I've succeeded with this before," and "Getting started is the hardest part, then it will get easier for me," to counteract stress.

The third step is to practice this *in vivo*, meaning in real life situations, while using the relaxation and cognitive techniques to minimize the stress response.[33] In addition to stress management, stress inoculation has also been helpful in anger management.

Cognitive Self-Talk

What we tell ourselves, our self-talk, has a tremendous impact upon how well we manage our stress. Stress can be generated from faulty conclusions, misinterpretations and expecting the worst. Some people claim that if they expect the worst, they won't feel disappointed or hurt, but in reality, they still feel the pain from their disappointment. Also, it is important to be careful what you expect because you may inadvertently make it happen, a phenomenon referred to as **self-fulfilling prophecy**.[34] Self-fulfilling prophecy can work for you or against you. If you expect that work will be boring and uninteresting, you will tend to portray a negative, unmotivated attitude and will probably have a miserable time. However, if you expect to enjoy yourself at work, you are more likely to go into work looking for challenge and making it more fun.

In order to change your cognitive distortions, you need to generate some rebuttals to your negative self-statements. This entails finding middle ground between all-or-nothing thinking by asking yourself, "What is the evidence?" that this statement is true and identifying some exceptions to this statement. Look for balance in your statements by asking yourself what is the opposite of this negative self-statement? Rather than telling yourself what you "should" do, ask yourself what do you "want" to do. Be specific instead of generalizing and avoid labeling yourself and others. Instead of telling yourself, "I'm lazy," you might say, "I wish I would have studied a few more hours for that test," Stick to the facts without blaming yourself or others. Question yourself as to how you know something is true and if you might be making an assumption or mind reading. Be mindful of your self-fulfilling prophecies. It may be wiser to acknowledge that you don't know or consider many different possible outcomes rather than to expect the worst.

Changing negative self-talk requires time, practice, and patience. We develop these patterns of thinking over years and they become almost automatic. It takes concentrated

---

> **Key Terms**
>
> **self-fulfilling prophecy** the tendency to make something more likely to happen as a result of your own expectations and attitudes.

Coping with the Stress in the Aftermath of 9/11

Certainly our country as a whole experienced a great deal of stress from the terrorist attacks of September 11, 2001. A poll of 560 adults conducted 3 to 5 days after Sept. 11 showed that 44 percent of adults reported one or more substantial symptoms of stress, such as having difficulty concentrating, having trouble falling or staying asleep, and feeling irritable or having angry outbursts. Children have also suffered increased stress from these events, reporting more nightmares and feeling more worried about their own safety since 9/11.

Researchers have found that people who used "active coping" strategies right after the attacks were experiencing fewer symptoms of stress than those who denied the events or avoided talking about them. Donating money or blood, attending memorials, and talking with people about their feelings after the attacks were some of the strategies that seemed to alleviate the stress people were feeling. Studies have also shown that there was an increase in the alcohol consumption, cigarette smoking and marijuana use among Manhattan residents after the September 11 terrorist attacks, providing evidence that people were avoiding having thoughts or feelings about these events and not coping well with the stress they were experiencing.

Many people reported feeling a decreased sense of security and felt increasingly vulnerable and threatened. With the continual warnings of further terrorist attacks, people's stress levels could not return to a normal level and were constantly in a state of high stress, leading to chronic stress. Many people reported that they felt hopeless about the future and began to question the meaning and purpose of their lives.

Disaster reactions tend to follow a predictable sequence of phases for community groups. The initial "heroic" phase involves concerns for survival and altruistic efforts to help overcome reactions such as fear, anger, confusion, and numbness. A "honeymoon" phase occurs next, characterized by outpourings of community and professional support and assistance. As the aftermath of the crisis extends in time, many sources of initial support may be withdrawn as agencies complete their initial goals and normal routines are reestablished. This has been identified as a "disillusionment" phase. This may be characterized by a loss of a sense of shared experience in the community, and a sense of a more pervasive disappointment, anger, resentment, and abandonment. The final phase of disaster adaptation is to mourn what was lost, to reestablish relationships, and reinvest one's energies into current life pursuits, relationships, and interests. This process can extend for years, depending on the magnitude of the losses sustained by individuals and communities. It is important to note that the honeymoon phase ends just at the point when persistent and severe post-traumatic stress reactions would be likely to emerge, about 1 to 3 months following the disaster.

Sometimes present loss or trauma can trigger past events. If you have been the victim of past abuse or trauma, the 9/11 terrorist attacks may have triggered these memories for you or made it more difficult to cope with the stress of these events.

What can you do to cope?

- Spend time with other people. Coping with stressful events is easier when people support each other.

- Talk about how you are feeling. Be willing to listen to others who need to talk about how they feel.
- Get back to your everyday routine. Familiar habits can be comforting.
- Take time to grieve if you need to. It is better to express your feelings rather than push them away or avoid them as feelings tend to emerge one way or another and it is better for you to have some say in how they are expressed.
- Ask for support and help from your family, friends, church, or other community resources. Join or develop support groups.
- Limit how much time you spend watching the news about the war or related events in order to avoid retraumatizing yourself.
- Find something positive you can do. Join efforts in your community to respond to this tragedy.
- Stay positive and watch your negative self-talk and expectations in terms of self-fulfilling prophecy.
- Get professional help if you continue to experience difficulties. College counseling centers offer excellent services in coping with grief and loss and trauma.

Sources: Vahvo D, Galea S, Resnick H, Ahern J, Boscarino J, Bucuvalas M, Gold J, Kilpatrick D. Increased Use of Cigarettes, Alcohol and Marijuana Around Manhattan: New York Residents After the September 11th Terrorist Attacks. *American Journal of Epidemiology* 155(11) 988–996, 2002; Welzant V and Loewenstein R. Psychiatry and the Aftermath of 9/11, Vol. 28, No. 2; Pg 1, 4–6, 2002.

effort to be aware of and change this way of thinking. Remember that your rebuttals need to be strong, nonjudgmental, and specific. Practice developing more flexible and balanced thinking about people, behavior, and situations.

As you can see, there are many different aspects to consider in managing stress, such as the physical, social, environmental, and psychological component of stress. As you think about how you can more effectively manage your stress level, you will need to practice and experiment to find the stress management techniques that will be most beneficial for you.

TALKING POINTS Think back to stressful times in your life. What were some positive ways you coped and what were some negative things you did to cope?

Taking Charge of Your Health

- Analyze your past successes in resolving stressful situations, noting the resources that were helpful to you.
- Prioritize your daily goals in a list that you can accomplish, allowing time for recreational activities.
- Counteract a tendency to procrastinate by setting up imaginary (early) deadlines for assignments and rewarding yourself when you meet those dates.
- Add a new physical activity, such as an intramural team sport, to your daily schedule.

- Replace a negative coping technique that you currently use, such as smoking, with an effective alternative, such as deep breathing, relaxation exercises, or yoga.
- List the positive aspects of your life, and make them the focus of your everyday thoughts.
- Explore the stress-reduction services that are available in your community, both on and off campus.

Summary

- Stress refers to physiological changes and responses your body makes in response to a situation. This can be a real or perceived threat.
- The fight or flight response is a physiological response to perceived, anticipated, or real threat: it causes the heart to race, breathing becomes labored, muscles are tense, the body sweats, and blood flow is constricted to the extremities and digestive organs and increases to the major muscles and brain.
- Chronic stress refers to remaining at a high level of physiological arousal too long and not being able to immediately react to the perceived or real threat.
- While too much stress can have a negative impact and cause some serious health problems, a moderate level of stress is positive and beneficial.
- Both eustress and distress elicit the predictable stress response also called the fight or flight response.
- The term *eustress* is assigned to the stress response when its presence is interpreted as being positive (such as stress experienced when riding a roller coaster).
- The term *distress* is assigned to the stress response when its presence is interpreted as being uncomfortable, threatening, or frightening.
- Yerkes-Dodson Law refers to a bell-shaped curve demonstrating that there is an optimal level of stress for peak performance. This law states that too little and too much stress is not helpful, while a moderate level of stress is positive and beneficial.
- Constant arousal and increased levels of adrenaline in your system will eventually wear down your body's immunological system. You will be less able to cope with stress, and so it takes less and less to cause a stress reaction.
- General Adaptation Syndrome is a sequenced physiological response to the presence of a stressor, involving the alarm, resistance, and exhaustion stages of the stress response.

- Students can experience unique types of stress such as homesickness relationship problems, test anxiety, speech anxiety, math anxiety, problems with learning, time management, procrastination, and perfectionism.
- When you are more stressed or anxious, you have a diminished ability to concentrate, recall information and for problem-solving activities.
- An overwhelming number of students identify time management as the reason for their academic success or failure. Setting priorities and goals, balancing academic life with your social life and finding time for sleeping, eating, exercising, and working along with studying is an essential aspect of managing your stress effectively.
- Procrastination means postponing something that is necessary to do to reach your goal. Typically there is a psychological aspect to procrastination, as we tend to delay doing things we don't want to do.
- While striving to do your best is an admirable quality, expecting to be perfect in everything you do and never making a mistake places a great deal of stress and pressure on yourself.
- Research has shown that stress can be related to having inadequate social interactions.
- To effectively manage your stress, you need to take into consideration environmental stressors such as the noise level, amount of light, and aesthetic quality of the space you inhabit. It is equally important to get adequate rest, nutrition, and exercise.
- Effective psychological tools for managing stress include progressive muscle relaxation, visualization, guided imagery, meditation, hypnosis, biofeedback, stress inoculation, and cognitive self-talk.
- Self-fulfilling prophecy is the tendency to make something more likely to happen as a result of your expectations and attitudes.

Review Questions

1. What is stress? How is it linked to your physical and psychological health?
2. What is the fight or flight response?
3. What are some of the long-term effects of chronic stress?
4. Describe the Yerkes-Dodson Law.
5. Explain the three stages of the General Adaptation Syndrome.
6. List at least five unique types of stress students can experience.
7. What are some ways to cope with test anxiety? Math anxiety? Speech anxiety?
8. What type of anxiety is one of the most common fears for people?
9. How does stress affect your ability to learn?
10. What do an overwhelming number of students identify as the reason for their academic success or failure?
11. Define procrastination, and explain how it relates to stress.
12. How can being perfectionistic cause stress?
13. How do social interactions affect your stress level?
14. List some environmental stressors, and explain how higher levels of stress have been linked to environmental factors.
15. Describe the relaxation response and how it is effective for stress management.
16. Name five psychological tools for stress management and explain how they work.
17. What is a self-fulfilling prophecy?

References

1. Selye H. *Stress Without Distress.* New American Library, 1975.
2. Selye H. *The stress of Life.* New York: The McGraw-Hill Co., 1976.
3. Holmes T and Rahe R. Social Readjustment Rating Scale. *Journal of Psychosomatic Research,* 11, 1967.
4. Girdano DA, Everly GS, Dusek DE. *Controlling Stress and Tension.* Allyn & Bacon, 1996.
5. Benson H and Allen R. How much stress is too much? *Harvard Business Review,* September/October, 1980.
6. Rowh M. *Coping with Stress in College.* New York: College Board Publications, 1989.
7. Raber M and Dyck G. *Managing Stress for Mental Fitness.* Menlo Park, CA: Crisp Publications, 1993.
8. Vandenbeele J. Affordable Care for Kids Squeezes College Students. *The Detroit News,* November 23, 2001.
9. Newman E. *No More Test Anxiety.* Los Angeles, CA: Learning Skills Publications, 1996.
10. Arem C. *Conquering Math Anxiety: A self-help workbook.* Pacific Grove: CA: Brooks/Cole Publishing Co., 1993.
11. Kahn N. *More Learning in Less Time.* Berkeley, CA: Ten Speed Press. 1992.
12. Lindzey G, Thompson R, and Spring B. *Psychology,* 3rd ed. New York: Worth Publishers, Inc., 1988.
13. Lakein A. *How to Get Control of Your Time and Your Life.* New York: New American Library, 1973.
14. Roberts M. *Living Without Procrastination.* Oakland, CA: New Harbinger Publications, 1995.
15. Hill MB, Hill DA, Chabot AE, and Barrall JF. A Survey of College Faculty and Student Procrastination. *College Student Journal* 12, 256–262, 1978.
16. Ferrari J, Johnson J, and McGown W. *Procrastination and Task Avoidance; Theory, Research and Treatment.* New York: Plenum, 1995.
17. Basco M. *Never Good Enough.* New York: Simon & Schuster, 1999.
18. Maslow AH. *Motivation and personality,* 2nd ed. New York: Van Nostrand, 1970.
19. Ferber R. *Solve Your Child's Sleep Problems.* New York: Simon & Schuster, 1985.
20. Saladin KS. *Anatomy and Physiology: the Unity of Form and Function.* McGraw-Hill, 2001.
21. Spear P, Penrod S, and Baker T. *Psychology: Perspectives on Behavior.* New York: John Wiley & Sons, 1988.
22. Lefcourt HM and Martin RA. *Humor and Life Stress: Antidote to Adversity.* Springer-Verlag, New York, 1986.
23. Asterita MF. *The Physiology of Stress.* New York: Human Sciences Press, 1985, p. 4–5.
24. Hugging Warms the Heart and Also May Protect It. *USA Today,* March 10, 2003.
25. Allen K, Shykoff BE, Izzo JL, Jr. Pet Ownership but Not ACE Inhibitor Therapy Blunts Home Blood Pressure Responses to Mental Stress. *Hypertension 2001,* October, 38(4), 815–20.
26. Goliszek AG. *Breaking the Stress Habit.* Winston-Salem, NC: Carolina Press, 1987.
27. Rosenthal NE. *Winter Blues.* New York: The Guilford Press, 1998.
28. Seligman M. *Learned Optimism.* New York: Simon & Schuster, 1990.
29. Wade C and Tavris C. *Psychology.* New York: Harper & Row Publishers, 1987.

30. Benson H. *The Relaxation Response.* New York: Avon, 1976.

31. Fanning P. *Visualization for Change.* Oakland, CA: New Harbinger Publications, Inc., 1988.

32. McKay M, Davis M, and Fanning P. *Thoughts and Feelings: the Art of Cognitive Stress Intervention.* Oakland, CA: New Harbinger Publications, 1981.

33. Jones RA. *Self-Fulfilling Prophecies.* Hillsdale, NJ: John Wiley & Sons, 1977.

As We Go to Press

Can our stress levels be regulated by the government? Jeff Peckman, an activist and author of the "Initiative for Safety Through Peace" or "Initiative 101" thought so. He was instrumental in putting a measure on the Denver ballot in the November 2003 election for a city ordinance to "ensure public safety by adopting and promoting stress reducing techniques or programs." His "anti-stress" legislation is the first of its kind in the nation, suggesting programs such as improving the nutritional quality of school meals, playing "peace promoting music" in elevators, waiting rooms, and offices, offering meditation, yoga and relaxation programs for voters, and developing other stressfree environments. He likened the city's obligation to reducing the public's stress level to hauling away trash in the city. Unfortunately, the measure received only 32% of the vote and didn't pass. Perhaps this ballot will pave the way for others to coordinate ways to reduce stress on a community level.

Source: "In Denver, stress is on the ballot" in USA Today, August 13, 2003. Telephone conversation on February 18, 2004 with Jeff Peckman.

managing work-related stress

When someone is introduced to you, the first thing you learn is the person's name. Next, you usually find out something about that person's occupation. Since Americans identify people with the jobs they perform, much of our self-identity is linked to our occupations. As a result, anything that threatens our job or job performance can be a threat to our sense of personal worth.

Job stress is becoming a part of everyday life. In a 1999 study for *The Wirthin Report,* 67% of the respondents reported that their work was very stressful or moderately stressful. Only 10 percent said that their work was not stressful. If left unchecked, employment-related stress can have negative effects on our feelings of well-being and the structure and function of our bodies. The cardiovascular and immune systems are particularly vulnerable to work-related stress.[1,2]

Sources of Job Stress

Since work-related stress can be a significant problem, it is important to identify what specific things can cause stress in the workplace, such as the following:

- Conflicts with colleagues, supervisors, or workers under your supervision
- Changes in work routine
- Deadlines
- Too much (or too little) responsibility
- Lack of control over work methods and planning
- Long work hours
- Repetitive tasks
- Excessive or rhythmic noise
- Poor time management or organization
- Working with hazardous equipment or substances
- Threat of pay reduction or unemployment
- Lack of necessary resources

Nearly everyone has to deal with these issues at one time or another in the workplace. Although these stressors may vary from job to job, and individuals may react to them in different ways, they still produce an effect.

Job Stress Among Older Workers

In general, older workers are hit hardest by job stress. Technological advances tend to cause more stress for them, especially workers who have been performing a similar routine for a long time and are suddenly forced to assimilate new technology into their daily work. Older workers are also prime targets for layoffs.[3] As a result, some are leaving the workforce at an earlier age than expected. This situation may produce both financial and psychological stress.

Stress in the Modern Workplace

Throughout the last twenty-five years, corporate mergers and buyouts have eliminated entire companies and thousands of jobs, new technology has caused a drastic increase in the pace of work, and heightened competition has forced individual employees to take on much heavier workloads. All of this adds up to increased stress.

Technology

Today's workers must deal with stressors that are unique to our time. The most obvious is the drastic increase in workplace technology. Workers must be more knowledgeable about the new machines they use, and so reeducation becomes necessary. Personal computers and computer networks, which are constantly increasing workplace efficiency and speed, also contribute to job stress. Getting more work done in a specified time means more profit for a company, but it also leads to the expectation that more work

will continue to be accomplished in less time. Therefore the person working at the computer may be asked to perform more and more tasks in a workday. The increased productivity resulting from computer use can lead to the elimination of many jobs, since one worker may now be able to do the work that was once done by two or more people.

The computer may also contribute to physical problems. Constant work on a keyboard places excess stress on the fingers, hands, and wrists. This, in turn, may contribute to arthritic conditions or *carpal tunnel syndrome.* The simple act of sitting at the computer for extended periods with the body in a fixed position puts stress on the muscles and bones of the back, neck, and limbs.[4]

Problems caused by repetitive motions, unusual body postures, or holding static joint positions over extended periods are referred to as *repetitive strain injuries* (RSIs).[5] The risk of developing RSIs is increased during periods of emotional stress or deadline pressure. RSIs can also develop because of improper placement of equipment (e.g., a keyboard). Company production goals based on quotas, such as counting workers' keystrokes, may influence employees to work through needed break periods to meet the expected work output.

Downsizing

The corporate practice of eliminating jobs to cut costs—downsizing—can contribute greatly to job stress.[3] This practice affects both rank-and-file workers and management; everyone is vulnerable. Often, cuts are made with little or no regard to an employee's years of service or experience (or senior employees are "let go" as a way of saving money). This lack of job security has been an important contributor to job stress over the last decade.

The fear of being unemployed and the difficult transition following unemployment causes workers and their families to develop a variety of stress-induced conditions, including anxiety and depression. These families also often display higher than normal rates of divorce and drug and alcohol abuse.

One extreme expression of the impact of work-related stress is death resulting from cardiovascular disease, particularly heart attack. As long ago as 1982, this trend was reported in the Swedish workforce.[6] Autopsies on these heart attack victims, some of whom were as young as 29, showed that no significant risk factors were present except for high levels of chemicals (e.g., epinephrine) that are released in response to stress. Other industrialized nations, including the United States, are observing signs of this trend in their workforces.

Downsizing has been a stated goal of many U.S. corporations and agencies, including IBM, Boeing, Apple Computer, and NASA. AT&T announced a "reduction in force" anticipated to be as high as 40,000 employees.

Competition

Although there are more than enough jobs being created to offset those lost through downsizing, many new jobs offer lower pay, fewer benefits, and less desirable working conditions. As a result, competition for good jobs is growing keener. A college education is no longer enough, More than 20% of adults hold at least a bachelor's degree, and over 40% of adults have some college experience. Workers whose jobs are cut are facing competition from new college graduates, who will often work for less money, and from others who have been laid off. New graduates are competing with displaced workers, who usually have a wealth of work experience.

This uncertainty in the workplace has led many people to broaden their knowledge to become more competitive within their chosen field or to change careers altogether. This has resulted in a booming business for colleges and universities. Many students face the challenge of succeeding at school while trying to raise a family or hold down a job. It is becoming increasingly common for students to attend classes either before or after working a full shift at a regular job. Job stress is thus compounded with classroom stress.

Reducing Work-Related Stress

Since work-related stress appears to be increasing in most professions, it is important to recognize the physical signs of stress and reduce job stress when possible. Here are a few things you can do to reduce the effects of work-related stress:

- *Recognize when stress is negatively affecting you.* Be able to identify early warning signs that you may be under excessive amounts of stress. Psychological signs may include anxiety, lack of interest, and irritability. Mental fatigue, physical exhaustion, and frequent illness may be physical manifestations of stress. Know yourself well enough to recognize when stressors are affecting you.
- *Control your environment when you can.* Not every work situation can be controlled, but managing some situations can help reduce stress. Try not to schedule stressful work activities in succession. Break larger jobs down into smaller parts. Rearrange your work area to keep things fresh.
- *Know the things you cannot control and deal with them.* Becoming angry or obsessed over a situation you can't do anything about only increases your stress level. Developing a flexible attitude toward situations on the job that are not flexible is a healthy approach.
- *Take a break.* Schedule some down time to keep yourself refreshed. If your breaks are scheduled for you, don't use them to get extra work done. When performing repetitive tasks, step away from the task whenever you can. If you work at a computer terminal, get up occasionally and move around.
- *Get some exercise.* Physical activity can be healthy for the mind and the body. Exercise can actually increase energy levels and strengthen physical resistance to stress.
- *Make your workplace safe.* Take safety precautions when possible. If safety equipment is available, use it. Staying safe on the job can prevent stressful situations that may occur because of an injury, such as missed work, decreased productivity, and physical pain.

If you notice that stress on the job is affecting you physically or mentally, see your family doctor or a qualified mental health professional as soon as possible. Work-related stress does not have to become an overwhelming factor in your life. Managing stress is an important skill that all employees must learn to master. Set aside time to assess your problems and devise strategies to deal with your stressful situations.

personal assessment

how stressed are you?

A widely used life stress scale called the Social Readjustment Rating Scale by Holmes and Rahe has been used to determine the degree of stress that you are experiencing due to life events over the past year. It also projects your chances of developing an illness- or stress-related health condition. Stress can lead to some serious health problems, and the more stress you have in your life, the more vulnerable you are to being susceptible to illness. Let's see how you score.

Life-Stress Scale

Check off the events which have happened to you **within the last year.** Then add up your total number of stress units for each life stress event. The number on the right hand side represents the amount, duration and severity of change required to cope with each item. See the point scale at the bottom of the inventory to determine your health risk associated with your stress level.

Life Event	Value	Score
Death of a partner	100	_____
Divorce	73	_____
Relationship separation	65	_____
Jail term	63	_____
Death of a family member	63	_____
Personal injury/illness	53	_____
Marriage	50	_____
Fired from job	47	_____
Reconciliation with partner	45	_____
Retirement	45	_____
Illness—family member	44	_____
Pregnancy	40	_____
Sexual difficulties	39	_____
Addition of a family member	39	_____
Change in financial situation	38	_____
Death of a close friend	37	_____
Change in job	36	_____
Frequent arguments with partner	35	_____
Mortgage over $10,000	31	_____
Foreclosure of mortgage/loan	30	_____
Change in work responsibilities	29	_____
Child leaving home	29	_____
Trouble with in-laws	29	_____
Outstanding personal achievement	28	_____
Begin or end school	26	_____
Partner begins/stops working	26	_____
Change in living conditions	25	_____
Change in personal habits	24	_____
Trouble with supervisor	23	_____
Change in work hours	20	_____
Change in residence	20	_____
Change in schools	20	_____
Change in recreation	19	_____
Change in church activities	19	_____
Change in social activities	18	_____
Mortgage/loan less than $10,000	17	_____
Change in sleeping habits	16	_____
Change in family visits	15	_____
Change in eating habits	15	_____
Vacation	13	_____
Christmas	12	_____
Minor violations of the law	11	_____
TOTAL SCORE		_____

What Is Your Health Risk?

Notice that positive events such as outstanding personal achievements, vacations, Christmas, can be as stressful as negative ones. Think of events in your life that are not listed on this inventory. For example, where would you put running in a marathon or going on a diet?

⇒ If your score was 150 points or less . . .
You are on reasonably safe and healthy ground. You have about a one-in-three chance of a health change in the next 2 years.

⇒ If your score was between 150–300 points . . .
You have about a 50/50 chance of developing an illness related to stress in the next 2 years.

⇒ If your score was 300 points or more . . .
You have a 90% chance of developing an illness due to stress that could seriously affect your health. You need to be very watchful in how you are managing your stress.

personal assessment

am i a perfectionist?

Below are some ideas that are held by perfectionists. Which of these do you see in yourself? To help you decide, rate how strongly you agree with each of the statements below on a scale from 0 to 4.

0	1	2	3	4
I do not agree		I agree somewhat		I agree completely

_____ 1.   I have an eye for details that others can miss.

_____ 2.   I can get lost in details and forget the real purpose of the task.

_____ 3.   I can get overwhelmed by too many details.

_____ 4.   It stresses me when people do not want to do things the right way.

_____ 5.   There is a right way and a wrong way to do most things.

_____ 6.   I do not like my routine to be interrupted.

_____ 7.   I expect a great deal from myself.

_____ 8.   I expect no less of others than I expect of myself.

_____ 9.   People should always do their best.

_____ 10.   I am neat in my appearance.

_____ 11.   Good grooming is important to me.

_____ 12.   I do not like being seen before I have showered and dressed.

_____ 13.   I do not like making mistakes.

_____ 14.   Receiving criticism is horrible.

_____ 15.   It is embarrassing to make mistakes in front of others.

_____ 16.   Sharing my new ideas with others makes me anxious.

_____ 17.   I worry that my ideas are not good enough.

_____ 18.   I do not have a great deal of confidence in myself.

_____ 19.   I'm uncomfortable when my environment is untidy or disorganized.

_____ 20.   When things are disorganized it is hard for me to concentrate.

_____ 21.   What others think about my home is important to me.

_____ 22.   I have trouble making difficult decisions.

_____ 23.   I worry that I may make the wrong decision.

_____ 24.   Making a bad decision can be disastrous.

_____ 25.   I often do not trust others to do the job right.

_____ 26.   I check the work of others to make certain it was done correctly.

_____ 27.   If I can control the process it will turn out fine.

_____ 28.   I am a perfectionist.

_____ 29.   I care more about doing a quality job than others do.

_____ 30.   It's important to make a good impression.

_____   **TOTAL SCORE**

Scoring

Add all thirty items together to get total score. If your score was less than 30, then you are probably not a perfectionist, although you may have a few of the traits. Scores from 31 to 60 suggest mild perfectionism. When you are stressed your score may be higher. Scores of 61 to 90 suggest moderate perfectionism. This probably means that perfectionism is causing you trouble in some specific areas but is not out of control. Scores higher than 91 suggest a level of perfectionism that could cause you serious problems.

Adapted from: _Never Good Enough_ by Monica Ramirez Basco.

chapter four

becoming physically fit

Online Learning Center Resources

www.mhhe.com/hahn7e

Log on to our Online Learning Center (OLC) for access to these additional resources:

- Chapter key terms and definitions
- Learning objectives
- Student interactive question-and-answer sites
- Self-scoring chapter quiz
- Online assessments
- Key term flash cards

Talking It Over

Fitness for Kids—A Great Start

Talking to kids about fitness isn't easy—especially if you're out of shape yourself. Here are some approaches to try:

- Be a good role model. Start getting in shape by walking. Tell your kids how much better you feel, and ask them to join you.
- When you buy gifts for your kids, choose items for active play, like a bike, rollerblades, a basketball, or a tennis racquet.

- Make time for play with your kids. Toss a football around in the backyard or throw a Frisbee with them. Take your kids to the pool and get in the water with them. Show them—and tell them—that being active together is fun.

CommunicationLinks

www.intelihealth.com
www.mayohealth.org

Eye on the Media

Magazines Feature Readers' Choice—Health News

In the past decade, popular magazines have initiated or greatly expanded their coverage of health issues. This is especially true for the magazines that cover national and international news. In fact, it is difficult to pick up a major news magazine (such as *Time, Newsweek,* or *U.S. News & World Report*) and *not* find one or two articles about health issues. Occasionally, these magazines have cover stories on topics such as fitness, obesity, smoking, prescription drugs, the environment, herbal supplements, growth and development, and sexuality.

This inclusion of health issues did not come about without careful consideration by the media moguls. Readers have been routinely surveyed by publishers about their preferences for topics. Since readers have reported that they want more coverage of health issues, magazine publishers have complied.

Fortunately, the health editors and writers for these major publications generally do an excellent job of preparing their news reports.

Eye on the Media *continued*

Most try to consult (and then quote) health researchers who are experts in their fields. Many reports in the popular news magazines present the results of health-related research that has been published in scientific journals or presented at professional meetings.

You, the consumer (reader), should be aware, however, that magazine articles may not give the most complete coverage of a health issue or may exaggerate the threat posed by certain diseases. Most health issues that are hot news items can be viewed from more than one perspective. Be inquisitive about finding out if there are conflicting views about stories that interest you. Find and read the original sources identified in the magazine article. Many of these original sources are available in your college library or on the Internet. If you have additional questions, ask professors, nutritionists, exercise physiologists, physical therapists, or physicians. Used in this way, magazine articles can provide an excellent first step in your quest to discover new information concerning your health.

TALKING POINTS If you had a strong reaction to a news magazine's treatment of a certain health issue, would you consider writing a letter to the editor expressing your opinion?

When your day begins early in the morning, then you go to class or work or immerse yourself in recreational activities, and your day does not end until after midnight, you must be physically fit to keep up the pace. Even a highly motivated college student must have a conditioned, rested body to maintain such a schedule.

OK, let's simplify things a bit. The paragraph above reflects how college health professors might view the value of fitness—it helps people function well enough to cope with their hectic lifestyles. But what motivates students to value **physical fitness**? Quite simply, students say that overall body fitness helps them look and feel better.

Many college students want to look in the mirror and see the kind of body they see in the media: one with well-toned muscles, a trim waistline, and no flabby tissue, especially on the arms and legs. Students become motivated to start fitness programs because they hope that they can build a better body for themselves. Through their efforts to do so, students usually start to feel better, both physically and mentally. They realize that change is possible, since they see it happening to their bodies with each passing week. "Go for it" and "Just do it" then become more than just sports marketing phrases; they become reminders that the activities that lead to fitness are a meaningful part of their lives. Fitness actually becomes fun (Figure 4-1).

Fortunately, you don't have to be a top-notch athlete to enjoy the health benefits of physical activity. In fact, even a modest increase in your daily **physical activity** level can be rewarding. The health benefits of fitness can come from regular participation in moderate **exercise,** such as brisk walking or dancing[1] (see HealthQuest Activities).

HealthQuest Activities

- The *How Fit Are You?* exercise in the Fitness module will help you determine your current level of fitness in four major areas: body composition, cardiorespiratory capacity, muscular fitness, and flexibility. Complete the series of questions about how much you exercise, what types of training you do, how intensely you exercise, and your body size. After you complete the questions and receive feedback, develop an individual plan for improving or maintaining your current fitness level.

- The *Exercise Interest Inventory* in the Fitness module allows you to rate your feelings about certain aspects of exercise. *HealthQuest* provides feedback about the activities and exercises you would most enjoy, based on your individual needs and preferences. First, write down the five fitness activities that you like best or those you participate in most often. After each one, indicate your motivation for engaging in that particular activity. For example, you could list "enjoyment," "habit," or "convenience." When you have completed the *Exercise Interest Inventory,* compare the two lists. Any surprises? What factors had you not considered to be influential in your choice of exercise?

Key Terms

physical fitness a set of attributes that people have or achieve that relates to the ability to perform physical activity.

physical activity any bodily movement produced by skeletal muscles that results in energy expenditure.

exercise a subcategory of physical activity; it is planned, structured, repetitive, and purposive in the sense that an improvement or maintenance of physical fitness is an objective.

Physical Activity Preferences
Among adults who say they exercise regularly, here are the activities they prefer:

- 25% — At least 20 minutes aerobic exercise
- 21% — Work out on home equipment
- 19% — Participate in sports
- 16% — Strength training
- 14% — Jog/run
- 11% — Work out at club/gym
- 5% — Work out with exercise video

Figure 4-1 Running or working out in a gym is not for everyone. Which physical activities fit your preferences and lifestyle?

Components of Physical Fitness

Physical fitness is characterized by the ability to perform occupational and recreational activities without becoming unduly fatigued and to have the capacity to handle unforeseen emergencies. The following sections focus on cardiorespiratory endurance, muscular strength, muscular endurance, flexibility, and body composition.

These characteristics of physical fitness can be categorized as health-related physical fitness. Other characteristics, such as speed, power, agility, balance, and reaction time are associated with what would be called performance-related physical fitness. Although the latter type is most important for competitive athletes, it is the former type that has the most relevance to general population. Thus, it is health-related physical fitness that this chapter will focus on.

Cardiorespiratory Endurance

If you were limited to improving only one area of your physical fitness, which would you choose—muscular strength, muscular endurance, or flexibility? Which would a dancer choose? Which would a marathon runner select? Which would an expert recommend?

The experts, exercise physiologists, would probably say that another fitness dimension is even more important than those listed above. They regard improvement of your heart, lung, and blood vessel function as the key focal point of a physical fitness program. **Cardiorespiratory endurance** forms the foundation for whole-body fitness.

Cardiorespiratory endurance increases your capacity to sustain a given level of energy production for a prolonged period. It helps your body to work longer and at greater levels of intensity.

Your body cannot always produce the energy it needs for long-term activity. Certain activities require performance at a level of intensity that will outstrip your cardiorespiratory system's ability to transport oxygen efficiently to contracting muscle fibers. When the oxygen demands of the muscles cannot be met, **oxygen debt** occurs. Any activity that continues beyond the point at which oxygen debt begins requires a form of energy production that does not depend on oxygen.

This oxygen-deprived form of energy production is called **anaerobic** (without oxygen) **energy production,**

Key Terms

cardiorespiratory endurance the ability of the heart, lungs, and blood vessels to process and transport oxygen required by muscle cells so that they can contract over a period of time.

oxygen debt the physical state that occurs when the body can no longer process and transport sufficient amounts of oxygen for continued muscle contraction.

anaerobic energy production the body's means of energy production when the necessary amount of oxygen is not available.

Cardiorespiratory fitness is essential for optimal heart, lung, and blood vessel function.

the type that fuels many intense, short-duration activities. For example, rope climbing, weight lifting for strength, and sprinting are short-duration activities that quickly cause muscle fatigue; they are generally considered anaerobic activities.

The key factor is if the energy demand of the activity exceeds the aerobic energy production capability. Thus, even activities that are typically considered to be aerobic (walking or cycling) can require anaerobic energy if the intensity is high enough.

If you usually work or play at low intensity but for a long duration, you have developed an ability to maintain **aerobic** (with oxygen) **energy production.** As long as your body can meet its energy demands in this oxygen-rich mode, it will not convert to anaerobic energy production. Thus fatigue will not be an important factor in determining whether you can continue to participate. Marathon runners, serious joggers, distance swimmers, cyclists, and aerobic dancers can perform because of their highly developed aerobic fitness. The cardiorespiratory systems of these aerobically fit people have developed a large capacity to take in, transport, and use oxygen.

Besides allowing you to participate in activities such as those mentioned, aerobic conditioning (cardiorespiratory endurance conditioning) may also provide certain structural and functional benefits that affect other dimensions of your life (see Discovering Your Spirituality on page 85). These recognized benefits (see the Star box on page 85) have received considerable documented support. It is now well accepted that regular physical activity that produces aerobic fitness will reduce the risk of heart disease, type 2 diabetes, osteoporosis, obesity, depression, and cancer of the breast and colon.[3]

Muscular Fitness

Muscular fitness is the term used to represent the capabilities of the skeletal muscles to perform contractions. The capacity of the muscles has two distinct yet integrated characteristics: muscular strength and muscular endurance. The strength of the muscle is related to its ability to perform at or near its maximum for a short period of time. Whereas the endurance of the muscle is related to its ability to perform at submaximal levels for a long period of time.

Muscular fitness is essential for your body to accomplish work. Your ability to maintain posture, walk, lift, push, and pull are familiar examples of the constant demands you make on your muscles to maintain or increase their level of contraction. The stronger you are, the greater your ability to contract muscles and maintain a level of contraction sufficient to complete tasks.

Muscular strength can be improved best by training activities that use the **overload principle.** By overloading, or gradually increasing the resistance (load, object, or weight) your muscles must move, you can increase your muscular strength. The following three types of training exercises are based on the overload principle.

> ### Key Terms
>
> **aerobic energy production** the body's means of energy production when the respiratory and circulatory systems are able to process and transport a sufficient amount of oxygen to muscle cells.
>
> **muscular strength** the component of physical fitness that deals with the ability to contract skeletal muscles to a maximal level; the maximal force that a muscle can exert.
>
> **overload principle** the principle whereby a person gradually increases the resistance load that must be moved or lifted; this principle also applies to other types of fitness training.

**Harnessing the Spirit:
The Saga of Lance Armstrong**

In July 2001, American cyclist Lance Armstrong won his third straight Tour de France, the most grueling cycling event in the world. As amazing as this feat may seem, an even bigger victory for Lance Armstrong was his conquest of cancer. In October 1996, Armstrong was diagnosed with advanced testicular cancer and given less than a 50% chance of survival. At the time of diagnosis, the cancer had already spread to his abdomen, lungs, and brain.

However, before starting aggressive cancer therapy, Armstrong declared himself "a cancer survivor, not a cancer victim." He convinced himself, his family, and his medical support team that he could beat the long odds facing him. He even established the Lance Armstrong Foundation (**www.laf.org**) before he had surgery and chemotherapy. He battled through his therapy without giving up hope that the cancer would be defeated.

Along the way, many doubted whether Armstrong would ever compete again at the world-class level. Armstrong proved his doubters wrong by winning not only the 1999 race, but also the 2000, 2001, 2002, and 2003 Tour de France races. He became a world celebrity and chronicled his battle with testicular cancer in his best-selling book *It's Not about the Bike: My Journey Back to Life* (Putnam) and followed this with a cycling training book called *The Lance Armstrong Performance Program: Seven Weeks to the Perfect Ride* (Rodale Press).

Clearly, Armstrong's powers of the mind and spirit worked to help him overcome his physical barriers. His success story has undoubtedly inspired others to take charge of their lives by doing their best to rise above mental and physical barriers to pursue the dreams that sometimes seem impossible.

Structural and Functional Benefits of Cardiorespiratory (Aerobic) Fitness

Aerobic fitness can help you do the following:

- Complete and enjoy your daily activities.
- Strengthen and increase the efficiency of your heart muscle.
- Increase the proportion of high-density lipoproteins in your blood.
- Increase the capillary network in your body.
- Improve **collateral circulation.**
- Control your weight.
- Stimulate bone growth.
- Cope with stressors.
- Ward off infections.
- Improve the efficiency of your other body systems.
- Bolster your self-esteem.
- Achieve self-directed fitness goals.
- Reduce negative dependence behavior.
- Sleep better.
- Recover more quickly from common illnesses.
- Meet people with similar interests.
- Receive reduced insurance premiums.

In **isometric** (meaning "same measure") **exercises,** the resistance is so great that your contracting muscles cannot move the resistant object at all. So your muscles contract against immovable objects, usually with increasingly greater efforts. Because of the difficulty of precisely evaluating the training effects, isometric exercises are not usually used as a primary means of developing muscular strength. These exercises can be dangerous for people with hypertension.

Isotonic resistance exercises, meaning *same-tension* exercises, are currently the most popular type of strength-building exercises and include the use of traditional free weights (dumbbells and barbells), as well as many resistance exercise machines. People who perform progressive resistance exercises use various muscle groups to move (or lift) specific fixed resistances or weights. Although during a given repetitive exercise the weight resistance remains the same, the muscular contraction effort required varies according to the joint angles in the range of motion. The greatest effort is required at one angle (sticking point) in the range of motion.

Isokinetic (meaning "same motion") **exercises** use mechanical devices that provide resistances that consistently overload muscles throughout the entire range of motion. The resistance will move only at a preset speed, regardless of the force applied to it. For the exercise to be effective, a user must apply maximal force.[4] Isokinetic training requires elaborate, expensive equipment.

Key Terms

collateral circulation the ability of nearby blood vessels to enlarge and carry additional blood around a blocked blood vessel.

isometric exercises muscular strength training exercises in which the resistance is so great that the object cannot be moved.

isotonic resistance exercises muscular fitness training exercises in which traditional barbells and dumbbells with fixed resistances are used.

isokinetic exercises muscular strength training exercises in which machines are used to provide variable resistances throughout the full range of motion.

Thus the use of isokinetic equipment may be limited to certain athletic teams, diagnostic centers, or rehabilitation clinics. The most common isokinetic machines are Cybex, Orthotron, Biodex, Mini-Gym, and Exergenie.

Which type of strength-building exercise (machines or free weights) is most effective? Take your choice, since all will help develop muscular strength. Some people prefer machines because they are simple to use, do not require stacking the weights, and are already balanced and less likely to drop and cause injury.

Other people prefer free weights because they encourage the user to work harder to maintain balance during the lift. In addition, free weights can be used in a greater variety of exercises than weight machines.

Muscular endurance can be improved by performing repeated contractions of a less than maximal level. This aspect of muscular fitness is most related to common physical activities (postural muscles, leaf raking, pushing a lawn mower). Although it is not viewed to be as glamorous as the muscular strength component, it is an important part of muscular fitness. Energy production requires that oxygen and nutrients be delivered by the circulatory system to the muscles. After these products are transformed into energy by individual muscle cells, the body must remove the potentially toxic waste by-products.

Amateur and professional athletes often wish to increase the endurance of specific muscle groups associated with their sports activities. This can be achieved by using exercises that gradually increase the number of repetitions of a given movement. However, muscular endurance is not the physiological equivalent of cardiorespiratory endurance. For example, a world-ranked distance runner with highly developed cardiorespiratory endurance and extensive muscular endurance of the legs may not have a corresponding level of muscular endurance of the abdominal muscles.

Flexibility

The ability of your joints to move through their natural range of motion is a measure of your **flexibility.** This fitness trait, like so many other aspects of structure and function, differs from point to point within your body and among different people. Not every joint in your body is equally flexible (by design), and over the course of time, use or disuse will alter the flexibility of a given joint. Certainly, gender, age, genetically determined body build, and current level of physical fitness will affect your flexibility.

Inability to move easily during physical activity can be a constant reminder that aging and inactivity are the foes of flexibility. Failure to use joints regularly will quickly result in a loss of elasticity in the connective tissue and

Guidelines for Static Stretching

Take the following precautions to reduce the possibility of injury during stretching:

- Warm up using a slow jog or fast walk before stretching.
- Stretch only to the point at which you feel tightness or resistance to your stretching. Stretching should not be painful. Hold the stretch for 10–30 seconds.
- Be sure to continue normal breathing during a stretch. Do *not* hold your breath.
- Use caution when stretching muscles that surround painful joints. Pain is an indication that something is wrong—it should not be ignored.

shortening of muscles associated with the joints. Benefits of flexibility include improved balance, posture, and athletic performance and reduced risk of low back pain.

As seen in young gymnasts, flexibility can be highly developed and maintained with a program of activity that includes regular stretching. Stretching also helps reduce the risk of injury. Athletic trainers generally prefer **static stretching** to **ballistic stretching** for people who wish to improve their range of motion. Guidelines for stretching are given in the Star box above.

Body Composition

Body composition is the analysis of what the body is made up of (muscle, bone, fat, water, minerals).[4] Of particular interest to fitness experts are percentages of body fat and fat-free weight. Health experts are especially concerned about the large number of people in our society who are

Key Terms

muscular endurance the aspect of muscular fitness that deals with the ability of a muscle or muscle group to repeatedly contract over a long period of time.

flexibility the ability of joints to function through an intended range of motion.

static stretching the slow lengthening of a muscle group to an extended stretch; followed by holding the extended position for 10 to 30 seconds.

ballistic stretching a "bouncing" form of stretching in which a muscle group is lengthened repetitively to produce multiple quick, forceful stretches.

Muscular fitness is important for both good health and optimal function.

overweight and obese. Increasingly, cardiorespiratory fitness trainers are recognizing the importance of body composition and are including strength-training exercises to help reduce body fat. (See Chapter 6 for further information about body composition, health effects of obesity, and weight management.)

Aging Physically

The period between 45 and 64 years of age brings with it a variety of subtle changes in the body's structure and function. When life is busy and the mind is active, these changes are generally not evident. Even when they become evident, they are not usually the source of profound concern. Your parents, older students in your class, and people with whom you will be working are, nevertheless, experiencing these changes.

- Decrease in bone mass and density
- Increase in vertebral compression
- Degenerative changes in joint cartilage

- Increase in adipose tissue—loss of lean body mass
- Decrease in capacity to engage in physical work
- Decrease in visual acuity
- Decrease in basal energy requirements
- Decrease in fertility
- Decrease in sexual function

For some midlife adults these health concerns can be quite threatening, especially for those who view aging with apprehension and fear. Some middle-aged people reject these physical changes and convince themselves they are sick. Indeed, *hypochondriasis* is much more common among midlife people than among young people.

Two medical conditions influenced by physical activity, osteoporosis and osteoarthritis, deserve careful examination and are discussed in the following sections.

Osteoporosis

Osteoporosis is a condition often seen in late middle-aged women. However, it is not fully understood why menopausal women are so susceptible to the increase in calcium loss that leads to fracture of the hip, wrist, and vertebral column. Half of all women over the age of 50 will likely suffer an osteoporosis-related fracture.

The endocrine system plays a large role in the development of osteoporosis. At the time of menopause, a woman's ovaries begin a rapid decrease in the production of *estrogen*, one of two main hormones associated with the menstrual cycle. This lower level of estrogen may decrease the conversion of the precursors of vitamin D into the active form of vitamin D, the form necessary for absorbing calcium from the digestive tract. As a result, calcium may be drawn from the bones for use elsewhere in the body.

Premenopausal women have the opportunity to build and maintain a healthy skeleton through an appropriate intake of calcium. Current recommendations are for an intake of 1200 mg of calcium per day. Three to four daily servings of low-fat dairy products should provide sufficient calcium. Adequate vitamin D must also be in the diet because it aids in the absorption of calcium.

Many women do not take in an adequate amount of calcium. Calcium supplements, again in combination with vitamin D, can be used to achieve recommended calcium levels. It is now known that calcium carbonate,

---

Key Terms

osteoporosis loss of calcium from the bone, seen primarily in postmenopausal women.

a highly advertised form of calcium, is no more easily absorbed by the body than are other forms of calcium salts.

In premenopausal women, calcium deposition in bone is facilitated by exercise, particularly exercise that involves movement of the extremities. Today, women are encouraged to consume at least the recommended servings from the milk group and engage in regular physical activity that involves the weight-bearing muscles of the legs, such as aerobics, jogging, or walking.

Postmenstrual women who are not elderly can markedly slow the resorption of calcium from their bones through the use of hormone replacement therapy (HRT). When combined with a daily intake of 1500 mg of calcium, vitamin D, and regular exercise, HRT almost eliminates calcium loss. Women will need to work closely with their physicians in monitoring the use of HRT because of continuing concern over the role of HRT and the development of breast cancer and the increased risk of coronary artery disease and stroke.

Osteoarthritis

Arthritis is an umbrella term for more than 100 forms of joint inflammation. The most common form is **osteoarthritis.** It is likely that as we age, all of us will develop osteoarthritis to some degree. Often called "wear and tear" arthritis, osteoarthritis occurs primarily in the weight-bearing joints of the knee, hip, and spine. In this form of arthritis, joint damage can occur to bone ends, cartilaginous cushions, and related structures as the years of constant friction and stress accumulate.

The object of current management of osteoarthritis (and other forms) is not to cure the disease but rather to reduce discomfort, limit joint destruction, and maximize joint mobility. Aspirin and nonsteroidal antinflammatory agents are the drugs most frequently used to treat osteoarthritis.

It is now believed that osteoarthritis develops most commonly in people with a genetic predisposition for excessive damage to the weight-bearing joints. Thus the condition seems to "run in families." Further, studies comparing the occurrence of osteoarthritis in those who exercise and those who do not demonstrate that regular movement activity may decrease the likelihood of developing this form of arthritis.

Developing a Cardiorespiratory Fitness Program

For people of all ages, cardiorespiratory conditioning can be achieved through many activities. As long as the activity you choose places sufficient demand on the heart and lungs, improved fitness is possible. In addition to the familiar activities of swimming, running, cycling, and aerobic dance, many people today are participating in brisk walking, rollerblading, cross-country skiing, swimnastics, skating, rowing, and even weight training (often combined with some form of aerobic activity) (see Learning from Our Diversity, p. 89). Regardless of age or physical limitations, you can select from a variety of enjoyable activities that will condition the cardiorespiratory system. Complete the Personal Assessment on pages 105–106 to determine your level of fitness.

Many people think that any kind of physical activity will produce cardiorespiratory fitness. Golf, bowling, hunting, fishing, and archery are considered to be forms of exercise. If performed regularly and for sufficient periods of time, they may enhance your health. However, they do not meet the requirements to be called exercise and would not necessarily lead to improved physical fitness. The American College of Sports Medicine (ACSM), the nation's premier professional organization of exercise physiologists and sport physicians has well-accepted guidelines for exercise training.[1, 6]

The ACSM's most recent recommendations for achieving cardiorespiratory fitness were released in 1998 and include four major areas: (1) mode of activity, (2) frequency of training, (3) intensity of training, and (4) duration of training. ACSM has also made recommendations for muscular fitness and flexibility training. These recommendations are summarized in the following sections. You may wish to compare your existing fitness program with these standards.

Mode of Activity

The ACSM recommends that the mode of activity be any continuous physical activity that uses large muscle groups and can be rhythmic and aerobic in nature. Among the activities that generally meet this requirement are continuous swimming, cycling, aerobics, basketball, cross-country skiing, rollerblading, step training (bench aerobics), hiking, walking, rowing, stair climbing, dancing, and running. Recently, water exercise (water or aqua aerobics) has become a popular fitness mode, since it is especially effective for pregnant women and elderly, injured, or disabled people. (The Focus On article on pages 102–103, provides more information about exercise during pregnancy.)

Key Terms

osteoarthritis arthritis that develops with age; largely caused by weight bearing and deterioration of the joints.

Learning from Our Diversity

A Different Kind of Fitness: Developmentally Disabled Athletes Are Always Winners in the Special Olympics

In America, as in many other countries around the world, physical fitness and athletic prowess carry a high degree of prestige, whereas lack of conditioning and poor sports performance often draw scorn and rejection. As anyone knows who's ever been picked last when sides were being chosen for a schoolyard game, few things are more damaging to youthful self-esteem than being the player nobody wants.

Some of these children blossom into accomplished athletes as they gain coordination or are inspired and guided by caring coaches. Others, lacking strong interest in sports, turn to less physical arenas in which they can excel—drama, debating, music, computers, science.

But what about people who want to be athletes at almost any cost, but who have no realistic hope of attaining the standards of athletic accomplishment set for those in top physical condition? The Joseph P. Kennedy Foundation created an arena in which these athletes could compete when it established the Special Olympics in 1968. Joseph Kennedy was the father of President John F. Kennedy, whose older sister Rosemary was virtually shut away from the world when her family discovered she was mentally disabled. Many people at that time shared the Kennedy's view that the kindest way to treat family members who were developmentally disabled was to "protect" them from stares and whispers by keeping them at home or placing them in institutions or residential facilities. Spearheaded by President Kennedy's sister Eunice Kennedy

Shriver, the Special Olympics was intended to change the old attitudes toward developmentally disabled people by giving them an opportunity to compete at their own level and to celebrate their victories publicly.

Now, nearly thirty years later, the Special Olympics holds both winter and summer games and boasts participation of more than 1 million developmentally disabled athletes in 140 countries around the world. The contests are open to athletes between the ages of eight and sixty-three, some of whom have proved wrong the specialists who claimed they would never walk, let alone compete internationally. "Mainstream" Olympic champions like figure-skating silver medalist Brian Orser and a host of well-known entertainers have attended opening-day ceremonies to cheer and inspire the special athletes.

But medals aren't what the Special Olympics is all about. No matter where a Special Olympian finishes in a contest, he or she is applauded and celebrated for the accomplishment of playing the game and seeing it through. The oath taken by each participant in the Special Olympics aptly states the credo of this remarkable group of athletes: "Let me win. But if I cannot win, let me be brave in the attempt."

In what ways other than physical conditioning do you think a developmentally disabled person might benefit from participating in the Special Olympics? What can the rest of us learn from these athletes' courage and perseverance?

Endurance games and activities, such as tennis, racquetball, and basketball, are fine as long as you and your partner are skilled enough to keep the ball in play; walking after the ball will do very little for you. Riding a bicycle is a good activity if you keep pedaling. Coasting will do little to improve fitness. Softball and football are generally less than sufficient continuous activities—especially the way they are played by weekend athletes.

Regardless of which continuous activity you select, it should also be enjoyable. Running, for example, is not for everyone—despite what some accomplished runners say! Find an activity you enjoy. If you need others around you to have a good time, get a group of friends to join you. Vary your activities to keep from becoming bored. You might cycle in the summer, run in the fall, swim in the winter, and play racquetball in the spring. To help you maintain your fitness program, see the suggestions in the accompanying Changing for the Better box on page 90.

Frequency of Training

Frequency of training refers to the number of times per week a person should exercise. The ACSM recommends three to five times per week. For most people, participa-

tion in fitness activities more than five times each week does not significantly further improve their level of conditioning. Likewise, an average of only two workouts each week does not seem to produce a measurable improvement in cardiorespiratory conditioning. Thus, although you may have a lot of fun cycling twice each week, do not expect to see a significant improvement in your cardiorespiratory fitness level from doing so.

Intensity of Training

How much effort should you put into an activity? Should you run quickly, jog slowly, or swim at a comfortable pace? Must a person sweat profusely to become fit? These questions all refer to **intensity** of effort.

> ### Key Terms
>
> **frequency** the number of exercise sessions per week; for aerobic fitness 3–5 days are recommended.
>
> **intensity** the level of effort put into an activity.

The ACSM recommends that healthy adults exercise at an intensity level of between 65% and 90% of their maximum heart rate (calculated by subtracting your age from 220). This level of intensity is called the **target heart rate (THR).** This rate refers to the minimum number of times your heart needs to contract (beat) each minute to have a positive effect on your heart, lungs, and blood vessels. This improvement is called the *training effect.* Intensity of activity below the THR will be insufficient to make a significant improvement in your fitness level.

Although intensity below the THR will still help you expend calories and thus lose weight, it will probably do little to make you more aerobically fit. On the other hand, intensity that is significantly above your THR will probably cause you to become so fatigued that you will be forced to stop the activity before the training effect can be achieved. For persons who are quite unfit, the 1998 ACSM recommendations permit intensity levels as low as 55%.

Choosing a particular THR between 65% and 90% of your maximum heart rate depends on your initial level of cardiorespiratory fitness. If you are already in relatively good physical shape, you might want to start exercising at 75% of your maximum heart rate. A well-conditioned person needs to select a higher THR for his or her intensity level, whereas a person with a low cardiorespiratory fitness level will still be able to achieve a training effect at a lower THR of 65% of maximum.

In the accompanying Star box, page 91, the younger person would need to participate in a continuous activity for an extended period while working at a THR of 160 beats per minute. The older person would need to function at a THR of 117 beats per minute to achieve a positive training effect.

Determining your heart rate is not a complicated procedure. Find a location on your body where an artery passes near the surface of the skin. Pulse rates are difficult to determine by touching veins, which are more superficial than arteries. Two easily accessible sites for determining heart rate are the *carotid artery* (one on either side of the windpipe at the front of your neck) and the *radial artery* (on the inside of your wrist, just above the base of the thumb).

You should practice placing the front surface of your index and middle fingertips at either of these locations and feeling for a pulse. Once you have found a regular pulse, look at the second hand of a watch. Count the number of beats you feel in a 10-second period. Multiply this number by 6. This number is your heart rate. With a little practice, you can become very proficient at determining your heart rate.

| Key Terms |

target heart rate (THR) the number of times per minute the heart must contract to produce a training effect.

Duration of Training

The ACSM recommends that the **duration** of training be between 20 and 60 minutes of continuous or intermittent aerobic activity. Intermittent activity can be accumulated in 10-minute segments throughout the day. This is especially helpful for persons who cannot take a single large chunk of time during the day to devote to an exercise program.

However, for most healthy adults the ACSM recommends moderate-intensity activity levels with longer duration times, perhaps 30 minutes to an hour. For healthy adults who train at higher intensity levels, the duration of training will likely be shorter, perhaps 20 minutes or more.[1] Adults who are unfit or have an existing medical condition should check with their fitness instructor or physician to determine an appropriate duration of training.

Resistance Training

Recognizing the important fact that overall body fitness includes muscular fitness, the ACSM recommends resistance training in its current standards. The ACSM suggests participation in resistance training two or three times a week. This training should help develop and maintain a healthy body composition—one with an emphasis on lean body mass. The goal of resistance training is not to improve cardiorespiratory endurance but to improve overall muscle strength and endurance. For some people (individuals with Type II diabetes) resistance training with heavy weights is not recommended because it can induce a sudden and dangerous increase in blood pressure. See the Changing for the Better box above for safety precautions to observe during strength training.

The resistance training recommended by the ACSM includes one set of 8 to 12 repetitions (10 to 15 for adults over age 50) of 8 to 10 different exercises. These exercises should be geared to the body's major muscle groups (legs, arms, shoulders, trunk, and back) and should not focus on just one or two body areas. Isotonic (progressive resistance) or isokinetic exercises are recommended. For the average person, resistance training activities should be done at a moderate-to-slow speed, use the full range of motion, and not impair normal breathing. With just one set recommended for each exercise, resistance training is not very time-consuming. The ACSM, however, indicates that multiple sets could provide greater benefits, if time is available.

Flexibility Training

To develop and maintain a healthy range of motion for the body's joints, the ACSM suggests that flexibility exercises be included in one's overall fitness program. Stretching can be done in conjunction with other cardiorespiratory or muscular fitness training or can be performed separately. It is important to note that if flexibility training is done separately, a general warm-up should be performed prior to stretching. For most

Key Terms

duration the length of time one needs to exercise at the THR to produce a cardiorespiratory training effect.

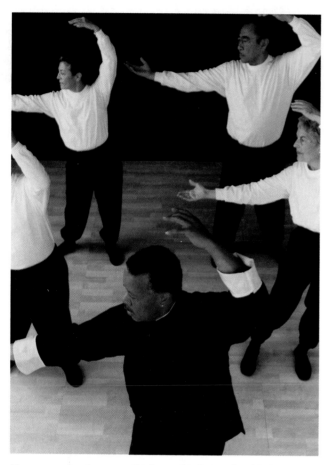

Group exercise classes can be fun and help people with their physical fitness program.

individuals, static stretching is the best type. Flexibility improvements can be obtained by training as little as two days per week; however, stretching is an activity that can be safely performed daily. ACSM recommends that a flexibility program should include all the major muscle and/or tendon groups. The intensity of each stretch should be at a position where you feel mild discomfort in the muscle. Each stretch should be held for 10 to 30 seconds and should be repeated three to four times per training session. Stretching should be done according to safe and appropriate techniques. (See the Guidelines for Static Stretching on page 86).

Warm-up, Conditioning, Cooldown

Each training session consists of three basic parts: the warm-up, the conditioning, and the cooldown.[4] The warm-up should last 10 to 15 minutes. During this period, you should begin slow, gradual, comfortable movements related to the upcoming activity, such as walking or slow jogging. All body segments and muscle groups should be exercised as you gradually increase your heart rate. Near the end of the warm-up period, the major

muscle groups should be stretched. This preparation helps protect you from muscle strains and joint sprains.

The warm-up is a fine time to socialize. Furthermore, you can mentally prepare yourself for your activity or think about the beauty of the morning sky, the changing colors of the leaves, or the friends you will meet later in the day. Mental warm-ups can be as beneficial for you psychologically as physical warm-ups are physiologically.

The second part of the training session is the conditioning phase, the part of the session that involves improving muscular fitness, cardiorespiratory endurance, and flexibility. Workouts can be tailor-made, but they should follow the ACSM guidelines discussed earlier in this chapter.

The third important part of each fitness session, the cooldown, consists of a 5- to 10-minute session of relaxing exercises, such as slow jogging, walking, and stretching. This activity allows your body to cool and return to a resting state. A cooldown period helps reduce muscle soreness.

Exercise for Older Adults

An exercise program designed for younger adults may be inappropriate for older people, particularly those over age fifty. Special attention must be paid to matching the program to the interests and abilities of the participants. Often, this is best achieved by having older individuals begin their exercise program under the supervision of a certified exercise professional. The goals of the program should include both social interaction and physical conditioning.

Older adults, especially those with a personal or family history of heart problems, should have a physical examination before starting a fitness program. This examination should include a stress cardiogram, a blood pressure check, and an evaluation of joint functioning. Participants should learn how to monitor their own cardiorespiratory status during exercise.

Well-designed fitness programs for older adults will include activities that begin slowly, are monitored frequently, and are geared to the enjoyment of the participants.[5] The professional staff coordinating the program should be familiar with the signs of distress (excessively elevated heart rate, nausea, breathing difficulty, pallor, and pain) and must be able to perform CPR. Warm-up and cooldown periods should be included. Activities to increase flexibility are beneficial in the beginning and ending segments of the program. Participants should wear comfortable clothing and appropriate shoes and should be mentally prepared to enjoy the activities.

A program designed for older adults will largely conform to the ACSM criteria specified in this chapter. Certainly, specific modifications or restrictions to the exercise program may be required due to health concerns that are more frequent in older adults. Also, because of possible joint, muscular, or skeletal problems, certain activities may

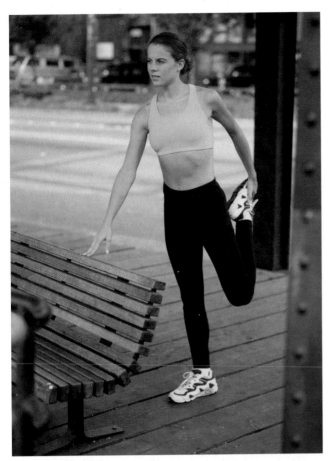

Stretching is important for flexibility and can be performed almost anywhere.

have to be done in a sitting position. Pain or discomfort should be reported immediately to the fitness instructor.

Fortunately, properly screened older adults will rarely have health emergencies during a well-monitored fitness program. Of course, for some older adults, individual fitness activities may be more enjoyable than supervised group activities. Either choice offers important benefits.

Low Back Pain

A common occurrence among adults is the sudden onset of low back pain. Four out of five adults develop this condition, at least once in their lifetime which can be so uncomfortable that they miss work, lose sleep, and generally feel incapable of engaging in daily activities. Many of the adults who have this condition will experience these effects two to three times per year.

Although low back pain can reflect serious health problems, most low back pain is caused by mechanical (postural) problems. As unpleasant as low back pain is, the symptoms and functional limitations usually subside within a week or two. The services of a physician, physical therapist, or chiropractor are not generally required.

By engaging in regular exercise, such as swimming, walking, and bicycling, and by paying attention to your back during bending, lifting, and sitting, you can minimize the occurrence of this uncomfortable and incapacitating condition. Commercial fitness centers and campus recreational programs are starting to offer specific exercise classes geared to muscular improvement in the lower back and abdominal areas.

Fitness Questions and Answers

Along with the six necessary elements to include in your fitness program, you should consider many additional issues when you start a fitness program.

Should I See My Doctor Before I Get Started?

This issue has probably kept thousands of people from ever beginning a fitness program. The hassle and expense of getting a comprehensive physical examination is an excellent excuse for people who are not completely sold on the idea of exercise. We should state that it is highly desirable to have regular checkups with your family physician as part of your overall health plan. However, the question still applies to many. The Surgeon General suggested that most adults can safely increase their activity level to a moderate amount without the need for a comprehensive medical evaluation. Individuals with chronic diseases should consult with their physician prior to increasing their activity level. If more vigorous forms of exercise are desired, then a medical exam is recommended for men over the age of 40 and women over the age of 50. It would also be recommended for individuals with more than one risk factor for coronary artery disease or if there were any other notable health problems. The American College of Sports Medicine would also recommend an exercise ("stress") test for these individuals.[6]

 TALKING POINTS If your screening tests indicate that you cannot start a vigorous fitness program, are you prepared to ask your doctor about alternative activities?

How Beneficial Is Aerobic Dance Exercise?

One of the most popular fitness approaches is aerobic exercise, including aerobic dancing. Many organizations sponsor classes in this form of continuous dancing and movement. The rise in popularity of televised and videotaped aerobic exercise programs reflects the enthusiasm for this form of exercise. Because extravagant claims are often made about the value of these programs, the wise consumer should observe at least one session of the activity before enrolling. Discover for yourself whether the program meets the criteria outlined earlier in this chapter: mode of activity, frequency, intensity, duration, resistance training, and flexibility training.

Street dancing, swing dancing, and Latino dancing are fast becoming some of the most popular aerobic exercises. Popularized by rap music, hip-hop music, and the growth of vigorous dancing in music videos, these forms of dancing provide an excellent way of having fun and maintaining cardiorespiratory fitness. Have you experienced the exhilaration that results from an hour or two of dancing?

What Are Low-Impact Aerobic Activities?

Because long-term participation in some aerobic activities (for example, jogging, running, aerobic dancing, and rope skipping) may lead to injury of the hip, knee, and ankle joints, many fitness experts promote low-impact aerobic activities. Low-impact aerobic dancing, water aerobics, bench aerobics, and brisk walking are examples of this kind of fitness activity. Participants still conform to the principal components of a cardiorespiratory fitness program. THR levels are the same as in high-impact aerobic activities.

The main difference between low-impact and high-impact aerobic activities is the use of the legs. Low-impact aerobics do not require having both feet off the ground at the same time. Thus weight transfer does not occur with the forcefulness seen in traditional high-impact aerobic activities. In addition, low-impact activities may include exaggerated arm movements and the use of hand or wrist weights. All of these variations are designed to increase the heart rate to the THR without undo strain on the joints of the lower extremities. Low-impact aerobics are excellent for people of all ages, and they may be especially beneficial to older adults.

In-line skating (rollerblading) is one of the fastest-growing participant fitness activities. This low-impact activity has cardiorespiratory and muscular benefits similar to those of running without the pounding effect that running can produce. However, it should be recognized that it requires both skill and balance. Rollerblading requires important safety equipment: sturdy skates, knee and elbow pads, wrist supports, and a helmet.

What Is the Most Effective Means of Fluid Replacement During Exercise?

Despite all the advertising hype associated with commercial fluid replacement products, for an average person involved in typical fitness activities, water is still the best fluid replacement. The availability and cost are unbeat-

able. However, when activity is prolonged and intense, commercial sports drinks may be preferable to water because they contain electrolytes (which replace lost sodium and potassium) and carbohydrates (which replace depleted energy stores). However, the carbohydrates in sports drinks are actually simple forms of sugar. Thus sports drinks tend to be high in calories, just like regular soft drinks. Regardless of the drink you choose, exercise physiologists recommend that you drink fluids before and at frequent intervals throughout the activity particularly in warm, humid environments.

What Effect Does Alcohol Have on Sport Performance?

It probably comes as no surprise that alcohol use is generally detrimental to sport performance. Alcohol consumption, especially excessive intake the evening before a performance, consistently decreases the level of performance. Many research studies have documented the negative effects of alcohol on activities involving speed, strength, power, and endurance.[7] Lowered performance appears to be related to a variety of factors, including impaired judgment, reduced coordination, depressed heart function, liver interference, and dehydration.

What Level of Physical Activity Is Necessary to Produce Fitness?

According to the surgeon general's report on physical activity and health,[8] moderate amounts of physical activity can produce significant health benefits, including lowering the risk of premature death, coronary heart disease, hypertension, colon cancer, and diabetes. Even a variety of simple activities, such as gardening, walking, raking

Choosing an Athletic Shoe

Aerobic Shoes

When selecting shoes for aerobic dancing, J. Lynn Reese, president of J. Lynn & Co. Endurance Sports, Washington, DC, advises the following:

- Check the width of the shoe at the widest part of your foot. The bottom of the shoe should be as wide as the bottom of your foot; the uppers shouldn't go over the sides.
- Look for leather or nylon uppers. Leather is durable and gives good support, but it can stretch. Nylon won't stretch and gives support, but it's not as durable. Canvas generally doesn't offer much support.
- Look for rubber rather than polyurethane or black carbon rubber soles. Treads should be fairly flat in the forefoot. If you dance on carpet, you can go with less tread; if you dance on gym floors, you may need more grab.

Basketball Shoes

What's most important when choosing a basketball shoe? John Burleson, of the Sports Authority, offers this advice:

- Cushioning. Cushioning is especially important in the forefoot area. Each shoe manufacturer has its own cushioning "system." For example, Nike has "Air," and Reebok promotes its "Hexalite" material, composed of hexagonal air chambers.
- Side support. Side support, also called lateral and medial support, is important for making quick directional changes.
- Fit of heel cup. Try on the shoe, and then put your little finger in behind the heel. It should fit snugly.
- Traction. Keep in mind the surface on which you play most often. More traction is needed on asphalt than on hardwood.
- Socks should be breathable and pull moisture away from the foot.
- "Rope" laces are more convenient than the more traditional flat laces because pulling on the ends will tighten up the laces on the whole shoe at once.

Running Shoes

Need new running shoes? Here's advice from Jeff Galloway, former Olympic runner and founder and president of Phidippides International aerobic sports stores, headquartered in Atlanta.

- Take time to shop, and find a knowledgeable salesperson. Good advice is crucial.
- Check the wear pattern on your old shoes to see whether you have floppy or rigid feet. Floppy-footed runners wear out their soles on the outside and inside edges; rigid-footed runners wear out soles predominantly on the outside edges. Floppy-footed runners can sacrifice cushioning for support; rigid-footed runners can sacrifice support for cushioning.
- Know whether your feet are curved or straight and whether you have high arches or are flatfooted. The shoe should fit the shape of your foot.

Walking Shoes

Have you joined the millions of people who walk for fitness? If so, and if you are ready for a pair of athletic walking shoes, shoe manufacturer Nike has the following advice for you:

- Note where most of your weight falls on your foot when you walk. Are you landing mostly on the heel or on the forefoot? This is where you will want cushioning.
- As with all other types of athletic shoes, take the time to find a knowledgeable salesperson who will provide good advice.
- Go for comfort. Stride in the different types of shoes at your typical walking pace and identify the shoes that are most comfortable.
- Choose shoes that are comfortable in the forefoot area, which will be carrying much of your weight.
- All-leather uppers are satisfactory for most walkers. If you are a serious walker, consider shoes with breathable uppers made of material such as mesh.

Crosstraining Shoes

Crosstraining shoes are a hybrid, an all-purpose shoe for those who participate in a variety of fitness activities, such as basketball, weight lifting, or light trail hiking. If you tend to specialize in one type of activity (such as basketball), consider buying shoes designed specifically for that activity (for example, high-top basketball shoes for ankle support). To shop for an all-purpose crosstraining shoe, Nike recommends that you keep the following points in mind: *(continued)*

---

leaves, or dancing, that consistently increase a person's daily activity levels can be as helpful for the majority of Americans as are activities such as jogging, swimming, and cycling.

What Are the Risks and Benefits of Androstenedione?

Androstenedione ("andro") and creatine have recently received much attention for their use as possible **ergogenic aids.** Ergogenic aids are supplements taken to improve

athletic performance.[9] Andro is a steroidlike precursor to the male hormone testosterone. When taken into the body, andro stimulates the body to produce more of its

> **Key Terms**
>
> **ergogenic aids** supplements that are taken to improve athletic performance.

- Once again, comfort is paramount. Try to simulate the activity when you try on the shoe, such as rolling from side to side for court sports, fast movement for walking or running, or walking an incline for light hiking.
- If you tend toward one activity (such as running), look for crosstraining shoes that support that activity (for example, heel and forefoot cushioning for running).
- If you intend to use the shoes for activities with lots of lateral movement, such as court sports or aerobic classes, look for good lateral support.

Aerobic Shoes (*below*)

Flexibility: More at ball of foot than running shoes; less flexible than court shoes or running shoes; sole is firmer than running shoes. Uppers: Most are leather or leather-reinforced nylon. Heel: Little or no flare. Soles: Rubber if you dance on wood floors; polyurethane for other surfaces. Cushioning: More than court shoes; less than running shoes. Tread: Should be fairly flat, especially on forefoot; may also have "dot" on the ball of the foot for pivoting.

Basketball Shoes (*above right*)

Soles: Can be made from rubber for durability, EVA for lightweight cushioning, or polyurethane, which is both lightweight and durable. Flexibility: Should be most flexible in the forefoot, for making jump shots. Cushioning: Should absorb shock in the ball of the foot, for landing from jump shots. Heel: A snug-fitting heel cup is essential to keep the ankle in place; the shoe can be high-, mid-, or low-cut, depending on the amount of ankle support desired. Tread: For playing

outdoors, the sole should be harder and the tread deeper; a smoother tread works well for playing on a court. Uppers: Can be made of leather for durability or nylon or other synthetics for breathability.

Running Shoes (*below*)

Heel: Flare gives foot broader, more stable base. Soles: Usually carbon-based for longer wear. Cushioning: More than court shoes, especially at heel. Tread: "Waffle" or other deep-cut tread for grip on many surfaces.

Walking Shoes

Cushioning: Can be forefoot and heel, or primarily forefoot or heel. Heel: May have some flare, similar to running shoes. Soles: Typically polyurethane for durability. Tread: Some tread for traction, but slightly flatter than running shoes.

Crosstraining Shoes

Cushioning: Can be forefoot and heel, or primarily forefoot or heel. Tread: Can be moderate to aggressive.

---

natural testosterone. Increased levels of testosterone help a person build lean muscle mass and recover from injury more quickly.

Andro's primary use as an ergogenic aid is to build muscle tissue, improve overall body strength, and boost performance, especially in anaerobic sports. Andro is banned by the National Football League (NFL), the National Collegiate Athletic Association (NCAA), and the IOC. The health concerns that most physicians attribute to andro are similar to those of anabolic steroids (see Figure 4-2).

St. Louis Cardinal baseball player Mark McGwire's admitted use of andro put this supplement in the national spotlight in the summer of 1998. That was the season when McGwire rocked the baseball world by surpassing Roger Maris's home run record by hitting seventy home runs. It is interesting, though, that during the 1999 baseball season McGwire opted to stop using andro but still managed to hit nearly seventy home runs.

What Are the Risks and Benefits of Creatine?

Creatine is an amino acid found in meat, poultry, and fish. In a person's body, creatine is produced naturally in the liver, pancreas, and kidneys. Typically, people get one to two grams of creatine each day from their food intake.[9] As an ergogenic aid, creatine performs its work in the muscles, where it helps restore the compound adenosine triphosphate (ATP). ATP provides quick energy for muscle contractions. It also helps to reduce the lactic acid buildup that occurs during physical exertion. This buildup causes a burning sensation that limits the amount of intense activity one can perform.

Early studies suggest that creatine can help athletes in anaerobic sports, which require short, explosive bursts of energy. However, the increase in performance has been small, the long-term health impacts are unknown, studies have been restricted to highly trained subjects (not recreational athletes), and damage to kidneys is possible with high dosages. Users are cautioned to consume ample amounts of water to prevent cramping and dehydration.

All in all, creatine is unlikely to prove as potentially dangerous as androstenedione. If additional studies should indicate that creatine can consistently improve performance, this substance might be banned by many sports federations. At the time of this writing, the safest, most prudent recommendation is for athletes to spend their time and energy improving their training programs rather than looking for a solution in a bottle.

How Worthwhile Are Commercial Health and Fitness Clubs?

The health and fitness club business is booming. Fitness clubs offer activities ranging from free weights to weight machines to step walking to general aerobics. Some clubs have saunas and whirlpools and lots of frills. Others have course offerings that include wellness, smoking cessation, stress management, time management, dance, and yoga. The atmosphere is friendly, and people are encouraged to have a good time while working out.

If your purpose in joining a fitness club is to improve your cardiorespiratory fitness, measure the program offered by the club against the ACSM standards. If your primary purpose is to meet people and have fun, request a trial membership for a month or so to see whether you like the environment.

Before signing a contract at a health club or spa, do some careful questioning. Find out when the business was established, ask about the qualifications of the employees, contact some members for their observations, and request a thorough tour of the facilities. You might even consult your local Better Business Bureau for additional information. Finally, make certain that you read and understand every word of the contract.

What Is Crosstraining?

Crosstraining is the use of more than one aerobic activity to achieve cardiorespiratory fitness. For example, runners may use swimming, cycling, or rowing periodically to replace running in their training routines. Crosstraining allows certain muscle groups to rest and injuries to heal. Also, crosstraining provides a refreshing change of pace for the participant. You will probably enjoy your fitness program more if you vary the activities.

What Are Steroids and Why Do Some Athletes Use Them?

Steroids are drugs that can be legally prescribed by physicians for a variety of health conditions, including certain forms of anemia, inadequate growth patterns, and chronic debilitating diseases. Steroids can also be prescribed to aid recovery from surgery or burns. **Anabolic steroids** are drugs that function like the male sex hormone testosterone. They can be taken orally or by injection.

Anabolic steroids are used by athletes who hope to gain weight, muscular size and strength, power, endurance, and aggressiveness. Over the last few decades, many bodybuilders, weightlifters, track athletes, and football players have chosen to ignore the serious health risks posed by illegal steroid use.

The use of steroids is highly dangerous because of serious, life-threatening side effects and adverse reactions. These effects include heart problems, certain forms of cancer, liver complications, and even psychological disturbances. The side effects on female steroid users are as dangerous as those on men. Figure 4-2 shows the adverse effects of steroid use.

Steroid users have developed a terminology of their own. Anabolic steroids are called "roids" or "juice." "Roid rage" is an aggressive, psychotic response to chronic steroid use. "Stacking" is a term that describes the use of multiple steroids at the same time.

Most organizations that control athletic competition (for example, the NCAA, The Athletics Congress, the

---

Key Terms

anabolic steroids drugs that function like testosterone to produce increases in weight, strength, endurance, and aggressiveness.

Figure 4-2 Effects of steroids on various parts of the body.

Brain
Increased hostility can lead to tranquilizer use, hypertension, psychological dependence, and eating compulsions; increases aggression, which makes injuries more probable

Face
Facial hair growth, body hair growth, and baldness in women; acne in both men and women

Throat
Deepening of voice in women

Chest
Breast growth in men; breast cancer and decreased breast size in women

Heart
High blood pressure, clogging of arteries

Liver and prostate
Liver cancer in men and women; prostate cancer in men

Genitals
Sterility or atrophied testicles in men; menstrual irregularities, enlarged genitals in women

Arms, chest, and legs
Helps stimulate muscle growth, decreases recovery time needed between workouts

NFL, and the IOC) have banned steroids and are testing athletes for illegal use. Many athletes finally seem to be getting the message and are steering clear of steroids.

TALKING POINTS If you suspected a young person you know was using steroids, what strategies would you use to encourage the person to change his or her behavior?

Are Today's Children Physically Fit?

Major research studies published during the last 10 years have indicated that U.S. children and teenagers lead very sedentary lives. Children ages 6 to 17 score extremely poorly in the areas of strength, flexibility, and cardiorespiratory endurance. In many cases, parents are in better shape than their children. A major consequence of these sedentary habits in children is obesity. The 1999–2000 National Health and Nutrition Examination Survey (NHANES) indicates that 15% of children and adolescents ages 6–19 years are overweight. Indeed from NHANES II (1976-80) to NHANES III (1988–1994), the prevalence of overweight nearly doubled among children and adolescents and has continued to rise. The seriousness of these data is revealed by the fact that most obese children become obese adults.

This information presents a challenge to educators and parents to emphasize the need for strenuous play activity. Television watching and parental inactivity were implicated as major reasons in these studies. For students reading this text who are parents or grandparents of young children, what can you do to encourage more physical activity and less sedentary activity?

TALKING POINTS What can you do to encourage children to become more active participants in physical activities?

How Does Sleep Contribute to Overall Fitness?

Although sleep may seem to be the opposite of exercise, it is an important adjunct to a well-planned exercise program. Sleep is so vital to health that people who are unable to sleep sufficiently (those with insomnia) or who are deprived of sleep experience deterioration in every dimension of their health. Fortunately, exercise is frequently associated with improvement in sleeping.

The value of sleep is apparent in a variety of positive changes in the body. Dreaming is thought to play an important role in supporting the emotional dimension of health. Problem-solving scenarios that occur during

Table 4.1 Common Injuries Associated with Physical Activity

Injury	Condition
Achilles tendinitis	A chronic tendinitis of the "heel cord," or muscle tendon, located on the back of the lower leg just above the heel. It may result from any activity that involves forcefully pushing off with the foot and ankle, such as in running and jumping. This inflammation involves swelling, warmth, tenderness to touch, and pain during walking and especially running.
Ankle sprains	Stretching or tearing of one or several ligaments that provide stability to the ankle joint. Ligaments on the outside or lateral side of the ankle are more commonly injured by rolling the sole of the foot downward and toward the inside. Pain is intense immediately after injury, followed by considerable swelling, tenderness, loss of joint motion, and some discoloration over a 24- to 48-hour period.
Groin pull	A muscle strain that occurs in the muscles located on the inside of the upper thigh just below the pubic area and that results from either an overstretch of the muscle or from a contraction of the muscle that meets excessive resistance. Pain will be produced by flexing the hip and leg across the body or by stretching the muscles in a groin-stretch position.
Hamstring pull	A strain of the muscles on the back of the upper thigh that most often occurs while sprinting. In most cases, severe pain is caused simply by walking or in any movement that involves knee flexion or stretch of the hamstring muscle. Some swelling, tenderness to touch, and possibly some discoloration extending down the back of the leg may occur in severe strains.
Patellofemoral knee pain	Nonspecific pain occurring around the knee, particularly the front part of the knee, or in the kneecap (patella). Pain can result from many causes, including improper movement of the kneecap in knee flexion and extension; tendinitis of the tendon just below the kneecap, which is caused by repetitive jumping; bursitis (swelling) either above or below the kneecap; and osteoarthritis (joint surface degeneration) between the kneecap and thigh bone. It may involve inflammation with swelling, tenderness, warmth, and pain associated with movement.
Quadriceps contusion "charley horse"	A deep bruise of the muscles in the front part of the thigh caused by a forceful impact or by some object that results in severe pain, swelling, discoloration, and difficulty flexing the knee or extending the hip. Without adequate rest and protection from additional trauma, small calcium deposits may develop in the muscle.
Shin splints	A catch-all term used to refer to any pain that occurs in the front part of the lower leg or shin, most often caused by excessive running on hard surfaces. Pain is usually caused by strain of the muscles that move the ankle and foot at their attachment points in the shin. It is usually worse during activity. In more severe cases it may be caused by stress fractures of the long bones in the lower leg, with the pain being worse after activity is stopped.
Shoulder impingement	Chronic irritation and inflammation of muscle tendons and a bursa underneath the tip of the shoulder, which results from repeated forceful overhead motions of the shoulder, such as in swimming, throwing, spiking a volleyball, or serving a tennis ball. Pain is felt when the arm is extended across the body above shoulder level.
Tennis elbow	Chronic irritation and inflammation of the lateral or outside surface of the arm just above the elbow at the attachment of the muscles that extend the wrist and fingers. It results from any activity that requires forceful extension of the wrist. Typically occurs in tennis players who are using faulty techniques hitting backhand ground strokes. Pain is felt above the elbow after forcefully extending the wrist against resistance or applying pressure over the muscle attachment above the elbow.

dreams seem to afford some carryover value in actual coping experiences. A variety of changes in physiological functioning, particularly a deceleration of the cardiovascular system, occurs while you sleep. The feeling of being well rested is an expression of the mental and physiological rejuvenation you feel after a good night's sleep.

The amount of sleep needed varies among people. In fact, for any person, sleep needs vary according to activity level and overall state of health. As we age, the need for sleep appears to decrease from the six to eight hours young adults require. Elderly people routinely sleep less than they did when they were younger. This decrease may be offset by the short naps older people often take during the day. For all people, however, periods of relaxation, daydreaming, and even an occasional afternoon nap promote electrical activity patterns that help regenerate the mind and body.

How Do I Handle Common Injuries That May Be Caused by My Fitness Activities?

For the most part, emergency care for injuries that pertain to the bones or muscles should follow the RICE acronym.[10] Depending on the type and severity of the injury, the importance of rest (R), ice (I) or cold application, compression (C), and elevation (E) cannot be overstated. Each type of injury identified in Table 4.1 has a particular RICE protocol to follow. Any significant injury should be reported to your college student health center, an athletic trainer, a physical therapist, or a physician. See the adjacent Star box on this page for exercise danger signs you should be aware of.

What Is the Female Athlete Triad?

In the early 1990s, the American College of Sports Medicine identified a three-part syndrome of disordered eating, **amenorrhea** (lack of menstruation), and osteoporosis as the female athlete triad.[11] The conditions of this syndrome appear independently in many women, but among female athletes they appear together. The female athlete triad is most likely to be found in athletes whose sport activities emphasize appearance (for example, diving, ice skating, or gymnastics).

Parents, coaches, athletic trainers, and teammates should be watchful for signs of the female athlete triad. This syndrome has associated medical risks, including inadequate fuel supply for activities, inadequate iron intake, reduced cognitive function, altered hormone levels, reduced mental health, early onset of menopause, increased likelihood of skeletal trauma, altered blood fat profiles, and increased vulnerability to heart disease.[11] Vitally important is an early referral to a physician who is knowledgeable about the female athlete triad. The physician will likely coordinate efforts with a psychologist, a nutritionist, or an athletic trainer to improve the health of the athlete and prevent recurrences.

What Are the Common Exercise Danger Signs?

- A delay of over one hour in your body's return to a fully relaxed, comfortable state after exercise.
- A change in sleep patterns.
- Any noticeable breathing difficulties or chest pains. Exercising at your THR should not initiate these problems. If these effects occur, consult a physician.
- Persistent joint or muscle pain. Any lingering joint or muscle pain might signal a problem. Seek the help of an athletic trainer, a physical therapist, or your physician.
- Unusual changes in urine composition or output. Marked color change in your urine could signal possible kidney or bladder difficulties. Drink plenty of water before, during, and after you participate in your activity.
- Anything unusual that you notice after starting your fitness program. Examples are headaches, nosebleeds, fainting, numbness in an extremity, and hemorrhoids.

Key Terms

amenorrhea cessation or lack of menstrual periods.

Taking Charge of Your Health

- Assess your level of fitness by completing the National Fitness Test on pages 105–106.
- Start a daily stretching program based on the guidelines in this chapter.
- Implement or maintain a cardiorespiratory fitness program that uses the most recent American College of Sports Medicine recommendations.
- Examine your athletic shoes to determine their appropriateness for the fitness activities you do (see Choosing an Athletic Shoe on pages 95–96).

- Monitor your physical activities for potential danger signs indicating that you should consult an athletic trainer, physical therapist, or physician.
- For 2 weeks, keep track of the amount of sleep you are getting. Determine whether this is enough sleep, and make adjustments accordingly.

Summary

- Physical fitness allows one to engage in life's activities without unreasonable fatigue.
- The health benefits of exercise can be achieved through regular moderate exercise.
- Fitness is composed of four components: cardiorespiratory endurance, muscular fitness, flexibility, and body composition.
- The American College of Sports Medicine's program for cardiorespiratory fitness has four components:

mode of activity, frequency of training, intensity of training, and duration of training.
- The target heart rate refers to the number of times per minute the heart must contract to produce a training effect.
- Training sessions should take place in three phases: warm-up, conditioning, and cooldown.
- Fitness experts are concerned about the lack of fitness in today's youth.

- Dancing, step aerobics, and rollerblading are currently popular aerobic activities.
- College students who are interested in fitness should understand the important topics of steroid use, crosstraining, fluid replacement, the female athlete triad, and proper sleep.

Review Questions

1. Identify the four components of fitness described in this chapter. How does each component relate to physical fitness?
2. What is the difference between anaerobic and aerobic energy production? What types of activities are associated with anaerobic energy production? With aerobic energy production?
3. List some of the benefits of aerobic fitness.
4. Describe the various methods used to promote muscular strength. How do "andro" and creatine differ?
5. What does the principle of overload mean in regard to fitness training programs?
6. Identify the ACSM's four components of an effective cardiorespiratory fitness program. Explain the important aspects of each component.
7. Under what circumstances should you see a physician before starting a physical fitness program?
8. Identify and describe the three parts of a training session.
9. Describe some of the negative consequences of anabolic steroid use.
10. How does adequate sleep help improve ones fitness?

References

1. American College of Sports Medicine. Position stand on the recommended quantity and quality of exercise for developing and maintaining cardiorespiratory and muscular fitness and flexibility in healthy adults. *Med Sci Sports Exerc* 30(6):975–991, 1998.
2. American Heart Association, Councils on Clinical Cardiology and Nutrition, Physical Activity and Metabolism. *Exercise and Physical Activity in the Prevention and Treatment of Atherosclerotic Cardiovascular Disease.* Circulation; 107:3109, 2003.
3. Casperson C, et al. Public Health Reports 100:126, 1985
4. Brubaker PH, Kaminsky LA, Whaley MH. Coronary Artery Disease. *Human Kinetics,* 2002.
5. An exercise prescription for older people. *Harvard Heart Letter* 8(10): 1–4, 1998.
6. American College of Sports Medicine. *Guidelines for Exercise Testing and Prescription.* 6th ed., Lippincott, Williams, and Wilkins, 2000.
7. Williams MH. Alcohol and sport performance, *Sports Science Exchange* 4(40): 1–4, 1992.
8. U.S. Department of Health and Human Services. *Physical activity and health: a report of the surgeon general,* 1996, Centers for Disease Control and Prevention, National Center for Chronic Disease Prevention and Health Promotion.
9. The creatine craze, *UC Berkeley Wellness Letter* 14(3):6, 1998.
10. Arnheim DD, Prentice WE. *Essentials of athletic training,* 1999, McGraw-Hill.
11. Stevens WC, Brey RA, Harris JE, Fowlkes-Godek S. The dangerous trio: a case study approach to the female athletic triad, *Athletic Therapy Today,* 2(2):30–36, 1997.

focus on

staying fit during pregnancy

Exercise is especially beneficial to pregnant women.

Like many other attitudes, our thinking on fitness during pregnancy has changed in recent years.[1] No longer is a pregnant woman treated as fragile. A woman needs to be quite careful when carrying a baby, but these days a doctor is more likely to advise against a sedentary lifestyle for a healthy pregnant woman. Exercise during pregnancy can increase a woman's muscle strength, making delivery of the baby easier and faster. Exercise can also help control her weight, making it easier to get back to normal weight after delivery. The baby may benefit from the mother's exercise program as well.

Importance of Exercise for Pregnant Women

Exercise in general is beneficial to the human body, and it is even more important for pregnant women to exercise regularly.[2] During pregnancy a woman's entire body undergoes many physical changes. Muscles are stretched, joints are loosened, and tissues are subjected to stress. If a woman is in good physiological condition, she is more likely to handle these changes with few complications.[3] The baby may also benefit: studies have shown that women who exercise during pregnancy tend to give birth to healthier babies.[2]

Types of Exercise

The types of exercises a woman should perform during pregnancy will vary with the individual and with the stage of pregnancy. General exercises that increase overall fitness and stamina should be practiced, as well as exercises that strengthen specific muscle groups. Muscles of the pelvic floor, for example, should be exercised regularly, since these muscles will be supporting most of the extra weight of the baby. The pelvic floor muscles are involved with control of the bladder and rectum and with controlling increases in pressure within the abdominal cavity resulting from pushing during labor.[3] General exercises for the pelvic floor muscles include Kegel exercises. These exercises involve the contraction of pelvic floor muscles, and they can be performed by squeezing and then relaxing the anal sphincter.[3] These exercises work on the sphincters (rings of muscle) that control the openings of the urethra and anus.

The abdominal muscles are responsible for supporting the load of the growing fetus in the front of the mother's body. They are also used for pushing during delivery. These muscles must be kept in good shape so they can adequately support the increased weight.[3] Muscles involved in maintaining good posture, such as the back and leg muscles, should also be exercised. Efficient breathing should be practiced as well.

A variety of exercises is available, including walking, swimming, stretching, and strengthening exercises.[2] Yoga and tai chi are also good forms of exercise for pregnant women. The muscles of the pelvic floor, abdomen, and back are especially subject to stress and strain during pregnancy and delivery, so certain exercises can also be performed to strengthen these muscles. Exercises can also be performed to speed up recovery after delivery.[4] Such postpartum exercises can be started in some cases within 24 hours after delivery. Exercises can even be started before conception if a pregnancy is anticipated.

Hydrotherapy is becoming a popular option for expectant mothers. Exercising in the water helps reduce stress on joints. Water also provides more resistance than air, so muscles get a better workout. No special equipment is needed, but various props such as weights or fans can be used to increase resistance. Immersion in water has also been shown to decrease blood pressure, reduce heart rate, and reduce tissue swelling in pregnant women.[5] Exercising in water may also reduce the risk for pregnant women of getting overheated or tired. The water must not be too warm, however, since water that is too hot (around 97.8° F or above) may damage the nervous system and brain of the fetus.[2]

Risks to the Fetus

Although exercise during pregnancy has definite advantages, there are some drawbacks that must be considered as well. Studies suggest that exercise can be harmful to the fetus in some cases. Women who undergo exercise for long periods may experience a prolonged increase in core body temperature (a condition called *hyperthermia*), which may in turn increase the body temperature of the fetus. It is thought that such increases in fetal temperature may in turn put the baby at risk for congenital malformations. It has been shown that fever-induced hyperthermia is related to congenital malformation in many mammals, and recent studies suggest that this may be true for humans as well.[5] If fever from illness can increase the expectant mother's core temperature enough to produce malformations in the fetus, then it is possible that an increase in the mother's core temperature resulting from prolonged exercise may have similar effects. Fortunately, exercise over short periods (15 minutes or less) is not likely to raise the mother's core temperature enough to cause problems.[5]

Exercising Safely

If the expectant mother exercised regularly before becoming pregnant, she may have to alter her exercise routine. Intense, high-impact workouts should be avoided in favor of moderate exercise, since very intense workouts may reduce blood flow to the fetus and deprive it of nutrients. Sports that involve sudden stops, such as basketball or tennis, should be avoided, and certain strenuous sports may eventually result in birth complications.[2] Exercises that involve lying on the back should not be performed after the first trimester of pregnancy, since they may reduce blood flow to the mother's heart and the heart of the fetus. Deep knee bends, sit-ups and toe touches should be avoided, as well as downhill skiing, rock climbing, and horseback riding.[6] Exercises should be chosen that minimize the risk of injury to the fetus and the mother. Because of the changes in the mother's weight distribution during the course of pregnancy, she should be especially aware of balance during workouts. Exercises that may put her at risk of losing her balance and falling should be avoided, especially during the last trimester.[2]

Once safety factors have been accounted for, the healthy pregnant woman still has an array of options to choose from for her exercise routine. As with any workout program, she should consult her physician before beginning. Her obstetrician can tell her which exercises will be most beneficial and can also give tips to reduce potential injury to her and her baby. The obstetrician can give the expectant mother guidelines concerning safe levels of exertion and duration times of exercise as well.

For Discussion . . .

Do you think exercise during pregnancy is a good idea or not? Do the benefits outweigh the risks?

References

1. Kaehler K, Tivers C. *Primetime pregnancy: the proven program for staying in shape before and after your baby is born,* 1997, Contemporary Books.
2. Marti J, Hine A. *The alternative health and medicine encyclopedia,* 1995, Gale.
3. Noble E. *Essential exercises for the childbearing year,* 1982, Houghton Mifflin.
4. Parr R, Rudnitsky DA. *Rob Parr's post-pregnancy workout,* 1997, Berkeley Publishing Group.
5. Cefalo RC, Moos M-K. *Preconceptional health care: a practical guide,* 1995, Mosby.
6. Williams, RD. Healthy pregnancy, healthy baby, *FDA Consumer* 33(2):18–23, 1999.

personal assessment

what is your level of fitness?

You can determine your level of fitness in thirty minutes or less by completing this short group of tests based on the National Fitness Test developed by the President's Council on Physical Fitness and Sports. If you are over 40 years old or have chronic medical disorders such as diabetes or obesity, check with your physician before taking this or any other fitness test. You will need another person to monitor your test and keep time.

Three-Minute Step Test

Aerobic capacity. Equipment: 12-inch bench, crate, block, or stepladder; stopwatch. Procedure: face bench. Complete 24 full steps (both feet on the bench, both feet on the ground) per minute for 3 minutes. After finishing, sit down, have your partner find your pulse within 5 seconds, and take your pulse for 1 minute. Your score is your pulse rate for 1 full minute.

Scoring standards (heart rate for 1 minute)

Age	18–29		30–39		40–49		50–59		60+	
Gender	F	M	F	M	F	M	F	M	F	M
Excellent	<80	<75	<84	<78	<88	<80	<92	<85	<95	<90
Good	80–110	75–100	84–115	78–109	88–118	80–112	92–123	85–115	95–127	90–118
Average	>110	>100	>115	>109	>118	>112	>123	>115	>127	>118

Sit and Reach

Hamstring flexibility. Equipment: yardstick; tape. Between your legs, tape the yardstick to the floor. Sit with legs straight and heels about 5 inches apart, heels even with the 15-inch mark on the yardstick. While in a sitting position, slowly stretch forward as far as possible. Your score is the number of inches reached.

Scoring standards (inches)

Age	18–29		30–39		40–49		50–59		60+	
Gender	F	M	F	M	F	M	F	M	F	M
Excellent	>22	>21	>22	>21	>21	>20	>20	>19	>20	>19
Good	17–22	13–21	17–22	13–21	15–21	13–20	14–20	12–19	14–20	12–19
Average	<17	<13	<17	<13	<15	<13	<14	<12	<14	<12

Arm Hang

Upper body strength. Equipment: horizontal bar (high enough to prevent your feet from touching the floor); stopwatch. Procedure: hang with straight arms, palms facing forward. Start watch when subject is in position. Stop when subject lets go. Your score is the number of minutes and seconds spent hanging.

Scoring standards (heart rate for 1 minute)

Age	18–29		30–39		40–49		50–59		60+	
Gender	F	M	F	M	F	M	F	M	F	M
Excellent	>1:30	>2:00	>1:20	>1:50	>1:10	>1:35	>1:00	>1:20	>:50	>1:10
Good	:46–1:30	1:00–2:00	:40–1:20	:50–1:50	:30–1:10	:45–1:35	:30–1:00	:35–1:20	:21–:50	:30–1:10
Average	<:46	<1:00	<:40	<:50	<:30	<:45	<:30	<:35	<:21	<:30

Curl-Ups

Abdominal and low back strength. Equipment: stopwatch. Procedure: Lie flat on upper back, knees bent, shoulders touching the floor, arms extended above your thighs or by your sides, palms down. Bend knees so that the feet are flat and 12 inches from the buttocks. Curl up by lifting head and shoulders off the floor, sliding hands forward above your thighs or the floor. Curl down and repeat. Your score is the number of curl-ups in 1 minute, without breaking a beat.

	Scoring standards (number in 1 minute)									
Age	18–29		30–39		40–49		50–59		60+	
Gender	F	M	F	M	F	M	F	M	F	M
Excellent	>45	>50	>40	>45	>35	>40	>30	>35	>25	>30
Good	25–45	30–50	20–40	22–45	16–35	21–40	12–30	18–35	11–25	15–30
Average	<25	<30	<20	<22	<16	<21	<12	<18	<11	<15

Push-Ups (Men)

Upper body strength. Equipment: stopwatch. Assume a front-leaning position. Lower your body until chest touches the floor. Raise and repeat for 1 minute. Your score is the number of push-ups completed in 1 minute, without breaking a beat.

	Scoring standards (number in 1 minute)				
Age	18–29	30–39	40–49	50–59	60+
Excellent	>50	>45	>40	>35	>30
Good	25–50	22–45	19–40	15–35	10–30
Average	<25	<22	<19	<15	<10

Modified Push-Ups (Women)

Upper body strength. Equipment: stopwatch. Assume a front-leaning position with knees bent up, hands under shoulders. Lower your chest to the floor, raise, and repeat. Your score is the number of push-ups completed in 1 minute, without breaking a beat.

	Scoring standards (number in 1 minute)				
Age	18–29	30–39	40–49	50–59	60+
Excellent	>45	>40	>35	>30	>25
Good	17–45	12–40	8–35	6–30	5–25
Average	<17	<12	<8	<6	<5

To Carry This Further . . .

Note your areas of strengths and weaknesses. To improve your fitness, become involved in a fitness program that reflects the concepts discussed in this chapter. Talking with fitness experts on your campus might be a good first step.

chapter five

Understanding nutrition and your diet

Chapter Objectives

After reading this chapter, you should be able to:

▮ name and describe the seven types of nutrients.

▮ describe saturated, monounsaturated, and polyunsaturated fats, and explain their effects on the human body.

▮ discuss the recent growth in fat-free foods and their possible advantages and disadvantages.

▮ define complete protein foods and incomplete protein foods, and give examples of each.

▮ describe three processes that vitamins help perform in the body.

▮ discuss the roles of minerals and water in the body.

▮ describe the benefits of soluble and insoluble fiber.

▮ describe the Food Guide Pyramid and the number of recommended servings for each food group in the pyramid.

▮ discuss seven recommendations in the *Dietary Guidelines for Americans*.

▮ describe foodbourne illnesses and strategies for preventing them.

▮ name three types of vegetarian diets and describe the advantages and disadvantages of each.

Online Learning Center Resources

www.mhhe.com/hahn7e

Log on to our Online Learning Center (OLC) for access to these additional resources:

- Chapter key terms and definitions
- Learning objectives
- Student interactive question-and-answer sites

- Self-scoring chapter quiz
- Online assessments
- Key term flash cards

Talking It Over

Food Fiction vs. Food Fact

When it comes to food and nutrition, there are many myths that people believe are true. Here are some of the most popular ones:

FICTION: If I don't eat fat, I won't get fat.
FACT: Overeating—consuming more calories than you need or expend—can lead to storing any type of food as fat, even salad!

FICTION: Pasta is bad and should be avoided.
FACT: Pasta is a good source of carbohydrate, an important source of energy, and protein, the fundamental structural material for every cell in your body. Both are essential!

FICTION: Fat is bad and should be avoided.
FACT: Fat provides the body with slow-releasing energy and helps it carry and absorb vitamins and essential nutrients. It also provides the body with a sense of satisfaction, which helps us to avoid overeating.

FICTION: Eating certain foods— such as celery or grapefruit—makes your body burn extra calories and helps you to lose weight.
FACT: No matter what you've eaten, digestion only burns a small percentage of calories consumed—not nearly enough to affect your weight.

FICTION: Eating after 8 P.M. is bad and causes weight gain.
FACT: It's not what time you eat, but what time you go to sleep that's important. When you are sleeping, your metabolism tends to be lower than when you are active and awake. Researchers suggest limiting food intake 2 to 3 hours before going to sleep for this reason. So if you go to sleep at midnight, you certainly may want a nutritious snack at 8 P.M.!

Eye on the Media

The Truth About Food Addiction

There is a lot of debate about whether we can be addicted to food. Certainly some chocolate lovers will tell you that they are "chocoholics," and must have their dose of daily chocolate or suffer miserably. But even though there may be a psychological dependence or issue with food (as we'll discuss in Chapter 6 on Weight Management), there is no evidence that people can become physiologically addicted to particular foods. Yet many popular diets—including Overeaters Anonymous, Sugar Busters, and the Carbohydrate Addicts Diet among others—are based on the premise that we can become addicted to food in the same way that we can become addicted to alcohol or drugs. What is the truth about food addiction?

Diet programs that are based upon an addiction model lack sufficient scientific support for their claims. These diets suggest that there is a biological craving for carbohydrates—especially white flour and refined sugar—and that we need more and more of these foods in order to satisfy this craving. But it is important to recognize the difference between a physiological need and psychological craving. A craving is based on your thoughts and feelings, while hunger is a biological or physiological process. While individuals with eating disorders or problems with compulsive overeating may experience psychological cravings, their cravings are not physiologically based.

Indeed, there are some similarities between overeating and substance abuse—such as obsessively thinking about the food or drug, having periods of fasting and bingeing, and experiencing problems in day-to-day functioning—but this is where the likeness ends. Because, while even an addict can live without alcohol or drugs, nobody can abstain from food. We don't build up tolerance to certain foods, nor do we go through physiological withdrawal when abstaining from certain foods similar to what is seen with drug or alcohol withdrawal and physical dependence.

A number of popular diets are predicated on the idea that one can be addicted to sugar or carbohydrates because of the insulin reaction that occurs in the body when one eats any food. The glycemic index measures how much a food provokes the body to release insulin into the blood, causing the body to convert blood sugar (glucose) into fat. A high level of insulin speeds up the conversion too quickly and the blood sugar level plummets, causing individuals to feel light-headed, tired, and hungry. The higher the glycemic index, the faster the insulin response.

Diets based on the addiction model (such as The Atkins' Diet, Sugar Busters, the Carbohydrate Addict's Diet, or The Zone diet) are based upon the theory that people who are addicted to carbohydrates are "insulin resistant," and have an insulin imbalance in which their bodies produce too much insulin, causing them to feel con-stantly hungry which in turn causes them to overeat. Foods high in sugar, corn syrup, and complex carbohydrates like potatoes and carrots have a high glycemic index, and this is the reason the food addiction diets suggest avoiding carbohydrates.

The premise behind these diets is problematic for a number of reasons. First, they fail to take into consideration that when these foods are eaten in combination with other foods, such as eating carrots or potatoes with meat, this insulin response is not provoked. Second, these diets treat all carbohydrates the same, but we know this is not the case. Simple carbohydrates such as refined sugar provoke an insulin release into the blood, but the complex carbohydrates such as whole grains, fruits, and vegetables do not, even though they too have a high glycemic index. Also problematic is these diets' reliance on high fat, high cholesterol meals that put you at risk for heart disease, colon cancer, and ketosis.

The best way to keep your insulin levels stable is to follow the food pyramid guide and avoid sugary foods and drinks. So don't be fooled by diets based on the myth of food addiction!

Sources: Hall R. *The Unofficial Guide to Smart Nutrition.* Foster City, CA: IDG Books Worldwide International, 2000.
Poston W and Haddock C. *Food as a Drug.* New York: The Haworth Press, Inc., 2000.

Healthy eating is important from the prenatal period throughout life, in order to maintain a high level of wellness. Food provides the body with the **nutrients** required to produce energy, repair damaged tissue, promote tissue growth, and regulate physiological processes.

Physiologically, these nutrients—carbohydrates, fat, protein, vitamins, minerals, dietary fiber, and water—are essential in adequate quantity. In addition, the production, preparation, serving, and sharing of food enriches our lives in other ways (see Discovering Your Spirituality).

Key Terms

nutrients elements in foods that are required for the energy, growth, and repair of tissues and regulation of body processes.

Types and Sources of Nutrients

Let's discuss the familiar nutrients first: carbohydrates, fats, and proteins. These three nutrients provide our bodies with **calories.** * Calories are used quickly by our bodies in energy metabolism, or they are stored in the form of glycogen or adipose (fatty) tissue. The other nutrient groups, which are not sources of energy for the body, will be discussed later.

Carbohydrates

Carbohydrates are various combinations of sugar units, or saccharides and are the major energy source for the body. Each gram of carbohydrate contains 4 calories. Since the average person requires approximately 2000 calories per day and about 60% of our calories come from carbohydrates, roughly 1200 calories per day come from carbohydrates.[1]

Carbohydrates occur in three forms, depending on the number of saccharide (sugar) units that make up the molecule. Those that contain only one saccharide unit are classified as *monosaccharides* (glucose, or blood sugar), those with two units are *disaccharides* (sucrose, or table sugar), and those with more than two units are *polysaccharides* (starches).

Americans now consume about 150 pounds of sweeteners each year—usually in colas, candies, and pastries, which offer few additional nutritional benefits.[2] For years, excess sugar intake was blamed for a number of serious health problems, including obesity, mineral deficiencies, behavioral disorders, dental cavities, diabetes mellitus, and cardiovascular disease. However, with the exception of dental cavities, current scientific data do not confirm that sugar itself directly causes any of these health problems. Today, it is recommended that no more than 10% of our total calories come from simple sugars.

Much of the sugar we consume is hidden. For example, it is an ingredient in foods such as ketchup, salad

---

> ### Key Terms
>
> **calories** units of heat (energy); specifically, one calorie equals the amount of heat required to raise the temperature of 1 gram of water by 1°C.
>
> **carbohydrates** chemical compounds composed of sugar units; the body's primary source of energy.

---

*The term "calorie" is used here to mean a kilocalorie (kcal), which is the accepted scientific expression of the energy value of a food.

dressings, cured meat products, and canned vegetables and fruits. High-fructose corn syrup, often found in these items, is a highly concentrated sugar solution.

Starches are complex carbohydrates composed of long chains of sugar units. However, these starches should not be confused with the adjective "starchy." When people talk about starchy foods, they usually mean complex carbohydrates, or "heavy" foods. True starches are among the most important sources of dietary carbohydrates. Starches are found primarily in vegetables, fruits, and grains. Eating true starches is overall very nutritionally beneficial because most starch sources also contain much-needed vitamins, minerals, plant protein, and water.

Fats

Fats (lipids) are an important nutrient in our diets, as they provide a concentrated form of energy (9 calories per gram). Fats provide a feeling of **satiety** and keep us from feeling hungry. Because fats take longer to leave your stomach than either carbohydrates or proteins do, our stomachs feel full for a longer period of time, decreasing our appetite. Fat also helps give food its pleasing taste, or *palatability.* Fats carry the fat soluble vitamins A, D, E, and K. Without fat, these vitamins would quickly pass through the body. Fat also insulates our bodies to help us retain heat.

Dietary sources of fat are often difficult to identify. The visible fats in our diet, such as butter, salad oils, and the layer of fat on some cuts of meat, represent only about 40% of the fat we consume. Most of the fat we eat is hidden in food.

At the grocery store, the fat content of some foods is expressed as a percentage of the product's weight. For example, the different types of milk available include skim milk (no fat), low-fat milk (½%), reduced-fat milk (1% to 2%),

Choosing Fats: A Balancing Act

Current dietary recommendations suggest that no more than 30% of a person's total calories (600 calories from the benchmark 2000 calorie/day intake) should come from fat. But what balance should there be among the three forms of dietary fat?

Current guidelines specify that no more than 8% to 10% of total calories (160 to 200 calories/day) should be supplied by saturated fat, such as butter. Nonunsaturated fat sources, such as olive oil, should be relied on for 15% of total calories (300 calories/day), with a maximum of 10% of daily calories derived from polyunsaturated fats. Individuals with elevated LDL cholesterol levels (see Chapter 10) should reduce their intake of saturated fat to 7% or less of their total caloric intake.

and whole milk (3% to 4%). The labeling term "reduced-fat" for 1% and 2% milk was introduced in 1997 to indicate that these types of milk are no longer considered "low-fat."

The current recommendation is that no more than 25% to 30% of our calories come from fat (see the adjacent Star box). The Changing for the Better box on page 111 offers suggestions on how to reduce the fat content in your diet. Children under 2 years of age, however, need a certain amount of fat in their diets for growth.[3] Check with your doctor before restricting the amount of fat in a young child's diet.

All dietary fat is made up of a combination of three forms of fat: saturated, monounsaturated, and polyunsaturated, based on chemical composition. Paying attention to the amount of each type of fat in our diet is important because of the known link to heart disease (see Chapter 10). Not all fats are created equal. **Saturated fats,** including those found in animal sources and vegetable oils to which hydrogen has been added (hydrogenated), becoming *trans-fatty acids,* need to be carefully limited in a healthy diet.

Concern over the presence of trans-fatty acids (an altered form of a normal vegetable oil molecule) is associated with changes detrimental to the cell mem-

Key Terms

satiety (suh TIE uh tee) a food's ability to cause a feeling of fullness.

saturated fats fats that promote cholesterol formation; they are in solid form at room temperature; primarily animal fats.

brane, including those cells lining the artery wall. Among the changes being suggested is an increase in calcium deposits.[4] This could result in a rough surface, leading to plaque formation (see Chapter 10).

Processing can change the structure of fat, making it more saturated. As a result, the oils become semisolid and more stable at room temperature. The term *trans* describes the chemical makeup of a fatty acid. Most trans-fatty acids come from hydrogenated oil, which is found in foods such as stick margarine, peanut butter, and crackers. They are popular in food manufacturing because they can extend the shelf life of the food: the oil stays mixed in the food and doesn't rise to the top, and the food doesn't become too soft at room temperature. Many foods are fried with these fats in the fast-food industry.[5]

Tropical Oils

Although all cooking oils (and fats such as butter, lard, margarine, and shortening) have the same number of calories by weight (9 calories per gram), some oils contain high percentages of saturated fats. All oils and fats contain varying percentages of saturated, monounsaturated, and polyunsaturated fats. However, the tropical oils—coconut, palm, and palm kernel—contain much higher percentages of saturated fats than do other cooking oils. Coconut oil, for example, is 92% saturated fat. Tropical oils can still be found in some brands of snack foods, crackers, cookies, nondairy creamers, and breakfast cereals, although they have been removed from most national brands. Do you check for tropical oils on the ingredients labels of the foods you select?

Cholesterol

There has been a great deal of focus and concern over cholesterol levels. **Cholesterol** is a white, fat-like substance, found in cells of animal origin. It is not found in any vegetable product, so products such as peanut butter and margarine that claim they are cholesterol free never had it in the first place. Cholesterol is used to synthesize cell membranes and also serves as the starting material for the synthesis of bile acids and sex hormones. Although we consume cholesterol in our diet, in such foods as shrimp and other shellfish, animal fat, and milk, you don't need to obtain cholesterol from external sources—the human liver can synthesize enough of the substance to meet the body's needs. It is important to note that some foods high in cholesterol may provide other important nutrients and could remain in a healthy diet on a modest basis. A high level of cholesterol has been reported to be a risk factor in the development of cardiovascular disease (see Chapter 10). There are a number of medical conditions that can give rise to high blood cholesterol such as liver disease, kidney failure, hypothyroidism, and diabetes. Certain medications,

(some diuretics, for example) can also raise blood cholesterol, irrespective of diet. Considerable evidence suggests that increased intake of saturated fats may increase serum (blood) cholesterol levels. Nutritionists recommend that people restrict their dietary intake of cholesterol to 300 mg or less per day. In other words, no more than 30% of your total caloric intake should come from fat, with 7–10% from saturated fats, 10–15% from monounsaturated fats, and 10% from polyunsaturated fats.

Trans fats can act like saturated fat, potentially raising LDL blood cholesterol levels and decreasing HDL cholesterol. In order to reduce your intake of trans fat, make sure you check the labels on foods to see if they list "partially hydrogenated vegetable oil" as one of the ingredients. Foods such as cakes, cookies, crackers, snack foods, stick margarine, vegetable shortening, and fried foods are most likely to have hydrogenated vegetable oil as one of the ingredients. This is also the reason nutritionists encourage us to use butter rather than stick margarine.

Key Terms

cholesterol a primary form of fat found in the blood; lipid material manufactured within the body and derived from dietary sources.

Low-Fat Foods

Low fat and low calorie are not the same but often people confuse the two. Fat-free, low-fat, or reduced-fat foods have been popular for many years with people thinking they can eat as much as they want of these foods. This is far from true as a fat-free or reduced-fat product may have as many if not more calories per serving than regular products. For example, two tablespoons of fat-free caramel topping is 103 calories, the same amount of homemade-with-butter caramel topping.[6] Because fat helps you to feel fuller for a longer period of time, individuals tend to eat more of the fat-free foods in order to feel satiated, thus consuming more calories. In general, the lower the fat, the higher the price tag as the food industry recognized that Americans are willing to pay more for reduced-fat and fat-free labels. However, this may be changing as people have realized that lower fat with potentially higher calories doesn't equal weight loss or healthy weight management. With Subway trading in cookies for a fruit roll and soda for a 100 percent juice carton in its kids-pak meals and McDonald's offering a piece of fresh fruit in lieu of French fries for its Happy Meals and touting salads for adult fare, the fast-food tide seems to be turning from supersized and superfat toward healthier choices.

Proteins

Proteins are found in every living cell. They are composed of chains of **amino acids.** Of the twenty naturally occurring amino acids, the body can synthesize all but *nine essential amino acids** from the foods we eat. A food that contains all nine essential amino acids is called a *com-*

plete protein food. Examples are animal products, including milk, meat, cheese, and eggs. A food source that does not contain all nine essential amino acids is called an *incomplete protein* food. Vegetables, grains, and *legumes* (peas or beans—including chickpeas, butter beans, soybean curd [tofu], and peanuts) are principal sources of incomplete protein. For some people, including vegan vegetarians (see page 132 and the Focus On article on pages 138–139), people with limited access to animal-based food sources, or those who have significantly limited their meat, egg, and dairy product consumption, it is important to understand how essential amino acids can be obtained from incomplete protein sources. This requires the careful selection of plant foods in combinations that will provide all of the essential amino acids, as shown in the following list:

- Sunflower seeds/green peas
- Navy beans/barley
- Green peas/corn
- Red beans/rice
- Sesame seeds/soybeans
- Black-eyed peas/rice and peanuts
- Green peas/rice
- Corn/pinto beans

When even one essential amino acid is missing from the diet, a deficiency can develop. Soybeans provide the same high quality protein equal to that of animal protein.[7] Furthermore, soybeans contain no cholesterol or saturated fat and can actually lower blood lipid levels, reducing the risk of heart disease.[8]

Protein primarily promotes growth and maintenance of body tissue. However, when caloric intake falls, protein is broken down and converted into glucose. This loss of protein can impede growth and repair of tissue. Protein also is a primary component of enzyme and hormone structure. It helps maintain the *acid-base balance* of our bodies and is a source of energy (4 calories per gram consumed). Nutritionists recommend that 12% to 15% of our caloric intake be from protein, particularly that of plant origin. The RDA for adults is 58 grams of dietary protein for men and 46 grams for women each day.

---

*Eight additional compounds are sometimes classified as amino acids, so some nutritionists believe that there are more than twenty amino acids.

> **Key Terms**
>
> **proteins** compounds composed of chains of amino acids; the primary components of muscle and connective tissue.
>
> **amino acids** the chief components of protein; can be manufactured by the body or obtained from dietary sources.

I have heard that incorporating fish into my diet is a good source of protein and part of healthy eating. However, I recently learned that fish may be toxic. Should I limit my intake of fish?

While it is true that fish is a good source of protein and other nutritional benefits, there has been some compelling research to suggest that the big fish, swordfish, halibut, tuna, red snapper, flounder, freshwater bass, grouper, trout, marlin, king mackerel, tilefish, shark, and freshwater bass have been associated with toxic levels of mercury by the people who consume them regularly, some of which had more than double the amount the EPA deemed safe. Memory lapses, hair loss, stomach cramps, headaches, muscle and joint aches, nausea, and dizziness are the symptoms people reported who had toxic levels of mercury from eating these fish. Physicians claim that within 6 months of avoiding eating fish, their patients' mercury levels decreased significantly, their hair stopped falling out, and their other symptoms subsided. Recent studies also suggest that mercury may raise the risk of heart attack, and some experts are

even drawing links between mercury levels and autism in children and Alzheimer's disease in adults. Pregnant women and infants are at even greater risk as mercury can be excreted through breast milk and has been found to lower IQ level, and may cause learning disorders and other developmental problems.

So should you swear off fish forever? No, not necessarily. It is suggested that women of childbearing age, pregnant women, nursing mothers, and children under 8 years old should select a variety of cooked fish and eat a maximum of 12 ounces a week. Women and children are also suggested to avoid the fish that were associated with high mercury levels and eat fish such as salmon, sole, catfish, shrimp, clams, scallops, and oysters. Orange roughy and sea bass should be limited to once a month for women and children.

Source: Jetter A. How safe is your food? *Reader's Digest*, 53–63, August 2003.

Vitamins

Vitamins are organic compounds that are required in small amounts for normal growth, reproduction, and maintenance of health. Vitamins differ from carbohydrates, fats, and proteins because they do not provide calories or serve as structural elements for our bodies. Vitamins are *coenzymes*. By facilitating the action of **enzymes,** vitamins help initiate a wide variety of body responses, including energy production, use of minerals, and growth of healthy tissue.

Vitamins can be classified as *water soluble* (capable of being dissolved in water) or *fat soluble* (capable of being dissolved in fat or lipid tissue). Water soluble vitamins include the B-complex vitamins and vitamin C. Most of the excess of these water soluble vitamins is eliminated from the body in the urine. The fat soluble vitamins are vitamins A, D, E, and K. Excessive intake of these vitamins causes them to be stored in the body in the adipose (fat) tissue. It is therefore possible to consume and retain too many of these vitamins, particularly vitamins A and D. Because excess fat soluble vitamins are stored in the body's fat, organs that contain fat, such as the liver, are primary storage sites.

Because water soluble vitamins dissolve quickly in water, it's important not to lose them during the preparation of fresh fruits and vegetables. One method is not to overcook fresh vegetables. The longer vegetables are steamed or boiled, the more water soluble vitamins will be lost. Some people save the water in which vegetables were boiled or steamed and use it for drinking or cooking. More vitamins are retained with microwave cooking than with stove top cooking.

To ensure adequate vitamin intake, a good approach is to eat a variety of foods. Unless there are special circumstances, such as pregnancy, lactation, infancy, or an existing health problem, nearly everyone who eats a reasonably well-rounded diet consumes enough vitamins to prevent deficiencies. People often think taking megadoses of vitamins such as vitamin C can be health-enhancing, but actually the reverse is true. Taking large doses of vitamin C from a dietary supplement can put a strain on your kidneys, causing kidney stones and diarrhea. Too much niacin, vitamin B6, and folate can also be harmful.[5]

 TALKING POINTS What would you say to a friend who is following a low-carbohydrate, high-fat weight loss diet to help that person see the potential pitfalls of the diet?

Some recommend that supplements be taken with food, since they're really components of food and help the body metabolize other food components. The fat-soluble

Key Terms

vitamins organic compounds that facilitate the action of enzymes.

enzymes organic substances that control the rate of physiological reactions but are not themselves altered in the process.

nutrients should be taken with a little oil or fat to enhance absorption. The water-soluble nutrients are easily absorbed without food, but may work better when taken with meals. In addition, some people complain of stomach upset when they take vitamins on an empty stomach.

Unfortunately, not all people eat a balanced diet based on a variety of foods. Recent studies suggest that a somewhat higher intake of vitamins A, C, and E for adults might reduce the risk of developing cancer, atherosclerosis, and depressed levels of high-density lipoprotein (HDL) cholesterol; however, several unanswered questions remain, including the amounts needed for effectiveness (see Chapter 10).[9]

Consuming an adequate amount of folic acid before and during pregnancy has been shown to reduce the incidence of birth defects. To ensure adequate folic acid intake (400 micrograms/day), in 1997 the Food and Drug Administration (FDA) began to require that bread and cereal products be supplemented with folic acid. The goal of this requirement is for pregnant women and women of childbearing age to receive at least 140 micrograms/day through dietary intake. Taking a daily multivitamin before and during pregnancy would easily provide the remaining amount of folic acid necessary to promote fetal neural tube closure (thus preventing spina bifida). Folic acid is also considered important in the prevention of cardiovascular disease.[10]

At the same time that many health experts are recommending some vitamin supplementation, the FDA has prohibited manufacturers of food supplements, including vitamins, from making *unsubstantiated claims* for the cure and prevention of disease. Supplement manufacturers fought against the implementation of this regulation by suggesting to the public that vitamins might become available only by prescription. This did not happen. Today, manufacturers of folic acid supplements may make claims about the product's ability to prevent neural tube defects in infants.

Minerals

Nearly 5% of the body is composed of inorganic materials, the *minerals.* Minerals function primarily as structural elements (in teeth, muscles, hemoglobin, and hormones). They are also critical in the regulation of body processes, including muscle contraction, heart function, blood clotting, protein synthesis, and red blood cell formation. Approximately twenty-one minerals have been recognized as essential for good health. Unlike vitamins, minerals are inorganic and can't be destroyed by heat or food processing.

Major minerals are those that exist in relatively high amounts in our body tissues. The RDA recommends taking 250 mg of each one daily. Examples are calcium, phosphorus, sulfur, sodium, potassium, and magnesium. Examples of **trace elements,** minerals seen in relatively small amounts in body tissues, include zinc, iron, copper, sele-

nium, and iodine. Trace elements are required only in small quantities, fewer than 20 mg daily of each, but they are essential for good health. As with vitamins, the safest, most appropriate way to prevent a mineral deficiency is to eat a balanced diet. However, calcium, a major mineral, can be taken as a supplement to help prevent osteoporosis.

Water

Water may well be our most essential nutrient, since without water most of us would die from the effects of **dehydration** in less than 1 week. We could survive for weeks or even years without some of the essential minerals and vitamins, but not without water. More than half our body weight comes from water. Water provides the medium for nutrient and waste transport, controls body temperature, and functions in nearly all of our body's biochemical reactions.

Most people seldom think about the importance of an adequate intake of water and fluids. The average adult loses about 10 cups of water daily through perspiration, urination, bowel movements, and breathing. Adults require about six to ten glasses a day, depending on their activity level and environment. People who drink beverages that tend to dehydrate the body (tea, coffee, and alcohol) should increase their water consumption. To see if you're drinking enough fluid, check your urine. A small amount of dark-colored urine can be an indication that you are not consuming enough fluid and need to drink more. Urine that is pale or almost colorless means you are most likely taking in enough fluids. Needed fluids are also obtained from fruits, vegetables, fruit and vegetable juices, milk, and noncaffeinated soft drinks. Excessive water consumption by infants, however, can dilute sodium stores in the body to dangerously low levels, possibly causing death.[11] Also, dentists are increasingly concerned about the abnormally high number of dental caries (cavities) seen in children who have consumed bottled water rather than fluoridated tap water.[12]

Fiber

Although not considered a nutrient by definition, **fiber** is an important component of sound nutrition. Fiber consists of plant material that is not digested but moves

---

Key Terms

trace elements minerals present in very small amounts in the body; micronutrient elements.

dehydration the abnormal depletion of fluids from the body; severe dehydration can be fatal.

fiber plant material that cannot be digested; found in cereal grains, fruits, and vegetables.

Figure 5-1 The USDA Food Guide Pyramid.

through the digestive tract and out of the body. Cereal, fruits, and vegetables all provide us with dietary fiber.

Fiber can be classified into two large groups on the basis of water solubility. *Insoluble* fibers are those that can absorb water from the intestinal tract. By absorbing water, the insoluble fibers give the stool bulk and decrease the time it takes the stool to move through the digestive tract. In contrast, *soluble* fiber turns to a "gel" in the intestinal tract and binds to liver bile, to which cholesterol is attached. Thus the soluble fibers may be valuable in removing cholesterol, which lowers blood cholesterol levels. How much fiber do you need? Adults should eat from 25 to 35 g of fiber each day; however, most American adults eat only 11 g per day. Fiber has many benefits, including helping to curb your appetite and prevent overeating because it is filling, requires more chewing, stays in the stomach longer, and absorbs water, adding to the feeling of fullness. Fiber also helps to slow the absorption of sugar from the intestines, thus steadying the blood sugar and slowing down the absorption of fat from the foods you eat. Consuming adequate amounts of fiber has an important effect on reducing serious medical problems because soluble fiber lowers LDL cholesterol and protects against cardiovascular disease while insoluble fiber protects against developing colon cancer.[13]

In recent years, attention has been given to three forms of soluble fiber—oat bran, psyllium (from the weed plantain), and rice bran—because of their ability to lower blood cholesterol levels.

Oat bran can lower cholesterol levels by five to six points in people whose initial cholesterol levels are moderately high. To accomplish this reduction, a daily consumption of oat bran equal to a large bowl of cold oat bran cereal or three or more packs of instant oatmeal would be necessary. Oatmeal can also be eaten as a cooked cereal or used in other foods, such as hamburgers, pancakes, or meatloaf.

The Food Groups

The most effective way to take in adequate amounts of nutrients is to eat a **balanced diet**—one that includes a wide variety of foods from different food groups. Over the past several decades, various methods of grouping foods have been used, identifying five, seven, four, and now (again) five food groups from which selections are to be made. Today, the U.S Department of Agriculture (USDA) Food Guide Pyramid outlines five groups for which recommendations have been established and an additional group (fats, oils, and sweets) for which no specific recommendations exist (Figures 5-1 and 5-2). Table 5.1 on page 117

> **Key Terms**
>
> **balanced diet** a diet featuring food selections from each of the levels of the Food Guide Pyramid.

Eating a balanced diet including fruits and vegetables is the best way to get all the necessary vitamins and minerals.

summarizes the major nutrients that each food group supplies, and Table 5.2 shows the adult recommended dietary allowances (RDAs). To determine whether you are eating a healthful diet balanced with choices from each food group, complete the Personal Assessment on page 141.

Fruits

Two to four daily servings from the fruit group are recommended for an adult. The important functions of this

USDA-recommended daily servings for 2- to 6-year-olds

SODA

Less fats, sweets

Milk
2

Meat
2

Vegetables
3

Fruit
2

Grains
6

Figure 5-2 Children's nutritional requirements are different from those of adults, but they do need to eat a variety of nutrient-dense foods. This pyramid shows what the USDA recommends for 2- to 6-year olds.

group are to provide vitamin A, vitamin C, complex carbohydrates, and fiber in our diets. At least one serving high in vitamin C should be eaten daily.

Vegetables

Three to five servings from the vegetable group are recommended for an adult. As with the fruit group, the important functions are to provide vitamin A, vitamin C, complex carbohydrates, and fiber. Foods included in this group are dark-green, yellow, and orange vegetables, canned or cooked vegetables, and tossed salads. **Cruciferous vegetables,** such as broccoli, cabbage, brussels sprouts, and cauliflower, may be especially important in the prevention of certain forms of cancer.[14]

Milk, Yogurt, and Cheese

This group contributes two primary nutritional benefits: high-quality protein and calcium (required for bone and tooth development). Foods included in this group are whole milk, reduced-fat milk, low-fat milk, fat-free milk, yogurt, cheese, and ice cream. The adult recommendation is 2 to 3 cups of milk or two to three equivalent servings from this group each day. Premenopausal women

Key Terms

cruciferous vegetables vegetables whose plants have flowers with four leaves in the pattern of a cross, such as broccoli.

Table 5.1 Guide to Daily Food Choices

Food Group	Serving	Major Contributions	Foods and Serving Sizes*
Milk, yogurt, and cheese	2 (adult[†]) 3 (children, teens, young adults, and pregnant or lactating women)	Calcium Riboflavin Protein Potassium Zinc	1 cup milk 1½ oz cheese 2 oz processed cheese 1 cup yogurt 2 cups cottage cheese 1 cup custard/pudding 1½ cups ice cream
Meat, poultry, fish, dry beans, eggs, and nuts	2–3	Protein Niacin Iron Vitamin B$_6$ Zinc Thiamin Vitamin B$_{12}$[‡]	2–3 oz cooked meat, poultry, fish 1–1½ cups cooked dry beans 4 T peanut butter 2 eggs ½–1 cup nuts
Fruits	2–4	Vitamin C Fiber	¼ cup dried fruit ½ cup cooked fruit ¾ cup juice 1 whole piece fruit 1 melon wedge
Vegetables	3–5	Vitamin A Vitamin C Folate Magnesium Fiber	½ cup raw or cooked vegetables 1 cup raw leafy vegetables
Bread, cereal, rice, and pasta	6–11	Starch Thiamin Riboflavin[§] Iron Niacin Folate Magnesium[‖] Fiber[‖] Zinc[‖]	1 slice of bread 1 oz ready-to-eat cereal ½–¾ cup cooked cereal, rice, or pasta
Fats, oils, and sweets		Foods from this group should not replace any from the other groups. Amounts consumed should be determined by individual energy needs.	

This is a practical way to turn the RDA into food choices. You can get all essential nutrients by eating a balanced variety of foods each day from the food groups listed here. Eat a variety of foods in each food group, and adjust serving sizes appropriately to reach and maintain desirable weight.

*May be reduced for children's servings.
[†] ≥ 25 years of age.
[‡] Only in animal food choices.

[‖] Whole grains especially.
[§] enriched.

should consume three to four daily servings from this group to provide maximal protection from osteoporosis.

Because of the general concern about saturated fat, cholesterol, and additional calories, low-fat and fat-free milk products are recommended in place of high-fat milk products. The Changing for the Better box on page 124 shows the differences in calories (per cup), fat content (in grams), and % Daily Value among types of milk currently available. Aside from differences in fat content, all forms of milk offer similar nutritional benefits.

Meat, Poultry, Fish, Dry Beans, Eggs, and Nuts

It's essential to make daily selections from the protein-rich group because of our daily need for protein, iron, and the B vitamins. Meats include all red meat (beef, pork, and game), fish, and poultry. Meat substitutes include eggs, cheese, dried peas and beans (legumes), and peanut butter. Eggs can also be used as meat substitutes; however, using only the separated egg whites provides

Table 5.2 Adult Recommended Dietary Allowances[1]

Category	Age (years)	Weight[2] (kg)	(lb)	Height[2] (cm)	(in)	Protein (g)	Vitamin A (μg RE)[3]	Vitamin D (μg)[4]	Vitamin E (μg α-TE)[5]	Vitamin K (μg)
Males	15–18	66	145	176	69	59	1000	10	10	65
	19–24	72	160	177	70	58	1000	10	10	70
	25–50	79	174	176	70	63	1000	5	10	80
	51+	77	170	173	68	63	1000	5	10	80
Females	15–18	55	120	163	64	44	800	10	8	55
	19–24	58	128	164	65	46	800	10	8	60
	25–50	63	138	163	64	50	800	5	8	65
	51+	65	143	160	63	50	800	5	8	65
Pregnant						60	800	10	10	65
Lactating	1st 6 Months					65	1300	10	12	65
	2nd 6 Months					62	1200	10	11	65

Vitamin C (mg)	Thiamin (mg)	Riboflavin (mg)	Niacin (mg NE)[6]	Vitamin B6 (mg)	Folate (μg)	Vitamin B12 (μg)	Calcium (mg)	Phosphorus (mg)	Magnesium (mg)	Iron (mg)	Zinc (mg)	Iodide (μg)	Selenium (μg)
60	1.5	1.8	20	2.0	200	2.0	1200	1200	400	12	15	150	50
60	1.5	1.7	19	2.0	200	2.0	1200	1200	350	10	15	150	70
60	1.5	1.7	19	2.0	200	2.0	800	800	350	10	15	150	70
60	1.2	1.4	15	2.0	200	2.0	800	800	350	10	15	150	70
60	1.1	1.3	15	1.5	180	2.0	1200	1200	300	15	12	150	50
60	1.1	1.3	15	1.6	180	2.0	1200	1200	280	15	12	150	55
60	1.1	1.3	15	1.6	180	2.0	800	800	280	15	12	150	55
60	1.0	1.2	13	1.6	180	2.0	800	800	280	10	12	150	55
70	1.5	1.6	17	2.2	400	2.2	1200	1200	320	30	15	175	65
95	1.6	1.8	20	2.1	280	2.6	1200	1200	355	15	19	200	75
95	1.6	1.7	20	2.1	260	2.6	1200	1200	340	15	16	200	75

[1]The allowances, expressed as average daily intakes over time, are intended to provide for individual variations among most normal people as they live in the United States under usual environmental stresses. Diets should be based on a variety of common foods to provide other nutrients for which human requirements have been less well defined. See text for detailed discussion of allowances and of nutrients not tabulated.

[2]Weights and heights of reference adults are actual medians for the U.S. population of the designated age, as reported by NHANES II. The use of these figures does not imply that the height-to-weight ratios are ideal.

[3]Retinol equivalents. 1 retinol = 1 μg retinol or 6 μg β-carotene.

[4]As cholecalciferol. 10 μg cholecalciferol = 400 IU of vitamin D.

[5]α-Tocopherol equivalents. 1 mg d-α tocopherol = 1 α-TE.

[6]1 NE (niacin equivalent) is equal to 1 mg of niacin or 60 mg of dietary tryptophan.

excellent protein without the accompanying fat (including cholesterol). The current recommendation for adults is 4 ounces total per day, preferably in two to three servings.

The fat content of meat varies considerably. Some forms of meat yield only 1% fat, but others may be as high as 40% fat. Poultry and fish are usually significantly lower in overall fat than red meat. The higher the grade of red meat, the more fat will be marbled throughout the muscle fiber and thus the higher will be its caloric value.

Bread, Cereal, Rice, and Pasta

The nutritional benefit from this group lies in its contribution of B-complex vitamins and energy (in the form of calories) to our diets. Some nutritionists believe that eating foods from this group also promotes protein intake, since many of them are prepared with foods in other groups and thus become complete-protein foods, such as macaroni and cheese, cereal and milk, and bread and meat sandwiches. Six to eleven servings

Food labels are comprised of a language all their own, defined by government regulation. It is important that you learn this language and know what is meant by these terms. Here are some translations of what is meant by the labels you read:

- Calorie-free = contains less than 5 calories per serving
- Low calorie = contains 40 calories or less per serving
- Reduced calorie = contains at least 25% fewer calories than regular versions of the food
- Lite or light = contains ⅓ fewer calories than regular versions of the product or no more than half the fat of the regular version of the product
- Fat free = contains less than 0.5 g of fat per serving

- Free = contains none or trivial amounts of a substance such as sodium, fat, cholesterol, calories, or sugars
- Low fat = contains 3 g or less per serving
- Reduced fat = at least 25% or less fat than regular versions of the food
- Cholesterol free = contains no more than 2 mg of cholesterol and 2 g or less of saturated fat per serving
- Low saturated fat = contains 1 g or less of saturated fat per serving
- Lean = contains fewer than 10 g of fat, 4 g of saturated fat, and 95 mg of cholesterol per serving or per 100 g of food
- Fresh = unprocessed, uncooked, unfrozen
- Healthy = contains no more than 3 g of fat, including 1 g of saturated fat and 60 mg of cholesterol per serving and must also contain at least 10% of RDA of either

vitamin A, vitamin C, calcium, iron, protein, or fiber. Must contain no more than 300 mg of sodium and there is no limit on sugar content
- Good source = serving must contain 10–19% of RDA of a particular nutrient
- High = serving contains 20% or more of the RDA of a particular nutrient
- More = serving contains 10% or more of the RDA of a particular nutrient than the regular food to which it is being compared
- Less = contains at least 25% less of the nutrient to which it is being compared
- Energy = refers to any product that contains calories, so any drink, except water, can meet this definition

---

daily from this group are recommended. Several daily servings of any **enriched** or whole-grain bread or cereal are recommended.

Fats, Oils, and Sweets

Butter, candy, colas, cookies, chips, and pastries fit into this food group. Such foods contribute little to healthful nutrition. Since they provide additional calories (generally from table sugar) and large amounts of salt and fat, they should be consumed in moderation. It's important to remember that cookies, crackers, and desserts called "fat free" or "low fat" may be high in sugar and calories. Many of the foods at the top of the food pyramid are known collectively as *junk foods*.

Healthy Pyramid Alternatives

While most people are aware of the food pyramid as a guideline for healthy eating, less than 40% of Americans actually follow it (see Table 5.3). Dr. Walter Willett has developed what he hopes will be accepted as the new food pyramid as he describes the current one as "built on shaky scientific ground." The Healthy Eating Pyramid (Figure 5-3) advises people to:

1. Select whole grains over the highly processed carbohydrates.
2. Choose monounsaturated and polyunsaturated fats over saturated fats and avoid trans fat.
3. Select deep green and colorful vegetables.

Table 5.3 Americans Are Not Following the Food Pyramid

	Current Guidelines	Actual Consumption
Fats, oils, sweets	use sparingly	36 teaspoons of added fats and sugar per day
Milk, yogurt, cheese	2–3 servings daily	1½ servings per day
Meat, poultry, fish, dry beans, eggs, nuts	2–3 servings daily	2 servings per day
Vegetable	3–5 servings daily	3 servings per day
Fruit	2–4 servings daily	1½ servings per day
Bread, cereal, rice, pasta	6–11 servings daily	7 servings per day

Source: USDA

| Key Terms |

enriched the process of returning to foods some of the nutritional elements (B vitamins and iron) removed during processing.

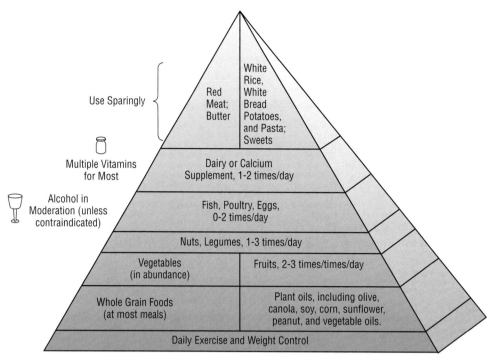

Figure 5-3 Healthy Eating Pyramid.

4. Choose protein sources such as nuts, legumes, fish, and poultry over red and processed meats.
5. Include physical activity.
6. De-emphasize dairy products and refined grains such as white bread and white rice.
7. Take a daily multivitamin for insurance.[15]

The food pyramid is released every 5 years by the USDA and is scheduled to publish the next set of dietary guidelines in February 2005. However, since its inception in 1992, the guidelines have changed to include more current information but have not actually been revised. It will be interesting to see if Dr. Willett's Healthy Eating Pyramid is adopted for the new dietary guidelines.

Fast Foods

Fast foods deliver a high percentage of their calories from fat, often associated with their method of preparation (e.g., frying in saturated fat). **Fat density** is a serious limitation of fast foods (Table 5.3). In comparison with the recommended standard (25% to 30% of total calories from fat), 40% to 50% of the calories in fast foods come from fats. Although many fast-food restaurants are now using vegetable oil instead of animal fat for frying (to reduce cholesterol levels), this change has not lowered the fat density of these foods. One average fast-food meal supplies over one-half the amount of fat needed in a day. In addition, fast foods are often high in sugar and salt.

But trends indicate that the fast-food tide may be beginning to shift. In 2000 Subway began heavily promoting its line of low-fat sandwiches with great success. Now larger chains like McDonald's, Burger King, Pizza Hut, and Wendy's are following Subway's lead, adding lower-fat sandwiches and salads to their menus.[16] The industry is also focusing on healthier options for children; for example, Wendy's has announced plans to test fruit cups and milk as options in its kids' meals, and McDonald's has begun testing white-meat-only Chicken McNuggets.

Phytochemicals

Certain physiologically active components are believed to deactivate carcinogens or function as antioxidants. Among these are the carotenoids (from green vegetables), polyphenols (from onions and garlic), indoles (from cruciferous vegetables), and the allyl sulfides (from garlic, chives, and onions). These *phytochemicals* may play an important role in sparking the body to fight and slow the development of some diseases such as cancer. At this time, however, the

> **Key Terms**
>
> **fat density** the percentage of a food's total calories that are derived from fat; above 30% is considered to be a high fat density.

Table 5.4 Fast Food: Fast, Convenient, Affordable—But Fattening

Menu Item	Calories	Calories from Fat	% Calories from Fat
Burgers			
McDonald's Hamburger	260	81	31%
Wendy's Jr. Hamburger	270	90	33%
Jack in the Box Hamburger	280	108	36%
Hardee's Hamburger	270	99	37%
McDonald's Cheeseburger	320	117	38%
Wendy's Jr. Cheeseburger	320	117	38%
Wendy's Plain Single Hamburger	360	144	39%
Jack in the Box Cheeseburger	330	135	42%
Burger King Cheeseburger	380	171	45%
Wendy's Jr. Bacon Cheeseburger	380	171	45%
McDonald's Quarter Pounder	420	189	45%
Wendy's Plain Double Hamburger	560	261	46%
McDonald's Big Mac	560	279	50%
McDonald's Quarter Pounder w/Cheese	530	270	51%
Hardee's Works Burger	530	270	51%
Burger King Double Cheeseburger	600	324	53%
Burger King Whopper	640	351	55%
Burger King Whopper with Cheese	730	414	56%
Jack in the Box Jumbo Jack	560	324	57%
Burger King Double Whopper	870	504	57%
Hardee's Monster Burger	1060	711	67%
Jack in the Box Ultimate Bacon Cheeseburger	1150	801	70%
Chicken Sandwiches			
Boston Market Plain Chicken Sandwich	430	45	9%
Chick-Fil-A Chargrilled Chicken Sandwich	280	27	11%
McDonald's Plain Grilled Chicken Deluxe	300	45	15%
Wendy's Grilled Chicken Sandwich	310	72	23%
Chick-Fil-A Chicken Sandwich	290	81	28%
Hardee's Grilled Chicken Sandwich	350	99	29%
Hardee's Chicken Fillet Sandwich	480	162	33%
Wendy's Breaded Chicken Sandwich	440	162	36%
KFC Original Recipe Chicken Sandwich	497	198	40%
McDonald's Crispy Chicken Deluxe	500	225	44%
Burger King Broiler	550	261	47%
Jack in the Box Chicken Sandwich	450	234	51%
Burger King Chicken Sandwich	710	387	55%
Jack in the Box Chicken Supreme	680	405	59%
Sub Sandwiches (6″)			
Subway Veggie Delite	237	27	11%
Blimpie Roast Beef	340	45	12%

continued

Table 5.4 Fast Food: Fast, Convenient, Affordable—But Fattening *continued*

Menu Item	Calories	Calories from Fat	% Calories from Fat
Subway Turkey Breast	289	36	12%
Blimpie Grilled Chicken	400	81	20%
Subway Steak & Cheese	398	90	23%
Blimpie Ham & Swiss	400	117	30%
Subway Cold Cut Trio	378	117	31%
Subway Meatball	419	144	34%
Blimpie Steak & Cheese	550	234	42%
Blimpie Tuna	570	288	51%
Subway Tuna	542	288	53%
French Fries			
Hardee's Medium	350	135	37%
Hardee's Small	240	90	38%
Dairy Queen Large	390	162	41%
Jack in the Box Regular	360	153	42%
Jack in the Box Jumbo	430	180	42%
McDonald's Super Size	540	234	43%
McDonald's Small	210	90	43%
Wendy's Biggie	460	207	43%
McDonald's Large	450	198	44%
Wendy's Small	260	117	46%
Burger King Medium	370	180	49%
Jack in the Box Seasoned Curly	420	216	52%
Jack in the Box Chili Cheese Curly	650	369	57%
Tacos, Burritos, Pitas (and related items)			
Taco Bell Bean Burrito	380	108	29%
Taco Bell Steak Soft Taco	200	63	30%
Wendy's Chicken Caesar Pita	490	153	33%
Taco Bell Gordita Fiesta (steak)	270	90	33%
Wendy's Garden Veggie Pita	390	135	36%
Taco Bell Burrito Supreme	440	162	39%
Wendy's Classic Greek Pita	430	171	40%
Taco Bell Beef Burrito Supreme	520	207	40%
Taco Bell Steak Fajita Wrap	460	189	41%
Long John Silver's Salsa Chicken Wrap	690	288	42%
Long John Silver's Tartar Fish Wrap	730	315	42%
Long John Silver's Cajun Chicken Wrap	730	324	44%
Taco Bell Gordita Santa Fe (beef)	380	180	47%
Jack in the Box Taco	190	99	53%
Taco Bell Taco Supreme	220	117	55%
Jack in the Box Monster Taco	290	162	55%
Taco Bell BLT Soft Taco	340	207	62%

Table 5.5 Making Better Fast Food Choices

Fast food meals can be high in calories, fat, cholesterol, and sodium. But it is still possible to eat fast food occasionally and follow a sensible diet. Take a look at how a few sample meals stack up against each other, and against the recommended daily intake for calories (2000–2700 per day), fat (no more than 50–80 g), cholesterol (no more than 300 mg), and sodium (no more than 1100–3300 mg).

	Poor choice	Sensible choice
Burger (McDonald's)	Quarter-pound burger with cheese, large fries, 16 oz soda	Hamburger, small fries, 16 oz diets soda
	1166 calories *51 g fat* *95 mg cholesterol* *1450 mg sodium*	*481 calories* *19 g fat* *30 mg cholesterol* *664 mg sodium*
Pizza (Domino's)	4 slices sausage and mushroom pizza, 16 oz soda	3 slices cheese pizza, 16 oz diet soda
	1000 calories *28 g fat* *62 mg cholesterol* *2302 mg sodium*	*516 calories* *15 g fat* *29 mg cholesterol* *1470 mg sodium*
Chicken (KFC)	2 pieces fried chicken (breast and wing), buttermilk biscuit, mashed potatoes with gravy, corn-on-the-cob, 15 oz soda	1 piece fried chicken (wing), mashed potatoes with gravy, cole slaw, 15 oz diet soda
	1232 calories *57 g fat* *157 mg cholesterol* *2276 mg sodium*	*373 calories* *19 g fat* *46 mg cholesterol* *943 mg sodium*
Taco (Taco Bell)	Taco salad, 16 oz soda	3 light tacos, 16 oz diet soda
	1057 calories *55 g fat* *80 mg cholesterol* *1620 mg sodium*	*420 calories* *15 g fat* *60 mg cholesterol* *840 mg sodium*

SOURCE: Adapted from "Fast Food Facts" from the office of the Minnesota Attorney General *http://www.olen.com/food/book.html*

exact mechanisms through which the various phytochemicals reduce the formation of cancer cells is not understood.[17] Although it is generally agreed that these foods are important in planning food selections, no precise recommendations regarding the amounts of various phytochemical-rich plants have been made.

Functional Foods

At the forefront of healthful nutrition is the identification and development of foods intended to affect a particular health problem or to improve the functional capability of the body. **Functional foods** contain not only recognized nutrients but also new or enhanced elements that impart medicine-like properties to the food. Alternative labels also exist for various subclasses of functional foods, such as *nutraceuticals,* or food elements that may be packaged in forms appearing more like medications (for example, pills or capsules), and *probiotics,* or foods that improve the microbial flora that reside within the human digestive tract.[18]

Examples of functional foods include garlic (believed to lower cholesterol), olive oil (thought to prevent heart disease), foods high in dietary fiber (which prevent constipation and lower cholesterol), and foods rich in calcium (which prevent osteoporosis). In addition, foods that contain high levels of vitamins A, C, and E—primarily fruits and vegetables—and provide the body with natural sources of antioxidants are functional foods.

Other functional foods are those that contain or are enriched with folic acid. These vitamin B–family foods aid in the prevention of spina bifida and other neural tube defects and the prevention of heart disease. Foods

> **Key Terms**
>
> **functional foods** foods capable of contributing to the improvement/prevention of specific health problems.

I've been drinking whole milk for years, and I enjoy it. Would changing to one of the lower-fat types really make a health difference?

The next time you're grocery shopping, choose milk that's one level lower in fat than the kind you usually buy. Then, if you still have some of the high-fat milk left, ask someone to give you a blind taste test. If you can't distinguish between the two, try switching to the lower-fat form. You'll not only reduce your exposure to saturated fat but also cut down on calories.

Milk's New Names

Old Name	Possible New Names	Total Fat [per cup] Grams	% Daily Value	Calories per cup
Milk	Milk	8.0 g	12%	150
Low-fat 2% milk	Reduce fat or less fat milk	4.7 g	7%	122
Not on the market	Light milk	4.0 g or less	6% or less	116 or less
Low-fat 1% milk	Low-fat milk	2.6 g	4%	102
Skim milk	Fat-free, skim, zero-fat; no-fat or nonfat milk	less than 0.5 g	0%	80

As you can see from the information above, the names assigned to various types of milk have recently undergone a big change.

that are rich in selenium are sometimes categorized as functional foods because of selenium's potential as an agent in cancer prevention. Most recently, the FDA has approved a "heart healthy" label for foods that are rich in soy protein.[19] All of the functional foods discussed here are approved to carry **health claims** on the basis of current FDA criteria.[20]

One category of functional foods being researched is vegetables that are genetically engineered to produce a specific biological element that is important to human health. An example is tomatoes that are high in lycopene. Another example, as described earlier, is a new type of margarine that can lower the level of and change the properties of blood cholesterol. Food technologists are interested in expanding the functional food family to include a greater array of health-enhancing food items.

The new USDA organic food labels went into effect in October 2002 to standardize regulations for foods grown without synthetic pesticides or other chemicals. Under the new USDA rules, organic means:

- Meat, poultry, and eggs are from animals given no growth hormones or antibiotics. Vitamin and mineral supplements are allowed. Livestock are given organic feed and live in conditions that allow for "exercise, freedom of movement and reduction of stress."
- Products are not genetically engineered or irradiated to kill germs.
- Crops are grown on land that has not been fertilized with sewage sludge or chemical fertilizers.
- Pests and plant disease are treated primarily with insect predators, traps, natural repellants, and other non-chemical methods.
- Weeds are controlled by mulching, mowing, hand weeding, or mechanical cultivation, not chemical herbicides.

There are different types of organic foods: "100% organic" meaning the food contains all organic ingredients, "organic" which means at least 95% of the product is organic, and "made with organic ingredients" which means at least 70% of the food is organic as defined above.

TALKING POINTS What fast-food restaurants are your favorites? Are you surprised at any of the information in this chapter regarding your favorite meals? Will you change your order next time you visit a fast-food restaurant?

Food Additives

Today many people believe that the food they consume is unhealthy because of the 2,800 generally recognized as safe (GRAS) **food additives** that can be put into food during production, processing, and preparation. But should these additives be banned?

Food additives refer to substances added to food to provide color or flavor, replace sugar or fat, or improve

> ### Key Terms
>
> **health claims** liable statements attesting to a food's contribution to the improvement/prevention of specific health problems.
>
> **food additives** chemical compounds intentionally added to our food supply to change some aspect of the food, such as its color or texture.

I am always in a hurry and don't have time to cook, and so a lot of my meals end up being fast food. Are there better choices I can make when eating on the run?

The typical American eats about three hamburgers and four orders of French fries each week so you aren't alone. With over 300,000 fast-food restaurants in the United States, fast food is definitely part of the American lifestyle. Here are some things to consider when eating at fast food restaurants:

- Don't supersize! Go for the "small" or "regular" size.
- Don't wait until you are starving because that leads to overeating and supersizing!
- Decide what you want to order ahead of time and don't be swayed by "value meal" or what "looks good."
- Choose salads, baked potatoes and whole grain bread over fried food.

- Order grilled instead of fried chicken or fish.
- Look for the "light" choices.
- Limit your condiments. Mustard, catsup, salsa, or low-fat or fat-free condiments and dressing are preferable to regular mayonnaise or high-fat dressings.
- For breakfast, choose cereal and milk or pancakes rather than a breakfast sandwich (which can have about 475 calories, 30 grams of fat, and 1,260 mg of sodium).
- Bring fast food from home! Buy portable foods at the grocery store to take with you that can be eaten quickly and easily such as portable yogurt, a banana or apple, low-fat granola bar, or breakfast bar.
- Order low-fat or skim milk or water instead of soda.
- Go to a variety of different kinds of fast-food restaurants so you aren't eating hamburgers every day and set a limit on how many meals you are going to eat out each week.

nutritional content, texture, or shelf life. Food additives must undergo FDA testing and approval to ensure that the benefits outweigh any risks associated with these additives. For example, emulsifiers help to give peanut butter a more consistent texture and prevent separation while stabilizers and thickeners can give ice cream a smooth, uniform texture. Preservatives such as antioxidants prevent apples from turning brown from exposure to air and fats and oils in baked goods from spoiling. The three most common additives are sugar, salt, and corn syrup.[21]

Food Labels

Since 1973, the FDA has required food manufacturers to provide nutritional information (labels) on products to which one or more nutrients have been added or for which some nutritional claim has been made. Originally, there was concern about whether the public could understand the labels and whether additional information would be required. So the FDA, in consultation with individual states and public interest groups, developed new labeling regulations. Revised labels began appearing on food packages in May 1993. The currently used label is shown in Figure 5-4. Specific types of information contained on this label are highlighted. (See also the HealthQuest Activities box on page 128.)

Foods that were not initially covered by the 1993 food labeling guidelines are gradually being assigned labels. For example, many single-ingredient meats are now being labeled. Processed meat, fish, and poultry products, such

Organic foods tend to be safer and healthier.

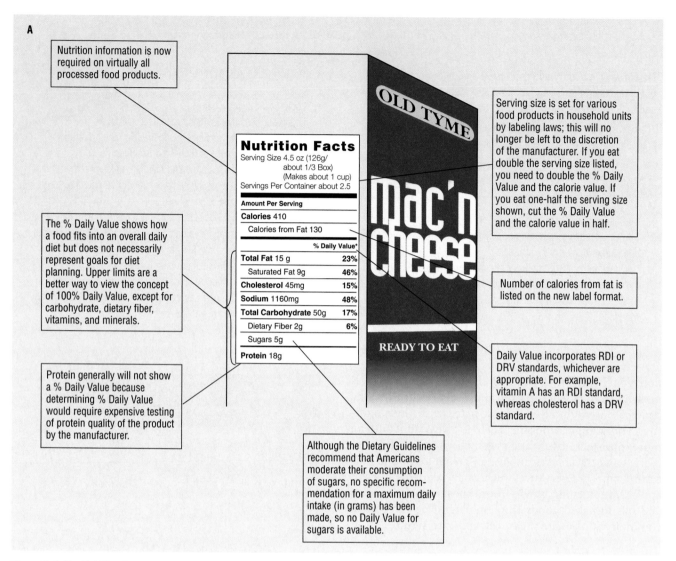

A

Nutrition information is now required on virtually all processed food products.

Nutrition Facts
Serving Size 4.5 oz (126g/ about 1/3 Box) (Makes about 1 cup)
Servings Per Container about 2.5

Amount Per Serving

Calories 410

Calories from Fat 130

	% Daily Value*
Total Fat 15 g	23%
Saturated Fat 9g	46%
Cholesterol 45mg	15%
Sodium 1160mg	48%
Total Carbohydrate 50g	17%
Dietary Fiber 2g	6%
Sugars 5g	
Protein 18g	

OLD TYME

mac'n cheese

READY TO EAT

Serving size is set for various food products in household units by labeling laws; this will no longer be left to the discretion of the manufacturer. If you eat double the serving size listed, you need to double the % Daily Value and the calorie value. If you eat one-half the serving size shown, cut the % Daily Value and the calorie value in half.

The % Daily Value shows how a food fits into an overall daily diet but does not necessarily represent goals for diet planning. Upper limits are a better way to view the concept of 100% Daily Value, except for carbohydrate, dietary fiber, vitamins, and minerals.

Number of calories from fat is listed on the new label format.

Protein generally will not show a % Daily Value because determining % Daily Value would require expensive testing of protein quality of the product by the manufacturer.

Daily Value incorporates RDI or DRV standards, whichever are appropriate. For example, vitamin A has an RDI standard, whereas cholesterol has a DRV standard.

Although the Dietary Guidelines recommend that Americans moderate their consumption of sugars, no specific recommendation for a maximum daily intake (in grams) has been made, so no Daily Value for sugars is available.

Figure 5-4 The Nutrition Facts panel on a current food label.

as hot dogs and chicken patties, must bear labels. Fresh fruits and vegetables are not required to be labeled, but many stores do so voluntarily.

Recent additions to the 1993 requirements include the labeling of fruit juices for pasteurization (unpasteurized juices can be a source of *Escherichia coli [E. coli]* contamination), the identification of milk from cows whose food has been enhanced with bovine growth hormone, and the issuing of specific criteria for legal use of the term "organic." Some supermarkets also label fresh and frozen poultry and seafood with information about how it was prepared and stored. This point-of-purchase labeling is voluntary. Beginning January 1, 2006, food makers will be required by the FDA to put the amount of trans fat on food labels, sparking some companies such as Frito-Lay and Kraft to start reducing and even eliminating trans fat from its products. Additionally, some restaurant menus now state the nutritional content of some selections and provide cautionary notes about their safe cooking.

Dietary Supplements

In 2000 it was estimated that Americans spent 17 billion dollars on a wide array of over-the-counter (OTC) products known collectively as *dietary supplements.* These nonprescription products are legally described as:[22]

- Products (other than tobacco) that are intended to supplement the diet, including vitamins, amino acids, minerals, glandular extracts, herbs, and other plant products such as fungi

B

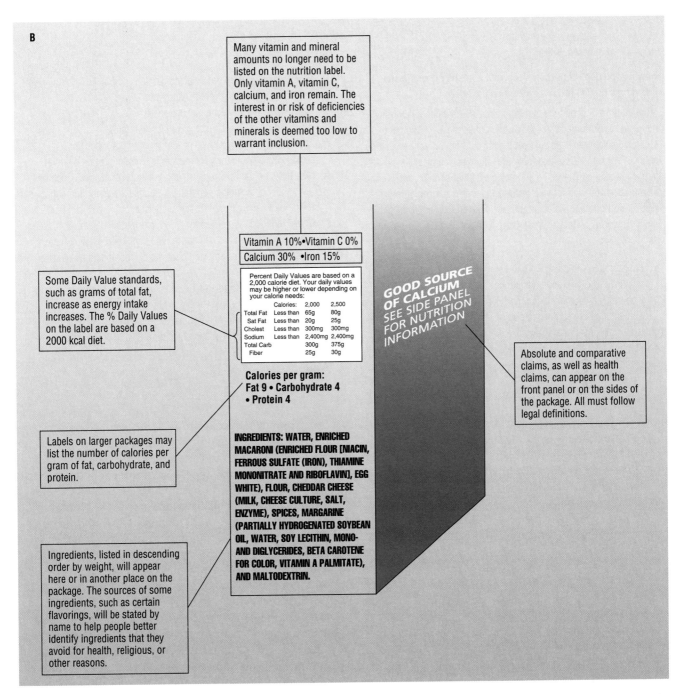

Many vitamin and mineral amounts no longer need to be listed on the nutrition label. Only vitamin A, vitamin C, calcium, and iron remain. The interest in or risk of deficiencies of the other vitamins and minerals is deemed too low to warrant inclusion.

Vitamin A 10%•Vitamin C 0%
Calcium 30% •Iron 15%

Percent Daily Values are based on a 2,000 calorie diet. Your daily values may be higher or lower depending on your calorie needs:

		Calories:	2,000	2,500
Total Fat	Less than		65g	80g
Sat Fat	Less than		20g	25g
Cholest	Less than		300mg	300mg
Sodium	Less than		2,400mg	2,400mg
Total Carb			300g	375g
Fiber			25g	30g

Some Daily Value standards, such as grams of total fat, increase as energy intake increases. The % Daily Values on the label are based on a 2000 kcal diet.

GOOD SOURCE OF CALCIUM SEE SIDE PANEL FOR NUTRITION INFORMATION

Absolute and comparative claims, as well as health claims, can appear on the front panel or on the sides of the package. All must follow legal definitions.

Calories per gram:
Fat 9 • Carbohydrate 4
• Protein 4

Labels on larger packages may list the number of calories per gram of fat, carbohydrate, and protein.

INGREDIENTS: WATER, ENRICHED MACARONI (ENRICHED FLOUR [NIACIN, FERROUS SULFATE (IRON), THIAMINE MONONITRATE AND RIBOFLAVIN], EGG WHITE), FLOUR, CHEDDAR CHEESE (MILK, CHEESE CULTURE, SALT, ENZYME), SPICES, MARGARINE (PARTIALLY HYDROGENATED SOYBEAN OIL, WATER, SOY LECITHIN, MONO- AND DIGLYCERIDES, BETA CAROTENE FOR COLOR, VITAMIN A PALMITATE), AND MALTODEXTRIN.

Ingredients, listed in descending order by weight, will appear here or in another place on the package. The sources of some ingredients, such as certain flavorings, will be stated by name to help people better identify ingredients that they avoid for health, religious, or other reasons.

Figure 5-4 *continued*

- Products that are intended for use by people to supplement the total daily intake of nutrients in the diet
- Products that are intended to be ingested in tablet, capsule, softgel, gelcap, and liquid form
- Products that are not in themselves to be used as conventional foods or as the only items of a meal or diet

Unlike prescription medications (see Chapter 15), dietary supplements have been available in the market-place for years almost without restriction. However, dietary supplements now must be deemed safe for human use on the basis of information supplied to the FDA by the manufacturers. In addition, the labels on these products cannot make a direct claim, with the exception of calcium and folic acid supplements, that they can cure or prevent illnesses. However, other materials with such claims may be displayed close to the dietary supplements themselves. Further, the labels on dietary supplements must remind consumers that the FDA has not required these products to undergo the rigorous research required of prescription medications and so the FDA cannot attest to their effectiveness. Beyond this, consumers are left to themselves to decide whether to purchase and use dietary supplements.

Probiotic products, dietary supplements with live bacteria, are gaining in popularity. Although probiotics have been around for over a century, some scientists are now saying that they may help prevent or treat almost any disease from kidney stones to cancer. Probiotics are "good bugs" and they work by making the environment in the digestive system inhospitable for harmful bacteria. The U.S. sales of probiotic supplements have increased 10 to 15% over the past 5 years, reaching $170 million in 2002. Actimel is one of the biggest sellers, claiming to "help to strengthen your body's natural defenses" and enhance your immune system. Yogurt is another way to get your daily dose of probiotics as it contains lactobacillus bulgaris.[23]

Easily accessible to anyone, over 15,000 different dietary supplements can be purchased in grocery stores, drugstores, and discount stores, through mail-order catalogs, and over the Internet. Because of the great demand for these products, major pharmaceutical companies are now entering the dietary supplement field. Whether this trend leads to the development of more effective products, or to a greater effort on the part of the FDA to demand proof of effectiveness, remains to be seen. By definition, supplements are not foods, but simply "supplements." Therefore they remain free from requirements to substantiate their claims of effectiveness (as now required for functional foods).

HealthQuest Activities

One of the most valuable consumer skills you can acquire is the ability to read and interpret food labels. The Food Labeling activity in the Nutrition and Weight Control module demonstrates the purpose and importance of food labels. A tutorial outlines the steps in reading a food label, explains the terms used on food labels, and helps you evaluate health claims. The activity also lets you plan a meal and have it critiqued, using food labels as resources to guide you. Choose a food not listed in the activity, and do a nutritional comparison of five different labels for that food. Compare the ingredients on each label to determine where the differences in nutrient content may be. Research the ingredients to find out their sources, other foods or substances that contain the ingredients, and the purpose for including each ingredient.

TALKING POINTS A friend asks you about the advantages and disadvantages of taking a dietary supplement. What would you point out to your friend?

Food Safety

Technological advances in food manufacture and processing have done much to assure that the food we eat is fresh and safe. Yet there is growing concern that certain recent developments may also produce harmful effects on humans. For example the preparation, handling, and storage of food, irradiation of foods, and genetic engineering of foods all contribute to the safety of our food in terms of food contamination.

Food Poisoning

Foodborne illness or food poisoning is the result of eating contaminated food. The symptoms of food poisoning can be easily mistaken for the flu—fatigue, chills, mild fever, dizziness, headaches, upset stomach, diarrhea, and severe cramps. Illness develops within 1 to 6 hours following ingestion of the contaminated food and recovering is fairly rapid.[24] Bacteria are the culprits for most cases of food poisoning which can be the result of food not being cooked thoroughly to destroy bacteria or not keeping food cool enough to slow their growth. In addition, nearly half of all cases of food poisoning can be prevented with proper hand washing so as to not contaminate food by viruses, parasites, or toxic chemicals.

Salmonella is the second most common foodborne illness and is found mostly in raw or undercooked poultry, meat, eggs, fish, and unpasteurized milk. *Clostridium perfringens*, also called the "buffet germ," grows where there is little to no oxygen and grows fastest in large portions held at low or room temperatures. For this reason, buffet table servings should be replaced often and leftovers should be refrigerated quickly. A third type of food poisoning is botulism which is rare but often fatal. It is caused from home-canned or commercially canned food that hasn't been processed or stored properly. Some warning signs are swollen or dented cans or lids, cracked jars, loose lids, and clear liquids turned milky.

Safe Handling of Food

It is important to handle food properly to avoid food poisoning. Frequent hand washing is at the top of the list of food safety tips. Bacteria live and multiply on warm, moist hands, and hands can inadvertently transport germs from one surface to another. It is also important to clean work surfaces with hot, soapy water and keep nonfood items such as the mail, newspapers, purses, off the countertops. There are some that advocate for use of antibacterial products while others maintain that if they are overused, these products can lose their effectiveness and bacteria then become resistant to them. Utensils, dishes, cutting boards, cookware, and towels and sponges need to be washed in hot, soapy water and rinsed well.[25]

Irradiation of Food

Due to the increasing concern about contaminated meat and meat products, the first irradiated meat, ground beef, arrived in American supermarkets in early 2000. Irradiated frozen chicken was introduced more recently. Irradiation is a process that causes damage to the DNA of disease-causing bacteria such as salmonella and E. coli as well as of insects, parasites, and other organisms so that they can't reproduce. While irradiated meat has much lower bacteria levels than regular meat, irradiation doesn't destroy all bacteria in meat. In fact, irradiation actually destroys fewer bacteria than does proper cooking.[24] There is also some concern that irradiation will lull consumers into a false sense of security so that they erroneously believe that they don't have to take the usual precautions in food handling and preparation. For example, undercooking, unclean work surfaces, unwashed cooking utensils, or improper storage can still cause contamination in the meat. Some also claim that irradiated meat has a distinct off-taste and smell likening it to "singed hair."

Safe Farming Techniques

In recent decades, there has been an increased push towards ensuring better treatment of animals raised for slaughter or dairy production in the United States. As a result of recent reforms, more than half of beef cattle in North America meet their end at slaughterhouses based on innovative designs that consider the fears and inclinations of herd animals. The cages of laying hens are nearly one third larger than the old ones and the practice of starving hens for weeks at a time to stimulate egg production is beginning to diminish in use. These reforms are important to ensure more humane treatment of these animals, but are also proving beneficial to human health and food quality. It has been suggested that there is an increase in the quality of meat when animals are treated humanely, with less bruising, improved tenderness, lower incidence of dark-cutting beef, and lessened occurrence of pale, soft, and dry pork. Furthermore, the taste of eggs is significantly better if they come from humanely treated hens.

One important component in these reforms—some of which have been government mandated and others voluntarily adopted by the agricultural industry—relates to the feed given to beef cattle. The spread of bovine spongiform encephalopathy, more commonly known as Mad Cow Disease, has largely been attributed to the use of animal feed containing the protein-rich by-products of slaughtered cows, including nerve tissue, the tissue most likely to harbor the disease. Such feed—which is believed to be the primary, if not the only, way the disease could be transmitted—was banned in the United States and Canada in August 1997.[26] While the disease had been restricted to European cows, a number of cases of Mad Cow detected in American cattle in

Learning from Our Diversity

Understanding Kosher Laws

Food has been part of many religious practices and customs for centuries. Some foods have symbolic meanings related to major life experiences, and ceremonies and religious rites involving food are associated with certain events. Understanding the dietary restrictions of your friends, classmates, and colleagues can help you to be more sensitive to their needs when dining out, or when you entertain at home.

While many religions have specific dietary restrictions, perhaps the most familiar are those that govern the diets of many Jews. Foods selected and prepared according to the "Rules of Kashruth" are referred to as kosher, meaning "fit or proper." These laws dictate that no pork or shellfish shall be consumed, and all other types of meat must be meticulously cleansed of all blood. Animals that may be eaten must be slaughtered in accordance with Jewish law, with one swift stroke of a sharp blade across the throat. This method kills the animal quickly and painlessly, and is widely held to be the most humane method of slaughter. The slaughter of sick or lame animals is strictly forbidden. Combining meat and milk is not permitted, and there must be at least 6 hours between the consumption of the two. Orthodox Jewish homes maintain two sets of dishes for serving meat and for dairy products. On Saturday, the Sabbath, no cooking occurs. Fasting (no food or water) for 24 hours occurs during Yom Kippur. During Passover, no leavened bread is consumed.

For many Jews, following a kosher diet is a not merely a matter of following tradition or of being aware of what they eat. The laws governing the kosher diet are an important part of Jewish law, spelled out in the Torah. Many of these laws are in essence guidelines for safe and sanitary food; indeed, the laws governing the butchering of animals are so humane and sanitary that the federal government exempts kosher butchers and slaughterhouses from many USDA regulations.[1] For this reason, many non-Jews choose to eat only kosher meat, noting that it is not only very safe to eat, but also tastes better.[2] In the wake of the first reported cases of Mad Cow Disease in the United States at the end of 2003, many more consumers began to seek kosher beef, noting that the kosher law prohibits the slaughter of cows that cannot walk, and does not allow animals to be killed by being struck or shot in the head, which can scatter infected brain tissue through the animal's bloodstream.[3] However, it is very important to recognize that the laws go far beyond practical health concerns, and that for observant Jews, observance of these laws represents an important part of their culture and faith.

[1] *Kashrut: Jewish Dietary Laws.* The Jewish Virtual Library. http://www.usisrael.org/jsource/Judaism/kashrut/html
[2] Fernau K. "Kosher foods appealing to healthy eaters." *The Arizona Republic,* September 17, 2003.
[3] Burros M. "Warily Searching for Safer Beef." *The New York Times,* December 31, 2003.

---

late 2003 encouraged the U.S. government to impose even stricter rules to protect the nation's beef supply from the disease, including banning the butchering of sick or injured cows, banning certain animal parts from the food supply, and increasing testing on suspect animals.[27]

Eliminating animal products from feed has also proven beneficial in hens. Many consumers choose only to eat poultry and eggs from free-range, vegetarian-fed chickens, for health and safety reasons. Several companies (such as Eggland's Best) claim that their vegetarian-fed hens produce eggs that have seven times more vitamin E than regular eggs, are lower in cholesterol, have a higher unsaturated/saturated fat ratio, and contain more omega-3 fatty acids than factory-farmed eggs.[28]

Interestingly, McDonald's Corporation has been one of the champions for animal welfare reform. Since 1997, the fast-food leader has required all of its meat producers to undergo animal welfare audits, and in 1999 they conducted 100 audits in the United States, and in 2002, they did 500 worldwide. Because McDonald's makes up such a formidable part of the meat industry, few companies could afford to lose its business by not complying with its animal welfare standards. Thus McDonald's has been instrumental in pushing the entire industry to change its production techniques.[29] The state of Florida has also been a forerunner in pushing for animal welfare in its recent passage of a measure outlawing slow stalls, where pregnant pigs are confined in stalls 2 feet wide and 7 feet long, unable to turn around or walk for much of their 115-day pregnancy.

Genetically Modified Foods

The success of American agriculture, in terms of food quality and marketability, has been based on the ability to genetically alter food sources to improve yield, reduce production costs, and introduce new food characteristics. Today, however, genetic technology is so sophisticated that changes are being introduced faster than scientists can fully evaluate the effects of these changes. Concerned individuals and agencies in the United States and abroad called for more extensive longitudinal research into safety issues and stricter labeling requirements for genetically modified foods. In January of 2001, the FDA determined that food companies did not need to label foods as having genetically modified components, although they could inform consumers that they are "derived through biotechnology." They

Table 5.6 Recommended Dietary Changes to Reduce the Risk of Diseases and Their Complications

Change in Diet:	Reduce Fats	Control Calories	Increase Starch* and Fiber	Reduce Sodium	Control Alcohol
Reduce risk of:					
Heart disease	√	√		√	
Cancer	√	√	√		√
Stroke	√	√		√	√
Diabetes	√	√	√		
Gastrointestinal disease†	√	√	√		√

*Starch refers to complex carbohydrates provided by fruits, vegetables, and whole-grain products.
†Primarily gallbladder disease (fat), diverticular disease (fiber), and cirrhosis (alcohol).

had argued that without these measures consumers would have been at risk for unrecognized problems. Read more about genetically modified foods at the end of the chapter.

Guidelines for Dietary Health

Although dietary guidelines have been issued on many occasions, the Dietary Guidelines for Americans are the most current and widely used guidelines. The newest version appeared in June 1, 2000 as the fifth edition of *Nutrition and Your Health: Dietary Guidelines for Americans*.[30] These guidelines are directed to healthy Americans 2 years of age and older and to the health professional, who can influence public dietary practices. Information contained in these guidelines came from a variety of sources, including the Surgeon General's Report on Nutrition and Health. The most recent dietary guidelines are shown in the adjacent Star box.

Table 5.6 shows how healthful dietary changes can lead to reduced chances of developing certain major diseases. Notice that a reduction in fat and better control of caloric intake are important factors in reducing the likelihood of chronic illness.

Almost all Americans could make changes that would bring them closer to meeting these guidelines. The Changing for the Better box on page 128 presents recommendations for making healthful food choices when eating out.

Vegetarian Diets

A *vegetarian diet* relies on plant sources for all or most of the nutrients needed by the body. This approach includes a range of diets from those that allow some animal sources of nutrients to those that exclude all animal sources. Studies show that vegetarians who eat a balanced diet don't seem to have any more iron-deficient problems than do meat eaters. Although the iron in plant food is not as well absorbed as the iron in animal food, vegetarians tend to eat more of iron-containing foods and more vitamin C foods which helps with the absorption of the iron.[22] In addition, vegetarians tend to get enough calcium from either dairy foods, tofu, beans, soybeans, calcium fortified cereals, and vegetables such as broccoli. There has been some concern about a vitamin B-12 deficiency as animal foods are the best source for B-12 and plant foods don't naturally contain the vitamin. However, soy foods such as some form of tempeh may contain vitamin B-12, although again this is not as biologically active as the source in animal foods. Many soy products are fortified with vitamin B-12 as well. It is important also to note that the liver stores so much B-12 that it would take years to become deficient in this vitamin.[22] Three types of vegetarian diets, beginning with the least restrictive, are summarized below.

Dietary Guidelines for Americans

- Aim for healthy weight.
- Exercise at least 30 minutes each day.
- Make food choices based on the U.S. Department of Agriculture *food pyramid* diagram.
- Eat a variety of grains daily, especially whole grains.
- Eat a variety of fruits and vegetables daily.
- Keep food safe to eat.
- Choose a diet that is low in saturated fat and cholesterol and moderate in total fat.
- Choose beverages and foods to moderate your intake of sugars.
- Choose and prepare foods with less salt.
- If you drink alcoholic beverages, do so in moderation.

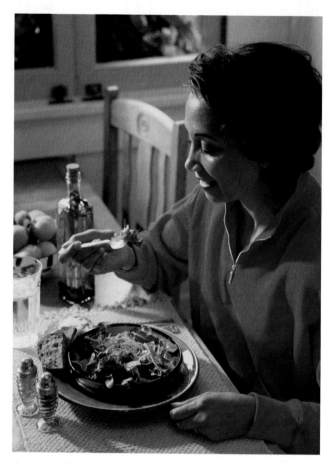

Over 12 million Americans are vegetarian.

TALKING POINTS What do you think about vegetarian diets? If you were to follow a vegetarian diet, which one would you be more likely to choose?

Ovolactovegetarian Diet

Depending on the particular pattern of consuming eggs (*ovo*) and milk (*lacto*) or using one but not the other, an **ovolactovegetarian diet** can be a very sound approach to healthful eating for adults (see Figure 5-5 for an Ovolactovegetarian Food Guide Pyramid). Ovolactovegetarian diets provide the body with the essential amino acids and limit the high intake of fats involved in more conventional diets. The exclusion of meat as a protein source lowers the total fat intake, and the consumption of milk or eggs allows an adequate amount of saturated fat to remain in the diet. The consistent use of vegetable products as the primary source of nutrients complies with the current dietary recommendations for an increase in overall carbohydrates, complex carbohydrates, and fiber. Most vegetarians in the United States fit into this category. Vegetarians who do consume dairy products face challenges when making food choices if they wish to avoid other animal products in their food.

Because most cheese is made with rennet, a coagulating agent that usually comes from stomachs of slaughtered newly born calves, many vegetarians eliminate cheese from their diet or opt for rennetless cheese. Vegetarian cheeses are manufactured using rennet from either fungal or bacterial sources. Similarly, yogurt is often made with gelatin derived from animal ligaments, skins, tendon, and bones (gelatin is also found in marshmallows, candy such as jelly beans and candy corn, poptarts, and a variety of other foods).

It has become somewhat easier to follow a vegetarian diet as stores have begun offering organic vegetarian items that do not contain these animal products. However, it can be difficult to avoid all animal products without being an avid reader and knowledgeable consumer. For example, McDonald's recently acknowledged it failed to disclose the use of beef flavoring in its fries and hash browns.

Lactovegetarian Diet

People who include dairy products in their diet but no other animal products, including eggs, are *lactovegetarians*. A **pesco-vegetarian** eats fish, dairy products, and eggs along with plant foods.

Vegan Vegetarian Diet

A **vegan vegetarian diet** is one in which not only meat but also other animal products, such as milk, cheese, and eggs, are removed from the diet. When compared with the ovolactovegetarian diet, the vegan diet requires a higher level of nutritional understanding to avoid nutritional inadequacies.

One potential difficulty is that of obtaining all of the essential amino acids. Since a single plant source does not contain all the essential amino acids, the vegan must learn to consistently employ a complementary diet. By carefully combining various grains, seeds, and legumes, amino acid deficiency can be prevented.

In addition to the potential amino acid deficiency, the vegan could have some difficulty in maintaining the necessary intake of vitamin B_{12}. Possible ramifications of

> ### Key Terms
>
> **ovolactovegetarian diet** a diet that excludes all meat but does include the consumption of eggs and dairy products.
>
> **pesco-vegetarian** a vegetarian diet that includes fish, dairy products, and eggs along with plant foods.
>
> **vegan vegetarian diet** a vegetarian diet that excludes all animal products, including eggs and dairy products.

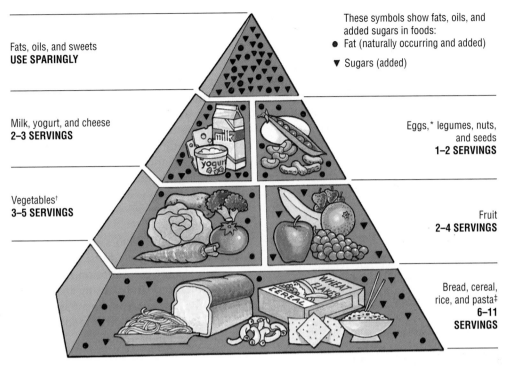

A Food Pyramid for Ovolactovegetarians¶,‖

* Lactovegetarians can omit eggs from this pyramid.
† Include one dark green or leafy variety daily.
‡ One serving of a vitamin- and mineral-enriched cereal is recommended.
¶ Contains about 75 g of protein and 1650 calories.
‖ Base serving sizes on those listed for the Food Guide Pyramid (see Chapter 5).

Figure 5-5 A food pyramid for ovolactovegetarians (vegetarians who include eggs and dairy products in their diet).

inadequate B$_{12}$ intake include depression, anemia, back pain, and menstrual irregularity. Vegans often have difficulty maintaining adequate intakes of iron, zinc, and calcium.[1] Calcium intake must be monitored closely by the vegan. In addition, vitamin D deficiencies can occur. Supplements and daily exposure to sunshine will aid in maintaining adequate levels of this vitamin.

Food Allergies

There is a difference between being intolerant to certain foods and being allergic to particular foods. **Food intolerance** means that a food upsets your intestines, usually due to an enzyme deficiency. A lactase deficiency, for example, causes lactose intolerance. Lactose intolerance affects 20% of Caucasian Americans, 75% of African Americans, and 50% of Hispanic Americans. Gluten intolerance (found in wheat, rye, barley, and perhaps oats) affects 1 out of every 150 Americans and can cause malnutrition, premature osteoporosis, colon cancer, thyroid disease, diabetes, arthritis, miscarriage, and birth defects.

A **food allergy** means that the body's disease fighting immune system is mistakenly called into action, creating unpleasant and sometimes life-threatening symptoms. Peanuts, milk, eggs, shellfish, tree nuts, fish, soy, and wheat account for 90% of food allergies. Eight percent of children and 2% of adults have food allergies. For some members of this group, food-based allergies may be serious or even life threatening.

Because food allergies generally develop slowly, initial symptoms may not be fully recognized or even associated

---

Key Terms

food intolerance an adverse reaction to a specific food which does not involve the immune system; usually caused by an enzyme deficiency.

food allergy a reaction in which the immune system attacks an otherwise harmless food or ingredient; allergic reactions can range from mildly unpleasant to life threatening.

with the food. It takes three exposures to the allergic food to obtain a significant food allergy reaction. The first time someone eats a food she or he is allergic to, they may have little to no reaction. The second time an individual eats this food, he or she will most likely have a more observable reaction such as breaking out in hives, itching, runny nose, burning in the mouth, and wheezing. The third exposure can bring on a full-blown reaction, which for peanut allergies, among others, can result in death within minutes. There is no cure for food allergies, and the treatment is to avoid these foods and for the food allergy person to carry an epi-pin (epinephrine) with him or her at all times.

Nutrition and the Older Adult

Nutritional needs change as adults age. Age-related changes to the structure and function of the body are primarily responsible for such altered nutritional requirements.

Changing for the Better

Do's and Don'ts for Food Safety

I keep reading about food poisoning and food contamination in restaurants and even from home cooked meals. Is there any way to lessen my chances of contracting food poisoning?

The following are some do's and don'ts for food safety:

1. Don't thaw food on the countertop—keep it in a covered container in the refrigerator or thaw it out in the microwave.
2. Don't leave food left out of the refrigerator for longer than 2 hours.
3. Don't use wooden cutting boards with deep grooves or knife scars.
4. Don't marinate food at room temperature—marinate in the refrigerator.
5. Do put groceries away as soon as you get home and don't make other stops first.
6. Do use two different plates for raw and grilled meat.
7. Do use different spoons to stir and taste the food.
8. Do refrigerate leftovers from restaurants immediately.
9. Do use different knives to cut raw meat and chop vegetables.
10. Do store food in an airtight container. Don't store food in open cans or on uncovered dishes.
11. Do wash fresh fruits and vegetables, even if you are throwing away the rind or peels, as cutting through the produce can carry bacteria from the outside surface to the inside of the produce.
12. Do rinse poultry and seafood in cold water.

Source: Duyff R. *American Dietetic Association Complete Food and Nutrition Guide,* 2nd edition. Hoboken, New Jersey: John Wiley & Sons, Inc., 2002.

These changes can involve the teeth, salivary glands, taste buds, oral muscles, gastric acid production, and peristaltic action. In addition, chronic constipation resulting from changes in gastrointestinal tract function can decrease the older adult's interest in eating.

The progressive lowering of the body's basal metabolism is another factor that will eventually influence the dietary patterns of older adults. As energy requirements fall, the body gradually senses the need for less food. In addition a tendency to decrease activity levels also occurs with aging. Because of this decreased need for calories, nutrient density—the nutritional value of food relative to calories supplied—is an important consideration for the elderly.

Psychosocial factors also alter the role of food in the lives of many older adults. Social isolation, depression, chronic alcohol consumption, loss of income, transportation limitations, and housing are lifestyle factors that can lessen the ease and enjoyment associated with the preparation and consumption of food. Consequently, a person's food intake might decrease.

International Nutritional Concerns

Nutritional concerns in the United States are centered on overnutrition, including fat density and excessive caloric intake. In contrast, in many areas of the world the main concern is the limited quantity and quality of food. Reasons for these problems are many, including the weather, the availability of arable land, religious practices, political unrest, war, social infrastructure, and material and technical shortages. Underlying nearly all of these factors, however, is unabated population growth.

To increase the availability of food to countries whose demand for food outweighs their ability to produce it, a number of steps have been suggested, including the following:

- Increase the yield of land currently under cultivation.
- Increase the amount of land under cultivation.
- Increase animal production on land not suitable for cultivation.
- Use water (seas, lakes, and ponds) more efficiently for the production of food.
- Develop unconventional foods through the application of technology.
- Improve nutritional practices through education.

Little progress is being made despite impressive technological breakthroughs in agriculture and food technology (such as a wide array of genetically modified seeds and soybean-enhanced infant foods), the efforts of governmental programs, and the support of the Food and

Agricultural Organization of the United Nations and the U.S. Department of Agriculture. Particularly in Third World countries, where fertility rates are two to four times higher than those of the United States, annual food production needs to increase between 2.7% and 3.9% to keep up with population needs. With the world population now at 6.1 billion, and projected to reach 9 billion by 2070 before dipping to 8.4 billion in 2100,[31] food production in the coming decades may need to be increased beyond these estimates.

Taking Charge of Your Health

Smart Supermarket Store Shopping

- Make a shopping list before you go and stick to it!
- Don't go grocery shopping when you are hungry.
- Shop just once a week, don't make special trips.
- Read the food labels and check for the percentage of fat, sodium, sugar, etc.
- Take note of the "sell by" or expiration date. The items stocked towards the back are usually the newest.
- For the single shopper, look for foods sold in single servings: juice, yogurt, frozen meals, soup, and pudding, for example.
- Buy fresh fruits and vegetables over canned and frozen. If buying canned or frozen fruits and vegetables, look for ones without added sugar, fats, salt, or sauces.
- Choose brown rice over white, whole wheat over white bread.
- Skip the ramen noodle soups as they are usually flash-cooked in oil and high in fat.
- Avoid giant muffins, bagels, and donuts, and select the smaller sized ones.

- Meat labeled "select" is leaner than meat graded "choice."
- Leaner cuts of beef are flank, sirloin, and tenderloin. The leanest pork is fresh, canned, cured and broiled ham, Canadian bacon, pork tenderloin, rib chops, and roast.
- Ground turkey and chicken can contain the skin which makes it higher in fat and calories. For a lower fat option, look for ground turkey or chicken. Ground turkey breast is lower still.
- Buy water-packed tuna and sardines rather than those packed in oil.
- Buy low-fat or fat-free milk rather than 2% or whole milk.
- Look for low-fat cheeses, sour cream, mayonnaise, and cream cheese which are labeled "part skim," "reduced fat," or "fat free."
- Buy canola oil rather than corn oil, or use nonstick cooking spray.
- Consider buying cholesterol-free or reduced cholesterol egg substitutes especially if you don't use eggs very often as they tend to last longer than fresh eggs.

Source: Kirby J. *Dieting for Dummies.* New York: Wiley Publishing Co., 1998.

Summary

- Carbohydrates, fat, and protein supply the body with calories.
- Carbohydrates differ on the basis of their molecular makeup, with sugars being the least complex and starches the most complex.
- Fat is important for nutritional health beyond serving as the body's primary means of storage of excess calories.
- Saturated fats, including trans-fatty acids, should be carefully limited because of their association with chronic diseases.
- Dietary intake of cholesterol should be limited through careful monitoring of food choices.
- The food pyramid provides important dietary guidelines for a balanced diet.
- Protein supplies the body with amino acids needed to construct its own protein.
- When few foods of animal origin are consumed, incomplete protein sources must be carefully balanced to provide complete protein in the diet.

- Vitamins serve as catalysts for body responses and are found in water soluble and fat soluble forms.
- The use of vitamin supplements is desirable for some people, but extensive use of food supplements can be dangerous.
- Minerals are incorporated into various tissues of the body and participate in regulatory functions within the body.
- An adequate amount of water and other fluids is required by the body daily and is obtained from a variety of food sources, including beverages.
- Fiber is undigestible plant material and has two forms, water soluble and water insoluble.
- Food allergies can be life threatening, and currently there is no cure for them. The most common food allergies are: peanut, milk, egg, shellfish, tree nuts, fish, soy, and wheat.
- Foods are currently classified into six groups, although recommendations regarding the needed

number of daily servings have been given for only five of them.

- Fat-free or low-fat foods can be more calorie dense than anticipated.
- Fast foods should play only a limited role in daily food intake because of their high fat density and their high levels of sugar and sodium.
- Phytochemicals, capable of protecting the body from carcinogens or free radicals, are now being identified in many types of vegetables.
- Functional foods are capable of assisting in the prevention of specific health conditions.
- Food additives enhance the overall quality and convenient use of our food supply.
- New food labels provide considerably more information for the consumer than labels used previously.

- Dietary supplements are taken by millions of Americans, although their effectiveness is uncertain.
- Controversy exists about the application of new food technologies such as irradiation, genetic engineering, and animal welfare.
- Current dietary recommendations focus on the role of fat, saturated fat, starch, and sodium in health and disease.
- Ovolactovegetarianism, lactovegetarianism, vegan vegetarianism, and pesco-vegetarianism are different forms of vegetarianism.
- Nutrient density plays an important role in the management of caloric intake for people of all ages, particularly older adults.
- A variety of factors contribute to malnourishment in many areas of the world.

Review Questions

1. Which nutrients supply the body with calories?
2. How do sugars differ structurally from starches?
3. What is the function of fat in nutritional health besides serving as the body's primary means of storage for excess calories? What is the basis of our current concern about saturated fats, cholesterol, and trans-fatty acids?
4. What is the principal role of protein in the body? How can complete protein be obtained by people who eat few or no animal products?
5. Which vitamins are water soluble and which are fat soluble? What is the current perception regarding the need for vitamin supplementation? Which vitamins are regarded as antioxidants?
6. What are food allergies and which are the most common ones?
7. What functions do minerals have in the body? What is a trace element?
8. What are the two principal forms of fiber, and how does each of them contribute to health?

9. How many glasses of water per day are currently recommended?
10. What method of grouping foods is now used?
11. What are the current dietary recommendations regarding fat, saturated fat, starch, and sodium intake?
12. How can fat-free or low-fat foods be both low in nutritional density and high in caloric density?
13. What are functional foods, and how are they different from dietary supplements? Which has been empowered by the FDA to make health claims?
14. What information can be obtained from our current food labels?
15. If additives were eliminated from our food, what lifestyle adjustments would the public be forced to make?
16. What are an ovolactovegetarian diet and semivegetarianism, and how do they differ from a vegan diet?
17. What is nutrient density, and how does it relate to the aging process?

References

1. Wardlaw GM, Kessel M. *Perspective in nutrition,* ed 5, McGraw-Hill, 2002.
2. Wardlaw GM. *Contemporary nutrition: issues and insights,* McGraw-Hill, 1999.
3. *Caring for your school-age child: 5–12,* American Academy of Pediatrics, 2001.
4. Kummerow FA, Zhou Q, Mahfouz MM. Effect of trans-fatty acids on calcium influx into human arterial endothelial cells, *Am J Clin Nutr* 70(5):832–838, 1999.
5. Duyff R. *American Dietetic Association Complete Food and Nutrition Guide,* 2nd edition, Hoboken, New Jersey: John Wiley & Sons, Inc. 2002.
6. National Institutes of Health. *Practical Guide to the Identification, Evaluation and Treatment of Overweight and Obesity in Adults,* 2001.

7. Young VR. Soy protein in relation to human protein and amino acid nutrition, *J Am Diet Assoc* 91, 828–835, 1991.

8. Anderson J, Johnstone R, Cook-Newell M. Meta-analysis of the effects of soy protein intake on serum lipids, *N Engl J Med* 333, 276–282, 1995.

9. Greenberg ER, Sporn MB. Antioxidant vitamins, cancer, and cardiovascular disease, *N Engl J Med* 334(18):1189–1190, 1996.

10. Jacques PF, et al. The effect of folic acid fortification on plasma folate and total homocysteine concentrations, *N Engl J Med* 340(19):1449–1454, 1999.

11. Scariati PD, et al. Water supplementation of infants in the first month of life, *Arch Pediatr Adolesc Med* 151(8):830–832, 1997.

12. Children, water, and fluoride: AAPD parent information, American Academy of Pediatric Dentistry.

13. Sears W. and Sears M. *The Family Nutrition Book,* New York: Little, Brown and Co., 1999.

14. American Cancer Society. *Cancer facts and figures—* The Association, 2001.

15. Marcus, Eric. On the Fast Track to Health. *Newsday,* p. B14, January 7, 2004.

16. Willett W. *Eat, Drink and Be Healthy,* New York: Free Press, 2001.

17. Waladkhani AR, Clemens MR. Effect of dietary phytochemicals on cancer, *Int J Mol Med* 1(4): 747–753, 1998.

18. Fransworth ER. What we are trying to do? *Medicinal Food News* 1(1):1–6, 1999.

19. FDA approves new health claim for soy protein and coronary heart disease [FDA talk paper], U.S. Food and Drug Administration Center for Food Safety and Applied Nutrition, October 20, 1999.

20. Kurtzweil P. Staking a claim to good health, *FDA Consumer,* November–December 1998.

21. Insel P, Turner E, Ross D. *Nutrition,* Sudbury, MA: Jones and Barlett Publishers, 2002.

22. Dietary Supplement Health and Education Act of 1994, U.S. Food and Drug Administration, Center for Food Safety and Applied Nutrition, 1 December 1995.

23. A bug for what's bugging you, in *USA Today,* D-1, July 9, 2003.

24. The Truth about Irradiated Meat, *Consumer Reports,* 34–37, August, 2003.

25. Williams S and Schlenker E. *Essentials of Nutrients and Diet Therapy,* 8th edition, St. Louis, MO: Mosby Inc., 2003.

26. Oppel RA, Jr. Infected Cow Old Enough to Have Eaten Now-Banned Feed. *The New York Times,* December 30, 2003.

27. Grady D. U.S. Imposes Stricter Safety Rules for Preventing Mad Cow Disease. *The New York Times,* December 31, 2003.

28. Corporate Website, *http://www.eggland.com*

29. Food Sellers Push Animal Welfare, *USA Today,* August 13, 2003.

30. U.S. Department of Agriculture, U.S. Department of Health and Human Services. June 2000.

31. Lutz W, Sanderson W, Scherbov S. The end of the world population growth, *Nature* 412(6846): 543–545, 2001.

As We Go to Press

How would you like to be part of an experiment in which all you eat for an entire month is McDonald's food? In our fast paced society, many people tend to eat out at fast-food restaurants much of the time eating on the run. Thirty-three year old filmmaker Morgan Spurlock decided to make a documentary called, SuperSize Me, to look at the potential consequences of America's tendency to order bigger portion sizes.

Spurlock supersized all of his orders and ate three meals a day at McDonald's for an entire month and filmed his experiences. At 6'2", Spurlock gained 25 lbs and his cholesterol went from 168 to 230 within the month. Typically 40–70% of the calories in fast-foods are from fat, so it is not hard to see how Spurlock had these results. After three weeks of this fast-food diet, he was complaining of "pounding headaches," his liver was at toxic levels, and his sex drive had dramatically decreased. Spurlock and his physicians were shocked at how rapidly he became dramatically ill.

Recently McDonald's announced it is phasing out Supersize fries and drinks in its more than 13,000 U.S. restaurants and will stop selling them altogether by year's end, except during promotions. McDonald's denied that the award winning documentary "SuperSize Me" nor the two lawsuits claiming McDonald's hid the health risks associated with eating Big Macs and Chicken McNuggets had anything to do with this decision. They contend that the move is part of their "Eat Smart, Be Active" initiative in an attempt to revive sales.

With obesity on the rise and 35% of food consumed by Americans eaten away from home, it is more important than ever to make healthy choices in eating out such as those suggested in the "Changing for the Better" box on page 125.

Sources: My Month at Mickey D's. *People* Magazine, February 9, 2004. McDonald's Menu to Go on Diet in 2005. *ABC News,* March 3, 2004.

genetically modified food

Chances are you've had it for breakfast. And lunch. And dinner. It is now virtually impossible for Americans to avoid eating genetically modified (GM) foods, or what the British tabloids call "Frankenfood."

Britain's Prince Charles proclaims that he would never eat the stuff and won't stand for it being grown on his land.[1] In Britain and throughout Europe, public fears about GM foods are running high and have provoked a trade war with the United States. Americans, however, appear only dimly aware of GM foods, and Kraft's million taco-shell recall in September 2000 didn't prove to be the tide-turning cataclysm that some GM critics had hoped for. The taco shells contained traces of corn meal from StarLink, a genetically engineered variety of corn that hadn't been approved for human consumption, but no one suffered harm from eating the shells. Nevertheless, in the worst-case scenario, allergens or other harmful substances, added to food by design or accident, could have found their way into our stomachs.[2]

Since the mid 1990s, armed with new knowledge about DNA and how it functions, scientists have been able to manipulate the genetic code of organisms that are food sources and have created new strains of plants and animals capable of growing larger in less time on less suitable soil. Some new plant strains can do this while also resisting insect pests.

Farmers have long engaged in "traditional genetics," favoring seeds from plants with the most desirable characteristics or crossbreeding closely related species. Scientists have tried to speed things up by exposing plants to chemicals and radiation. These ongoing experiments produce hundreds of mutations among genes, some of which may be useful.

Genetic engineering, in contrast, is very specific. It allows scientists to select a single gene for a single characteristic and insert that stretch of DNA into another organism, or even another species. The ability to crossbreed diverse forms of life has had a profound effect on U.S. agriculture and on the food we purchase in the grocery store. An example is the Flavr-Savr tomato, developed by Calgene to soften more slowly, meaning it can stay on the vine longer and develop a fuller taste. Its longer shelf life also reduces waste.

The percentage of genetically modified seed is now estimated to approach 40% to 60% of all U.S. planting, designed either to make the crops resistant to weedkillers or to produce their own pesticides. Bioengineered corn and soybeans in particular are used as ingredients in a wide range of processed food, from soft drinks and beer to chips and breakfast cereal. Genetically modified organisms are fed to farm animals. Even health-food products like tofu and canola oil often contain genetically modified ingredients.

What Are the Potential Health Risks?

Genetically engineered crops hold down food production costs and reduce the need for pesticides and herbicides. Modified foods in the works are more nutritious and flavorful, and productive grains, drought-resistant crops, caffeine-free coffee beans, and even plants that produce drugs and vaccines have been developed.

While the potential benefits of higher-yielding GM food and a new revolution in agricultural practices appear indisputable, serious concerns have also arisen. Biotechnology foes warn that we do not know enough about the way genes operate and interact to be sure of the outcome of any modification. They worry that alterations could accidentally lead to substances that are poisonous or that trigger allergies.

Critics fear that the use of DNA from plant viruses and bacteria in the modification of crops may also somehow trigger disease. They also argue that antiobiotic-resistant genes could be passed to the microorganisms that make us sick. If this happened, we might not have the drugs necessary to fight back.[3]

Environmental concerns are also an issue. The green lobby (that is, environmentalists working in the political arena) is worried about genes that confer herbicide and insect resistance. They believe some of these genes could "escape" and be transferred to other crops, resulting in the emergence of "superweeds." They fear this leakage could cause the disappearance of familar species of insects and birds as food chains are damaged.

In addition, the corporations at the forefront of GM food production are also the world's biggest producers of agrochemicals. Critics claim these companies are trying to handcuff farmers by attempting to tie them into deals where they have little choice but to buy the GM seed and the designer chemicals to go with it.

How Do Bioengineers Counter These Objections?

The biotechnology industry claims that there is no evidence of any GM food causing serious ill effects. Proponents point out that many of our conventional food products have gotten to grocery stores only after their non-GM, raw ingredients have been treated to remove undesirable or toxic substances.[3]

While genetic modification may result in the emergence of new allergens, so too may conventional plant breeding, say GM defenders. The new technology holds out the possibility of engineering such problems out of food, however.

Use of DNA from plant viruses and bacteria presents minimal risk, precisely because we are not plants. Further, genetic modifications allow us to improve the flavor, texture, nutritional value, and shelf life of food. It could boost the vitamin content of fruits and vegetables, incorporate anticancer substances, and reduce our exposure to less healthy fats and oils. A recent example of genetically engineered food is "miracle" rice with higher levels of vitamin A, developed with the hope that rice with boosted nutritional value will stave off illness in developing countries.

Proponents also argue that GM technology offers a chance to recover biodiversity, since GM crops will require fewer chemicals that have low toxicity, are rapidly degraded, and stay in the soil rather than being washed into streams and rivers. At the same time these crops will produce higher yields, reducing pressure on remaining uncultivated habitats. Scientists also are investigating plants that may be modified to produce new plastics and biofuels that would be kinder to the environment than oil-based products.

Some companies are bowing to perceived consumer pressure by shying away from genetically modified ingredients. Baby food manufacturers Gerber and Heinz have removed themselves from the debate by saying no to genetically modified corn and soybeans, at least for now. Frito-Lay (owned by PepsiCo) stopped using engineered corn in its chips. McDonald's has asked suppliers to stop shipping genetically altered potatoes, as has McCain Foods, the world's largest producer of french fries.[4]

Many of these companies are not actually abandoning biotechnology, however. PepsiCo, Frito-Lay's parent company, still uses corn syrup made from GM crops for its soft drinks. And McDonald's still cooks its fries in oil made from genetically altered corn and soy.[4] According to big food producers, GM crops are so pervasive, there's simply no method to segregate them from other crops. In many instances, food manufacturers may not even know which genetically modified ingredients are contained in their products. As Pillsbury has noted in a written statement, "Many of our products contain food ingredients derived from soy (soy oil, soy protein, soy sauce) and corn (corn starch, corn oil, high fructose corn syrup), all of which could have been produced using genetic modification. Since soy and corn are managed as commodity ingredients in the United States, it is possible that traditional and genetically modified products could become commingled during harvest, storage, and processing."[1]

Nobody, from farmers to grain handlers to Kraft Foods executives, could explain how StarLink got mixed into corn meal meant for taco shells. And critics were more alarmed that the tests that detected its presence were administered not by Kraft or others along the production line, nor by government inspectors, but by a private company working for the Genetically Engineered Food Alert, a volunteer coalition of biotechnology skeptics and foes.[2]

Kraft now favors a more aggressive federal policy on testing GM foods and assuring their purity, including a requirement that developers of new crops provide an easy-to-use test for identifying GM material in food products. Since grain handlers claim it's not possible to fully segregate one type of corn from all others, Kraft also proposes that the government ban the planting of any food crop not certified for humans.[2] That a major food company is proposing such steps suggests that the food industry is realizing that growing public unease about GM food demands something more than companies' assurances about its safety.

Britain, Japan, Australia, Italy, and a dozen other nations currently require labels on foods containing genetically altered ingredients. U.S. regulators so far have rejected pressure for similar labeling requirements (with the exception of organic food products), saying the foods are no different from those grown with conventional crops. The Food and Drug Administration is expected to issue voluntary labeling guidelines for U.S. companies that wish to say a food does or does not contain GM ingredients. Critics, however, say that consumers need a clear choice at the grocery store. In response, Greenpeace has issued a "shopping list" that includes thousands of brand-name cereals, snacks, frozen dinners, and other foods that contain genetically altered corn, soybeans, and other ingredients. The "True Food Shopping List" is posted on the Internet (**www.truefoodnow.org**), along with a list of foods that do not contain gene-spliced ingredients, to help American consumers avoid genetically engineered food.

In Western society, our overriding concern is quality, safety, and consumers' rights to make informed choices about what they eat, yet Americans readily accept drugs and medicines that have been modified and rarely think twice about swallowing a pill for the slightest ailment, often seizing on new research before it has been proven. If foods can be modified to improve the quality of our lives, do you object to biotechnology being applied to agriculture?

For Discussion . . .

Should labeling of genetically modified foods be required? Why or why not? Do you think a moratorium should be imposed on GM crops until long-term studies prove them safe, or do you believe the potential nutritional and environmental benefits outweigh the risks?

References

1. Longman PJ. The curse of Frankenfood. *U.S. News & World Report,* 26 July 1999.
2. Editorial. Taco-shell recall—a mishap that could have been worse. *Minneapolis-St. Paul Star Tribune,* 29 September 2000.
3. Genetically-modified Q&A, *BBC News,* 6 April 1999. **http://news.bbc.co.uk**
4. Schueller G. Seeds of change: understanding the GM food revolution. *Environmental News Network* 29 September 2000. **http://enn.com**

personal assessment

rate your plate

Take a closer look at yourself—your current food decisions and your lifestyle. Think about your typical eating pattern and food decisions.

Do You . . .

	Usually	Sometimes	Never
Consider nutrition when you make food choices?	❑	❑	❑
Try to eat regular meals (including breakfast), rather than skip or skimp on some?	❑	❑	❑
Choose nutritious snacks?	❑	❑	❑
Try to eat a variety of foods?	❑	❑	❑
Include new-to-you foods in meals and snacks?	❑	❑	❑
Try to balance your energy (calorie) intake with your physical activity?	❑	❑	❑

Now for the Details

Do You . . .

	Usually	Sometimes	Never
Eat at least 6 servings* of grain products daily?	❑	❑	❑
Eat at least 3 servings* of vegetables daily?	❑	❑	❑
Eat at least 2 servings* of fruits daily?	❑	❑	❑
Consume at least 2 servings* of milk, yogurt, or cheese daily?	❑	❑	❑
Go easy on higher-fat foods?	❑	❑	❑
Go easy on sweets?	❑	❑	❑
Drink 8 or more cups of fluids daily?	❑	❑	❑
Limit alcoholic beverages (no more than 1 daily for a woman or 2 for a man)?	❑	❑	❑

Score Yourself

Usually = 2 points
Sometimes = 1 point
Never = 0 points

If you scored . . .

24 or more points—Healthful eating seems to be your fitness habit already. Still, look for ways to stick to a healthful eating plan—and to make a "good thing" even better.

16 to 23 points—You're on track. A few easy changes could help you make your overall eating plan healthier.

9 to 15 points—Sometimes you eat smart—but not often enough to be your "fitness best."

0 to 8 points—For your good health, you're wise to rethink your overall eating style. Take it gradually—step by step!

Whatever your score, make moves for healthful eating. Gradually turn your "nevers" into "sometimes" and your "sometimes" into "usually."

Adapted from *The American Dietetic Association's Monthly Nutrition Companion: 31 Days to a Healthier Lifestyle,* Chronimed Publishing, 1997.

Sample Serving Sizes
Bread, cereals, rice, and pasta group—6 to 11 servings daily:
1 slice (1 oz.) enriched or whole-grain bread
½ hamburger roll, bagel, English muffin, or pita
½ cup cooked rice or pasta
1 ounce (1 cup) ready-to-eat cereal

Vegetable group 1—3 to 5 servings daily:
½ cup chopped raw, non-leafy vegetables
½ cup cooked vegetables
1 small baked potato (3 ounces)
¾ cup vegetable juice

Fruit group—2 to 4 servings daily:
1 medium fruit (apple, orange, banana, peach)
¾ cup fruit juice
½ cup canned, frozen, or cooked fruit

Milk, yogurt, and cheese group—2 to 3 servings daily:
1 cup milk, buttermilk, or yogurt
1½ ounces natural cheese (cheddar, mozzarella, Swiss)
1 cup frozen yogurt

Meat, poultry, fish, beans, eggs, and nuts group—2 to 3 servings daily:
2 to 3 ounces cooked lean meat, poultry, or fish
½ cup cooked legumes (equals 1 ounce meat)
1 egg (equals 1 ounce meat)

Fats, oils, and sweets—use sparingly:
sugars
salad dressings
oils
cream
butter
soft drinks

*Serving sizes vary depending on the food and food group

personal assessment

are you feeding your feelings?

Sometimes people use food as a way of coping with their emotions and problems. To identify how you might be using food as a coping strategy and what feelings you tend to associate with eating, complete the following inventory.

1 = Never

2 = Rarely

3 = Occasionally

4 = Often

5 = Always

1. _____ Do you eat when you are angry?
2. _____ When you feel annoyed, do you turn to food?
3. _____ If someone lets you down, do you eat to comfort yourself?
4. _____ When you are having a bad day, do you notice that you eat more?
5. _____ Do you eat to cheer yourself up?
6. _____ Do you use food as a way of avoiding tasks you don't want to do?
7. _____ Do you view food as your friend when you are feeling lonely?
8. _____ Is food a way for you to comfort yourself when your life seems empty?
9. _____ When you are feeling upset, do you turn to food to calm yourself down?
10. _____ Do you eat more when you are anxious, worried, or stressed?
11. _____ Does eating help you to cope with feeling overwhelmed?
12. _____ Do you eat more when you are going through big changes or transitions in your life?
13. _____ Do you reward yourself with food?
14. _____ When you think you have done something wrong, do you punish yourself by eating?
15. _____ When you are feeling badly about yourself, do you eat more?
16. _____ When you feel discouraged about your efforts to improve yourself, do you eat more, thinking "what's the use of trying"?

_____ TOTAL SCORE

Interpretation

If you scored between . . .

0–13   You don't eat to cope with your emotions. Your eating may not be related to your emotional state. However, you may avoid eating when you are upset or having trouble coping with your feelings. You may run away from food rather than running to food to cope.

14–66   Although you fall in the average range, you may use food to deal with specific situations or feelings such as anger, loneliness, or boredom. See the breakdown of scores below to identify how you may be using food to cope with particular feelings.

67 and above   You run to food to cope with your emotions, and you may want to consider developing other ways of appropriately expressing your feelings.

If you answered "4" or "5" to most of questions #1–#4, this can be indicative of eating when you are angry.

If you answered "4" or "5" to most of questions #5–#8, this can be indicative of eating when you are lonely or bored.

If you answered "4" or "5" to most of questions #9–#12, this can be an indication that you are a stress eater.

If you answered "4" or "5" to most of questions #13–#16, this can be an indication that you are using food to cope with feelings of low self-esteem and self-worth.

chapter six

maintaining a healthy weight

Online Learning Center Resources

www.mhhe.com/hahn7e

Log on to our Online Learning Center (OLC) for access to these additional resources:

- Chapter key terms and definitions
- Learning objectives
- Student interactive question-and-answer sites
- Self-scoring chapter quiz
- Online assessments
- Key term flash cards

Talking It Over

Is Fat a Feeling?

Have you ever said or heard someone say, "I feel fat"? Is fat a feeling? Typically "fat" refers to our weight and body composition and is not a feeling such as anger, happiness, or sadness. However, we often say that we feel fat when we are feeling one of these emotions. When you are "feeling fat," think about how you felt the day before. If you felt better yesterday and your weight has not changed, why are you feeling fatter and worse today? Most likely, there is something bothering you other than your weight and appearance—sometimes it seems easier to focus on something concrete and physical (such as weight) rather than on emotions that are less tangible and obvious. Perhaps you are really feeling unloved, hurt, angry, annoyed, bored, overwhelmed, or stressed.

When you are "feeling fat" or "having a fat day," you might ask yourself, "What is bothering me? What am I upset about?" It might be helpful to write in a journal about your feelings or talk with a trusted friend or family member about your feelings.

Eye on the Media

Buy or Bye to Quick and Easy Weight Loss

What's on TV tonight? A minute of channel surfing tells you that it's bodies—bodies conditioned through athletics, dance, or grueling training and drug enhancement, or bodies thinned to anorexic proportions to show off the latest fashions. Tune in to the cable medical channel and watch a liposuction procedure being done to remove excess fat. Or watch a program in which "ordinary people" volunteer to have their bodies made over to be "rock star bodies" in a 3-month period.

Commercials for weight loss products and procedures abound on television and in newspapers and magazines; people are further bombarded with email offers and Internet pop-up ads promoting various weight loss products. With all of these ads, it's important to look carefully at the small print disclaimers that say "results may vary" or "results not typical." The Federal Trade Commission (FTC) has issued a warning to be

Eye on the Media *continued*

wary of advertisements for weight loss products and services that make "grossly exaggerated claims" such as "I lost 120 pounds in 7 weeks and didn't change my eating habits at all. I just took this diet pill." The FTC recently reviewed 300 weight loss ads and found that 55% made claims that were likely very false or lacked adequate proof. Since 1990, the agency has filed 93 cases against false and misleading weight loss claims involving over-the-counter drugs, supplements, weight loss programs, and exercise equipment. The report states, "The problem is getting worse not better."

In addition, lawsuits have been filed against The Health Laboratory of North American which produces Berry Trim because it has been sending letters to unsuspecting people advertising a weight loss drug with a hand-written note using the person's first name saying "Try this, it works!" as a marketing tool. The envelope has no return address and is postmarked from California. Often the receiver erroneously believes that a friend or neighbor has sent this ad and feels humiliated and embarrassed. One obese woman who received such a letter didn't come out of her house for 5 days, saying that she didn't want to encounter the person who sent this to her, and didn't know who sent it.

Advertising encourages the belief in American culture that we can transform or recreate ourselves quickly and effortlessly in days by using this cream, taking that pill, following this diet program, or joining that gym. In our fast-paced society of fast food, fast track jobs, and drive-through services, we have come to expect to lose weight fast and are tempted by these promises. That's just what the weight loss industry is hoping for, and why they spend so much money on advertising. Americans spend $50 billion each year on weight loss programs and products, many of which do not even work. It is estimated that it costs an average of $84 for each pound lost and a total of $500 a year. It is important to recognize that there is no magic pill or 10-day solution for weight loss. Healthy weight management is a life long process.

Kilbourne J. *Can't Buy My Love.* New York: Simon & Schuster Inc., 1999. Weight Loss Deception Found, *USA Today,* September 18, 2002.

Berrry Trim's Dirty Little Trick, National Council Against Fraud Newsletter, Sept–Oct 1989, Volume 12, issue #5.

Weight management has become an obsession in American culture as well as a significant health problem. In the United States, obesity has risen at an epidemic rate during the past 20 years. One of the national health objectives for the year 2010 is to reduce the prevalence of obesity among adults to less than 15%. Research indicates that the situation is worsening rather than improving. According to the National Center for Chronic Disease Prevention and Health Promotion, an estimated 61% of U.S. adults are either overweight or obese. In 2000 38.8 million American adults met the criteria for obesity. Children are affected as well. There are nearly twice as many overweight children and almost three times as many overweight adolescents as there were 20 years ago.[1,2]

When the body is supplied with more energy than it can use, the result is an excess of energy (or a **positive caloric balance**) stored in the form of fat. This continuous buildup of fat can eventually lead to obesity. The average caloric intake for Americans has increased by 10% over the past two decades. Additionally, nearly two-thirds of Americans are not physically active on a regular basis and 25% are completely sedentary.[3] In fact, in a recent study conducted by the RAND Institute, it was found that in terms of chronic conditions, obesity is a more powerful risk factor than poverty, heavy drinking, or smoking.[4]

Regardless of this issue, few experts question the real dangers to health and wellness from obesity.[5] Among the health problems caused by or complicated by obesity are increased surgical risk, hypertension, various forms of heart disease, stroke, type 2 diabetes, several forms of cancer, deterioration of joints, complications during pregnancy, gallbladder disease, and an overall increased risk of mortality[6] (see Star box on page 148). Obesity is so closely associated with these chronic conditions that medical experts now recommend that obesity itself be defined and treated as a chronic disease.

Body Image and Self-Concept

Although physicians focus on obesity, in our image-conscious society, being overweight is also a problem. The media tell people that being overweight is undesirable and that they should conform to certain ideal **body images** (such as being tall, thin, and "cut" with muscular definition). For example, the average actress and model is thinner than 95% of the female population and weighs 23% less than the average woman.[7] The average American woman is 5'4", 143 pounds, and wears a size 10–12. The average model is 5'10" and 110 pounds.[8] Today's lean but muscular version of

---

Key Terms

positive caloric balance caloric intake greater than caloric expenditure.

body image our subjective perception of how our body appears.

Studies show that mirrors can make us more self conscious, critical and conforming.

perfection is a very demanding standard for both women and men to meet (see Discovering Your Spirituality).

People may become dissatisfied and concerned about their inability to achieve these ideals. The scope of this dissatisfaction is evident in a study of over 800 women, which revealed that nearly half were unhappy with their weight, muscle tone, hips, thighs, buttocks, and legs.[9] When this type of dissatisfaction exists, people begin to question their attractiveness, and their self-esteem tends to decline.

In comparison with being overweight, little media attention has been paid to being underweight. However, the body image problems experienced by some extremely thin people can be equally distressing.

Overweight and Obesity Defined

What's the difference between overweight and obesity? Doctors usually define **overweight** as a condition in which a person's weight is 1%–19% higher than normal, as defined by a standard height/weight chart. **Obesity** is usually defined as a condition in which a person's weight is 20% or more above normal weight. "Morbid obesity" refers to being 50% to 100% above normal weight, more

than 100 pounds over normal weight, or sufficiently overweight to interfere with health or normal functioning.[10]

Some clinicians and laymen continue to use standard height-weight tables to determine when weight is excessive. However, more precise techniques to determine body composition are currently available. Several of these techniques, including waist-to-hip ratio (*healthy body weight*), body mass index, "BOD POD" assessment, electrical impedance, skinfold measurements, and hydrostatic weighing, are described in the following section.

Determining Weight and Body Composition

Some of the techniques used to determine overweight and obesity are common and are routinely used by the general public. Others are expensive and of limited availability.

Height-Weight Tables

Height and weight tables were originally developed in 1983 to assist people in determining the relationship between their weight and desirable standards. Nearly every version of these tables has come under criticism for not considering variables such as gender, age, frame size,

> **Key Terms**
>
> **overweight** a condition in which a person's excess fat accumulation results in a body weight that exceeds desirable weight by 1% to 19%.
>
> **obesity** a condition in which a person's body weight is 20% or more above desirable weight as determined by standard height/weight charts.

and body composition. Some versions were thought to be too rigorous in establishing cutoff points for ideal or **desirable weight,** and others were deemed too generous. Although still available, these tables are being gradually replaced by other assessment techniques.

 TALKING POINTS If a friend or close family member were dangerously overweight or obese, how would you express your concern?

Healthy Body Weight

You can determine your **healthy body weight** by using the weight guidelines (Table 6.1) found in the *Dietary Guidelines for Americans.*[11] This assessment involves converting two body measurements, the waist and the hip circumferences, into a waist-to-hip ratio (WHR) that can then be applied to weight ranges for people of particular ages and heights. An acceptable WHR, for women is near the lower end of each weight range, and for men it is at the higher end of each weight range.

To make a WHR determination, follow these steps:

1. Measure around your waist near your navel while you stand relaxed (not pulling in your stomach).
2. Measure around your hips, over the buttocks where the hips are largest.
3. Divide the waist measurement by the hip measurement.

For example, a woman with a 25-inch waist and 36-inch hips has a WHR of .69, which is well within a healthy range. Women with a WHR of less than .80 generally have a body weight that falls within the healthy range for their age and height; men with a WHR of less than .90 will also probably fall within the range considered healthy for their age and height.

Health Risks of Obesity

Each of the diseases listed below is followed by the percentage of cases for which obesity is a contributing factor:

Colon cancer 10%

Breast cancer 11%

Hypertension 33%

Heart disease 70%

Diabetes (type 2, non–insulin-dependent) 90%

As these statistics show, being obese greatly increases your risk of many serious, and even life-threatening, chronic conditions.

Table 6.1 Healthy Weight: Recommended Guidelines

Height+	Weight*	
	19–34 years	35 years and over
5'	97–128	108–138
5'1"	101–132	111–143
5'2"	104–137	115–148
5'3"	107–141	119–152
5'4"	111–146	122–157
5'5"	114–150	126–162
5'6"	118–155	130–167
5'7"	121–160	134–172
5'8"	125–164	138–178
5'9"	129–169	142–183
5'10"	132–174	146–188
5'11"	136–179	151–194
6'	140–184	155–199
6'1"	144–189	159–205
6'2"	148–195	164–210
6'3"	152–200	168–216
6'4"	156–205	173–222
6'5"	160–211	177–228
6'6"	164–216	182–234

*Without clothes.
+Without shoes.

Note: The higher weights in the ranges generally apply to men, who tend to have more muscle and bone mass; the lower weights more often apply to women, who generally have less muscle and bone mass.

This new system was developed because of the growing concern over the relationship between the amount of fat located around the waist, the spare tire, and the development of several serious health problems. As a point of interest, the *Dietary Guidelines for Americans* do not use WHR as a clinical marker for the treatment of obesity; instead they use only waist circumference. The risk of health problems such as heart disease and diabetes increases at a waist measurement of 35 inches for women and 40 inches for men, regardless of height.[12]

Key Terms

desirable weight the weight range deemed appropriate for people, taking into consideration gender, age, and frame size.

healthy body weight body weight within a weight range appropriate for a person with an acceptable waist-to-hip ratio.

Body Mass Index

Another method for assessing healthy body weight is the **body mass index (BMI).** BMI is calculated metrically as weight divided by height squared (kg/m^2).[13] The BMI does not reflect body composition (fat versus lean tissue) or consider the degree of fat accumulated in the central body cavity. It is, nevertheless, widely used in determining obesity. Overweight is defined for women with a BMI over 27.3 and 27.8 for men. Individuals are considered obese when BMI is 30.0 or above. Severe or morbid obesity is when the BMI is greater than 40.[10]

An alternative method of determining the BMI is to use a **nomogram,** such as that shown in Figure 6-1 on page 148. Like the BMI, the nomogram requires information about both weight and height.

Once the BMI has been obtained, its relationship to a desirable BMI for persons of various ages can be determined by using Table 6.2 on this page.

BOD POD (Body Composition System)

The newest method of determining body composition involves the use of the **BOD POD,** an egg-shaped chamber that uses computerized pressure sensors to determine the amount of air displaced by the person's body (larger people displace more air than smaller people). From this measure, you can then calculate the person's body density and percentage of body fat.[14] Additional techniques in which highly accurate but expensive technology is used to determine body composition, including *computed tomography (CT)*

Table 6.2 Desirable Body Mass Index in Relation to Age

Age Group (years)	BMI (kg/m²)
19–24	19–24
25–34	20–25
35–44	21–26
45–54	22–27
55–65	23–28
>65	24–29

Key Terms

body mass index (BMI) a mathematical calculation based on weight and height; used to determine desirable body weight.

nomogram a graphic means of finding an unknown value.

BOD POD body composition system used to measure body fat through air displacement.

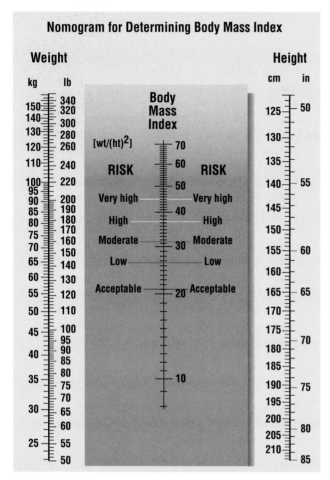

Nomogram for Determining Body Mass Index

Weight

Height

| kg | lb | | cm | in |

Body Mass Index

[wt/(ht)²]

RISK

RISK

Very high — Very high

High — High

Moderate — Moderate

Low — Low

Acceptable — Acceptable

Figure 6-1 To use this nomogram, place a ruler or other straightedge between the body weight in kilograms or pounds (without clothes) located on the left-hand column and the height in centimeters or in inches (without shoes) located on the right-hand column. The BMI is read from the middle of the scale and is in metric units.

Body fat determination using skinfold calipers. Skinfold measurements are used in equations that calculate body fat density and percent body fat.

scans, magnetic resonance imaging (MRI), infrared light transmission, and *neutron activation,* may become common ways of measuring body composition in the future.[15]

Skinfold Measurements

Skinfold measurements are another way to measure body composition. In this assessment procedure, constant-pressure **calipers** are used to measure the thickness of the layer of fat beneath the skin's surface, the *subcutaneous fat layer.* These measurements are taken at key places on the body. Through the use of specific formulas, skinfold measurements can be used to calculate the percentage of body fat. The percent body fat value can also be used in determining desirable weight.[15] It should be noted that there are some drawbacks to this type of measure. First, body fat calipers may require someone else to perform the

test as it is sometimes difficult to get an accurate measurement on yourself. Second, skinfolds are notoriously hard to locate precisely, and just a few millimeters off can make a significant difference.[16]

Young adult men normally have a body fat percentage of 10% to 15%. The normal range for young adult women is 22% to 25%. When a man's body fat is higher than 20% and a woman's body fat is above 30%, they are considered to be obese. The higher percentage of fat typically found in women is related to preparation for pregnancy and breastfeeding.

Hydrostatic Weighing

Hydrostatic (underwater) *weighing* is another precise method of determining the relative amounts of fat and lean body mass that make up body weight. A person's percentage of body fat is determined by comparing the underwater weight with the body weight out of water and dry. The need for expensive facilities (a tank or pool) and experienced technicians makes the availability and cost of this procedure limited to small-scale application, such as a large research university or teaching hospital.

Appearance

While it may seem as though the simplest method of determining one's body size is to look in the mirror, for most people this is not an accurate measure. Research shows that most women are dissatisfied with their appearance or

Key Terms

calipers a device used to measure the thickness of a skinfold from which percent of body fat can be calculated.

body image and perceive themselves as needing to lose an average of 10–15 pounds when in actuality they are in a healthy weight range. Body dissatisfaction is endemic to young women in Western culture as evidenced by the rate of dieting in the United States, starting at a young age. In fact, on any given day, 50% of 10 year olds are on a diet, two-thirds of high school women, and a third of all adult women are dieting.[17] There is also an important difference between one's internal concept of memory of one's body and actual body perception, and this is particularly problematic for people with eating disorders.

Most people use scales to determine their weight, but scales can be highly inaccurate, as evidenced by weighing yourself on a variety of scales and weighing different amounts. Also, you will probably weigh less in the morning when you first wake up and more in the evening, after having eaten during the day. So if you are using a scale to monitor your weight, you need to do so on the same scale, at the same time of day, and with approximately the same weight of clothing. Also, remember that muscle weighs more than fat, which explains why some toned and muscular athletes can weigh as much as someone who is sedentary and overweight. In general, risk of disease increases with a higher percentage of body fat, not weight.

In extreme cases, a clinical condition referred to as "body dysmorphic disorder" (BDD) may develop. BDD is a secret preoccupation with an imagined or slight flaw in one's appearance. Sometimes, people become almost completely fixated on concerns regarding body image, leading to repeatedly weighing themselves and checking in mirrors throughout the day, compulsively dieting and exercising, and undergoing cosmetic surgery.[21] These attempts to achieve the perfect body may lead to psychological dysfunction such as not wanting to leave the house because of imagined defects.

Causes of Obesity

There is still an ongoing debate as to the causes of obesity. Genetic, physiological, metabolic, environmental, psychological, and other factors may all play a part. In the past decade, the overall prevalence of obesity has increased so that currently one-third of all Americans are obese. Moreover, in the last 20 years, the number of obese children in the United States has doubled to one in five children.[18] Genetics, dietary practice, and activity level seem to all play a role in this dramatic increase.

There are four additional factors that seem to play a significant role in the prevalence of obesity: sex, age, socioeconomic status, and race. As biology only accounts for 33% of the variation in body weight, the environment can also exert an enormous influence. According to the Centers for Disease Control, prevalence rates for obesity in women is 35% and 31% among men and is found mainly in the 20–55 age group. Among women, obesity is strongly associated with socioeconomic status, being twice as common among those with lower socioeconomic status as it is among those with higher status.[19] Although prevalence among black and white men does not differ significantly, obesity is far more common among black than among white women, affecting 60% of middle-aged black women compared with 33% of white women.

While the precise cause of obesity remains unclear, we do know that obesity is a complex condition caused by a variety of factors. Until we are sure what causes obesity, it makes sense that it is difficult to develop effective ways of managing weight.

Genetic Factors

Through years of research, we do know that heredity plays a major role in the development of body size and obesity. Based on studies comparing both identical and fraternal (nonidentical) twins raised together and separately, it's evident that both environment and genetics influence obesity. In fact, it is estimated that heredity accounts for 25% to 40% of the development of obesity.[10] Women have a higher percentage of body fat than do men and this seems stable across cultures and dietary habits.[20]

There is also some speculation about population differences and prevalence of obesity suggesting that some groups possess a "thrifty genotype."[21] For example, the differences in diabetes and obesity rates in Native Americans as compared with European Americans prompted some to consider that some groups of people have survived periods of feast and famine by increased efficiency in energy storage and expenditure through a particular genotype. However, no specific thrifty gene or genotype has been identified.

There is a complex interplay of genetic factors that very likely influence the development of obesity as more than 250 genes may play a role in obesity. There has been promising research exploring how the leptin gene influences obesity. The leptin gene, referred to as the "fat gene" was discovered in the mid 1990s to influence satiety or the feeling of fullness in mice.[22] When the leptin gene was faulty in mice, it produced lower leptin levels, and the mice experienced excessive weight gain. However, when the leptin gene was normal, the leptin levels were higher and the mice were able to maintain normal weight. It has been theorized that leptin resistance may be involved in weight gain and the maintenance of excessive weight, but much more research needs to be conducted in this area.[23]

Physiological and Hormonal Factors

Building on this new information about the genetic and neuropsychological basis of obesity, researchers have identified centers for the control of eating within the hypothalamus of the central nervous system (CNS). These centers—the feeding center for hunger and the satiety center for fullness—tell the body when it should begin consuming food and when food consumption should stop. It takes 20 minutes on average for these signals to go from the stomach to the brain to relay the message "stop eating."

There are also hormonal factors that influence obesity. Obesity can be caused by a condition called **hypothyroidism,** in which the thyroid gland produces an insufficient amount of thyroxin, a hormone that regulates metabolism. Over five million Americans have this common medical condition and as many as 10% of women may have some degree of thyroid hormone deficiency. In such individuals, the underactive thyroid makes burning up food difficult and so weight gain is common. As we acquire greater understanding of the hormones and neurotransmitters that influence hunger and satiety, drugs designed to influence their actions will be developed. Some of these drugs already exist and will be described later in this chapter.

The effects of hormonal changes on eating can be seen each month just before a woman's menstrual cycle, as many women say that they crave salty and sugary foods during this time. Pregnancy brings about another host of hormonal and metabolic changes. During a normal pregnancy, a woman requires an extra 300 calories a day to support the developing fetus and supportive tissues, and to fuel her elevated maternal metabolic rate. In addition, pregnant women will typically develop approximately 9 extra pounds of adipose tissue which will be used as an energy source during lactation. The average woman is expected to gain between 25 to 35 pounds during pregnancy.[10] Many women express concern about their ability to lose this weight following the birth of the child, and some women do gain much more than the recommended amount of weight. However, the majority of women lose their pregnancy weight within 6 months to a year after having a baby. Nevertheless, obesity is one of the most frequent causes for complications in pregnancy. The mother is considered obese if at the beginning of her pregnancy her BMI is over 25. Women who are obese during pregnancy have a much higher risk of hypertension and gestational diabetes. Obesity has also been associated with infertility, poor pregnancy outcomes and miscarriage.[10]

Typically, breast-feeding can help women to burn more calories and return to their prepregnancy weight, although extra fat may linger, as nature intended this to be a store of energy for breast-feeding. Breast-feeding requires an additional 500 calories a day.[10] Mothers who breast-feed tend to lose more weight when their babies are 3 to 6 months old than formula-feeding mothers who consume fewer calories.[24]

Metabolic Factors

Traditional theory has suggested that the energy expenditure and energy storage centers of the body possess a genetically programmed awareness of the body's most physiologically desirable weight, called **set point.**[25] However, the term *set point* is somewhat misleading in that it does not refer to a certain number or point but a weight range that the body is genetically programmed to maintain. When the body falls below its natural set point, one's metabolism reacts by slowing down the body's functioning in order to conserve energy. In other words, the body will sense that it is not receiving enough calories to maintain healthy functioning and so it will send calories to essential areas of the body and use the energy as efficiently as possible. Alternatively, when someone consumes more calories than is needed, the body will begin to increase the rate of metabolism in an effort not to gain weight above the set point. The process of storing or burning more energy to maintain the body's "best" weight is called **adaptive thermogenesis.** This process also explains the reason that 90% of people who go on any diet gain all their weight back plus more within a year of going off the diet. When dieting, people reduce their caloric intake which in turn lowers their metabolism. When they discontinue the diet, they typically eat more calories and foods with higher fat content on a lowered metabolism. This is a good formula for weight gain. In addition, dieters tend to lose muscle and regain their weight as fat.

There is a great deal of debate on how an individual's set point can be altered. The number of fat cells in the body, the blood level of insulin, and regions of the brain such as the hypothalamus all seem to play a role in determining set point. Certain drugs such as amphetamines and other diet pills and herbal supplements can act on the brain to temporarily lower the set point. However, once these drugs are discontinued, the set point returns to the previous level or perhaps an even higher level and weight increases as a result. Healthier and more permanent methods of changing one's set point are through regular exercise and healthy eating patterns. In fact, a recent study

---

Key Terms

hypothyroidism A condition in which the thyroid gland produces an insufficient amount of the hormone thyroxin.

set point A genetically programmed range of body weight, beyond which a person finds it difficult to gain or lose additional weight.

adaptive thermogenesis The physiological response of the body to adjust its metabolic rate to the presence of food.

of 8,000 successful dieters found that the majority of them used "my own diet and exercise regimen" and did not follow any formal weight reduction program.[26]

The body's requirement for energy to maintain basic physiological processes decreases progressively with age. This change reflects the loss of muscle tissue as both men and women age. This loss of muscle mass eventually alters the ratio of lean body tissue to fat. As the proportion of fat increases, the energy needs of the body are more strongly influenced by the lower metabolic needs of the fat cells.[27] This excess energy is then stored in the fat cells of the body. A gradual decrease in caloric intake and a conscious effort to expend more calories can effectively prevent this gradual increase in weight leading to obesity.

Social and Cultural Factors

There are also ethnic differences related to the incidence of obesity and cultural differences regarding what is seen as a healthy weight. African American, American Indian and Hispanic American women have the highest risk of becoming overweight, according to the Centers for Disease Control. In fact, the results of a national study showed that more than half of all African American and Hispanic women in the United States are above what is considered a healthy body weight. The statistics are startling: 66% of African American women are overweight and 33% are obese. For Caucasian women, 49% are considered overweight and 24% obese. Only one minority group, Asian Americans, has a lower rate of obesity than the general population.

Obesity is second only to tobacco as the leading cause of premature deaths and disproportionately affects women of color and women of lower socioeconomic classes. On the positive side, African American women report less pressure to be thin than their white counterparts and tend to be less self-conscious about their weight.[28] Acculturation also has a significant impact on the rates of obesity—the more an ethnic group has adapted to and absorbed Western culture, the higher the rate of obesity within that group.[29]

Socioeconomic status is also an important influence on obesity, particularly in women. Upper socioeconomic women tend to be thinner than lower socioeconomic women, while among men there is not such a pattern.[30] Interestingly, higher obesity levels are also related to marriage, parenthood, and geographical location as married men, parents, and people living in rural areas tend to have a higher incidence of obesity.[31]

Environmental Factors

Certainly environmental factors such as the smell or sight of freshly made cookies, or an advertisement for a candy bar can affect your eating habits. Even the clock signaling it is "time to eat" can encourage us to eat even when we aren't hungry. While this may seem adaptive and helpful in regulating our food intake, Dr. Kelly D. Brownell, a professor of psychology at Yale and an expert on eating disorders, has gone so far as to label American society a "toxic environment" when it comes to food. Researchers contend that the local environment has a powerful effect on eating. Factors such as portion size, price, advertising, the availability of food, and the number of food choices presented all can influence the amount the average person consumes. For example, moviegoers will eat 50% more popcorn if given an extra-large tub of popcorn instead of a container one size smaller, even if the popcorn is stale. If a tabletop in the office is stocked with cookies and candy, co-workers tend to nibble their way through the workday, even if they are not hungry. One study showed that when the candy was in plain sight on workers' desks, they ate an average of nine pieces each. Storing the candy in a desk drawer reduced consumption to six pieces, as compared to putting the candy a couple of yards from the desk, cutting the number to three pieces per person.[32] In response to these and other findings, many public schools have begun offering only healthy foods in their cafeterias, replacing soft drinks, candy, and chips with juice, milk, fruit, and granola bars.

Packaging and price can also influence the amount people consume, a concept of which advertisers, restaurants, and grocery stores are well aware. Dropping the price of the low-fat snacks by even a nickel resulted in dramatically increased sales. In contrast, stickers signaling low-fat content or cartoons promoting the low-fat alternatives had little influence over which snacks were more popular. This is not only true of food but also with beverages, as people tend to drink *more* from short, wide glasses than from thinner, taller ones, thinking they are drinking less.[32]

Having more choices also appears to make people eat more. In one study, people ate more when offered sandwiches with four different fillings than they did when they were given sandwiches with their single favorite filling. In another study, participants who were served a four-course meal with meat, fruit, bread, and a pudding, ate 60% more food than those served an equivalent meal of only their favorite course. Even the cup holders in automobiles have grown larger to make room for giant drinks. It is important to note that these findings were seen in people of all body sizes, not just with people who are overweight or obese as is often the misconception. However, there does seem to be a difference in the age of the individuals studied. One study found that 3 year olds who were served three different portion sizes of macaroni and cheese for lunch on three different days ate the same amount each time. Five-year-olds, however, ate more when more was put in front of them.[32]

Declaring War on Overweight

With the majority of adult Americans being overweight, some experts have declared war on the food industry and advocate treating obesity in a similar way to smoking. The food industry produces 3,800 calories a day for every adult and child in the United States, which far exceeds the recommended caloric requirements.[1] Not only are people consuming too many calories each day, but they are also overfeeding their pets. Studies show that at least 25% of dogs and cats in the Western world are obese and are at greater risk for developing obesity related health problems such as diabetes and heart disease.[2] It has been suggested that strategies used to decrease cigarette smoking be used to encourage healthier and smaller food choices. For example, a "fat tax" (also called the "Twinkie tax") on junk food has been suggested to subsidize the price of healthier foods so they cost less. Others suggest putting warning labels on the nutritional packaging for junk food similar to the warning labels on cigarettes. Legislators have discussed requiring fast-food and other restaurants to post calories and fat content on their menus. Some individuals are fighting back using the court system. McDonald's, Wendy's, Burger King, and Kentucky Fried Chicken were taken to court by a 270-pound maintenance worker who held them responsible for his obesity-related health problems; the suit, however, was dismissed.

Some companies are responding to this outcry by changing their packaging pricing, and options. For example, McDonald's plans to test a Happy Meal with an option of a piece of fresh fruit instead of the French fries that usually accompanies it. Kraft Foods, the nation's largest food company, plans to reduce the portion sizes, fat, and calories of many of its foods. Frito Lay has set a goal of eliminating all trans fatty acids from its chips and snacks.

Some speculate that there may be an increasing movement against the food industry, particularly against unhealthy foods, in regulating television commercials and advertising, and even perhaps prohibiting children from being able to buy junk food, again similarly to what has been done in the past 30 years with the tobacco industry.

[1]Nestle M. *Food Politics: How the Food Industry Influences Nutrition and Health.* Los Angeles, California: University of California Press, 2002.
[2]Fatter Cats and Dogs Are a Sizeable Problem. *USA Today,* September 9, 2003.

TALKING POINTS Do you think there should be more regulation of the food industry? If so, what recommendations would you make? What food would you include for regulation and how should this be determined?

Psychological Factors

Psychological factors related to overeating refer to the reasons people eat rather than due to physiological hunger. Individuals with eating disorders often report that they don't know when they are hungry and often eat when they are not hungry and don't eat when they have a biological reason for doing so. Why do people eat if not in response to hunger? Frequently people eat in response to their emotions such as eating to comfort themselves, when bored, tired, stressed, or depressed. Some people say they use food as a way of coping with hurt, sadness, and anger, suppressing their feelings and putting food on top of them. Others eat out of habit, and associate food with certain activities such as eating popcorn at a movie, eating chips in front of the television, or having dessert after dinner. There are certainly many associations with chocolate when feeling down as a way of cheering yourself up. Food is also part of celebrations, holidays, family bonding, and a mainstay of socialization. It is difficult to think about social activities we engage in that don't involve food in some way.

Many people develop relationships with food that substitute for real human relationships. Comments like "Food is my best friend" or "A great meal is better than sex" are indicative to the degree to which many people rely on food to fill their needs. As we'll learn in our discussion of eating disorders later in the chapter, psychological issues with food can become serious, even life-threatening problems.

HealthQuest Activities

The *Stages of Change* activity in the Nutrition and Weight Control module assesses your readiness to follow a diet containing appropriate levels of fats, carbohydrates, and proteins. It outlines concrete steps you can take to maintain healthy intake levels of these nutrients. The feedback for this activity is provided separately for each of these three dietary areas. You may address all three areas or choose among them. Develop a strategy for overcoming unhealthful eating habits, and keep an ongoing account of your progress. Record your mood, activity level, schedule, and any other factors that may affect your eating behavior. Then write down several ways to lessen the effects of such events on your eating behavior.

Dietary Practices

Many researchers believe that the number of fat cells a person has will be initially determined during the first 2 years of life. Babies who are overfed will develop a greater number of fat cells than babies who receive a balanced diet of appropriate, infant-sized portions. When these children reach adulthood, they will have more fat cells; this increase can result in five times as many fat cells in obese people as in people of normal weight. Dieting only reduces the size of fat cells, not the number of fat cells. People who have an abnormally high number of fat cells are biologically limited in their ability to lose weight.

Another way people can become obese is with a pattern of overeating over a long period of time. If an infant's cries for food are immediately responded to, that child will be more likely to learn what the sensation of hunger is and the appropriate response. If crying unrelated to hunger is responded to by offering a cookie or candy, that child will learn to soothe himself or herself with food. Studies show that children become confused about what hunger is and how to satisfy it if their hunger needs are neglected or overindulged in infancy.[33]

Some of the first power struggles between parents and their children revolve around issues of food. A child who has little power in her life can exert power and control through her refusal to eat certain foods and demanding other foods and when she wants to eat. Parents who use food as a reward for good behavior: "If you get an "A" on your test, I will treat you to ice cream," as punishment: "You weren't behaving so you can't have dessert," or as a guilt trip: "Don't waste food. Clean your plate. Children are starving in the world," may inadvertently be creating negative dietary practices that will continue on throughout the child's life. Interestingly, research has shown that children are extraordinarily adept at meeting their nutritional needs when left to their own devices. One study allowed children to eat whatever they wanted for a week. Did they always pick high-fat, high-sugar foods? No. Actually, when we look at each day's intake, they didn't eat a balanced diet. However, when one takes the full week into consideration, they met their nutritional needs perfectly.

Not only does what your parents say to you have a tremendous influence on your eating behavior, but what they do themselves, their own eating practices, can have even a greater impact. Children are exposed to different foods and model what their parents eat. If a parent makes comments such as, "I shouldn't eat that because I will get fat" or doesn't eat fruits or vegetables, or sits down with a bag of chips in front of the television every night, the child will probably do the same. In the same vein, when parents exercise regularly, eat a balanced diet, and make positive comments about their weight, children tend to mimic this behavior.

Inactivity

When weight management experts are asked to identify the single most important reason that obesity is so high in today's society, they are most certain to point to inactivity. People of all ages tend to be less active and burn fewer calories than did their ancestors only a few generations ago.

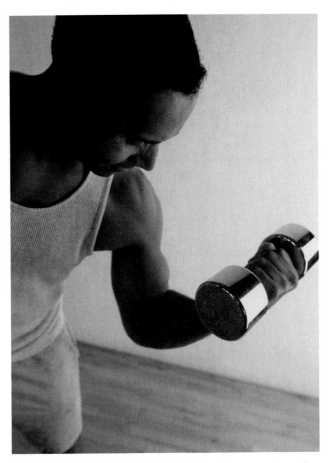

The most important component of weight management is regular exercise.

Both adults and children spend less time devoted to exercise as a result of longer work hours at sedentary jobs, a decline in physical education programs in school, and increased participation in sedentary recreational activities, such as browsing the Internet, playing video games, and watching television. In addition, many of the laborsaving devices and increased automation in the home and workplace have contributed to increased inactivity. According to some studies, nearly two-thirds of Americans are not physically active on a regular basis and 25% are completely sedentary.[3] It is not surprising that as inactivity becomes the norm, so does overweight.

 TALKING POINTS What were the messages you received in childhood regarding food? What positive and negative eating habits have you learned from your family?

Caloric Balance

Any calories consumed in excess of those that are used by the body are converted to fat. We gain weight when our energy input is greater than our energy output. On the

Figure 6-2 Caloric balance: energy input equals energy output, some of which comes from physical activity.

Energy Needs of the Body

What are our energy needs? How many calories should we consume (or burn) to achieve a healthy weight? Although there are rough estimates for college-aged men (2500 to 3300 calories daily) and women (approximately 2500 calories daily), we all vary in our specific energy needs. These needs are based on three factors: (1) basal metabolic rate (also referred to as resting energy expenditure, or REE), (2) activity requirements, and (3) the thermic effect of food.

Basal Metabolism

Of the three factors that determine energy needs, basal metabolism uses the highest proportion (50% to 70%) of the total calories required by each person. **Basal Metabolic**

other hand, we lose weight when our energy output is greater than our energy input (Figure 6-2). Weight remains constant when caloric input and output are equal. In such situations, our bodies are said to be in *caloric balance*.

Rate (BMR) is a measure of resting energy expenditure that is taken upon awakening, 10–12 hours after eating, or 12–18 hours after significant physical activity. A closely related construct, resting metabolic rate (RMR), is often used interchangeably with BMR. In comparison with the BMR, the RMR is measured at rest, without the stringent control on physical activity required as with measuring BMR. RMR measures the calories needed for functioning such as blood circulation, respiration, brain activity, muscle function, body temperature, and heart beat.[34]

Basal metabolism changes as people age. For both males and females, the BMR is relatively high at birth and

---

Key Terms

basal metabolic rate (BMR) the amount of energy, expressed in calories, that the body requires to maintain basic functions.

Table 6.3 Calories Expended during Physical Activity

To determine the number of calories you have spent in an hour of activity, simply multiply the *calories per hour per pound* column by your weight (in pounds). For example after an hour of archery a 120-pound person will have expended 209 calories; a 160-pound person, 278 calories; and a 220-pound person, 383 calories.

Activity	Calories/Hour/Pound	Activity	Calories/Hour/Pound
Archery	1.74	Marching (rapid)	3.84
Basketball	3.78	Painting (outside)	2.10
Baseball	1.86	Playing music (sitting)	1.08
Boxing (sparring)	3.78	Racquetball	3.90
Canoeing (leisure)	1.20	Running (cross-country)	4.44
Climbing hills (no load)	3.30	Running	
Cleaning	1.62	11 min 30 sec per mile	3.66
Cooking	1.20	9 min per mile	5.28
Cycling		8 min per mile	5.64
5.5 mph	1.74	7 min per mile	6.24
9.4 mph	2.70	6 min per mile	6.84
Racing	4.62	5 min 30 sec per mile	7.86
Dance (modern)	2.28	Scrubbing floors	3.00
Eating (sitting)	0.60	Sailing	1.20
Field hockey	3.66	Skiing	
Fishing	1.68	Cross-country	4.43
Football	3.60	Snow, downhill	3.84
Gardening		Water	3.12
Digging	3.42	Skating (moderate)	2.28
Mowing	3.06	Soccer	3.54
Raking	1.44	Squash	5.76
Golf	2.34	Swimming	
Gymnastics	1.80	Backstroke	4.62
Handball	3.78	Breaststroke	4.44
Hiking	2.52	Free, fast	4.26
Horseback riding		Free, slow	3.48
Galloping	3.72	Butterfly	4.68
Trotting	3.00	Table tennis	1.86
Walking	1.14	Tennis	3.00
Ice hockey	5.70	Volleyball	1.32
Jogging	4.15	Walking (normal pace)	2.16
Judo	5.34	Weight training	1.90
Knitting (sewing)	0.60	Wrestling	5.10
Lacrosse	5.70	Writing (sitting)	0.78

continues to increase until the age of 2. Except for a slight rise at puberty, the BMR will then gradually decline throughout life.[35] If people fail to recognize that their BMR decreases as they grow older (2% per decade), they might also fail to adjust their food intake and activity level accordingly. Thus they may gradually put on unwanted pounds as they grow older.

Activity Requirements

Each person's caloric *activity requirements* vary directly according to the amount of their daily physical activity.

For example, sedentary office workers require a smaller daily caloric intake than construction workers, lumberjacks, or farm workers do.

Physical activity that occurs outside the workplace also increases caloric needs. Sedentary office workers may be quite active in their recreational pursuits. Active employees may spend their off hours lounging in front of the TV. It's important to closely examine the total amount of work or activity an individual engages in to accurately estimate that person's caloric requirements. Physical activity uses 20% to 40% of caloric intake. See Table 6.3 on this page for a breakdown of caloric expenditures for various activities.

Thermic Effect of Food

Thermic effect of food (TEF) refers to the amount of energy our bodies require for the digestion, absorption, and transportation of food. This energy breaks down the bonds that hold complex food molecules together, resulting in smaller nutritional units that can be distributed throughout the body. The amount of TEF burned varies for different types of food, with some food such as fat requiring less energy to convert to energy stores and others such as protein and carbohydrates requiring more. The TEF peaks in about 1 hour after eating and accounts for approximately 10% of total energy expenditure.[36]

Lifetime Weight Control

Obesity and frequent fluctuation in weight are thought to be associated with higher levels of morbidity and mortality. So it is highly desirable to maintain your weight and body composition at or near optimum levels. Although this may be a difficult goal to achieve, it is not unrealistic when practiced on a consistent basis. The following are some keys to success:

- *Exercise:* Caloric expenditure through regular exercise, including cardiovascular exercise and strength training, is a key to maintaining a healthy weight and body composition (see Chapter 4).
- *Dietary modification:* Plan meals around foods that have moderate levels of fat and are low in total fat and saturated fat and high in complex carbohydrates. Many nutritionists are concerned about the safety of high-fat diets and ultra-low-fat diets for long-term weight management.
- *Lifestyle support:* In addition to committing yourself to a lifestyle that features regular physical activity and careful food choices, build a support system that will nurture your efforts. Inform your family, friends,

classmates, and coworkers that you intend to rely on them for support and encouragement.

- *Problem solving:* Reevaluate your current approaches to dealing with stressors. Replace any reliance on food as a coping mechanism with nonfood options, such as exercise or talking with friends or family members.
- *Redefinition of health:* Think about health and wellness (see Chapter 2) in a manner that reinforces the importance of prevention and self-care, rather than waiting to become sick or incapacitated before paying attention to your diet and activity level.

These suggested lifestyle choices will make a significant contribution to preventing a weight problem later.

Weight Management Techniques

Weight loss occurs when the calories consumed are less than the energy the body needs for physiological maintenance and activity. This may sound overly simplified and certainly the $50 billion-a-year weight loss industry would like us to think it is much more complicated than this.

Weight loss followed by weight gain may be less healthy and certainly more frustrating than maintaining body weight, even at weight above the desirable levels. When a diet or weight loss strategy fails, the person, not the diet, is blamed. This causes people to jump to another weight loss method and then another, and a vicious cycle has begun. However, a commitment to a lifestyle change of eating in healthy ways and engaging in regular exercise seems to be the most effective strategy for weight loss and weight maintenance. It is also important to set a goal to lose not more than 2 pounds a week because the body tends to lose muscle rather than fat if the weight loss occurs too rapidly. Many people also complain of "hanging skin" after a rapid, drastic weight loss, which can then require cosmetic surgery to rectify.

A number of approaches to weight loss can be pursued. How do dieters know when they have succeeded? Figure 6-3 on page 159 shows how Americans measure their progress at losing weight. The Personal Assessment at the end of this chapter will help you evaluate your food habits in relation to healthy weight (page 179) and how you feel about your body image (page 181).

Key Terms

thermic effect of food (TEF) the amount of energy our bodies require for the digestion, absorption, and transportation of food.

Dropping a clothing size

Don't know, 1.1%

Other, 2.8%

48.8%

34.1%

Feeling more energetic

Being able to avoid fattening foods, 6.5%

Getting compliments, 9.7%

Figure 6-3 How do Americans measure success when it comes to losing weight? Most say dropping a clothing size is the best indicator that their diet is working.

Dietary Alterations

A diet that reduces caloric intake is the most common approach to weight loss. The choice of foods and the amount of food are the two factors that distinguish the wide range of diets currently available. It's important to note, however, that dieting alone usually does not result in long-term weight loss. Effective and lasting weight loss requires a lifestyle change, not just going on a diet for a specific time period only to return to your old patterns of eating. This is the problem many people face, as they go on strict diets and overly restrict their calories. Because the diet is so restrictive and demanding, it is impossible to continue to follow it for very long and so people return to their previous eating patterns. In addition, people tend to overeat the foods they denied themselves while dieting because they feel deprived and the forbidden food seems even more alluring (see Figure 6-4). This can also lead to binge eating. Thus diets tend not to work in the long run (see Changing for the Better on page 163).

Balanced Diets Supported by Portion Control

For nutritional health, a logical approach to weight loss and subsequent weight maintenance is to establish a nutritionally sound balanced diet (moderately-low in fat, low in saturated fat, and high in complex carbohydrates) that controls portions. Many people are confused about the difference between a portion size and a serving size. Diet scales or food models can assist in gaining an understanding of portion sizes. However, a simple way of measuring one serving size is to think of a serving as equal to the size of the palm of your hand or your fist. This is not to say that this is all you need to eat for a meal, as the food pyramid recommends that we eat six to eleven servings of grains, three to five servings of vegetables, two to four servings of fruit, two to three servings of milk, and two to three servings of meat each day (see Focus On page 175).

TALKING POINTS Have you ever tried to lose weight? What methods were effective for you? What is the longest time you have stuck to a particular weight management strategy?

Fad Diets

Many people use fad diets in an attempt to lose weight quickly. Currently there are over 150 popular diets, often promoted by people who claim to be nutrition experts (see Changing for the Better on page 163). With few exceptions,

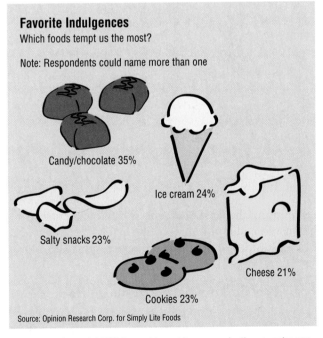

Favorite Indulgences
Which foods tempt us the most?

Note: Respondents could name more than one

Candy/chocolate 35%

Ice cream 24%

Salty snacks 23%

Cheese 21%

Cookies 23%

Source: Opinion Research Corp. for Simply Lite Foods

Figure 6-4 Late night kitchen raids and too many daytime snacks can compromise a healthy diet. Which foods are the most difficult for you to resist?

Table 6.4 Advantages and Disadvantages of Selected Diets

Type of Diet	Advantages	Disadvantages	Examples
Limited food choice diets	Reduce the number of food choices made by the users Limited opportunity to make mistakes Almost certainly low in calories after the first few days	Deficient in many nutrients, depending on the foods allowed Monotonous—difficult to adhere to Eating out and eating socially are difficult Do not retrain dieters in acceptable eating habits Low long-term success rates No scientific basis for these diets	Banana and milk diet Fitonics for Life diet Kempner rice diet The New Beverly Hills Diet Fit for Life Summer sizing
Restricted-calorie, balanced food plans	Sufficiently low in calories to permit steady weight loss Nutritionally balanced Palatable Include readily available foods Reasonable in cost Can be adapted from family meals Permit eating out and social eating Promote a new set of eating habits May employ a point system	Do not appeal to people who want a "unique diet" Do not produce immediate and large weight losses	Weight Watchers Diet Prudent Diet (American Heart Association) Eating Thin for Life Take Off Pounds Sensibly (TOPS) Overeaters Anonymous Jenny Craig
Fasting starvation diet	Rapid initial loss	Nutrient deficient Danger of ketosis >60% loss is muscle <40% loss in fat Low long-term success rate	ZIP Diet 5-Day Miracle Diet Hollywood Diet
High-carbohydrate diet	Emphasizes grains, fruits, and vegetables High in bulk Low in cholesterol	Limits milk, meat Nutritionally very inadequate for calcium, iron, and protein	Quick Weight Loss Diet Pritikin Diet Hilton Head Metabolism Diet
High-protein, low-carbohydrate diets	Rapid initial weight loss because of diuretic effect Very little hunger Usually include all the meat, fish, poultry, and eggs you can eat Occasionally permit milk and cheese in limited amounts Prohibit fruits, vegetables, and any bread or cereal products	Too low in carbohydrates Deficient in many nutrients—vitamin C, vitamin A (unless eggs are included), calcium, and several trace elements High in saturated fat, cholesterol, and total fat Extreme diets of this type could cause death Impossible to adhere to these diets long enough to lose any appreciable amount of weight	Dr. Stillman's Quick Weight Loss Diet Calories Don't Count by Dr. Taller Dr. Atkin's New Diet Revolution Scarsdale Diet Air Force Diet The Carbohydrate Addict's Life Span Program Mastering the Zone Diet South Beach Diet The Carbohydrate Addict's Diet Sugar Busters

continued

these approaches are both ineffective and potentially dangerous. In addition, some involve significant expense. A brief assessment of a variety of popular diet plans is presented in Table 6.4.

High-Protein/Low-Carbohydrate Diets

Currently, the most popular diets are those that reduce carbohydrate intake to an extremely low level, while permitting an almost unlimited consumption of animal protein (meat), with its accompanying high fat content. As indicated in Table 6.4, these diets, such as *Dr. Atkins' New Diet Revolution, Mastering the Zone,* and *Sugar Busters,* involve potential problems, particularly if followed for long periods.

The restriction of calories is the basis of all diets. Some suggest limiting the consumption of fat, others sugar, or the caloric intake is dangerously low for all food groups. Many diet plans, such as the Atkins' Diet, advocate the restriction of carbohydrates which can cause ketosis. When the carbohydrate calories are limited, intake of fat

Table 6.4 Advantages and Disadvantages of Selected Diets—continued

Type of Diet	Advantages	Disadvantages	Examples
		Dangerous for people with kidney disease Weight lost, which is largely water, is rapidly regained Expensive Unpalatable after first few days Difficult for dieter to eat out Unattractive side effects (e.g., bad breath) May require potassium and calcium supplements	Protein Power Get Skinny on Fabulous Food (with modifications)
Low-calorie, high-protein supplement diets	Usually a premeasured powder to be reconstituted with water or a prepared liquid formula Rapid initial weight loss Easy to prepare—already measured Palatable for first few days Usually fortified to provide recommended amount of micronutrients Must be labeled if >50% protein	Usually prescribed at dangerously low calorie intake of 300 to 500 cal Overpriced Low in fiber and bulk—constipating in short amount of time	Metracal Diet Cambridge Diet Liquid Protein Diet Last Chance Diet Oxford Diet Genesis New Direction
High-fiber, low-calorie diets	High satiety value Provide bulk	Irritating to the lower colon Decreases absorption of trace elements, especially iron Nutritionally deficient Low in protein	Pritikin Diet F Diet Zen Macrobiotic Diet
Protein-sparing modified fast <50% protein: 400 Cal	Safe under supervision High-quality protein Minimize loss of lean body mass	Decreases BMR Monotonous Expensive	Optifast Medifast
Premeasured food plans	Provide prescribed portion sizes—little chance of too small or too large a portion Total food programs Some provide adequate calories (1200) Nutritionally balanced or supplemented	Expensive Do not retrain dieters in acceptable eating habits Preclude eating out or social eating Often low in bulk Monotonous Low long-term success rates	Nutri-System Carnation Plan

usually increases. This high fat diet can cause an increase in blood ketones from fat breakdown and too few carbohydrates. Ketosis can cause the blood to become too acidic and dehydration can occur. The body requires a minimum of 50–100 grams of carbohydrate per day to avoid ketosis.[34] Low-carbohydrate diets are characterized by initial rapid weight loss which is appealing to most people, but this loss is primarily due to water and not fat loss. Complications associated with low-carbohydrate, high-protein diets include dehydration, electrolyte loss, calcium depletion, weakness due to inadequate dietary carbohydrate, nausea due to ketosis, vitamin and mineral deficiencies, and possible kidney problems. The risk of coronary heart disease may be higher in those who stay on the diet a long time, due to the increased consumption of foods high in saturated fat and cholesterol.

Controlled Fasting

In cases of extreme obesity, some patients are placed on a complete fast in a hospital setting. The patient consumes

Learning from Our Diversity

Pyramid Power—Mediterranean Style

In Chapter 5 we explored the components of the USDA Food Guide Pyramid, which is designed to help Americans make healthful food choices in appropriate quantities. As you'll recall, we're encouraged to enjoy relatively more servings of bread, cereal, rice, pasta, fruits, and vegetables (located on the first and second levels of the pyramid), while eating fewer servings of meat and dairy products and restricting our intake of fats, oils, and sweets (which occupy the narrower top levels of the pyramid).

Did you know there's another food pyramid that points the way to nutritious food selections that are essential to successful weight control? It's called the Mediterranean Pyramid, and some nutritionists believe it offers the best diet for good health (see the illustration below). Like the USDA Food Guide Pyramid, the Mediterranean Pyramid emphasizes a diet based on grains, fruits, and vegetables. The Mediterranean Pyramid recommends eating red meat just a few times a month and allows generous amounts of olive oil. The USDA Pyramid likewise calls for limited consumption of lean read meat, but it urges sparing consumption of all fats, including olive oil. Another important difference between these two pyramids is that the Mediterranean Pyramid calls for limited consumption of alcohol, which may reduce the risk of coronary heart disease; the USDA Pyramid makes no such recommendation.

Here are some of the other reasons many nutritionists advocate a diet based on Mediterranean favorites:

Greens: Dark leafy greens are rich in antioxidant vitamins, which may help guard against cancer and heart disease and possibly prevent damage to the eyes. Greens are also excellent sources of calcium, iron, and the B vitamin folic acid, which research shows can reduce the risk of neural tube (spinal cord) defects in fetuses. Folic acid may also reduce the risk of heart disease and stroke.

Legumes: Like dark leafy greens, legumes such as garbanzo beans (chick peas), cannellini beans, and red kidney beans are rich in folic acid and iron. What's more, they're high in protein, making them low-fat, no-cholesterol alternatives to meat. And they're great sources of soluble fiber, which can help reduce levels of blood cholesterol.

Garlic: Also shown to be effective in lowering blood cholesterol even when eaten in small quantities, garlic is a traditional staple of Mediterranean cuisine that adds flavor without contributing either fat or sugar.

Olive oil: For centuries, olive oil has been the fat of choice in Mediterranean cooking. Unlike butter and lard, animal products that are loaded with saturated fat, olive oil is a monounsaturated fat, which some studies suggest may reduce the risk of atherosclerosis.

Do you know any students of Mediterranean descent, such as those of Italian, Greek, or Turkish ancestry, who follow a diet based on the Mediterranean Pyramid? If so, what foods do they typically eat? Using the pyramid structure, make a diagram of your current food choices, with those you consume the most at the bottom and those you eat least at the top. How close is your diet to that recommended by the USDA Food Guide Pyramid? The Mediterranean Pyramid?

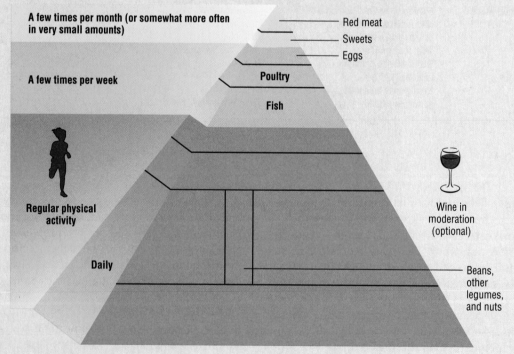

The Mediterranean Food Pyramid.

Changing for the Better

Tips for Losing Weight Successfully

I've tried all kinds of diets, and nothing seems to work for me. I've got to lose weight, but I can't face another failure. What should I do?

- Keep a log of the times, settings, reasons, and feelings associated with your eating.
- Set realistic long-term goals (for example, loss of 2 pounds a week instead of 5 pounds per week).
- Don't completely deprive yourself of enjoyable foods (occasionally reward yourself with a small treat).
- Realize that the sacrifices you're making are important for your health and happiness.
- Eat slowly. It takes about 20 minutes for your brain to recognize satiety signals from your body.
- Put more physical activity into your daily routine (take stairs instead of elevators or park in the distant part of a parking lot, for example).
- Reward yourself when you reach your goals (with new clothes, sporting equipment, a vacation trip).
- Share your commitment to weight loss with your family and friends so that they can support your efforts.
- Keep careful records of your daily food consumption and weekly weight change.
- Be prepared to deal with occasional plateaus and setbacks in your quest for weight loss.
- Remember that moderately-low fat, low saturated fat, and high–complex carbohydrate meals in combination with regular physical activity are the basis for these strategies.
- See this as a lifestyle change, not a short-term diet.

Changing for the Better

Choosing a Diet Plan

I've been trying to find a good diet plan, but I'm confused by all the promotional materials. How can I recognize a sensible approach to weight loss?

- Make sure the program incorporates a balanced diet, an exercise program, and behavior modification.
- Beware of inflexible plans, such as those that require you to eat certain foods on certain days.
- Avoid plans that allow fewer than 1200 calories a day which is the minimum needed to get essential nutrients.
- Make sure the recommended rate of weight loss does not exceed 2 pounds per week.
- Avoid programs that promote vitamins, pills, shots, gimmicks, gadgets, or brand-name diet foods.
- Look for a statement of approval by a reputable nutrition expert or institution.
- Beware of diets that promise fast, easy, or effortless weight loss or "a new secret formula."
- Choose a plan that teaches you how to keep the weight off once you've lost it.

only water, electrolytes, and vitamins. Weight loss is substantial because the body is quickly forced to begin **catabolism** of its fat and muscle tissues. Sodium loss, a negative nitrogen balance, and potassium loss are particular concerns.

Today, some people regularly practice unsupervised modified fasting for short periods. Solid foods are removed from the diet for a number of days. Fruit juice, water, protein supplements, and vitamins are used to minimize the risks associated with total fasting. However, unsupervised short-term fasting that is done too frequently can be dangerous and is not generally recommended.

Weight-Reduction Programs

In virtually every area of the country, at least one version of the popular weight-reduction programs, such as TOPS (Take Off Pounds Sensibly), Jenny Craig, Nutri Sure

Losers, and Weight Watchers, can be found. These programs generally feature a format consisting of (1) a well-balanced diet emphasizing portion control and moderate fat, low–saturated fat, and high–complex carbohydrate foods, (2) specific weight loss goals to be attained over a set period of time, (3) encouragement from supportive leaders and fellow group members, (4) emphasis on regular physical activity, and (5) a maintenance program (follow-up program). The Changing for the Better box above presents some guidelines for choosing a weight loss program.

In theory, these programs offer an opportunity to lose weight for people who cannot or will not participate in a physical activity program. But their effectiveness is very limited. In fact, the limited success of these programs and the difficulty that working people have in attending meetings have resulted in falling enrollment and the development of home-based programs, such as hospital-based

> **Key Terms**
>
> **catabolizing** the metabolic process of breaking down tissue for the purpose of converting it to energy.

Table 6.5 The Real Cost of Dieting

Plan	Annual Cost
Weight Watchers	$709
Over the counter diet pills	$500
Nutritional counseling	$450–$1200
Physician supervised weight loss program	$2,000–$3,5000
Prescription diet pills	$1,090–$1,343
Gastric bypass surgery	$20,000–$25,000

Source: Chatzky JS. The real costs of diets, *USA Weekend*, December 2002.

wellness programs, YMCA and YWCA programs, and Weight Watchers. All these programs are costly when compared with self-directed approaches, especially when the program markets its own food products (see Table 6.5).

Diet and Physical Activity

Most Americans attempting to lose weight fail to include a physical activity component in their dietary approach. How much exercise is enough? New studies suggest that Americans should engage in at least 45 minutes a day, 5 times a week of moderately intense aerobic exercise. Also weight training has become a more important factor in weight management. As with most things, too much or too little exercise is not beneficial. As will be discussed in the next chapter, some people with eating disorders tend to over-exercise which results in diminishing returns.

Physical Intervention

A second approach to weight loss involves techniques and products designed to change basic eating patterns. Some are self-selected and self-applied, and others must be administered in an institutional setting by highly trained professionals.

Hunger- and Satiety-Influencing Products

Many overweight people want to lessen their desire to eat or develop a stronger sense of when they have eaten enough. Today, many dieters are confused about the safety of pharmaceutical approaches to weight loss, including both over-the-counter (OTC) and prescription drugs.

Until recently, **phenylpropanolamine (PPA)** was incorporated into many OTC weight-loss products. Discontinuation of its use is based on its adverse effects on conditions such as hypertension, diabetes, glaucoma, and thyroid disease. PPA can also be found in some OTC and

prescription cold and cough medications. The FDA recommends that consumers not use any products containing PPA due to its association with higher risk for stroke.

The FDA also continues to advise against using OTC weight loss products containing the recently banned ephedrine (*ma huang* and Chinese ephedra). Because they are categorized as dietary supplements, the FDA can't regulate these products to ensure that they meet certain standards or are safe and effective. Many people see these supplements as safe because they are "natural," and yet they can be more dangerous and deadly than prescription medications because they are not inspected as to the purity and accuracy of the contents or the potency of the ingredients. A recent review showed that the use of herbal supplements increased by 370% between 1990 and 1997. Ephedrine, found in most herbal diet pills, has been linked to heart attacks, strokes, hepatitis, headache, tremors, anxiety, extreme irritability, and insomnia in consumers of all ages. Metabolife, an herbal diet supplement that contains ephedra which was recently banned by the FDA, has sold 50 million bottles in the last 5 years, about 101,000 pills an hour. In 2003 the death of 23-year-old Baltimore Orioles pitcher Steve Bechler was linked to an ephedra supplement, prompting the FDA to reexamine the supplement. Ephedra was banned by the FDA in late 2003.[37]

Some prescription medications have been shown to produce serious side effects. Two such medications, phentermine and fenfluramine, have been prescribed for patients who wanted to lose weight. Both drugs affect levels of serotonin, the neurotransmitter associated with satiety. This popular combination, referred to as *phenfen*, gradually raised concern among health experts because of the side effects it produced in people with angina, glaucoma, and high blood pressure. In addition, reports began to surface that some patients had developed a rare but potentially lethal condition called *pulmonary hypertension*.

During the mid-1990s, a new serotonin-specific weight loss drug, *dexfenfluramine* (Redux), was approved for use in the United States. Results among patients who used the drug, in combination with dietary modification and exercise, seemed impressive during the initial months of its widespread use. However, some patients began to take dexfenfluramine with fenfluramine in an attempt to

> ### Key Terms
>
> **phenylpropanolamine (PPA)** (fen ill pro pan **ol** ah meen) the active chemical compound still found in some over-the-counter diet products.

find a new combination that would be even more effective than phen-fen or Redux used alone, and death resulted in some cases.

Thus, two combinations of three serotonin-specific drugs were in vogue in early 1997. However, by May of 1997, there were reports of weight loss patients with newly diagnosed heart valve damage who had been using these drug combinations. In some cases, damage was correctable only by valve-replacement surgery. Accordingly, in September 1997, the FDA requested voluntary withdrawal of fenfluramine and dexfenfluramine from the market.[38] Manufacturers responded by ceasing all distribution of the drugs. Phentermine remains on the market and is used in combination with various antidepressants, such as Prozac, Zoloft, and Paxil.

Soon after reports of the initial concern over the use of phentermine and fenfluramine, the FDA approved another serotonin-specific obesity drug, sibutramine (Meridia) even though an advisory committee within the FDA recommended against approving it. Meridia acts on serotonin in the body similarly to how phenfen and redux functioned and, like its predecessors, has been linked to heart attacks, high blood pressure, strokes, and death; however, it still remains on the market in the United States. Italy recently pulled Meridia from the market following reports of deaths linked to this drug.

A non–serotonin-influencing drug, *orlistat* (Xenical), has recently been approved. Unlike the serotonin-specific drugs, orlistat reduces fat absorption in the small intestine by about 30%. The drug is intended for use among people who are 20% or more above ideal weight. It could cause a 10% loss of body weight without significant dietary restriction. Some concern exists about the lack of absorption of fat soluble vitamins among people taking the drug. Additionally, anal leakage may accompany the drug's use, particularly following meals with high fat content.

Surgical Measures

When a person is morbidly obese and weight loss is critical, surgical intervention may be considered. A *gastrointestinal* or *bariatric surgery* is a major operation in which a portion of the small intestine is bypassed in an attempt to decrease the body's ability to absorb nutrients. Candidates for this surgery include those with a BMI above 40 or about 100 pounds overweight for men and 80 pounds overweight for women. People with a BMI between 35–40 who suffer from type 2 diabetes or life-threatening cardiopulmonary problems may also be candidates for surgery. Although this procedure can produce a major weight loss, it is associated with many unpleasant side effects (including diarrhea and liver damage) and various nutritional deficiencies.

Gastric Band Surgery

This is a surgical procedure in which a gastric band is implanted around the stomach, dividing the stomach into upper and lower parts. The band can be tightened or loosened by inflating or deflating the hollow connection tubing which is filled with liquid. After implantation, a small amount of food fills the top of the stomach and keeps the individual feeling full for longer periods of time, dramatically reducing food intake. The surgery takes around 2 hours and involves the risks associated with major surgery. The band is permanent and some potential side effects are vomiting and nausea, and excess food may back up into the esophagus. Typically, weight loss is somewhat slower with this type of surgery as compared to bypass surgery.

Gastroplasty, or stomach stapling, is a surgical procedure that involves sealing off a sizable portion of the stomach with surgical staples or recently approved adjustable implanted stomach bands. The resulting reduced capacity of the stomach decreases the amount of food it can hold. Patients feel full more quickly after eating a small meal. This procedure carries the general risks associated with surgery, involves the expense of a major surgical procedure, and is sometimes reversible. It is also possible to loosen the staples through overeating, negating the effects of the surgery.

Liposuction

Another form of surgical weight loss management is *liposuction*, or *lipoplasty*. In this procedure, a physician inserts a small tube through the skin and vacuum aspirates away fat cells.

Liposuction is basically a cosmetic procedure. Possible infection, pain and discomfort, bruising, swelling, discoloration, abscesses, and unattractive changes in body contours are possible outcomes of liposuction.[39] Therefore people considering this procedure should carefully investigate all its aspects, including the training and experience of the surgeon, to determine whether it is appropriate for them.

Body Wraps

Although not a surgical procedure or a weight loss technique, *body wrapping* is another form of body contouring. In this procedure, various areas of the body are tightly wrapped with 6-inch strips of materials soaked in a solution of amino acids, which is claimed to draw toxins out of the underlying tissue, shrink fatty deposits, diminish cellulite, lighten stretch marks, and eliminate inches of fat. Once the wrapping is removed, the newly-contoured body area may remain this way for 4 to 10 weeks. Although the secret to the success of a particular spa's body wrapping approach is supposed to lie in its uniquely formulated soaking solution, the contouring effect probably

I hear all kinds of things I should do to control my weight, such as not eat after 5 P.M., don't eat snacks, skip breakfast. Is this correct?

There are lots of myths and misunderstandings about maintaining a healthy weight. Here are a few tips to follow:

- Eat every 2–3 hours to avoid overeating at your next meal. Choose small, nutritious, low-fat snacks.
- Eat slowly to allow yourself to enjoy your food and to allow your brain to register satiety before getting overly full.
- Wait 20 minutes before getting a second helping or adding food to your plate once you have finished your meal. It takes this long for the message to get to your brain from your stomach to communicate that you are full.

- Balance low-fat food with the number of calories you are consuming. Sometimes fat free means high caloric intake.
- Eat foods with high water content (for example watermelon) and remember to drink water with your meals.
- Avoid eating 2–3 hours before bedtime and be aware of the kinds of foods you are eating before bed such as chips, ice cream, and candy.
- Exercise in the morning if possible as this will start your metabolism going. Exercise aerobically for 45 minutes, five times a week.
- Incorporate weight training into your exercise regime at least three times a week.
- Eat breakfast! This will get your metabolism going in the morning and help you to avoid overeating later in the day.

results from dehydration of underlying tissue and redistribution of extracellular fluids through pressure from the wrapping.

Eating Disorders

Some people have medically identifiable, potentially serious difficulties with body image, body weight, and food selection. Among these disorders are two that are frequently seen among college students—anorexia nervosa and bulimia nervosa. In addition, binge eating and disordered eating are also found in college populations. These topics are included in this chapter because most eating disorders begin with dieting. However, most eating disorders also involve inappropriate food choices and psychological issues (discussed in Chapters 2 and 5).

In the United States, conservative estimates indicate that after puberty 5 to 10 million females and 1 million males are struggling with eating disorders such as anorexia, bulimia, or binge eating disorder. It is estimated that approximately 8% of college women will develop an eating disorder, and the population most at risk for developing bulimia is college freshmen women. Ninety to 95% of people with eating disorders are women, although the prevalence of eating disorders in men is on the rise. Athletes such as dancers, gymnasts, swimmers, runners, and wrestlers are at risk for developing eating disorders because of the focus on weight and appearance for successful performance. In fact, any group in which success is influenced by weight or attractiveness is at risk for the development of an eating disorder, such as those involved in the performance arts, theatre, television, and modeling.

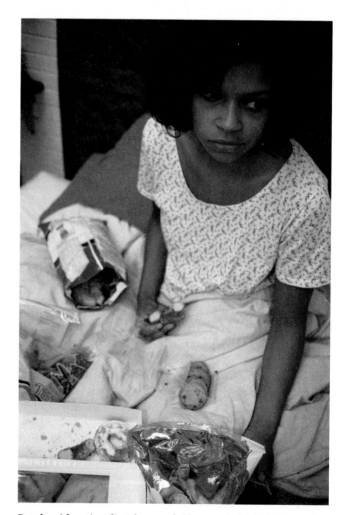

People with eating disorders use food to cope with feeling out of control, stressed, upset or bored.

Recognizing Anorexia Nervosa and Bulimia Nervosa

The American Psychological Association uses the following diagnostic criteria to identify anorexia nervosa and bulimia

Anorexia	Bulimia
• Body weight is 15% or more below desirable weight • Fear of weight gain • Distorted body image • In women, the absence of 3 or more menstrual periods (younger girls may not start); In men, sex hormones decrease	• Binge eating two or more times a week for at least 3 months • A lack of control over bingeing • Engaging in inappropriate compensatory behavior purging two or more times a week for at least 3 months to prevent weight gain • Overly concerned about body image

Characteristic symptoms include the following. Note that it is unlikely that all the symptoms will be evident in any one individual.

Anorexia	Bulimia
• Looks thin and keeps getting thinner • Skips meals, cuts food into small pieces, moves food around plate to appear to have eaten • Loss of menstrual periods and possible infertility • Wears baggy clothes in an attempt to disguise weight loss and to keep warm • Significant hair loss • Extreme sensitivity to cold • Dizziness, lightheadedness, headaches • Withdrawn, irritable, depressed • Insomnia • Decreased sex drive • Dehydration, kidney dysfunction • Fatigue, loss of energy • Decreased concentration • Lanugo (fine downy body hair) • Heart irregularities, heart failure	• Bathroom use immediately after eating • Eating in secret • Excessive time (and money) spent food shopping • Shopping for food at several stores instead of one store • Menstrual irregularities and possible fertility problems • Excessive constipation • Swollen and/or infected salivary glands, sore throat • Bursting blood vessels in the eyes • Dental erosion in teeth and gums • Dehydration and kidney dysfunction • Significant hair loss; dry, brittle hair and nails • Increased acne and skin problems • Heart irregularities, heart failure

Anorexia Nervosa

Anorexia nervosa is an eating disorder in which a person denies his or her own feelings of hunger and avoids food, with marked weight loss occurring. Anorexics tend to run from food in the relentless pursuit of thinness although they perceive themselves as never thin enough. To meet the diagnostic criteria for anorexia nervosa, the individual has an intense fear of gaining weight, even though he or she weighs less than 85% of the expected weight for his/her age, gender, and height, and, in females, menstruation ceases for at least three consecutive months.[40] In addition, people with anorexia perceive themselves as overweight and much larger than what they look like in reality. Anorexics lose their ability to recognize when they are hungry and have difficulty eating even if they want to do so. Depression, irritability, with-

drawal, perfectionism, and low self-esteem are some of the psychological problems associated with anorexia. In addition, anorexics tend to feel cold most of the time because they have very little body fat (2–10%) and also suffer from lightheadedness, dizziness, insomnia, hair loss,

> ### Key Terms
>
> **anorexia nervosa** an eating disorder in which the individual weighs less than 85% of their expected weight for his or her age, gender, and height, has an intense fear of gaining weight, and in females, menstruation ceases for at least 3 consecutive months. People with anorexia perceive themselves as overweight, even though they are underweight.

muscle cramps, stress fractures, fatigue, decreased memory and concentration, and gastrointestinal problems. More serious complications include heart and kidney failure, hypothermia, osteoporosis, infertility, and, in 25% of cases, death.

As with other eating disorders, anorexia nervosa also involves a sense of feeling out of control in one's life and attempting to find control through food and weight loss. It is not a coincidence that anorexia nervosa typically begins around puberty: Most individuals with anorexia have a fear of growing up and all that goes with being an adult, such as financial responsibility, sexual relationships, leaving one's family, and becoming more autonomous and independent.

Anorexia often begins with dieting, but may also begin as a result of an illness such as the stomach flu, a relationship that breaks up, or after dental surgery in which it might be expected that one would temporarily eat less. However, anorexics will tell you that the disorder begins to take on a life of its own after what started as wanting to lose a few pounds turns into losing 15% or more of body weight and still not feeling satisfied with one's appearance. Friends and family might initially encourage the person on his or her weight loss and say complimentary things about his or her appearance, but soon become concerned when the person's weight continues to dramatically decrease.

Anorexia has become more common as changing cultural ideals for beauty have changed. Our standards have gone from Marilyn Monroe who was a voluptuous 5′5″, 128-pound woman to Kate Moss who has been reported to be 5′7″ and 105 pounds.[7] Now the "lollipop look" is considered the "in look" in Hollywood, with actresses and models having stick-thin bodies, making their heads seem huge.

Denial of problems plays a major role in eating disorders in which the individual refuses to acknowledge that there is anything wrong, even though she is becoming thinner and wasting away, and family and friends are expressing great concern. While anorexia nervosa is considered a serious medical and psychological disorder, some anorexics argue that "Anorexia is a lifestyle not a disorder." These heated debates and discussions often occur through pro-anorexia websites. With names like "Thinspiration," "Stick Figures," and "Anorexic and Proud," these pro-anorexia forums have become very popular and deadly in the past few years. These websites show computer-enhanced pictures of models and actresses like Calista Flockhart and Lara Flynn Boyle, making them appear thinner and more skeletal than they really are.[41]

Messages on these websites include tips for how to starve, how to purge, ways of hiding one's disorder, and encouragement to lose more weight. There has been a push among health providers, educators, and health organizations to eliminate these types of websites, and they have been somewhat successful. However, these sites are purported to still exist, although more disguised and underground than in the past.[42]

Most recently, the three groups that have traditionally been overlooked in the incidence of anorexia are women of color, female athletes (see the Female Athlete Triad in Chapter 4), and men. The research shows a significant increase in the incidence of anorexia among these three groups. More focus has been given to anorexia among women of color, and it has been proposed that this group might be more vulnerable to developing eating disorders than Caucasian women because of ethno-cultural identity issues. It has been suggested that the more pressure women of color feel to fit into the dominant culture's standards of beauty and thinness, the more likely they are to develop eating disorders.

Often female athletes are not diagnosed with eating disorders because the symptoms of anorexia, absence of menses, low body fat and weight, and osteoporosis, referred to as the "female athletic triad" are not uncommon among athletes and don't necessarily signify the presence of an eating disorder.

The prevalence of anorexia nervosa (as well as bulimia nervosa, which we'll cover later) has traditionally been very low in men as compared with women. Today, however, the incidence of both conditions is increasing in men as they begin to feel some of the same pressures that women feel to conform to the weight and body composition standards imposed by others. The "lean look" of young male models serves as a standard for more and more young men, whereas the requirements to "make weight" for various sports drives others. Runners, jockeys, swimmers, and gymnasts frequently must lose weight quickly to meet particular standards for competition or the expectations of coaches and trainers. Researchers report that men are less inclined than women to admit that they may have an eating disorder, thinking it is a "women's illness." Thus they are less likely to seek treatment. In addition, physicians tend not to suspect men as having eating disorders, and so they go untreated.

Fortunately, psychological treatment in combination with medical and dietary interventions can return the person with anorexia nervosa to a more life-sustaining pattern of eating. The person with anorexia needs to receive the care of professionals experienced in the treatment of this disorder. It is not uncommon for this treatment to take 3 to 5 years. If others, including friends, coworkers, roommates, and parents observe this condition, they should consult a health care provider for assistance.

Resources for Anorexia and Bulimia Treatment

Local Resources

- College or university health centers
- College or university counseling centers
- Comprehensive mental health centers
- Crisis intervention centers
- Mental health associations

Organizations and Self-Help Groups

American Anorexia/Bulimia Association, Inc.
165 W. 46th St., Suite 1108, New York,
NY 10036
www.aabainc.org

Anorexia Nervosa and Associated Disorders, Inc.
P.O. Box 7, Highland Park, IL 60035
(847) 831-3438

Anorexia Nervosa and Related Eating Disorders, Inc.
P.O. Box 5102, Eugene, OR 97405
(541) 344-1144

Bulimia Anorexia Nervosa Association
300 Cabana Road, East, Windsor, Ontario,
Canada N9G 1A3
(519) 969-2112

Eating Disorders Awareness and Prevention, Inc.
www.edap.org

Laureate Eating Disorders Program
P.O. Box 470207
Tulsa, OK 74147
(800) 322-5173

www.laureate.org

National Institute of Mental Health
Eating Disorders Information Page
www.nimh.nih.gov/publicat/eatdis.htm

National Eating Disorder Association
603 Stewart St., Suite 803,
Seattle, WA 98101
(206) 382-3587
www.nationaleatingdisorders.org

TALKING POINTS What would you do if you suspected a friend of yours had an eating disorder? Would you share your concern with him or her? If so, what would you say?

Bulimia Nervosa

While anorexics are underweight, people with **bulimia nervosa** often are of a normal weight. These individuals use food and weight as a way of coping with stress, boredom, conflict in relationships, and low self-esteem. It is not uncommon in our society to comfort ourselves with food, to have social activities based around food, and to eat as a way of procrastinating a dreaded activity. However, people with bulimia take this to the extreme, engaging in recurrent bingeing, consuming unusually large amounts of food and feeling out of control with their eating.[40]

While anorexics run away from food, bulimics run to food to cope with their emotions, problems, and stress. Because they feel so guilty, ashamed, and anxious about the food they have consumed, people with bulimia **purge** by self-induced vomiting, taking an excessive number of laxatives and diuretics, excessively exercising or fasting. There is a strong preoccupation with weight, calories, and food among sufferers of bulimia. Most people with bulimia constantly count calories, weigh themselves throughout the day, and frequently make negative statements concerning different parts of their bodies, primarily focusing on the thighs, stomach, and waist. As with anorexia, bulimia is associated with depression, isolation, anxiety, perfectionism, and low self-esteem. Dental erosion, hair loss, esophageal lesions, blood in the vomit and stools, loss of voluntary gag reflex, kidney damage, heart failure, gastrointestinal problems, ketosis, edema, infertility, parotid gland swelling, depression, and insomnia are just some of the medical problems associated with bulimia nervosa.

As has been mentioned previously, bulimia often begins around age 17 to 18 years of age when young adults are separating from their families and are forging lives of their own. There may be some conflict around issues of independence, autonomy, and relationships with family. There is a higher incidence of bulimia than anorexia, although some bulimics may have had anorexia in the past. There is also a higher rate of bulimia among female college students as compared to their peers who are not attending colleges. Treatment for bulimia nervosa involves nutritional counseling, psychological treatment, and consultation with a physician. Often people with bulimia can recover from this disorder within a year of beginning treatment.

Key Terms

bulimia nervosa an eating disorder in which individuals engage in episodes of bingeing, consuming unusually large amounts of food and feeling out of control, and engaging in some compensatory purging behavior to eliminate the food.

purging using vomiting, laxatives, diuretics, enemas, or other medications, or means such as excessive exercise or fasting to eliminate food.

Binge Eating Disorder

Binge eating disorder is the newest term for what was previously referred to as compulsive overeating. Binge eaters use food to cope in the same way that bulimics do and also feel out of control and unable to stop eating during binges. People with this disorder report eating rapidly and in secret or may snack all day. They tend to eat until they feel uncomfortably full, sometimes hoarding food and eating when they aren't physically hungry.[40] Like people with bulimia, they feel guilty and ashamed of their eating habits and have a great deal of self-loathing and body hatred. People who have binge eating disorder do not engage in purging behavior and this is what differentiates it from bulimia nervosa. Typically, binge eaters have a long history of diet failures, feel anxious, are socially withdrawn from others, and are overweight. Heart problems, high blood pressure, joint problems, abnormal blood sugar levels, fatigue, depression, and anxiety are associated with binge eating. The treatment of this eating disorder involves interventions similar to those described for treating bulimia nervosa.

Chewing and Spitting Out Food Syndrome

Chewing and spitting out one's food without swallowing it has also been used as a method for weight loss or weight management. This is a common eating disorder and falls within the "Eating Disorder Not Otherwise Specified" diagnosis. It differs from bulimia nervosa and researchers contend that chewing and spitting out food without swallowing may indicate a more severe eating disorder.[43]

Night Eating Syndrome

Night eating syndrome has not yet been formally defined as an eating disorder. The signs and symptoms of this syndrome include: eating more than half of one's daily food intake after dinner and before breakfast, feeling tense, anxious, and guilty while eating, difficulty falling or staying asleep at night, and having little to no appetite in the morning. Unlike binge eating, night eating involves eating throughout the evening hours rather than in short episodes. It is important to note that there is a strong preference for carbohydrates among night eaters. Some researchers speculate that night eating may be an unconscious attempt to self-medicate mood problems because eating carbohydrates can trigger the brain to produce so-called "feel good" neurochemicals. Research is underway in examining the underlying causes of this syndrome and developing subsequent treatment interventions. It seems likely that a combination of biological, genetic, and psychological factors contribute to this problem.

Treatment for Eating Disorders

The treatment for eating disorders is multimodal and multidimensional involving nutritionists, psychologists, physicians, family, and friends. There are different treatment modalities such as individual, group, and family counseling. Sometimes treatment requires in-patient hospitalization to medically stabilize the individual. In extreme cases, a feeding tube may be inserted to treat starvation, especially if the person refuses to eat. Behavioral modification and cognitive therapy are utilized in counseling people with eating problems. Medications such as antidepressants are often used to decrease obsessive-compulsive behavior, reduce anxiety, alleviate depression, and improve mood. Some medications can stimulate or reduce appetite as well. There is some debate over the efficacy of using an addictions model, similar to the twelve-step Alcoholics Anonymous philosophy, with eating disorders. Overeaters Anonymous utilizes this model in helping people with eating problems and many hospital programs employ this model in their treatment programs. While there seems to be some overlap with substance abuse problems such as denial of problems, feeling out of control of one's behavior, and using food or drugs or alcohol to cope with problems, this is where the similarities end as obviously one needs food to live which is not the case with drugs and alcohol.

Underweight and Undernourished

For some young adults, the lack of adequate body weight is a serious concern, particularly for those who have inherited a tendency to thinness. These people would likely fall into a BMI category (see page 150) of less than 18.5 and be from 10% to 20% below normal on a standard height-weight table. Males tend to be particularly concerned with too thin a body type, preferring a lean, muscular V-shape appearance.

Nutritionists believe that the healthiest way to gain weight is to increase the intake of calorie-dense food. These foods are characterized by high fat density resulting from high levels of vegetable fats (polyunsaturated fats). Foods that meet this requirement are dried fruits,

> **Key Terms**
>
> **binge eating disorder** an eating disorder formerly referred to as compulsive overeating disorder; binge eaters use food to cope in the same way that bulimics do and also feel out of control, but do not engage in compensatory purging behavior.

bananas, nuts, granola, and cheeses made from low-fat milk. These foods should be consumed later in a meal so that the onset of satiety that quickly follows eating fat-rich foods does not occur. The current recommendation is to eat three calorie-dense meals of moderate size per day, interspersed with two or three substantial snacks. Using the Food Guide Pyramid (see Chapter 5, page 115) as a guide, **underweight** people should eat the highest number of recommended servings for each group.

A second component of weight gain for those who are underweight is an exercise program that uses weight-training activities intended to increase muscle mass. As detailed in Chapter 4, the use of anabolic drugs without highly competent medical supervision has no role in healthful weight gain. In addition, carefully monitored aerobic activity should be undertaken in sessions that adequately maintain heart-lung health. At the same time, unnecessary activity that expands calories should be restricted. See Chapter 4 to review the female athlete triad and its relationship to underweight.

For those who cannot gain weight, even by using these approaches, a medical evaluation may offer an ex-planation. If no medical reason can be found, the person must begin to accept the reality of his or her unique body type.

When individuals fall below 80% of their desirable weight on standard height-weight tables and display BMI rates from 16 to 10, it is highly probable that they are not only underweight but, more important, *undernourished*.[44] This condition suggests clinically significant deficiencies in both the quantity of food being consumed and its nutritional value. Whether the undernourishment is associated with anorexia nervosa, other medical conditions characterized by weight loss (such as irritable bowel disease), or poverty or famine, affected people are in danger of death from starvation.

Key Terms

underweight a condition in which the body is below the desirable weight.

Taking Charge of Your Health

- Investigate the resources available on your campus that you could use to determine your healthy weight and body composition profile.
- Evaluate your eating behaviors to find out if you are using food to cope with stress. If you are, develop a plan to use nonfood options, such as exercise or interaction with friends or family members, to deal with stress.
- Formulate a realistic set of goals for changing your weight and body composition in a time frame that allows you to do so in a healthful way.

- Establish a daily schedule that lets you make any necessary dietary and physical activity adjustments.
- Keep a daily journal of your weight-management efforts.
- Monitor your progress toward meeting your weight-management goals.
- Design a reward system for reaching each goal.
- Learn to accept your body, including the imperfections.
- Focus on other aspects of yourself, besides your appearance.

Summary

- Weight management has become an obsession in American culture as well as a significant health problem; an estimated 61% of U.S. adults are either overweight or obese.
- The average caloric intake for Americans has increased over the past two decades while the majority of Americans are not physically active on a regular basis.
- Doctors usually define "overweight" as a condition in which a person's weight is 1% to 19% higher than "normal," as defined by a standard height/weight chart. Obesity is usually defined as a condition in which a person's weight is 20% or more above normal

weight. "Morbid obesity" refers to being 50%-100% over normal weight, more than 100 pounds over normal weight, or sufficiently overweight to interfere with health or normal functioning.
- Some of the methods for assessing one's weight are: Body Mass Index, current height and weight tables, waist to hip ratios, electrical impedance, BOD POD, skinfold measurements, hydrostatic weighing, and medical scales.
- Basal Metabolic Rate (BMR) is a measure of resting energy expenditure that is taken upon awakening, 10–12 hours after eating, or 12–18 hours after significant physical activity.

- Thermic effect of food (TEF) refers to the amount of energy our bodies require for the digestion, absorption, and transportation of food.
- There are four factors that seem to play a significant role in the prevalence of obesity: sex, age, socioeconomic status, and race.
- Hypothyroidism is a condition in which the thyroid gland produces an insufficient amount of a hormone called thyroxin.
- The energy expenditure and energy storage centers of the body possess a genetically programmed awareness of the body's most physiologically desirable weight called set point.
- The process of storing or burning more energy to maintain the body's "best" weight is called adaptive thermogenesis.
- Lower socioeconomic status, married men, parents, and people living in rural areas are associated with a higher incidence of obesity.
- Environmental factors such as portion size, price, advertising, the availability of food, and the number of food choices presented all can influence the amount the average person consumes.
- Psychological reasons for eating refer to eating not out of hunger but as a way of coping with feelings, as a way of socializing and celebrating with others, and due to associating certain activities with eating.
- Weight management experts identify inactivity as the single most important reason that obesity is so high in today's society.
- Weight loss occurs when the calories consumed are less than the energy the body needs for physiological maintenance and activity.

- The primary types of weight management techniques include dietary alterations, surgical interventions, medications, weight loss programs, and physical activity.
- A commitment to a lifestyle change of eating in healthy ways and engaging in regular aerobic exercise seems to be the most effective strategy for weight loss and weight maintenance.
- Anorexia nervosa is a psychological condition in which the individual weighs less than 85% of his/her expected weight for his/her age, gender, and height, in women menstruation ceases for at least 3 consecutive months; and there is an intense fear of gaining weight. People with anorexia perceive themselves as overweight, even though they are underweight.
- People with bulimia nervosa often are of a normal weight. These individuals use food and weight as a way of coping with stress, boredom, conflict in relationships, and low self-esteem. People with bulimia engage in recurrent bingeing on unusually large amounts of food and feeling out of control with their eating.
- Binge eaters use food to cope in the same way that bulimics do and also feel out of control and unable to stop eating during binges but do not engage in inappropriate compensatory purging behaviors.
- The treatment for eating disorders is multimodal and multidimensional involving nutritionists, psychologists, physicians, family, and friends.

Review Questions

1. What percentage of U.S. adults are either overweight or obese?
2. How has the average caloric intake and physical activity level for Americans changed over the past two decades?
3. Define overweight, obesity, and morbid obesity.
4. List at least four of the methods used for assessing weight.
5. Define Basal Metabolic Rate (BMR).
6. Describe the thermic effect of food (TEF) and how it relates to the BMR.
7. What are four factors that seem to play a significant role in the prevalence of obesity?
8. Describe hypothyroidism and its impact on weight management.
9. Define set point.
10. The process of storing or burning more energy to maintain the body's "best" weight is called what?
11. What are two factors associated with a higher incidence of obesity?
12. Give four examples of how environmental factors can influence the amount the average person consumes.
13. Describe at least two psychological reasons for eating.
14. What is the single most important reason that obesity is so high in today's society, according to the experts?
15. How does weight loss occur?
16. Give examples of four different types of weight management techniques.
17. What is the most effective strategy for weight loss and weight maintenance?

18. Describe the symptoms of anorexia nervosa.
19. Describe the symptoms of bulimia.
20. How is binge eating disorder different from bulimia nervosa?

21. Discuss some of the components for effective treatment for eating disorders.

References

1. National Center for Chronic Disease Prevention and Health Promotion. Defining Overweight and Obesity, September 2002.
2. National Research Council, *Diet and Health: Implications for Reducing Chronic Disease Risk.* Washington, DC: National Academy Press: 1989.
3. Harvard Women's Health Watch: Panel issues new guidelines for healthy eating. *Harvard Medical School,* November 2002, Volume 10 (3).
4. Sturm R, Wells KB. Does obesity contribute as much to morbidity as poverty or smoking? *Public Health* 115 (3), 229–235, 2001.
5. Crowley LV. *Introduction to Human Disease,* ed 4, Jones & Bartlett, 1996.
6. Field AE, et al. Impact of overweight on the risk of developing common chronic disease during a 10-year period. *Arch Intern Med* 161 (13), 1581–1586, 2001.
7. Poulton T. *No Fat Chicks.* Secaucus, N.J. Carol Publishing Group, 1997.
8. Maine M. *Body Wars.* Carlsbad, CA: Gurze Books, 2000.
9. Cash T, Henry P. Women's body images: the results of a national survey in the U.S.A. *Sex Role Res* 33(1), 19–29, 1995.
10. Brownell KD and Fairburn CG. *Eating Disorders and Obesity: A Comprehensive Handbook.* New York: Guilford Press. 1995.
11. U.S. Department of Agriculture/U.S. Department of Health and Human Services. Nutrition and your health: dietary guidelines for Americans. *Home and Garden Bulletin,* 232, 2000.
12. Waist Management, Gauging Your Risk. *Consumer Reports,* p. 48, August 2003.
13. Roche AF. Anthropometric methods: new and old, what they tell us. *Int J Obess* 8 (5), 509–523, 1984.
14. Dempster P, Aitkens S. A new air displacement method for the determination of human body composition. *Medical Science Sports Exercise* 27 (2), 1692–1697, 1995.
15. International Health Racquet and Sportsclub Association. BOD POD Body Composition System to Descend on San Francisco's *IHRSA CONVENTION* as reported in the 29th Anniversary Exhibition in San Francisco's Moscone Convention Center, March 22–24, 2001.
16. Benardot, D. Nutrition for Serious Athletes. Atlanta, GA: Human Kinetics, 2000.
17. Thelen MH, Powell AL, Lawrence C, and Kuhnent ME. Eating and body image concerns among children. *Journal of Consulting and Clinical Psychology* 21, 41, 46, 1992.
18. Troiano RP, Flegal KM, Kuczmarski RJ, Campbell SM, and Johnson CL. Overweight prevalence and trends for children and adolescents. *Archives of Pediatrics and Adolescent Medicine* 149, 1085–1091, 1995.
19. Sobal J. Obesity and socioeconomic status: A framework for examining relationships between physical and social variables. *Medical Anthropology* 13, 231–247, 1991.
20. Wadden TA and Stunkard AJ. *Handbook of Obesity Treatment.* New York: Guilford Press, 2002.
21. Halaas J, et al. Weight-reducing effects on the plasma protein encoded by the obese gene. *Science* 269 (5223), 543–546, 1995.
22. Folsom AR, Jensen MD, Jacobs DR, Hilner JE, Tsai AW, and Schreiner PJ. Serum leptin and weight gain over eight years in African American and Caucasian young adults. *Obesity Research* 7 (1), 1–8, 1999.
23. Sakurai, T et al. Orexins and orexin receptors: A family of hypothalamic neuropeptides and G protein-coupled receptors that regulate feeding behavior. *Cell,* 92(4): 573–585, 1998.
24. LaLeche International. The Womanly Art of Breastfeeding, 1997.
25. Set Point: What your body is trying to tell you. *National Eating Disorders Information Centre Bulletin* 7(2), June, 1992.
26. The truth about dieting. *Consumer Reports,* 26–31 June, 2002.
27. Saladin KS. *Anatomy & Physiology: the unity of form and function.* Dubuque, IA: William C. Brown/ McGraw-Hill, 1998.
28. Sorbara M and Geliebter A. Body image disturbance in obese outpatients before and after weight loss in relation to race, gender and age of onset of obesity. *Internal Journal of Eating Disorders,* 416–423, May, 2002.
29. Stunkard AJ and Wadden TA. *Obesity: Theory and Therapy.* New York: Raven Press, 1993.
30. Sobal J and Stunkard AJ. Socioeconomic status and obesity: A review of the literature. *Psychological Bulletin* 105, 260–275, 1989.

31. Sobal J, Rauschenbach B, and Frongillo E. Marital status, fatness and obesity. *Social Science and Medicine* 35, 915–923, 1992.
32. Goode E. Obesity in America. *The New York Times,* August 19, 2003.
33. Weight Watchers. *Stop Stuffing Yourself: 7 Steps to Conquering Overeating.* New York: Wiley Publishing Inc., 1998.
34. Insel P, Turner RE, Ross D. *Nutrition.* Sudbury, MA: Jones and Bartlett Publishers, 2002.
35. Ganong WF. *Review of Medical Physiology,* 18th ed. Appleton & Lange, 1997.
36. Wardlaw GM. *Perspectives in Nutrition,* 4th ed. McGraw-Hill, 1999.
37. Ephedra Ban Puts Herb Industry on Notice. *The New York Times,* December 31, 2003.
38. Center for Drug Evaluation and Research, U.S. Food and Drug Administration: FDA announces withdrawal of fenfluramine and dexfenfluramine. *News Release* #97–32, September 15, 1997.
39. Grazer FM and de Jong RH. Fatal outcomes from liposuction; census survey of cosmetic surgeons. *Plastic Reconstructive Surgery* 105 (1) 436–446, 2000.
40. *Diagnostic and Statistical Manual of Mental Disorders IV TR.* Washington, D.C., American Psychiatric Association, 2000.
41. Gotthelf M. The new anorexia outrage. *Self Magazine,* 82–84. August 2001.
42. Lilenfeld L. Academy members debate over pro-anorexia websites. *Academy of Eating Disorders Newsletter,* June 2001.
43. *Update:* Chewing and Spitting Out Food. *Eating Disorders Review,* July/August, 2002.
44. Ferro-Luzzi A, James WP. Adult malnutrition, simple assessment techniques for use in emergencies. *Br J Nutr* 75 (1) 3–10, 1996.

As We Go to Press

How healthy is the Atkins' diet? There are some who argue that Robert Atkins, author of the book *"Dr. Atkins' New Diet Revolution,"* died from complications related to his diet. On April 8th, 2003, Atkins slipped on the ice, hit his head, and died on April 17th. The medical examiner's report stated that Atkins had a history of heart trouble, including congestive heart failure and high blood pressure. Dr. Atkins weighed 258 lbs and was 6 feet in height at the time of his death, which would put him in the obese category according to the Centers for Disease Control and Prevention. When he was admitted to the hospital, he weighed 195 lbs, which is considered overweight.

Atkins had suffered cardiac arrest in 2002, and there is speculation that this is a direct result of following his own diet which is high in fat and protein. In fact, the Atkins' diet allows up to two-thirds of one's daily intake to be from fat, more than double the U.S. Department of Agriculture's Food Pyramid Guide. Critics of the Atkins' diet have warned for years that following this diet can result in high cholesterol levels, cardiovascular problems, and hypertension.

However, Veronica Atkins, his widow, claims his death was "completely unrelated to his diet or any diet", and the weight gain had been attributed to retaining 60 lbs of fluid after he entered the hospital, while in a coma after his fall. Furthermore, some claim that Atkins suffered from cardiomyopathy, a disease of the heart muscle that may have been caused by virus.

While the jury is out on how much Atkins' diet contributed to his own death, if at all, it remains to be seen if the renewed interest in the Atkins' diet will produce an accompanying increase in the incidence of heart disease and hypertension in the years to come.

Sources: Did the Atkins Diet Fail Dr. Atkins?, People Magazine, February 23, 2004. Atkins obesity report sparks new round in diet fight, The Seattle Times, February 11, 2004.

are you a victim of portion distortion? learning to control serving sizes

Americans love to live large. According to social scientists, this is part of our national psyche that is directly traceable to our wide-spaced national boundaries, ample open space, and rags-to-riches dreams. Buying into this myth is beneficial when it motivates people to stretch themselves in areas of personal growth and achievement. When it comes to eating, however, the living-large philosophy puts Americans on a collision course with a variety of health risks and hinders their weight control efforts.[1]

A Supersized Trend

The trend toward supersized food portions is nothing new. Restaurants have long used large portions to lure value-seeking customers. The trend reversed for a while during the health-conscious 1980s, when meat consumption was coincidentally at an all-time high. Large serving sizes are enjoying a revival, however, as part of the current wellness backlash, which includes such risky behaviors as cigar smoking and increased consumption of hard liquor.

Fast-food chains target bargain-hungry consumers weary of wellness warnings. In an attempt to fend off competition within the industry as well as from new steak houses, ethnic eateries, full-service delis, and take-out restaurants, the fast-food industry is selling—and customers are buying—oversized portions of traditional favorites, such as burgers, fries, fried chicken, and pizza, in record numbers. Typically these supersized portions cost just pennies more than the standard-size serving. Another fattening sales strategy is to offer combo meals—essentially the addition of a large order of fries and a giant drink to popular menu items for under fifty cents.[1,2,3]

Serving Size Recommendations

As with many health-related issues, portion control embodies many contradictions. The USDA has standardized food portions, which are used to develop labeling laws and the Food Guide Pyramid (FGP) serving size recommendations. The average American, accustomed to gigantic servings when dining out, finds serving sizes on food labels surprisingly puny and, on the other hand, the number of servings of produce and grains suggested on the FGP surprisingly high (see the table comparing typical with recommended serving sizes).[4] Record numbers of low-fat and low-calorie foods are available, yet Americans are fatter than ever (average body weight has increased 7.5 pounds in the last decade).[1] Gourmets tend to favor small portions of fine food, whereas homestyle cooking enthusiasts prefer an abundance of food, especially meat and starch. Yet both groups are sporting wider waistlines.

Americans aren't entirely to blame for their ignorance of serving sizes. The USDA's standardization of serving sizes seems anything but standard to the average consumer. Food manufacturers and restaurant managers have been happy to ignore the USDA's advice and give cost-sensitive consumers the supersized servings they desire. According to USDA standards, the amount of food that constitutes a serving varies. Some serving sizes are based on volume and others on weight. For example, one-half of a three-inch-diameter bagel and one-half cup of cooked rice both constitute one serving from the grain, bread, and pasta group of the FGP. Three ounces of cooked chicken, one-half cup of cooked dried beans, or two tablespoons of peanut butter constitute one serving from the meat group. Even a single food, such as broccoli, can have different serving sizes depending on how it's prepared: According to the FGP, one serving of a fruit or vegetable equals one cup if eaten raw but only one-half cup if it's cooked.[4]

Despite pressure from the Nutrition Labeling and Education Act of 1990, food manufacturers continue to package foods in nonstandard sizes. They are simultaneously producing giant versions of trendy carbohydrate-rich foods, such as mega-muffins, behemoth bagels, and miniature versions of favorite high-fat snacks like mini-cheese-filled Ritz crackers and bite-sized Oreos.

Food companies also persist in packaging multiple servings of certain foods, particularly snack foods, in what appear to be single-serving containers. For instance, the USDA identifies a serving of soda as six ounces, but the typical soda can contains twelve ounces. This extra serving is inconsequential if you're drinking diet soda, but regular soda adds sixty-five calories, or roughly five teaspoons of sugar. Small packages of candy, chips, and cookies often exhibit this same deceptive packaging.[4]

The Portion-Distortion Trend Takes Shape

Well-meaning health care experts are partly to blame for this supersized servings trend. During the late 1980s and early 1990s, many of them urged people to eat less fat and more carbohydrates. The selling point for giving up favorite high-fat foods was that "you can eat more food for fewer calories." The underlying reasoning was sound—gram for gram, fat has twice as many calories as carbohydrates. Unfortunately, portion-ignorant Americans took this advice too literally and began devouring triple-sized tortillas, muffins, pretzels, bagels, and platters of pasta.

Letting someone else do the cooking doesn't make weight management any easier. Obesity experts identify dining out as a serious liability for diet-conscious diners. Presently, Americans spend more than 40% of every food dollar in restaurants.[5] Chic restaurants, featuring small portions of artistically prepared food, are blossoming on every corner in large cities, but in the suburbs and the heartland, the trend is fast-food chains, take-out shops, casual restaurants, and convenience foods, including frozen meals, packaged mixes, and full-service deli items.[3]

More than 80% of all dining-out dollars are spent at family-friendly eateries. Prices at these establishments are relatively low, but thanks to the supersized portions, calories tend to be high.[6]

Gourmets aren't faring any better when it comes to waist whittling. The small portions served in fine restaurants are no guarantee of low-calorie ingredients. Furthermore, just being in a restaurant, confronted with an overwhelming number of appealing food choices, causes many people to order more courses than they typically eat when dining at home. How often have you ordered an appetizer or felt overly full but still fallen prey to the dessert cart when it arrived at your table? Obesity experts believe this tendency to be seduced by the sight and smell of food partly explains the lack of healthy food choices on fast-food menus. Responding to consumer demand, McDonald's, Burger King, Taco Bell, and Kentucky Fried Chicken all added a variety of low-fat choices to their menus but found that, once on-site, their patrons were still ordering fries, burgers, full-fat burritos, or breaded and fried chicken. Paradoxically, the larger-portion items were selling better than the standard-sized versions of these foods. These chains have quietly been phasing out or significantly reducing their healthy menu options since early 1993.[7] For example, McDonald's replaced its McLean with a triple cheeseburger that has significantly more calories than the Big Mac. Kentucky Fried Chicken's skinless, roasted chicken was replaced by popcorn chicken, a breaded, deep-fried dish that has been breaking sales records.

Even diet-conscious diners who stick to heart-healthy menu choices can fall into calorie traps. A recent trip to an Olive Garden restaurant revealed that the pasta dishes on the heart healthy menu were large enough to feed three or four healthy hearts! Furthermore, they were accompanied by enough cheesy garlic breadsticks, soup or salad, to destroy anyone's best diet efforts. And Olive Garden is no exception. According to restaurant surveys conducted by the Center for Science in the Public Interest, most restaurants serve portions big enough for two to three people.[2]

Shrinking Your Serving Sizes

How can you make healthy choices when eating out? Putting into practice the American Dietetic Association's 1997 National Nutrition Month campaign theme "All Foods Can Fit" is one option.[7] This slogan is based on the idea that a balanced lifestyle can lead to a balanced body weight. Educating yourself about dietary balance and serving sizes is a first step. The FGP provides a pattern for overall dietary balance and even allows you to

Typical Serving Sizes vs. USDA Food Guide Pyramid Official Serving Sizes

Food	Typical Serving Size and Number of Calories	Official Serving Size and Number of Calories
Popcorn	Movie theater serving (small) 7 cups—400 calories	3 cups—160 calories
Muffins	Restaurant serving ¼ lb. (4 oz)—430 calories	⅛ lb. (2 oz)—190 calories
French fries	McDonald's Super Size Fries 3 cups (6 oz)—540 calories	1½ cups (3 oz)—220 calories
Soft drinks	Can 1½ cups (12 oz)—140 calories 7-Eleven Double Gulp 8 cups (64 oz)—800 calories	1 cup (8 oz)—100 calories
Steak	Restaurant serving of sirloin steak About ½ lb. cooked 7 oz—410 calories	About ⅓ lb. cooked 3 oz—170 calories

A Rule of Thumb for Serving Sizes

Use the parts of your hand to estimate serving sizes when it's not possible or convenient to use a food scale or measuring cups and spoons.

1 thumb = 1 ounce of cheese

1 thumb tip = 1 teaspoon of foods such as mayonnaise, peanut butter, and sugar

3 thumb tips = 1 tablespoon

1 fist = 1 cup of pasta, rice, or vegetables

1 or 2 handfuls = 1 ounce of a snack food (1 handful of small foods, such as nuts, or 2 handfuls of larger foods, such as chips and pretzels)

1 palm (minus the fingers) = 3 ounces of meat, fish, or poultry

include small amounts of sweets and fatty treats.[4] The FGP booklet supplies tables of food choices and serving size information. Learning to guesstimate sizes is also essential. You may need to use measuring cups and spoons and a food scale at home until you get the gist of it. A variety of mnemonic devices for estimating serving sizes are also available. The "Rule of Thumb for Serving Sizes" shown above is an easily learned, readily available approach. Other techniques include limiting meat servings to the size of a deck of cards or cassette tape, envisioning a tennis ball to estimate one-cup servings, and thinking of a one-half cup serving as the size of two Ping-Pong balls. Books featuring attractive photographs are available to assist parents and teachers in teaching children to recognize the sizes of portions of various types of food.[8]

Additional lifestyle changes may also be necessary. Learning to eat more slowly will allow you to feel satisfied with a smaller portion of food because your brain will have time to receive the signal that you have eaten. You should avoid other activities while eating so that you're fully aware of what and how much you're consuming. Dining out less frequently or dividing all restaurant portions in two and packaging up half before beginning to eat can also help. Accepting the fact that planned activity is an essential element of weight control and learning how much activity it takes to burn off a slice of cake is also important. Remember, there are 3,500 calories in a pound of body fat. Each mile you walk expends about 100 calories, so you would need to walk thirty-five miles to lose one pound of fat.

In essence, Americans can have their cake and eat it too, but it takes practice and persistence to become adept at balancing it all.

For Discussion . . .

What foods do you often consume in supersized portions? Would you be satisfied with smaller servings? Do you tend to order more courses and eat past the point of satiation when you dine in a restaurant because you're treating yourself or because you want to be sure to get your money's worth? What factors do you think are driving the "wellness backlash"?

References

1. Califano J. Nation's "supersize" trend leading to supersized people. *The New York Times* 1996 Nov 24: F8.
2. Liebman B, Hurley J. One size doesn't fit all. *Nutrition Action Healthletter* 1996; 23(9):10–12.
3. Mowma P. What will customers want in 1996 and beyond? *Restaurants USA* 1995 December: P35.
4. The Food Guide Pyramid. U.S. Department of Agriculture. *Home & Garden Bulletin* 1992; 232.
5. Critser, G. *Fat Land* New York: Houghton Mifflin Co. 2003.
6. National Restaurant Association. *Dining trends, 1996, quarterly reports.*
7. Woodburg R. The great fast-food pig-out. *Time* 1993; 141(26):51.
8. Hess MA. *Portion photos of popular foods.* Marketplace: The American Dietetic Association, 1997. **www.eatright.org/catalog**

personal assessment

how many calories do you need?

Resting Energy Requirement (RER)

Women
3–10 years 22.5 × weight (kg) + 499
10–18 years 12.2 × weight (kg) + 746
18–30 years 14.7 × weight (kg) + 496
30–60 years 08.7 × weight (kg) + 829
>60 years 10.5 × weight (kg) + 596

Men
3–10 years 22.7 × weight (kg) + 495
10–18 years 17.5 × weight (kg) + 651
18–30 years 15.3 × weight (kg) + 679
30–60 years 11.6 × weight (kg) + 879
>60 years 13.5 × weight (kg) + 487

Activity Energy Requirement (AER)
At bed rest: 1.20
Low activity (walking): 1.30
Average activity: 1.50–1.75
High activity: 2.0

Instructions: Calculate your resting energy requirement based on your sex, age, and weight. Then multiply your RER by your AER to determine how many calories you need each day to maintain your weight.

Example: Woman
   24 years
   120 lbs = 54.5 kg
   High activity
   (RER) × (AER) = Total Energy Requirement
   14.7 × 54.5 (kg) + 496 × 2.0 = 2594 calories/day
Note: 1 kg = 2.2 lbs.

Data from *Energy and protein requirements: report of a joint FAO/WHO/UNU expert consultation.* Technical Report Series 724. World Health Organization, 1985; Zeam FJ: *Clinical nutrition and dietetics,* 1991, Macmillan.

personal assessment

body love or body hate?

When you catch a glimpse of yourself in a mirror, do you smile at what you see or grimace? The following quiz will help you to assess your body self-esteem associated with your appearance. Please answer using the following rating scale:

1 = Rarely or never

2 = Sometimes

3 = Almost always or always

Add up your scores to determine your total score, and look at the summary below for an interpretation of your scores.

_____ 1. I worry about my weight and weighing "too much."

_____ 2. I prefer to eat by myself and not with other people.

_____ 3. My mood is determined by the scale and how I feel about my appearance.

_____ 4. I make negative comments about my appearance to myself and others.

_____ 5. I think I look less attractive on days that I haven't exercised.

_____ 6. I have a difficult time accepting compliments about my appearance from others.

_____ 7. I compare myself to other women and find myself lacking.

_____ 8. I ask other people how I look.

_____ 9. I avoid social situations, activities, and events involving food.

_____ 10. I feel more anxious about my body in the summertime because of the need to wear bathing suits and clothing suitable for warmer temperatures.

_____ **TOTAL SCORE**

Interpretation:

If you scored between 10 and 15, you have positive body self-esteem and are accepting of yourself and your appearance.

If you scored between 16 and 23, you scored in the average range. While you are in good company, feeling about your body the way most people do, you may want to reframe your body image and develop more of an appreciation for your body and appearance.

If your score was between 24 and 30, you have poor or low body self-esteem. Your self-esteem in general is probably driven by how you see yourself, and you may be putting too much emphasis on your appearance and are too self-critical. You may feel as though you never are thin enough or look good enough and can always find a flaw when looking in the mirror. In order to improve your body self-esteem, you need to focus on other aspects of yourself, focus on the positive aspects of your body, and be more accepting of yourself and less perfectionistic.

chapter seven

making decisions about drug use

Online Learning Center Resources

www.mhhe.com/hahn7e

Log on to our Online Learning Center (OLC) for access to these additional resources:

- Chapter key terms and definitions
- Learning objectives
- Student interactive question-and-answer sites

- Self-scoring chapter quiz
- Online assessments
- Key term flash cards

Talking It Over

Legalization of Marijuana

Discussions about the legalization of marijuana frequently focus on the following points. *Pros:*

1. Marijuana is a natural plant product.
2. People should be allowed to use or not use marijuana.
3. Many more harmful drugs than marijuana are available.
4. The government spends too much time, energy, and taxpayer money enforcing marijuana laws.
5. The "high" of marijuana is enjoyable and harmless.

Cons:

1. The possession, use, and distribution of marijuana are illegal.
2. Marijuana use is related to several significant health concerns.
3. Marijuana is a gateway drug.
4. Marijuana use keeps certain users from undertaking productive activities.
5. In combination with other drugs or medicines, marijuana use is dangerous. Where do you stand on this issue?

CommunicationLinks

www.samhsa.gov
www.drugfreeamerica.org

Eye on the Media

Do Media Scare Tactics Keep People from Using Drugs?

The media has tried to frighten people in many ways to keep them away from unhealthy behaviors. Bloody films showing the aftermath of a prom night car crash have been used to scare teenagers about dangerous drinking and driving behaviors. The late Frank Zappa, founder of the alternative music group the Mothers of Invention, warned young people in the early 1970s not to use stimulants (speed) because doing so would cause them "to turn out like your parents," a frightening thought for many counter-culture youth. More recently, television ads have featured celebrities speaking out against drug use.

Posters produced by both government and private health agencies have depicted cigarette smokers as filthy, wrinkled old men and women. Many of these posters are eye-catching in an almost humorous way. They grab the observer's attention and send the clear message that "this could happen to YOU." Advertisements for drug and alcohol rehabilitation facilities have shown alcoholics drowning in a sea of alcohol, drug users being confronted by their families, and employees caught by a drug screening test. The message is that miserable life situations can be changed if people are willing to get help.

It's difficult to measure the effectiveness of these approaches to drug prevention. Many people recall these media presentations, so they do make an impression. But, given the many variables involved in drug-taking behavior—family influence, inherited predispositions, life events and situations, drug availability, and peer influence—it's impossible to pinpoint the influence of a single media event. These scare tactics seem to be especially effective among people who have already made the decision not to use drugs. They remind these people how dangerous it is to use drugs. For people who are thinking about starting drug use, these messages may be beneficial, since they portray drug use in a negative light.

For hard-core drug users, though, it's unlikely that scare tactics will be effective. These people tend to lead chaotic lives, may never see the ads, and often remain in denial about their addiction. Nonusers and individuals leaning away from drug use are more likely to be influenced by this approach. Despite the fact that these ad campaigns are highly visible and costly, they seem to have only limited influence in drug prevention.

Effects of Drugs on the Central Nervous System

To better understand the disruption caused by the actions of psychoactive drugs, a general knowledge of the normal functioning of the nervous system's basic unit, the **neuron,** is required.

Changing for the Better

Coping with Family and Work Stress

Sometimes the pressures of being a college student, a family member, a parent, and an employee are too much, and I wonder how I'll get through the day. How can I stay healthy and drug-free?

Keep the lines of communication open. Work to communicate effectively with your friends, family members, and employers.

Recognize that trying to escape through drug use only makes situations worse. Realize that using drugs in stressful situations only masks the underlying problems you face.

Discuss your concerns with a trusted friend. Sometimes the person who knows you and your situation best can offer helpful guidance and support during difficult times.

Remember that you are a role model to your children. Because young children look to their parents for guidance, your ability to cope without drugs during stressful times will send an important message to your children.

Seek professional help as soon as possible. Many agencies and support groups are ready to help people who are having personal difficulties with family or work situations. Most large employers have Employee Assistance Programs that can be valuable resources. A campus counseling center or a local mental health association is another good source of assistance. It's up to you, though, to make the decision to seek these services. Don't hesitate to help yourself.

First, stimuli from the internal or external environment are received by the appropriate sensory receptor, perhaps an organ such as an eye or an ear. Once sensed, these stimuli are converted into electrical impulses. These impulses are then directed along the neuron's **dendrite,** through the cell body, and along the **axon** toward the *synaptic junction* near an adjacent neuron. On arrival at the **synapse,** the electrical impulses stimulate the production and release of chemical messengers called *neurotransmitters.*[1] These neurotransmitters transmit the electrical impulses from one neuron to the dendrites of adjoining neurons. Thus neurons function in a coordinated fashion to send information to the brain for interpretation and to relay appropriate response commands outward to the tissues of the body.

The role of neurotransmitters is critically important to the relay of information within the system. A substance that has the ability to alter some aspect of transmitter function

Key Terms

neuron (NOOR on) a nerve cell.

dendrite (DEN drite) the portion of a neuron that receives electrical stimuli from adjacent neurons; neurons typically have several such branches or extensions.

axon the portion of a neuron that conducts electrical impulses to the dendrites of adjacent neurons; neurons typically have one axon.

synapse (sinn APS) the location at which an electrical impulse from one neuron is transmitted to an adjacent neuron; also referred to as a *synaptic junction.*

1. Normal nerve activity

Neurotransmitter (green dots) delivers message to receptors and returns to cell

Synapse

Receptors

2. Drug interference

Alters deactivation, allowing continuous stimulation

Allows continuous slow release of neurotransmitter

Produces an altered neurotransmitter

Blocks the release of the stimuli completely

Direction of impulse

Dendrite

Stimuli

Axon

Synapse

Message sent to brain

Figure 7-1 This illustration depicts the disruption caused by the action of psychoactive drugs on the central nervous system. Neurotransmitters are chemical messengers that transfer electrical impulses across the synapses between nerve cells. Psychoactive drugs interrupt this process, thus disrupting the coordinating functioning of the nervous system.

has the potential to seriously disrupt the otherwise normally functioning system. Psychoactive drugs are capable of exerting these disruptive influences on the neurotransmitters. Drugs "work" by changing the way neurotransmitters work, often by blocking the production of a neurotransmitter or forcing the continued release of a neurotransmitter (see Figure 7-1).

Addictive Behavior

Experts in human behavior view drug use and abuse as just one of the many forms of addictive behavior. Such behavior includes addictions to shopping, eating, gambling, sex, television, video games, and work, as well as to alcohol or other drugs.

 TALKING POINTS How would you tell a friend that her video game playing is becoming an addiction that needs to be controlled?

The Process of Addiction

The process of developing an addiction has been a much-studied topic. Three common aspects of addictive behavior are exposure, compulsion, and loss of control.

Exposure

An addiction can begin after a person is exposed to a drug (such as alcohol) or a behavior (such as gambling) that he or she finds pleasurable. Perhaps this drug or behavior temporarily replaces an unpleasant feeling or sensation. This initial pleasure gradually, or in some cases quickly, becomes a focal point in the person's life.

Compulsion

Increasingly, the person spends more energy, time, and money pursuing the drug use or behavior. At this point in the addictive process, the person can be said to have a compulsion for the drug or behavior. Frequently, repeated exposure to the drug or behavior continues despite negative consequences, such as the gradual loss of family and friends, unpleasant physical symptoms resulting from taking a drug, or problems at work.

During the compulsion phase, a person's normal life often degenerates while she or he searches for increased pleasures from the drug or the behavior. An addicted person's family life, circle of friends, work, or study patterns become less important than the search for more and better "highs." The development of tolerance and withdrawal are distinct possibilities. (These terms are discussed later in the chapter.)

Why some people develop compulsions and others do not is difficult to pinpoint, but addiction might be influenced by genetic makeup, family dynamics, physiological processes, personality type, peer groups, and available resources for help.

Loss of Control

Over time, the search for highs changes to a desire to avoid the effects of withdrawal from the drug or behavior.

Drug abuse of all types remains a significant problem as we enter the twenty-first century.

Addicted people lose their ability to control their behavior. Despite overwhelming negative consequences (for example, deterioration of health, alienation of family and friends, or loss of all financial resources), addicted people continue to behave in ways that make their lives worse. The person addicted to alcohol continues to drink heavily, the person addicted to shopping continues to run up heavy debts, and the person addicted to food continues to eat indiscriminately. This behavior reflects a loss of control over one's life. Frequently, a person has addictions to more than one drug or behavior.

Intervention and Treatment

The good news for people with addictions is that help is available. Within the last two decades, much attention has been focused on intervention and treatment for addictive behavior. Many people with drug problems can be helped through programs such as those described in the Changing for the Better box on page 187. These programs often include inpatient or outpatient treatment, family counseling, and long-term aftercare counseling.

It is common for people in aftercare treatment for addictive behavior to belong to a self-help support group, such as Alcoholics Anonymous, Gamblers Anonymous, or Sex Addicts Anonymous. These groups are often listed in the phone book or in the classified section of the newspaper.

Drug Terminology

Before discussing drug behavior, it's important to become familiar with some basic terminology. Much of this terminology originates from the field of *pharmacology,* or the study of the interaction of chemical agents with living material.

What does the word *drug* mean? Each of us may have different ideas about what a drug is. Although a number of definitions are available, we will consider a drug to be "any substance, natural or artificial, other than food, that by its chemical or physical nature alters structure or function in the living organism."[1] Included in this broad definition is a variety of psychoactive drugs, medicines, and substances that many people do not usually consider to be drugs.

Psychoactive drugs alter the user's feelings, behavior, perceptions, or moods when using stimulants, depressants, hallucinogens, opiates, or inhalants. (The Changing for the Better box on page 188 suggests ways to improve your mood without resorting to drug use.) Prescription medications function to heal unhealthy tissue as well as to ease pain, prevent illness, and diagnose health conditions. Although some psychoactive drugs are used for medical reasons, as in the case of tranquilizers and some narcotics, the most commonly prescribed medicines are antibiotics, hormone replacement drugs, sulfa drugs, diuretics, oral contraceptives, and cardiovascular drugs. Legal substances not usually considered to be drugs (but which certainly are drugs) include caffeine, tobacco, alcohol, aspirin, and other over-the-counter (OTC) preparations. These substances are used so commonly in our society that they are rarely perceived as true drugs.

For organizational reasons, this chapter primarily deals with psychoactive drugs. Alcohol is covered in Chapter 8. The effects of tobacco are discussed in Chapter 9. Prescription and OTC drugs and medicines are explored further in Chapter 15. Anabolic steroids, drugs used primarily for increasing muscle growth, are discussed in Chapter 4.

Routes of Administration

Drugs generally enter the body through one of four methods: ingestion, injection, inhalation, and absorption.

> ### Key Terms
>
> **psychoactive drug** any substance capable of altering feelings, moods, or perceptions.

It's tempting to reach for a pill when I feel down, but I don't want to get into that habit. What can I do to improve my mood without using drugs?

Talk with a trusted friend. Confide your feelings to a close, trusted friend or family member. By opening up to another person, you'll gain insights into how you can get beyond your negative feelings without resorting to drug use.

Get moving. Go for a walk, ride your bike, or swim a few laps. Physical activity is a natural way to enhance your mood. Nearly every college provides recreation programs such as aerobics, swimming, dancing, or weight lifting.

Give yourself a break. If you're tired, take a quick power nap. If you're overworked, set aside some personal time—just for yourself. Read, watch TV, surf the net, or phone an old friend. Decide what you like to do, and then do it. You'll return to your responsibilities with renewed enthusiasm.

Do volunteer work. One way to feel good is to help others. Teach reading to adults, become a Big Brother or Big Sister, work in a soup kitchen, or drive a van for the elderly in your community.

Reexamine your spiritual health. Many people find comfort by making connections to their spiritual life. Through activities such as meditation, spiritual reflection, and renewal of faith, people often gain reassurance and a sense of calmness.

Restructure your daily activities. If you have one hectic day after another but feel as though you're not accomplishing anything, try reorganizing your daily activities. Experiment with new patterns. Plan to get sufficient sleep, eat regular meals, and set aside specific times for work, family activities, and pleasure. Find out what works best for you.

Seek professional guidance. If you've tried these strategies but your mood still isn't improving, consider seeking professional help. This important first step is up to you. Visit your college health center or counseling center, and talk with people who are trained to help you learn how to become a happier person.

Ingestion, or oral administration, is the entry of drugs through the mouth and into the digestive tract. *Injection* refers to the use of a needle to insert a drug into the body. With *inhalation,* the drug enters the body through the lungs. *Absorption* refers to the administration of a drug through the skin or mucous membranes.

Dependence

Psychoactive drugs have a strong potential for the development of **dependence.** When users take a psychoactive drug, the patterns of nervous system function are altered. If these altered functions provide perceived benefits for the user, the drug use may continue, perhaps at increasingly larger dosages. If persistent use continues, the user can develop a dependence on the drug. Pharmacologists have identified two types of dependences: physical and psychological.

A person can be said to have developed a *physical dependence* when the body cells have become reliant on a drug. Continued use of the drug is then required because body tissues have adapted to its presence.[2] The person's body needs the drug to maintain homeostasis, or dynamic balance. If the drug is not taken or is suddenly withdrawn, the user develops a characteristic **withdrawal illness.** The symptoms of withdrawal reflect the attempt by the body's cells to regain normality without the drug. Withdrawal symptoms are always unpleasant (ranging from mild to severe irritability, depression, nervousness, digestive difficulties, and abdominal pain) and can be life-threatening, as in the case of abrupt withdrawal from barbiturates or alcohol. In this chapter the term *addiction* is used interchangeably with physical dependence.

Continued use of most drugs can lead to **tolerance.** Tolerance is an acquired reaction to a drug in which continued intake of the same dose has diminishing effects.[2] The user needs larger doses of the drug to receive previously felt sensations. The continued use of depressants, including alcohol, and opiates can cause users to quickly develop a tolerance to the drug.

For example, college seniors who have engaged in 4 years of beer drinking usually recognize that their bodies have developed a degree of tolerance to alcohol. Many such students can vividly recall the initial and subsequent sensations they felt after drinking. For example,

---

Key Terms

dependence general term that refers to the need to continue using a drug for psychological and/or physical reasons.

withdrawal illness uncomfortable, perhaps toxic response of the body as it attempts to maintain homeostasis in the absence of a drug; also called *abstinence syndrome.*

tolerance an acquired reaction to a drug; continued intake of the same dose has diminished results.

five beers consumed during a freshman social gathering might well have resulted in inebriation, but if these same students continued to drink beer regularly for 4 years, five beers would probably fail to produce the response they experienced as freshmen. Seven or eight beers might be needed to produce such a response. Clearly, these students have developed a tolerance to alcohol.

 TALKING POINTS Some of your friends have started making a contest of beer drinking. How would you tell them you think this is dangerous without sounding preachy?

Tolerance developed for one drug may carry over to another drug within the same general category. This phenomenon is known as **cross-tolerance.** The heavy abuser of alcohol, for example, might require a larger dose of a preoperative sedative to become relaxed before surgery than the average person would. The tolerance to alcohol "crosses over" to the other depressant drugs.

A person who possesses a strong desire to continue using a particular drug is said to have developed a *psychological dependence.* People who are psychologically dependent on a drug believe that they need to consume the drug to maintain a sense of well-being. They crave the drug for emotional reasons despite having persistent or recurrent physical, social, psychological, or occupational problems caused or worsened by the drug use. Abrupt withdrawal from a drug by such a person would not trigger the fully expressed withdrawal illness, although some unpleasant symptoms of withdrawal might be felt. The term *habituation* is often used interchangeably with psychological dependence.

Drugs whose continued use can quickly lead to both physical and psychological dependence are depressants (barbiturates, tranquilizers, and alcohol), narcotics (the opiates, which are derivatives of the Oriental poppy: heroin, morphine, and codeine), and synthetic narcotics (Demerol and methadone). Drugs whose continued use can lead to various degrees of psychological dependence and occasionally to significant (but not life-threatening) physical dependence in some users are the stimulants (amphetamines, caffeine, and cocaine), hallucinogens (LSD, peyote, mescaline, and marijuana), and inhalants (glues, gases, and petroleum products).

Drug Misuse and Abuse

So far in this chapter we have used the term *use* (or *user*) in association with the taking of psychoactive drugs. At this point, however, it is important to define *use* and to introduce the terms **misuse** and **abuse.** [1] By doing so, we can more accurately describe the ways in which drugs are used.

The term *use* is all-encompassing and describes drug-taking in the most general way. For example, Americans use drugs of many types. The term *use* can also refer more narrowly to misuse and abuse.

Drug Classifications

Drugs can be categorized according to the nature of their physiological effects. Most psychoactive drugs fall into one of six general categories: stimulants, depressants, hallucinogens, cannabis, narcotics, and inhalants (Table 7.1).

Stimulants

In general, **stimulants** excite or increase the activity of the central nervous system (CNS). Also called "uppers," stimulants alert the CNS by increasing heart rate, blood pressure, and the rate of brain function. Users feel uplifted and less fatigued. Examples of stimulant drugs include caffeine, amphetamines, and cocaine. Most stimulants produce psychological dependence and tolerance relatively quickly, but they are unlikely to produce significant physical dependence when judged by life-threatening withdrawal symptoms. The important exception is cocaine, which seems to be capable of producing psychological dependence and withdrawal so powerful that continued use of the drug is inevitable in some users.

Caffeine

Caffeine, the tasteless drug found in chocolate, some soft drinks, coffee, tea, some aspirin products, and OTC "stay-awake" pills, is a relatively harmless stimulant when consumed in moderate amounts.[3] (Visit the Focus on Health website **www.mhhe.com/hahn7e** for a table listing the caffeine content in some products.) Many coffee drinkers believe that they cannot start the day successfully without the benefit of a cup or two of coffee in the morning.

For the average healthy adult, moderate consumption of caffeine is unlikely to pose any serious health threat.

Key Terms

cross-tolerance transfer of tolerance from one drug to another within the same general category.

misuse inappropriate use of legal drugs intended to be medications.

abuse any use of a legal or illegal drug in a way that is detrimental to health.

stimulants psychoactive drugs that stimulate the function of the central nervous system.

Table 7.1 Psychoactive Drug Categories

Drugs	Trade or Common Names	Medical Uses	Possible Effects
Stimulants			
Cocaine*	Coke, crack, gin, girlfriend, girl, double bubble, California cornflakes, caballo, bouncing powder, flake, snow	Local anesthetic	Increased alertness, excitation, euphoria, increased pulse rate and blood pressure, insomnia, loss of appetite
Amphetamines	Biphetamine, Delcobese, Desoxyn, Dexedrine, mediatric, methamphetamine (ice), black Mollies, aimies, amps, bam, beans, benz	Hyperactivity, narcolepsy, weight control	
Phendimetrazine	Prelu-2		
Methylphenidate	Ritalin, Methidate		
Other stimulants	Adipex, Bacarate, Cylert, Didrex, Ionamin, Plegine, PreSate, Sanorex, Tenuate, ephedra		
Depressants			
Chloral hydrate	Noctec, Somnos	Hypnotic	Slurred speech, disorientation, drunken behavior without odor of alcohol
Barbiturates	Amobarbital, Butisol, phenobarbital, phenoxbarbital, secobarbital, Tuinal, blockbusters, black bombers	Anesthetic, anticonvulsant, sedative, hypnotic	
Glutethimide	Doriden	Sedative, hypnotic	
Methaqualone	Optimil, Parest, Quaalude, Somnafec, Sopor	Sedative, hypnotic	
Benzodiazepines	Ativan, Azene, Clonopin, Dalmane, diazepam, Librium, Serax, Tranxene, Valium, Verstran	Antianxiety, anticonvulsant, sedative, hypnotic	
GHB	Gamma-hydroxybutyrate (G, liquid ecstasy, Georgia Home Boy)[1]	None	Unconsciousness, seizures, amnesia, vomiting, coma
Other depressants	Equanil, Miltown, Noludar, Placidyl, Valmid	Antianxiety, sedative	
Hallucinogens			
LSD	Acid, microdot, brown dot, cap, California sunshine, brown bomber	None	Delusions and hallucinations, poor perception of time and distance
Mescaline and peyote	Mesc, buttons, cactus, chief	None	
Amphetamine variants (designer drugs)	2,5-DMA, DOM, DOP, MDA, MDMA, PMA, STP, TMA, clarity, chocolate chips, booty juice	None	
Phencyclidine	Angel dust, hog, PCP, AD, boat, black whack, amoeba, angel hair, angel smoke	Veterinary anesthetic	
Phencyclidine analogs	PCE, PCPy, TCP	None	Euphoria, relaxed inhibitions, increased appetite, disorientation
Other hallucinogens	Bufotenin, DMT, DET, ibogaine, psilocybin	None	
Cannabis			
Marijuana	Acapulco gold, black Bart, black mote, blue sage, bobo, butterflowers, cannabis-T, cess, cheeba, grass, pot, sinsemilla, Thai sticks	Under investigation	Euphoria, relaxed inhibitions, increased appetite, disoriented behavior
Tetrahydrocannabinol	THC	Under investigation	
Hashish	Hash	None	
Hashish oil	Hash oil	None	
Narcotics			
Opium	Dover's powder, paregoric, Parapectolin, cruz, Chinese tobacco, China	Analgesic, antidiarrheal	Euphoria, drowsiness, respiratory depression, constricted pupils, nausea
Morphine	Morphine, Pectoal syrup, emsel, first line	Analgesic, antitussive	
Codeine	Codeine, Empirin compound with codeine, Robitussin A-C	Analgesic, antitussive	
Heroin	Diacetylmorphine, horse, smack, courage pills, dead on arrival (DOA)	Under investigation	
Hydromorphone	Dilaudid	Analgesic	Intoxication, excitation, disorientation, aggression, hallucination
Meperidine (pethidine)	Demerol, Pethadol	Analgesic	
Methadone	Dolophine, Methadone, Methadose	Analgesic, heroin substitute	
Other narcotics	Darvon,† Dromoran, Fentanyl, LAAM, Leitine, Levo-Dromoran, Percodan, Tussionex, Talwin,† Lomotil	Analgesic, antidiarrheal, antitussive	
Inhalants			
Anesthetic gases	Aerosols, petroleum products, solvents	Surgical anesthetic	Intoxication, excitation, disorientation, aggression, hallucination, variable effects
Vasodilators (amyl nitrite, butyl nitrite)	Aerosols, petroleum products, solvents	None	

*Designated a narcotic under the Controlled Substances Act.
†Not designated a narcotic under the Controlled Substances Act.
[1] Project GHB. What is GHB? www.projectghb.org/what_is_ghb.htm, accessed 15 May 2003.

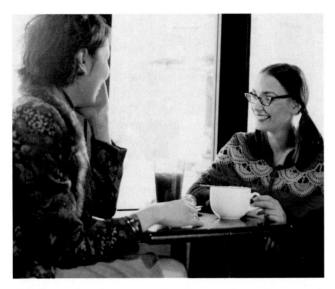

Coffeehouses have become popular places to relax, work, or spend time with friends.

However, excessive consumption (equivalent to ten or more cups of coffee daily) could lead to anxiety, diarrhea, restlessness, delayed onset of sleep or frequent awakening, headache, and heart palpitations. Pregnant women are advised to consume caffeine sparingly.[4]

Amphetamines

Amphetamines produce increased activity and mood elevation in almost all users. The amphetamines include several closely related compounds: amphetamine, dextroamphetamine, and methamphetamine. These compounds do not have any natural sources and are completely manufactured in the laboratory. Medical use of amphetamines is limited primarily to the treatment of obesity, **narcolepsy,** and **attention deficit hyperactivity disorder (ADHD).**

Amphetamines can be ingested, injected, or snorted (inhaled). At low-to-moderate doses, amphetamines elevate mood and increase alertness and feelings of energy by stimulating receptor sites for two naturally occurring neurotransmitters. They also slow the activity of the stomach and intestine and decrease hunger. In the 1960s and 1970s, in fact, amphetamines were commonly prescribed for dieters. Later, when it was discovered that the appetite suppression effect of amphetamines lasted only a few weeks, most physicians stopped prescribing them. At high doses, amphetamines can increase heart rate and blood pressure to dangerous levels. As amphetamines are eliminated from the body, the user becomes tired.

When chronically abused, amphetamines produce rapid tolerance and strong psychological dependence. Other effects of chronic use include impotence and episodes of psychosis. When use is discontinued, periods of depression may develop.

Today the abuse of amphetamines is a more pressing concern than it has been in the recent past because of the sharp increase in abuse of methamphetamine. Known by a variety of names and forms, including "crank," "ice," "crystal," "meth," "speed," "crystal meth," and "zip," methamphetamine is produced in illegal home laboratories.[5]

Ice Crystal meth, or ice, is among the most dangerous forms of methamphetamine. Ice is a very pure form of methamphetamine that looks like rock candy.[6] When smoked, the effects of ice are felt in about seven seconds as a wave of intense physical and psychological exhilaration. This is due to the drug telling the brain to release large amounts of dopamine.[7] This effect lasts for several hours (much longer than the effects of *crack*) until the user becomes physically exhausted. Chronic use leads to nutritional difficulties, weight loss, reduced resistance to infection, and damage to the liver, lungs, and kidneys. Psychological dependence is quickly established. Withdrawal causes acute depression and fatigue but not significant physical discomfort.

Ephedra Health professionals are warning people about the dangers of using any over-the-counter herbal supplement containing ephedra. Also known as *ma huang,* ephedra is an amphetamine-like drug that can be especially dangerous for people with hypertension or other

Key Terms

narcolepsy (nar co LEP see) a sleep disorder in which a person has a recurrent, overwhelming, and uncontrollable desire to sleep.

attention deficit hyperactivity disorder (ADHD) above-normal rate of physical movement; often accompanied by an inability to concentrate well on a specified task; also called *hyperactivity.*

cardiovascular disease. Presently, ephedra is used in many over-the-counter decongestants and asthma drugs. However, in these products, warning labels indicate possible harmful side effects and drug interactions. Some herbal products that contain ephedra are promoted as weight-control aids.[8] At the time of this writing, some states were banning ephedra as a weight-control aid.

Ritalin A prescription stimulant drug that has surged in popularity in recent years is Ritalin. This drug is typically prescribed to children and adolescents (and increasing numbers of young adults) to help them focus attention if they are hyperactive or cannot concentrate. Ritalin can be abused when the drug is shared among friends (see Star box). Critics of Ritalin use argue that it is being over-prescribed to treat a variety of problems, when a preferred course would be to identify and treat root causes of the problems. Supporters respond that Ritalin has enabled youth to succeed in school.

Cocaine

Cocaine, perhaps the strongest of the stimulant drugs, has received much media attention. It is the primary psychoactive substance found in the leaves of the South American coca plant.[9] The effects of cocaine are brief—from 5 to 30 minutes (Figure 7-2). Regardless of the form in which it is consumed, cocaine produces an immediate, near-orgasmic "rush," or feeling of exhilaration. This euphoria is quickly followed by a period of marked depression. Used only occasionally as a topical anesthetic, cocaine is usually inhaled (snorted), injected, or smoked (as *freebase* or crack). There is overwhelming scientific evidence that users quickly develop a strong psychological dependence using cocaine.

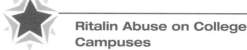

There is considerable evidence that physical dependence also rapidly develops. Cocaine users risk a weakened immune system making them "more susceptible to infections, including HIV."[10] However, physical dependence on cocaine does not lead to death upon withdrawal.

Freebasing

Freebasing and the use of crack cocaine are the most recent techniques for maximizing the psychoactive effects of

Figure 7-2 Cocaine's effects on the body.

① **The nose:** as cocaine is snorted, nasal vessels immediately constrict and prohibit about 40% of the drug from entering the body. The remaining 60% enters the bloodstream.

② **The heart:** electrical impulses that regulate rhythmic pumping are impaired. Beating becomes irregular (arrhythmia). The heart can no longer supply itself with enough oxygenated blood.

③ **The brain:** dopamine and norepinephrine are released into the brain, producing a feeling of euphoria and confidence. Electrical signals to the heart are distorted, heart rate and pulse increase. A seizure may occur, causing coma and breathing stoppage.

④ **The heart:** blood circulation is out of control. The heart may simply flutter and stop, or it can be pumping so little oxygenated blood to the brain that the brain dies and the heart stops beating.

Intravenous injection of cocaine results in an almost immediate high for the user.

the drug. Freebasing first requires that the common form of powdered cocaine (cocaine hydrochloride) be chemically altered (alkalized). This altered form is then dissolved in a solvent, such as ether or benzene. This liquid solution is heated to evaporate the solvent. The heating process leaves the freebase cocaine in a powder form that can then be smoked, often through a water pipe. Because of the large surface area of the lungs, smoking cocaine facilitates fast absorption into the bloodstream.

One danger of freebasing cocaine is the risk related to the solvents used. Ether is a highly volatile solvent capable of exploding and causing serious burns. Benzene is a known carcinogen associated with the development of leukemia. Clearly, neither solvent can be used without increasing the level of risk normally associated with cocaine use. This method of making smokeable cocaine led to a new epidemic of cocaine use, smoking crack.

Crack

In contrast to freebase cocaine, crack is made by combining cocaine hydrochloride with common baking soda. When this pastelike mixture is allowed to dry, a small rocklike crystalline material remains. This crack is heated in the bowl of a small pipe, and the vapors are inhaled into the lungs.[9] Some crack users spend hundreds of dollars a day to maintain their habit.

The effect of crack is almost instantaneous. Within 10 seconds after inhalation, cocaine reaches the CNS and influences the action of several neurotransmitters at specific sites in the brain. As with the use of other forms of cocaine, convulsions, seizures, respiratory distress, and cardiac failure have been reported with this sudden, extensive stimulation of the nervous system.

Within about 6 minutes, the stimulating effect of crack becomes completely expended, and users frequently become depressed. Dependence develops within a few weeks, since users consume more crack in response to the short duration of stimulation and rapid onset of depression.

Intravenous administration has been the preferred route for cocaine users who are also regular users of heroin and other injectable drugs. Intravenous injection results in an almost immediate high, which lasts about 10 minutes. A "smoother ride" is said to be obtained from a "speedball," the injectable mixture of heroin and cocaine (or methamphetamine). This type of mixture can be volatile and even fatal.[11]

Depressants

Depressants (or sedatives) sedate the user, slowing down CNS function. Drugs included in this category are alcohol (see Chapter 8), barbiturates, and tranquilizers. Depressants produce tolerance in abusers, as well as strong psychological and physical dependence.

Barbiturates

Barbiturates are the so-called sleeping compounds that function by enhancing the effect of inhibitory neurotransmitters. They depress the CNS to the point where the user drops off to sleep or, as is the case with surgical anesthetics, the patient becomes anesthetized. Medically, barbiturates are used in widely varied dosages as anesthetics and for treatment of anxiety, insomnia, and epilepsy.[2] Regular use of a barbiturate quickly produces tolerance—eventually such a high dose is required that the user still feels the effects of the drug throughout the next morning. Some abusers then begin to alternate barbiturates with stimulants, producing a vicious cycle of dependence. Other misusers combine alcohol and barbiturates or tranquilizers, inadvertently producing toxic or even lethal results. Abrupt withdrawal from barbiturate use frequently produces a withdrawal syndrome that can involve seizures, delusions, hallucinations, and even death.

Methaqualone (Quaalude, "ludes," Sopor) was developed as a sedative that would not have the dependence properties of other barbiturates.[1] Although this did not happen, Quaaludes were occasionally prescribed for anxious patients. Today, compounds resembling Quaaludes are manufactured in home laboratories and sold illegally so that they can be combined with small amounts of alcohol for an inexpensive, drunklike effect.

Tranquilizers

Tranquilizers are depressants that are intended to reduce anxiety and to relax people who are having problems managing stress. They are not specifically designed to produce sleep but rather to help people cope during their waking hours. Such tranquilizers are termed *minor tranquilizers,* of which diazepam (Valium) and chlordiazepoxide (Librium) may be the most commonly prescribed examples. Unfortunately, some people become addicted to these and other prescription drugs[12] (see the Focus On article on page 203).

Some tranquilizers are further designed to control hospitalized psychotic patients who may be suicidal or who are potential threats to others. These *major tranquilizers* subdue people physically but permit them to remain conscious. Their use is generally limited to institutional settings. All tranquilizers can produce physical and psychological dependence and tolerance.

"Date Rape" Depressants "Date rape" drugs or club drugs are commonly used on college campuses. These drugs are usually slipped into the drink of an unsuspecting woman and can result in a coma or even death.

Common "date rape" drugs include GHB (gamma hydroxybutyrate), also known as G, liquid ecstasy, Easy Lay, and Georgia Home Boy, and Rohypnol ("roophies"). When these drugs are consumed they cause a drunklike or sleepy state that can last for hours. During this time is when unsuspecting individuals are taken advantage of, against their will and sometimes against their knowledge.

High school and college students should not accept drinks from people they do not know. This recommendation extends to all parties where drinkers do not know what has been added to the punch or other drinks.[13]

Congress passed the 1996 Drug-Induced Rape Prevention and Punishment Act and it is now a federal crime to give someone a drug, without the user's knowledge, to aid in sexual assault. The maximum penalty for this crime is 20 years in prison and a $250,000 fine.[2] GHB (G, liquid ecstasy) and ketamine (K, Special K, Cat) are additional depressants that are being used as date rape drugs.[14] These drugs should serve as a reminder to all partygoers to keep an extremely careful watch over any drink in their possession.

Hallucinogens

As the name suggests, hallucinogenic drugs produce hallucinations—perceived distortions of reality. Also known as *psychedelic* drugs or *phantasticants,* **hallucinogens** reached their height of popularity during the 1960s. At that time, young people were encouraged to use hallucinogenic drugs to "expand the mind," "reach an altered state," or "discover reality." Not all of the reality distortions, or "trips," were pleasant. Many users reported "bummers," or trips during which they perceived negative, frightening distortions.

Hallucinogenic drugs include laboratory-produced lysergic acid diethylamide (LSD), mescaline (from the peyote cactus plant), and psilocybin (from a particular genus of mushroom). Consumption of hallucinogens seems to produce not physical dependence but mild levels of psychological dependence. The development of tolerance is questionable. *Synesthesia,* a sensation in which users report hearing a color, smelling music, or touching a taste, is sometimes produced with hallucinogen use.

The long-term effects of hallucinogenic drug use are not fully understood. Questions about genetic abnormalities in offspring, fertility, sex drive and performance, and the development of personality disorders have not been fully answered. One phenomenon that has been identified and documented is the development of *flashbacks*—the unpredictable return to a psychedelic trip that occurred months or even years earlier. Flashbacks are thought to result from the accumulation of a drug within body cells.

LSD

The most well-known and powerful hallucinogen is lysergic acid diethylamide. LSD ("acid") is a drug that helped define the counterculture movement of the 1960s. During

---

Key Terms

hallucinogens psychoactive drugs capable of producing hallucinations (distortions of reality).

---

the 1970s and the 1980s, this drug lost considerable popularity. LSD use has made a comeback, with studies reporting that 6.6% of high school seniors[15] and 14.7% of young adults age 18–20[16] had experimented with LSD. Fear of cocaine and other powerful drugs, boredom, low cost, and an attempt to revisit the culture of the 1960s are thought to have increased LSD's attractiveness to today's young people.

LSD is manufactured in home laboratories and frequently distributed in blotter paper decorated with cartoon characters.[17] Users place the paper on their tongue or chew the paper to ingest the drug. LSD can produce a psychedelic (mind-viewing) effect that includes altered perception of shapes, images, time, sound, and body form. Synesthesia is common to LSD users. Ingested in doses known as "hits," LSD produces a 6- to 9-hour experience.

Although the typical doses ("hits") today are about half as powerful as those in the 1960s, users still tend to develop high tolerance to LSD. Physical dependence does not occur. Not all LSD trips are pleasant. Hallucinations produced from LSD can be frightening and dangerous. Users can injure or kill themselves accidentally during a bad trip. Dangerous side effects include panic attacks, flashbacks, and occasional prolonged psychosis.

Designer Drugs

In recent years, chemists who produce many of the illicit drugs in home laboratories have designed versions of drugs listed on **FDA Schedule 1.** These *designer drugs* are similar to the controlled drugs on the FDA Schedule 1 but are sufficiently different so that they escape governmental control. The designer drugs are either newly synthesized products that are similar to already outlawed drugs but against which no law yet exists, or they are reconstituted or renamed illegal substances. Designer drugs are said to produce effects similar to their controlled drug counterparts.

People who use designer drugs do so at great risk because the manufacturing of these drugs is unregulated. The neurophysiological effect of these homemade drugs can be quite dangerous. So far, a synthetic heroin product (MPPP) and several amphetamine derivatives with hallucinogenic properties have been designed for the unwary drug consumer.

DOM (STP), MDA (the "love drug"), and ecstasy (MDMA or "XTC") are examples of amphetamine-derivative, hallucinogenic designer drugs. These drugs produce mild LSD-like hallucinogenic experiences, positive feelings, and enhanced alertness. They also have a number of potentially dangerous effects. Experts are particularly concerned that ecstasy can produce strong psychological dependence and can deplete serotonin, an important excitatory neurotransmitter associated with a state of alertness. Permanent brain damage is possible.[2]

Phencyclidine

Phencyclidine (PCP, "angel dust") has been classified variously as a hallucinogen, a stimulant, a depressant, and an anesthetic. PCP was studied for years during the 1950s and 1960s and was found to be an unsuitable animal and human anesthetic.[18] PCP is an extremely unpredictable drug. Easily manufactured in home laboratories in tablet or powder form, PCP can be injected, inhaled, taken orally, or smoked. The effects vary. Some users report mild euphoria, although most report bizarre perceptions, paranoid feelings, and aggressive behavior. PCP overdose may cause convulsions, cardiovascular collapse, and damage to the brain's respiratory center.

In a number of cases the aggressive behavior caused by PCP has led users to commit brutal crimes against both friends and innocent strangers. PCP accumulates in cells and may stimulate bizarre behavior months after initial use.

Cannabis

Cannabis (marijuana) has been labeled a mild hallucinogen for a number of years. However, most experts now consider it to be a drug category in itself. Marijuana produces mild effects like those of stimulants and depressants. The implication of marijuana in a large number of traffic fatalities makes this drug one whose consumption should be carefully considered. Marijuana is actually a wild plant (*Cannabis sativa*) whose fibers were once used in the manufacture of hemp rope. When the leafy material and small stems are dried and crushed, users can smoke the mixture in rolled cigarettes ("joints"), cigars ("blunts"), or pipes. The resins collected from scraping the flowering tops of the plant yield a marijuana product called *hashish*, or *hash*, commonly smoked in a pipe.

The potency of marijuana's hallucinogenic effect is determined by the percentage of the active ingredient tetrahydrocannabinol (THC) present in the product. The concentration of THC averages about 3.5% for marijuana, 7% to 9% for higher-quality marijuana (sinsemilla), 8% to 14% for hashish, and as high as 50% for hash oil.[2] Today's marijuana has THC levels that are higher than in past decades.

THC is a fat-soluble substance and thus is absorbed and retained in fat tissues within the body. Before being excreted, THC can remain in the body for up to a month. With the sophistication of today's drug tests, trace

---

Key Terms

FDA Schedule 1 a list of drugs that have a high potential for abuse but no medical use.

Table 7.2 Effects of Marijuana

Short-Term Effects	Long-Term Effects
• Increased heart rate and blood pressure	• Lung damage
• Feeling of elation	• Increased risk of bronchitis
• Drowsiness and sedation	• Emphysema
• Increased appetite	• Lung cancer
• Red eyes	• Heart attack[2]
• Food cravings	• Loss of motivation and short-term memory
• Slow reaction time	• Increased panic or anxiety
• Feelings of depression, excitement, paranoia, panic, and euphoria	• May become tolerant to marijuana
• Problems with attention span, memory, learning, problem-solving, and coordination	• Damage to lungs, immune system, and reproductive organs
• Sleeplessness[1]	• Can remain in the body for up to a month
	• Can cause birth defects
	• Five times more damaging to the lungs than tobacco products[3]

[1]Miller A: Campus Alcohol and Drug Resource Center, University of Florida; Health Education of Ball State University. 1 March 2002.
[2]Stronger Marijuana Is Major Health Risk. *The Independent,* 1 February 2001.
[3]Sternberg S: Pot smoking linked to sudden heart attacks. *USA Today,* 3 March 2000.

metabolites of THC can be detected for up to 30 days after consumption.[2] It is possible that the THC that comes from passive inhalation of high doses (for example, during an indoor rock concert) can also be detected for a short time after exposure.

Once marijuana is consumed, its effects vary from person to person (see Table 7.2 above). Being "high" or "stoned" or "wrecked" means different things to different people. Many people report heightened sensitivity to music, cravings for particular foods, and a relaxed mood. There is consensus that marijuana's behavioral effects include four probabilities: (1) users must learn to recognize what a marijuana high is like, (2) marijuana impairs short-term memory, (3) users overestimate the passage of time, and (4) users lose the ability to maintain attention to a task.

The long-term effects of marijuana use are still being studied. Chronic abuse may lead to an **amotivational syndrome** in some people. The irritating effects of marijuana smoke on lung tissue are more pronounced than those of cigarette smoke, and some of the over 400 chemicals in marijuana are now linked to lung cancer development. In fact, one of the most potent carcinogens, benzopyrene, is found in higher levels in marijuana smoke than in tobacco smoke. Marijuana smokers tend to inhale deeply and hold the smoke in the lungs for long periods. It is likely that at some point the lungs of chronic marijuana smokers will be damaged.

Thai sticks are a potent form of marijuana.

Key Terms

metabolite a breakdown product of a drug.

amotivational syndrome behavioral pattern characterized by lack of interest in productive activities.

Long-term marijuana use is also associated with damage to the immune system and to the male and female reproductive systems and with an increase in birth defects in babies born to mothers who smoke marijuana. Chronic marijuana use lowers testosterone levels in men, but the effect of this change is not known. The effect of long-term marijuana use on a variety of types of sexual behavior is also not fully understood.

Because the drug can distort perceptions and thus perceptual ability (especially when combined with alcohol), its use by automobile drivers clearly jeopardizes the lives of many innocent people.

The only medical uses for marijuana are to relieve the nausea caused by chemotherapy, to improve the appetite in AIDS patients, and to ease the pressure that builds up in the eyes of glaucoma patients. However, a variety of other drugs, many of which are nearly as effective, are also used for these purposes. In May 2001, the U.S. Supreme Court ruled unanimously against the distribution of marijuana in medical clinics.

Narcotics

The **narcotics** are among the most dependence-producing drugs. Medically, narcotics are used to relieve pain and induce sleep. On the basis of origin, narcotics can be subgrouped into the natural, quasisynthetic, and synthetic narcotics.

Natural Narcotics

Naturally occurring substances derived from the Oriental poppy plant include opium (the primary psychoactive substance extracted from the Oriental poppy), morphine (the primary active ingredient in opium), and thebaine (a compound not used as a drug). Morphine and related compounds have medical use as analgesics in the treatment of mild to severe pain.

Quasisynthetic Narcotics

Quasisynthetic narcotics are compounds created by chemically altering morphine. These laboratory-produced drugs are intended to be used as analgesics, but their benefits are largely outweighed by a high dependence rate and a great risk of toxicity. The best known of the quasisynthetic narcotics is heroin. Although heroin is a fast-acting and very effective analgesic, it is extremely addictive. Once injected into a vein or "skin-popped" (injected beneath the skin surface), heroin produces dreamlike euphoria and, like all narcotics, strong physical and psychological dependence and tolerance.

As with the use of all other injectable illegal drugs, the practice of sharing needles increases the likelihood of transmission of various communicable diseases, including HIV (see Chapter 12). Abrupt withdrawal from heroin use is rarely fatal, but the discomfort during **cold turkey** withdrawal is reported to be overwhelming. The use of heroin has increased during the last decade. The purity of heroin has improved while the price has dropped. Cocaine abusers may use heroin to "come down" from the high associated with cocaine.

Synthetic Narcotics

Meperidine (Demerol) and propoxyphene (Darvon), common postsurgical painkillers, and methadone, the drug prescribed during the rehabilitation of heroin addicts, are *synthetic narcotics*. These opiate-like drugs are manufactured in medical laboratories. They are not natural narcotics or quasisynthetic narcotics because they do not originate from the Oriental poppy plant. Like true narcotics, however, these drugs can rapidly induce physical dependence. One important criticism of methadone rehabilitation programs is that in some cases, they merely shift the addiction from heroin to methadone.

OxyContin OxyContin, also known as hillybilly heroin, Oxy, Oxycotton, is a time-released legal prescription drug used to treat individuals with moderate to severe pain.[19] Illegal use of OxyContin brought national attention when individuals in rural areas of the country were found abusing this drug. Now abuse of OxyContin is continuing to spread across the country.[20] Classified as a narcotic drug, OxyContin is an addictive controlled substance with an addiction potential similar to morphine. This prescription drug is considered extremely dangerous as an illicit drug. Some methods of usage that increase the likelihood of dangerous effects, including death, are chewing the tablets, snorting crushed tablets, and dissolving the tablets in water and then injecting the drug. When OxyContin is not taken in tablet form, the controlled-release dosage is defeated and the user has a high potential of receiving a lethal dose due to the drug being released immediately into one's system.[21] Many other long-term consequences of OxyContin abuse are physical dependence and severe respiratory depression that may lead to death. Common withdrawal symptoms include restlessness, muscle and bone pain, insomnia, diarrhea, vomiting, cold flashes with

---

> **Key Terms**
>
> **narcotics** opiates; psychoactive drugs derived from the Oriental poppy plant; narcotics relieve pain and induce sleep.
>
> **cold turkey** immediate, total discontinuation of use of a drug; associated withdrawal discomfort.

goose bumps, and involuntary leg movements.[20] The FDA continues to monitor the abuse of OxyContin and has approved the strongest warning labels for this drug with the intent of changing prescription practices as well as increasing the physician's focus on the potential for abuse.[21]

Inhalants

Inhalants are a class of drugs that includes a variety of volatile (quickly evaporating) compounds that generally produce unpredictable, drunklike effects in users and feelings of euphoria.[22] Users of inhalants may also have some delusions and hallucinations. Some users may become quite aggressive. Drugs in this category include anesthetic gases (chloroform, nitrous oxide, and ether), vasodilators (amyl nitrite and butyl nitrite), petroleum products and commercial solvents (gasoline, kerosene, plastic cement, glue, typewriter correction fluid, paint, and paint thinner), and certain aerosols (found in some propelled spray products, fertilizers, and insecticides).

Most of the danger in using inhalants lies in the damaging, sometimes fatal effects on the respiratory and cardiovascular systems. Furthermore, users may unknowingly place themselves in dangerous situations because of the drunklike hallucinogenic effects. Aggressive behavior might also make users a threat to themselves and others.

Combination Drug Effects

Drugs taken in various combinations and dosages can alter and perhaps intensify effects.

A **synergistic drug effect** is a dangerous consequence of taking different drugs in the same general category at the same time. The combination exaggerates each individual drug's effects. For example, the combined use of alcohol and tranquilizers produces a synergistic effect greater than the total effect of each of the two drugs taken separately. In this instance a much-amplified, perhaps fatal sedation will occur. In a simplistic sense, "one plus one equals four or five."

When taken at or near the same time, drug combinations produce a variety of effects. Drug combinations have additive, potentiating, or antagonistic effects. When two or more drugs are taken and the result is merely a combined total effect of each drug, the result is an **additive effect.** The sum of the effects is not exaggerated. In a sense, "one plus one plus one equals three."

When one drug intensifies the action of a second drug, the first drug is said to have a **potentiated effect** on the second drug. One popular drug-taking practice during the 1970s was the consumption of Quaaludes and beer. Quaaludes potentiated the inhibition-releasing, sedative effects of alcohol. This particular drug

HealthQuest Activities

Drug abuse can occur with illegal drugs or with over-the-counter or prescription drugs. Complete the assessment activity *Drugs: Are You at Risk?* in the Other Drugs module to raise your awareness of the many decisions you make about drugs. What is your overall risk score? Do you think the score is accurate? Do you think your score reflects campuswide drug use? What are the causes of drug abuse, and what can be done to prevent it?

combination produced an inexpensive but potentially fatal drunklike euphoria in the user.

An **antagonistic effect** is an opposite effect one drug has on another drug. One drug may be able to reduce another drug's influence on the body. Knowledge of this principle has been useful in the medical treatment of certain drug overdoses, as in the use of tranquilizers to relieve the effects of LSD or other hallucinogenic drugs.

Society's Response to Drug Use

During the last 25 years, society has responded to illegal drug use with growing concern. Most adults see drug abuse as a clear danger to society. This position has been supported by the development of community, school, state, and national organizations directed toward the reduction of illegal drug use. These organizations have included such diverse groups as Parents Against Drugs,

Key Terms

inhalants psychoactive drugs that enter the body through inhalation.

synergistic drug effect (sin er JIST ick) heightened, exaggerated effect produced by the concurrent use of two or more drugs.

additive effect the combined (but not exaggerated) effect produced by the concurrent use of two or more drugs.

potentiated effect (poe TEN she ay ted) phenomenon whereby the use of one drug intensifies the effect of a second drug.

antagonistic effect effect produced when one drug reduces or offsets the effects of a second drug.

Partnership for a Drug-Free America, Mothers Against Drunk Driving (MADD), Narcotics Anonymous, and the U.S. Drug Enforcement Administration. Certain groups have concentrated their efforts on education, others on enforcement, and still others on the development of laws and public policy. Famous people, such as athletes, are also speaking out against drug use (see Learning from Our Diversity on page 186).

The personal and social issues related to drug abuse are very complex. Innovative solutions continue to be devised. Some believe that only through early childhood education will people learn alternatives to drug use. Starting drug education in the preschool years may have a more positive effect than waiting until the upper elementary or junior high school years. Recently, the focus on reducing young people's exposure to **gateway drugs** (especially tobacco, alcohol, and marijuana) may help slow down the move to other addictive drugs. Some people advocate harsher penalties for drug use and drug trafficking, including heavier fines and longer prison terms.

Others support legalizing all drugs and making governmental agencies responsible for drug regulation and control, as is the case with alcohol. Advocates of this position believe that drug-related crime and violence would virtually cease once the demand for illegal products is reduced. Sound arguments can be made on both sides of this issue. What's your opinion?

In comparison with other federally funded programs, the "war on drugs" is less expensive than farm support, food stamps, Medicare, and national defense. However, it remains to be seen whether any amount of money spent on enforcement, without adequate support for education, treatment, and poverty reduction, can reduce the illegal drug demand and supply. The United States now spends nearly $18 billion annually to fight the drug war. About $11 billion is spent on law enforcement (supply reduction) and $6 billion on education, prevention, and treatment (demand reduction).[23,24]

Drug Testing

Society's response to concern over drug use includes the development and growing use of drug tests. Most of the specimens come from corporations that screen employees for commonly abused drugs. Among these are amphetamines, barbiturates, benzodiazepines (the chemical bases for prescription tranquilizers such as Valium and Librium), cannabinoids (THC, hashish, and marijuana), methaqualone, opiates (heroin, codeine, and morphine), and PCP. With the exception of marijuana, most traces of these drugs are eliminated by the body within a few days after use. Marijuana can remain detectable up to 30 days after use.

How accurate are the results of drug testing? At typical cutoff standards, drug tests will likely identify 90% of recent drug users. This means that about 10% of recent users will pass undetected. (These 10% are considered false negatives.) Nonusers whose drug tests indicate drug use (false positives) are quite rare. (Follow-up tests on these false positives would nearly always show negative results.) Human errors are probably more responsible than technical errors for inaccuracies in drug tests.

Recently, scientists have been refining procedures that use hair samples to detect the presence of drugs. These procedures seem to hold much promise, although certain technical obstacles remain. Watch for refinements in hair-sample drug testing in the near future.

Most Fortune 500 companies, the armed forces, various government agencies, and nearly all athletic organizations have already implemented mandatory drug testing. Corporate substance abuse policies are being developed, with careful attention to legal and ethical issues.

Do you think that the possibility of having to take a drug test would have any effect on college students' use of drugs?

College and Community Support Services for Drug Dependence

Students who have drug problems and realize they need help might select assistance based on the services available on campus or in the surrounding community and the costs they are willing to pay for treatment services.

One approach to convince drug-dependent people to enter treatment programs is the use of *confrontation*. People who live or work with chemically dependent people are being encouraged to confront them directly about their addiction. Direct confrontation helps chemically dependent people realize the effect their behavior has on others. Once chemically dependent people realize that others will no longer tolerate their behavior, the likelihood of their entering treatment programs increases significantly. Although effective, this approach is very stressful for family members and friends and requires the assistance of professionals in the field of chemical dependence. These professionals can be contacted at a drug treatment center in your area.

Key Terms
gateway drug an easily obtainable legal or illegal drug that represents a user's first experience with a mind-altering drug.

Treatment

Comprehensive drug treatment programs are available in very few college or university health centers. College settings for drug dependence programs are more commonly found in the university counseling center. At such a center the emphasis will probably be not on the medical management of dependence but on the behavioral dimensions of drug abuse. Trained counselors and psychologists who specialize in chemical dependence counseling will work with students to (1) analyze their particular concerns, (2) establish constructive ways to cope with stress, and (3) search for alternative ways to achieve new "highs" (see the Personal Assessment on page 207).

 TALKING POINTS Do you think that confronting a friend about her cocaine use would prompt her to get help?

Medical treatment for the management of drug problems may need to be obtained through the services of a community treatment facility administered by a local health department, community mental health center, private clinic, or local hospital. Treatment may be on an inpatient or outpatient basis. Medical management might include detoxification, treatment of secondary health complications and nutritional deficiencies, and therapeutic counseling for chemical dependence.

Some communities have voluntary health agencies that deliver services and treatment programs for drug-dependent people. Check your telephone book for listings of drug-treatment facilities. Some communities have drug hot lines that offer advice for people with questions about drugs. (See the Changing for the Better box on page 187 for a list of anti–drug abuse organizations and hot line numbers.)

Costs of Treatment for Dependence

Drug-treatment programs that are administered by colleges and universities for faculty and students usually require no fees. Local agencies may provide either free services or services based on a **sliding scale.** Private hospitals, physicians, and clinics are the most expensive forms of treatment. Inpatient treatment at a private facility may cost as much as $1000 per day. Since the length of inpatient treatment averages 3 to 4 weeks, a patient can quickly accumulate a very large bill. However, with many types of health insurance policies now providing coverage for alcohol and other drug dependencies, even these services may not require additional out-of-pocket expenses.

> **Key Terms**
>
> **sliding scale** a method of payment by which patient fees are scaled according to income.

Taking Charge of Your Health

- Assess your knowledge of drug use by completing the Personal Assessment on page 205.
- Calculate the amount of caffeine you consume daily. If you're drinking more than three cups of caffeinated beverages per day, develop a plan to reduce your overall intake.
- Prepare a plan of action to use if someone you know needs professional assistance with a drug problem.

- Identify five activities that can provide you with a drug-free high.
- Analyze your drug use patterns (if any), and assess the likelihood that you might fail a preemployment drug test.
- Assess your lifestyle for addictive behaviors that do not involve drugs, such as overexercising or watching too much TV. Develop a plan to moderate these activities and achieve more balance in your life.

Summary

- A drug affects the CNS by altering neurotransmitter activity on the neuron.
- Drug use, drug abuse, tolerance, and dependence are important terms to understand.
- Drugs enter the body through ingestion, injection, inhalation, or absorption.
- Drugs can be placed into six categories: stimulants, depressants, hallucinogens, cannabis, narcotics, and inhalants.

- Combination drug effects include synergist, addictive, potentiated, and antagonistic effects.
- Drug testing is becoming increasingly common in our society.
- Drug abuse has a devastating effect on society.
- Society's response to drug abuse has been widely varied and has included education, enforcement, treatment, testing, and the search for drug-free ways to achieve highs.

Review Questions

1. Describe how neurotransmitters work.
2. Identify and explain the three steps in the process of addiction.
3. How is the term *drug* defined in this chapter? What are psychoactive drugs? How do medicines differ from drugs?
4. Define the four routes of administration. Select a drug that reflects each of the ways drugs enter the body.
5. Explain what *dependence* means. Identify and explain the two types of dependence.
6. Define the word *tolerance*. What does *cross-tolerance* mean? Give an example of cross-tolerance.
7. Differentiate between drug misuse and drug abuse.
8. List the six general categories of drugs. For each category, give several examples of drugs and explain the effects they would have on the user. What are designer drugs?
9. Why do students without a prescription take Ritalin? What are the side effects and health risks of abusing Ritalin?
10. What is the active ingredient in marijuana? What are its common effects on the user? What are the short- and long-term effects of marijuana use?
11. Explain the terms *synergistic effect, additive effect, potentiated effect,* and *antagonistic effect.*
12. How accurate is drug testing?

References

1. Shier D, Butler J, Lewis R. *Hole's Human Anatomy and Physiology,* 9th ed. McGraw-Hill, 2002.
2. Ray O, Ksir C. *Drugs, society, and human behavior,* 9th ed. McGraw-Hill, 2002.
3. The Coffee Science Information Centre. *Caffeine* (online). Available: **http://www.cosic.org/caffeine/stimulanteffects/,** accessed 25 May 2003.
4. *Caffeine.* Johns Hopkins InteliHealth online newsletter, November 10, 1998. Available: **www.intelihealth.com** accessed 25 May 2003.
5. National Institute on Drug Abuse. National Institutes of Health: *Methamphetamine.* **www.nida.nih.gov/Infofax/methamphetamine. html,** accessed 17 March 2001.
6. U.S. Department of Justice. Drug Enforcement Administration: *Methamphetamine.* **www.usdoi.gov/dea/concern/meth.htm,** 31 December 2001.
7. Frackelmann K. Breaking bonds of addiction: Compulsion traced to part of the brain. *USA Today.* 18 April 2002.
8. Ephedra Education Council. *Ephedra Supported by Science—A Ban Is Not, Industry Tells FDA.* 8 April 2003.
9. U.S. Department of Justice. *Drugs of Concern.* **www.dea.gov,** October 2000.
10. Cocaine Weakens Immune System. *Boston Herald,* 7 March 2003.
11. Pinger RR, Payne WA, Hahn DB, Hahn EJ. *Drugs: issues for today,* 3rd ed. McGraw-Hill, 1998.
12. Health-Nexus: *Depressants* (online). Available: **www.health-nexus.com/depressants.htm.** 10 June 2003.
13. National Institute on Drug Abuse. NIDA InfoFacts: *Rohypnol and GHB* (online). Available: **www.nida.nih.gov/InfoFax/RohypnolGHB.html.** 10 June 2003.
14. National Institute on Drug Abuse. *Club drugs: community drug alert bulletin: some facts about club drugs.* **www.clubdrugs.org,** accessed 22 May 2003.
15. Johnston LD, O'Malley PM, Bachman JG. *Monitoring the Future: National Survey Results on Drug Use, 1975–2001.* University of Michigan Institute for Social Research (online). Available: **www.monitoringthefuture.org/pubs/monographs/vol1_2001.pdf,** accessed 22 May 2003.
16. Substance Abuse and Mental Health Services Administration (SAMHSA). *2001 National Household Survey on Drug Abuse.* **www.samhsa.gov/oas/nhsda/2k1nhsda/vol1/toc.htm,** accessed 22 May 2003.
17. Leinwand D. A strange new world of teenage drug use: the lowdown on the hippest highs. *USA Today.* 28 February 2001.
18. National Institute on Drug Abuse. NIDA InfoFacts: *PCP (Phencyclidine).* **www.nida.nih.gov/InfoFax/pcp.html.** 10 June 2003.
19. OxyContin Questions and Answers. Drug Information. U.S. Food and Drug Administration, Center for Drug Evaluation and Research. **www.fda.gov/cder/drug/infopage/oxycontin/oxycontin-qa.htm,** 25 July 2001.
20. OxyContin. OxyContin Addiction and Treatment and Rapid Detox Services (online). Available: **www.oxycontin-detox.com/index-overture-kw-oxycontin.html,** accessed 14 July 2003.
21. FDA Strengthens Warnings for OxyContin. U.S. Food and Drug Administration. **www.fda.gov/bbs/topics/ANSWERS/2001/ANS01091.html,** 25 July 2001.

22. Frackelmann K. Inhalants' hidden treat: Access makes huffing popular but kids can recover with help. *USA Today.* 25 June 2002.

23. **www.whitehousedrugpolicy.gov/publications/policy/04budget/exec_sum.pdf,** February 2003 accessed 21 May 2003.

24. Keen J. Bush plans hit on drug abuse: White House goal is to reduce 'crisis' by 25% in five years. *USA Today.* 13 February 2002.

As We Go to Press

In late December 2003 the Food and Drug Administration (FDA) announced its plans to soon ban the sale of dietary supplements containing ephedra. Until this date, Illinois and New York were the only states that had already banned the sale of ephedra.

This consumer alert was issued to warn consumers about the health risks of ephedra and to urge them not to purchase or consume ephedra products. Ephedra dietary supplements have been used to aid in weight control, to increase energy, and to enhance athletic performance. Health risks such as high blood pressure, heart problems, stroke, and stress on the circulatory system have been the result of consuming ephedra products.

As we go to press, on February 6, 2004, the FDA published its final rule banning ephedra. This ban becomes effective 60 days after the ruling. Once the ban is in effect, manufacturers and distributors may no longer market or sell ephedra products. Any violations of this rule will result in criminal prosecution.

focus on

prescription drug abuse

Lucy, a 35-year-old mother of two, seems like a typical suburban homemaker. She attends church regularly, belongs to the PTA, and volunteers at the local battered women's shelter. Her husband is a well-respected businessman, and her children are honor students at the local high school. Life seems perfect for Lucy and her family, at least on the outside. But Lucy has a secret that few outside her family know about.

Lucy's children and husband regularly come home to a disheveled household, finding Lucy passed out somewhere in the house or on the back porch. Lucy's mood swings are unpredictable. One day, she will be a loving, devoted wife and mother; the next, she will talk rapidly and endlessly to whomever she can get to listen; sometimes, her speech will slur and she will seem incoherent. All this usually occurs whenever a stressful or unpleasant situation comes up in her life with which she cannot cope. Lucy's family never knows what to expect from one day to the next. The children have moved in and out of the home to live with their grandparents dozens of times over the past several years, and Lucy's husband has threatened her with divorce. Lucy has been to inpatient detoxification programs three times, only to "fall off the wagon" whenever a stressful event occurs.

You would probably guess that Lucy is an alcoholic or an illegal drug addict; however, Lucy's drugs of choice are all legal and all readily available to her from any one of a number of reputable physicians she visits. She uses a combination of drugs that range from sedatives to tranquilizers to antidepressants. Lucy is a prescription drug addict. Her suppliers are unwitting physicians who have no idea that she is seeing other doctors.

In 1999, an estimated 9 million people (12 and older) are using prescription drugs for nonmedical reasons. Prescription drug misuse and abuse is common in older adults. This population is given prescription medications three times more

frequently than the general population.[1] According to the Prescription Drugs Research Report, it is estimated that 17% of adults (60 and older) are abusing prescription medications.[2]

According to the Drug Enforcement Administration, 12 of the top 20 most abused controlled substances are prescription drugs.[3] These drugs fall into the following categories:

- *Opioids.* These drugs are narcotics typically prescribed to relieve acute or chronic pain. Common prescription drugs include Demerol, Darvocet, Vicodin, and drugs with codeine.
- *Stimulants.* These drugs affect the central nervous system and increase mental alertness, decrease fatigue, and produce a sense of well-being. They are usually prescribed for appetite suppression, attention deficit disorder, and narcolepsy. Common prescription drugs include Dexedrine, Ritalin, Fastin, and Cyclert.
- *Sedatives.* These drugs depress the central nervous system and are frequently used to treat anxiety, panic disorder, and insomnia. Some are dispensed for either daytime or nighttime use. Common prescription drugs include Xanax, Valium, Ativan, Dalmane, and Ambien.[4]

Under certain conditions, nearly anybody could wind up abusing a prescription drug, but there are particular groups of people who are at high risk for prescription drug abuse. People with a family history of depression, smokers, and excessive drinkers are more likely to become addicted to prescription drugs, as are those with a history of abusing illegal drugs. Stress from traumatic experiences can also make a person more likely to abuse prescription drugs, and people who are hyperactive, obese, or who suffer from chronic pain are also at risk. Health care professionals are considered to be a high-risk group, and older people have a greater tendency to abuse prescription drugs.[2]

A patient can become physiologically dependent on a drug, which is considered to be a more manageable condition than addiction. Physiological dependence, involving the body's adaptation to a drug over time, is considered a temporary, benign condition. Physiological dependence is usually treated by gradual reductions in use of the drug, and although there may be withdrawal symptoms during this period, there is not normally a relapse afterward. The gradual reduction in dosage can be handled with medical supervision, and the patient does not normally need to enter a substance abuse program. Addiction involves a continued need to use a drug for psychological effects or mood alteration, and the patient goes to great lengths to obtain the drug even if its effects become harmful. Addiction is considered a chronic, complex problem and is usually handled with specific chemical dependence treatment.

Abuse is often caused or continued because of deliberate deception on the part of the patient, but misuse of a prescription drug can start innocently enough. A patient may be receiving several prescriptions that have the same effect, or a patient may have several doctors prescribing the same medication. Prescription drugs may react with each other and cause different effects than intended. Sometimes communication problems between patient and physician cause errors in prescription dispensation. The patient may unintentionally use the prescription incorrectly. One of these situations or a combination of factors can start prescription drug abuse.[5] Often a single prescription drug, such as a painkiller or sedative, is enough to start the process of dependence.

Older people are considered at high risk for prescription drug abuse for several reasons. The process of aging or the transition to retirement can leave a person with symptoms of depression or anxiety, and illnesses can also increase as a person gets older.[5] Many people see multiple doctors as they get older and thus may wind up getting several prescriptions for the same drug under different brand names without realizing it. Sometimes physicians give older patients the same dosages as younger patients.[6] Body functions slow and change with age, and when this occurs, the duration and intensity of drug effects can change as well.[5] Such conditions can increase the risk of drug abuse among the elderly.

If addiction starts, older people may then resort to the same tactics as any prescription drug addict. They may begin to "doctor-hop" (moving from one doctor to the next without informing the doctors) to get multiple prescriptions, or they may go to an emergency room to get a quick fix of a particular drug. Patients may also hoard pills or swap pills with friends to cut costs and ensure availability of their drug of choice.

Health care professionals are also at high risk for prescription drug abuse. Physicians are five times more likely than the general population to take sedatives or tranquilizers without another doctor's supervision. The high stress of the job and the availability of drugs are both believed to be contributing factors to abuse among health care professionals. However, studies suggest that those physicians who are psychologically sound had little problem handling the stress of their jobs and generally resisted the temptation of readily available drugs. Those physicians considered to have psychological problems were more likely to be abusers.[7]

Effects of Abuse

As abuse of a drug continues, the tolerance of the body to that drug increases, which can lead to stronger self-dosing. As use increases, the detoxification process can become more difficult. In some cases, people refuse to believe they are addicted, and older people who are isolated from others do not even realize they are hooked.[8] Physicians may inadvertently promote the abuse by failing or refusing to acknowledge the signs of addiction in a patient.

If a person admits he or she has a problem with a drug, the recovery process can begin. Trying to kick the habit without professional help may only make things worse. If the person tries to cut back or stop use of the drug, withdrawal symptoms may occur. These symptoms include pain, nausea, sleeplessness, nervousness, irritability, hallucinations, and confusion, and can be quite severe. In short, recovery from prescription drug abuse becomes as difficult as recovery from abuse of illegal drugs. For these reasons, professional help is usually necessary for a full recovery from prescription drug abuse.

If you or someone you know is abusing prescription drugs, help is available. Many hospitals that sponsor detoxification programs for alcoholics and illegal drug addicts also have programs for individuals who are addicted to prescription drugs. Often, insurance will cover the costs of these programs. After detoxification the individual will need to continue recovery through a program such as Alcoholics Anonymous (the principles used for recovery from alcoholism are also applicable to recovery from drug addiction) or Narcotics Anonymous. These organizations can be found in the white pages of the phone book.

If the addicted person has family or close friends who are being seriously affected by addiction issues, they may want to try Al-Anon, Alateen, or Adult Children of Alcoholics support groups. Finally, individual or family counseling may be of value in helping to sort out emotional issues that lie behind the addiction. A certified addictions counselor may be the most helpful person to an addict, or the family may choose a psychiatrist, psychologist, or social worker who has knowledge of addiction issues.

You also might wish to get additional information by going on-line to **www. prescriptionabuse.org**.[9] This website was created by a man whose wife was a former prescription drug addict. The site offers education, hope, and recovery approaches for abusers and their families.

Although prescription drug addicts will always be "recovering" rather than "recovered," they can still lead relatively normal lives with proper physical and psychological treatment. However, there are no quick fixes or easy answers. Recovery is an ongoing process for both the addict and his or her family.

For Discussion . . .

Do you know of anyone who has intentionally abused prescription drugs? Have you ever taken a prescription drug in a different way than it was prescribed? Have you ever taken someone else's prescription drug? If so, why did you take it? Can you think of a case where use of another person's prescription drug can be justified?

References

1. Leshner A: National Institute on Drug Abuse. *Prescription Drugs: Abuse and Addiction* (online). Available: **www.nida.nih.gov/ResearchReports/Prescription/ Prescription. html,** accessed 30 May 2003.

2. Botsford C: The NCADI Reports. *Prescription Drug Abuse Explodes in America.* 4 May 2001.

3. Colvin R: *Prescription drug abuse: the hidden epidemic: A guide to coping and understanding,* 1995, Addicus Books.

4. National Institute on Drug Abuse: *Research Report Series—Prescription Drugs: Abuse and Addiction.* **http:// www.nida.nih.gov/ResearchReports/ Prescription/prescription2.html,** accessed 3 June 2003.

5. Fackelmann K: Older but not wise to addiction: More seniors are getting hooked on prescription drugs as a way to deal with anxieties of old age. *USA Today.* 24 July 2001.

6. Snider V: U.S. Department of Health and Human Services and SAMHSA's National Clearinghouse for Alcohol and Drug Information. *Monitoring Prescription Drug Use Among Older Adults Can Prevent Misuse,* 15 April 2003.

7. Lott D: Physician—Treat Thyself? *Psychiatric Times.* December 2001; 18(12).

8. Hittenger ME: Substance Abuse and the Elderly (online): **www. fullspectrumrecovery.com/articles/ uploaded/Substance%220Abuse% 20and%20the%Eld pdf,** accessed 3 June 2003.

9. **www.prescriptionabuse.org,** accessed 3 June 2003.

personal assessment

test your drug awareness

1. What is the most commonly used drug in the United States?
   (a) heroin
   (b) cocaine
   (c) alcohol
   (d) marijuana

2. Name the three drugs most commonly used by children.
   (a) alcohol, tobacco, and marijuana
   (b) cocaine, crack, alcohol
   (c) heroin, inhalants, marijuana

3. Which drug is associated with the most teenage deaths?
   (a) heroin
   (b) cocaine
   (c) alcohol
   (d) marijuana

4. By the eighth grade, how many kids have tried at least one inhalant?
   (a) one in one hundred
   (b) one in fifty
   (c) one in twenty five
   (d) one in five
   (e) one in two

5. "Crack" is a particularly dangerous drug because it is
   (a) cheap.
   (b) readily available.
   (c) highly addictive.
   (d) all of the above.

6. Fumes from which of the following can be inhaled to produce a high?
   (a) spray paint
   (b) model glue
   (c) nail polish remover
   (d) whipped cream canisters
   (e) all of the above

7. People who have not used alcohol and other drugs before their 20th birthday:
   (a) have no risk of becoming chemically dependent.
   (b) are less likely to develop a drinking problem or use illicit drugs.
   (c) have an increased risk of becoming chemically dependent.

8. A speedball is a combination of which two drugs?
   (a) cocaine and heroin
   (b) PCP and LSD
   (c) valium and alcohol
   (d) amphetamines and barbiturates

9. Methamphetamines are dangerous because use can cause
   (a) anxiety/nervousness/irritability.
   (b) paranoia/psychosis.
   (c) loss of appetite/malnutrition/anorexia.
   (d) hallucinations.
   (e) aggressive behavior.
   (f) all of the above.

10. How is marijuana harmful?
    (a) It hinders the user's short-term memory.
    (b) Students may find it hard to study and learn while under the influence of marijuana.
    (c) It affects timing and coordination.
    (d) All of the above

Source: *A parent's guide to prevention*, U.S. Department of Education.

Answers to Personal Assessment

1. c
2. a
3. c
4. d
5. d
6. e
7. b
8. a
9. f
10. d

personal assessment

getting a drug free high

Experts agree that drug use provides only short-term, ineffective, and often destructive solutions to problems. We hope that you have found (or will find) innovative, invigorating drug-free experiences that make your life more exciting. Circle the number for each activity that reflects your intention to try that activity. Use the following guide:

1 No intention of trying this activity
2 Intend to try this within 2 years
3 Intend to try this within 6 months
4 Already tried this activity
5 Regularly engage in this activity

1. Learn to juggle	1	2	3	4	5
2. Go backpacking	1	2	3	4	5
3. Complete a marathon race	1	2	3	4	5
4. Start a vegetable garden	1	2	3	4	5
5. Ride in a hot air balloon	1	2	3	4	5
6. Snow ski or water ski	1	2	3	4	5
7. Donate blood	1	2	3	4	5
8. Go river rafting	1	2	3	4	5
9. Learn to play a musical instrument	1	2	3	4	5
10. Cycle 100 miles	1	2	3	4	5
11. Go skydiving	1	2	3	4	5
12. Go rockclimbing	1	2	3	4	5
13. Play a role in a theater production	1	2	3	4	5
14. Build a piece of furniture	1	2	3	4	5
15. Solicit funds for a worthy cause	1	2	3	4	5
16. Learn to swim	1	2	3	4	5
17. Overhaul a car engine	1	2	3	4	5
18. Compose a song	1	2	3	4	5
19. Travel to a foreign country	1	2	3	4	5
20. Write the first chapter of a book	1	2	3	4	5

TOTAL POINTS _____

Interpretation

61–100   You participate in many challenging experiences
41–60   You are willing to try some challenging new experiences
20–40   You take few of the challenging risks described here

To Carry This Further . . .

Looking at your point total, were you surprised at the degree to which you are aware of alternative activities? What are the top five activities, and can you understand their importance? What activities would you add to this list?

chapter eight

taking Control of alcohol use

Online Learning Center Resources

www.mhhe.com/hahn7e

Log on to our Online Learning Center (OLC) for access to these additional resources:

- Chapter key terms and definitions
- Learning objectives
- Student interactive question-and-answer sites
- Self-scoring chapter quiz
- Online assessments
- Key term flash cards

Talking It Over

Getting a Friend Into Treatment

Someone close to you has a drinking problem. What can you do to help this person get professional help?

- Talk with an alcohol or drug treatment counselor to learn what to expect.
- Confront your friend when both of you are sober.
- Express genuine concern for your friend's life.
- Point out specific situations when your friend's alcohol-related behavior was dangerous to him or her and to other people.
- Tell your friend where he or she can go to find help. Have names, phone numbers, and addresses ready.
- Offer to accompany your friend to a counselor or treatment center.
- Tell your friend that "now—this minute—is the time to get into treatment." Be persistent. Also be ready to transport your friend immediately, before his or her denial begins.

CommunicationLinks
www.way2hope.org/
www.aca-usa.org/

Eye on the Media

TV Ads Target Drunk Driving

The first successful national campaign against drunk driving, "Designated Driver," began in 1998. Besides targeting specific audiences and using well-timed and strategically placed public service announcements, its developers convinced TV producers and writers to work references to the designated driver into the dialogue of their shows. Gradually, the message got through to young people. It does make sense to plan to have someone else drive if you're not going to be up to it. The designated-driver approach is still considered a good idea on college campuses today.

In contrast, the "Campaign for Alcohol Free Kids," relied heavily on dramatic graphics, such as grisly photos of car crash scenes on prom night.[1] Although the overall visual impact was powerful, the campaign lacked a practical element. Worse, the ads seemed to be preaching.

The Ad Council's "Friends Don't Let Friends Drive Drunk" is based on the idea that we all have responsibility for each other. If someone is your friend, you want to take care of that person. So don't let your friend do something dangerous.[2] Here the message is practical, not preachy.

The "You Drink & Drive, You Lose" campaign, a part of the National Public Education Campaign, targets two high-risk groups, 21- to 34-year-olds and repeat offenders. The message is simple: Make the right choice—don't drink and drive. The "Don't Lose It!" TV spot focuses on the fact that it's inconvenient to be stopped but the time spent at the checkpoint is for your own safety. It seems to be saying: "Sure, you're in a hurry, but this is important. So be patient." The graphics range from a serious-looking police officer talking to a motorist to hands locked in handcuffs.

What the successful campaigns have in common is a message that is simple, believable, and acceptable. Rather than scolding or preaching, the ads emphasize the fact that you have a choice and ask you to make the right choice.

"Road Predators," an American Public Television special that aired in December 1999, touched off strong controversy. Funded by the Century Council, a corporation backed by a group of U.S. distillers, the program used tragic accounts of alcohol-related accidents to dramatize the fact that innocent people lose their lives, families are shattered, and billions of dollars are spent because of drunk drivers. The contrast between the life of the featured victim (a good and caring schoolteacher) and that of the drunk driver (an aimless man who spends most of his time drinking) was highlighted.

Beer manufacturers became angry. To them, the show suggested that drinking beer and driving is the problem, not drinking *any* type of alcohol and driving. Why, they wondered, was there no sign of hard liquor in the show? Other critics argued that by focusing on hard-core drinkers, the program implied that the problem of drunk driving is limited to a small group. What about bias? According to *The Wall Street Journal* ("Brewers Attack Drunken-Driving Special," Dec. 14, 1999, p. B8), the special's producer first claimed that the Century Group had had no input into its content but later conceded that it had supplied news clippings as background and had recommended that certain people be interviewed. As for accuracy, the deputy district attorney who tried the case said that it was not true that the drunk driver "very likely won't be required to complete" his 15-year sentence, as the program said. The producer responded that this was probably "a little dramatic license" on the writer's part. The sophisticated and expensive advertising for the special included an elaborate spread in *Newsweek* (Dec. 6, 1999), with an 8-page booklet featuring the drunk driver and the victim.

What is the motivation for an alcohol industry group to fund a campaign to discourage drunk driving? How do such campaigns compare with the tobacco industry's efforts to discourage smoking among teenagers? How effective do you think each kind of ad campaign is?

---

[1] Campaign for Alcohol Free Kids: Who We Are (online). **www.alcoholfreekids.com/au_who_ we_are.html** accessed 13 June 2003.

[2] Website Information: Ad Council. **www.adcouncil. org/** accessed 13 June 2003.

The push for zero tolerance laws, the tightening of standards for determining legal intoxication, and the growing influence of national groups concerned with alcohol misuse show that our society is more sensitive than ever to the growing misuse of alcohol.

People are concerned about the consequences of drunk driving, alcohol-related crime, and lowered job productivity. National data indicate that per capita alcohol consumption has gradually dropped in the United States since the early 1980s.[1] Alcohol use remains the preferred form of drug use for most adults (including college students), but as a society, we are increasingly uncomfortable with the ease with which alcohol can be misused.

Choosing to Drink

Clearly, people drink alcoholic beverages for many different reasons. Most people drink alcohol because it is an effective, affordable, and legal substance for altering the brain's chemistry. As **inhibitions** are removed by the influence of alcohol, behavior that is generally held in check

is expressed (Figure 8-1). At least temporarily, drinkers become a different version of themselves—more outgoing, relaxed, and adventuresome.

 TALKING POINTS If alcohol did not make people more outgoing, relaxed, and adventuresome, then do you think they would consume as much?

Alcohol Use Patterns

From magazines to billboards to television, alcohol is one of the most heavily advertised consumer products in the country.[2] You cannot watch television, listen to the radio, or read a newspaper without being encouraged to buy a

Key Terms

inhibitions inner controls that prevent a person from engaging in certain types of behavior.

Figure 8-1 Negative consequences of alcohol use as reported by college students. (*Occurred at least once in past year; year 2001 statistics from national sample of over 54,444 undergraduates from 131 colleges in U.S.) (Core Institute. 2001 Statistics on Alcohol and Other Drug Use on American College Campuses (online). Available: **www.siu.edu/departments/coreinst/public_html/recent.html** accessed 16 June 2003.)

particular brand of beer, wine, or liquor. The advertisements create a warm aura about the nature of alcohol use. The implications are clear: alcohol use will bring you good times, handsome men or seductive women, exotic settings, and a chance to forget the hassles of hard work and study.

With the many pressures to drink, it's not surprising that most adults drink alcoholic beverages. Two-thirds of all American adults are classified as drinkers. Yet one in three adults does not drink. In the college environment, where surveys indicate that 85% to 90% of all students drink, it's difficult for many students to imagine that every third adult is an abstainer. Although many college students assume that drinking is a natural part of their social life, others are making alternative choices (see Discovering Your Spirituality box on page 213).

Alcohol consumption figures are reported in many different ways, depending on the researchers' criteria. Various sources support the contention that about one-third of adults 18 years of age and older are abstainers, about one-third are light drinkers, and one-third are moderate-to-heavy drinkers. As a single category, heavy drinkers make up about 10% of the adult drinking population. Students who drink in college tend to classify themselves as light-to-moderate drinkers. It comes as a shock to students, though, when they read the criteria for each drinking classification. According to the combination of quantity of alcohol consumed per occasion and the frequency of drinking, these criteria are established as shown in Table 8.1.

Two-thirds of American adults are classified as drinkers. Only one-third choose to abstain from alcohol.

Table 8.1 Criteria for Drinking Classifications

Classification	Alcohol-Related Behavior
Abstainers	Do not drink or drink less often than once a year
Infrequent drinkers	Drink once a month at most and drink small amounts per typical drinking occasion
Light drinkers	Drink once a month at most and drink medium amounts per typical drinking occasion, or drink no more than three to four times a month and drink small amounts per typical drinking occasion
Moderate drinkers	Drink at least once a week and small amounts per typical drinking occasion or three to four times a month and medium amounts per typical drinking occasion or no more than once a month and large amounts per typical drinking occasion
Moderate/heavy drinkers	Drink at least once a week and medium amounts per typical drinking occasion or three to four times a month and large amounts per typical drinking occasion
Heavy drinkers	Drink at least once a week and large amounts per typical drinking occasion[1]

NOTE: Small amounts = One drink or less per drinking occasion
Medium amounts = Two to four drinks per drinking occasion
Large amounts = Five or more drinks per drinking occasion (binge drinking)
Drink = 12 fluid oz of beer, 5 fluid oz of wine, or 1.5 fluid oz of 80 proof distilled spirits[2]
1. U.S. Department of Health and Human Services: *Fourth Special Report to the U.S. Congress,* Washington, D.C., 1981, DHHS Pub No. ADM 81-1080.
2. Dufour M (1999): What is Moderate Drinking? Defining "Drinks" and Drinking Levels. *Alcohol Research and Health* 23(1), 5–14.

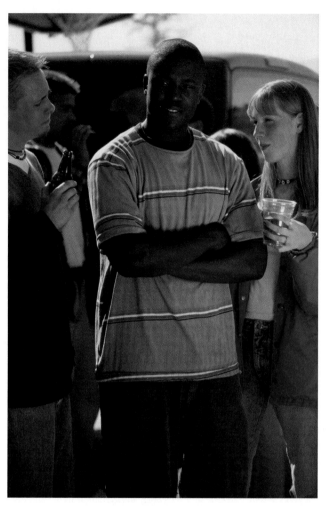

Mature adults know how to enjoy alcohol responsibly and understand how to decline alcohol use when they don't want to drink.

Moderate Drinking Redefined

Alcohol Research and Health defines moderate drinking as no more than two drinks each day for most men and one drink each day for women. A drink is defined as one 12-ounce regular beer, 5 ounce glass of wine, or 1.5 ounce 80 proof distilled spirits.[3] These cutoff levels are based on the amount of alcohol that can be consumed without causing problems, either for the drinker or society. (The gender difference is due primarily to the higher percentage of body fat in women and to the lower amount of an essential stomach enzyme in women.) Elderly people are limited to no more than one drink each day, again due to a higher percentage of body fat.

These consumption levels are applicable to most people. Indeed, people who plan to drive, women who are pregnant, people recovering from alcohol addiction, people under age 21, people taking medications, and those with existing medical concerns should not consume alcohol. Additionally, although some studies have shown that low levels of alcohol consumption may have minor psychological and cardiovascular benefits, nondrinkers are not advised to start drinking.

Binge Drinking

Alcohol abuse by college students usually takes place through *binge drinking.* This practice refers to the consumption of five drinks in a row, at least once during the previous 2-week period. College students who fit the category of "heavy drinkers" rarely consume small amounts of alcohol each day but instead binge on alcohol 1 or 2 nights a week. Some students openly admit that they plan to "get really drunk" on the weekend. They plan to binge drink.

 TALKING POINTS How do you tell a friend that you think he has a drinking problem?

Binge drinking can be dangerous. Drunk driving, physical violence, property destruction, date rape, police arrest, and lowered academic performance are all closely associated with binge drinking. The direct correlation between the amount of alcohol consumed and lowered

What's a Social Life without Alcohol?

When was the last time you went to a get-together where alcoholic drinks weren't served? It's probably been years. Socializing and drinking are connected in our consciousness in many ways. For instance, it's Friday night after a hard week and your friends ask you to join them for a beer. Why not? It'll be fun. Or you're invited to a party and want to bring something. How about a bottle of wine? That's easy and always appreciated.

Associating drinking with fun is something that many people, including college students, do. For various reasons, though, some college students are choosing to plan their fun around activities that don't involve drinking. Instead of going to a bar for a beer, they find a coffee shop and have a latte. Or they order soda with their pizza (not bad!). Others have discovered that they can get something that tastes great and is actually healthy at a juice bar.

What happens, though, when you go to a party and everyone else seems to be drinking? Choose something nonalcoholic—club soda, juice, soda, or water. (You probably won't be the only one doing this.) If someone gives you trouble about your choice, be firm. Just say that's what you want. You don't need to explain. And you don't have to say "yes" to be nice.

But maybe you want to drink at a party because it loosens you up and makes it easier to talk to people. How will you start a conversation without a drink to relax you? Think about how you talk easily and naturally with the people in your drama group or one of your favorite classes. You've got things in common, so it's easier to do. When you meet someone new at a party, look for common interests. You may feel self-conscious at first. But soon you'll forget about the fact that he or she is a stranger because you'll be involved in what you're talking about. Without that drink, you'll actually be more yourself.

Some students are making the commitment to be active instead of sitting around and drinking. They're going backpacking, joining a cycling group, taking an exercise class, or playing a team sport. What they're discovering is that it feels good—physically and mentally. They're socializing, doing something they enjoy, and getting in better shape. Think about something you've always wanted to try, and get going on it.

Making the choice to have fun without alcohol doesn't mean cutting yourself off from your friends. (If they're real friends, they'll respect your choice.) It's all about deciding what's right for you and making a commitment to that choice.

---

academic performance results in impaired memory, verbal skill deficiencies, and altered perceptions.[4] Frequently, the social costs of binge drinking are very high, especially when intoxicated people demonstrate their level of immaturity. How common is binge drinking on your campus?

In response to the personal dangers and campus trauma associated with binge drinking, colleges and universities are fighting back. Some colleges are conducting local alcohol education campaigns that feature innovative posters and materials displayed on campus. In the future, expect to see increasing efforts to reduce binge drinking on your campus to make it a safer environment.

For many students who drink, the college years are a time when they will drink more heavily than at any other time in their life (Figure 8-2). Some will suffer serious consequences as a result (Figure 8-1). These years will also mark the entry into a lifetime of problem drinking for some.

The Nature of Alcoholic Beverages

Alcohol (also known as *ethyl alcohol* or *ethanol*) is the principal product of **fermentation.** In this process, yeast cells act on the sugar content of fruits and grains to produce alcohol and carbon dioxide.[5]

The alcohol concentration in beverages such as whiskey, gin, rum, and vodka is determined through a process called **distillation.** These distilled beverages are

expressed by the term *proof,* a number that is twice the percentage of alcohol by volume in a beverage. Thus 70% of the fluid in a bottle of 140 proof gin is pure alcohol. Most proofs in distilled beverages range from 80 to 160. The familiar pure *grain alcohol* that is often added to fruit punches and similar beverages has a proof of almost 200.

The nutritional value of alcohol is extremely limited. Alcoholic beverages produced today through modern processing methods contain nothing but empty calories—about 100 calories per fluid ounce of 100-proof distilled spirits and about 150 calories for each 12-ounce bottle or can of beer.[6] Clearly, alcohol consumption is a significant contributor to the additional pounds that many college students accumulate. Pure alcohol contains only simple carbohydrates; it has no vitamins and minerals and no fats or protein.

Key Terms

fermentation a chemical process whereby plant products are converted into alcohol by the action of yeast cells on carbohydrate materials.

distillation the process of heating an alcohol solution and collecting its vapors into a more concentrated solution.

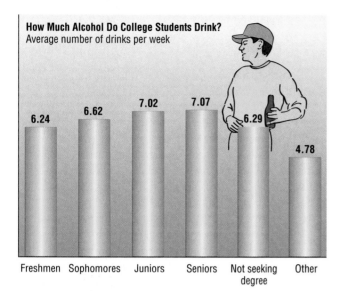

How Much Alcohol Do College Students Drink?
Average number of drinks per week

Freshmen 6.24 Sophomores 6.62 Juniors 7.02 Seniors 7.07 Not seeking degree 6.29 Other 4.78

Figure 8-2 Average number of alcoholic drinks consumed by college drinkers (year 2001 statistics from national sample of over 54,444 undergraduates from 131 colleges in U.S.).
(Core Institute. 2001 Statistics on Alcohol and Other Drug Use on American College Campuses (online). Available: **www.siu.edu/departments/coreinst/public_html/recent.html** accessed 16 June 2003.)

"Lite" beer and low-calorie wines have been introduced in response to concerns about the number of calories that alcoholic beverages provide. They are not low-alcohol beverages but merely low-calorie beverages. Only beverages marked "low alcohol" contain a lower concentration of alcohol than the usual beverages of that type. Recently, manufacturers have introduced a new form of beer called low carbohydrate beer (see Star box).

The popular new ice beers actually contain a higher percentage of alcohol than other types of beer. This is due to a production process that chills the fermented mixture sufficiently to allow ice crystals to form. When the ice crystals are removed, the beer contains a higher percentage of alcohol.

The Physiological Effects of Alcohol

First and foremost, alcohol is classified as a drug—a very strong CNS depressant. The primary depressant effect of alcohol occurs in the brain and spinal cord. Many people think of alcohol as a stimulant because of the way most users feel after consuming a serving or two of their favorite drink. Any temporary sensations of jubilation, boldness, or relief are attributable to alcohol's ability as a depressant drug to release personal inhibitions and provide temporary relief from tension.

Low Carbohydrate Beer

Many dieters in the United States consume low carbohydrate diets with the hope of shedding and keeping off unwanted pounds. Carbohydrates, which include a variety of sugars and starches, serve as a major dietary source of energy. Recently beer brewers have launched low carbohydrate beers for the diet-conscious consumers. These beers contain as few as 2.6 grams of carbohydrates per 12-ounce bottle of beer. Most regular beers contain between 3.2 grams to 6.6 grams of carbohydrates per 12-ounce serving. Ice beers may contain as many as 32 grams of carbohydrates per 12-ounce serving. Although these new low carbohydrate beers are similar in alcohol and calorie content to other beers, the carbohydrate content is lower. The brewers do state that there has been no health or weight loss claims attributed to this new type of beer. These beers let the consumer drink, yet keep carbohydrate intake to a minimum.

Factors That Influence the Absorption of Alcohol

The **absorption** of alcohol is influenced by several factors, most of which can be controlled by the individual. These factors include the following:

- *Strength of the beverage.* The stronger the beverage, the greater the amount of alcohol that will accumulate within the digestive tract.
- *Number of drinks consumed.* As more drinks are consumed, more alcohol is absorbed.
- *Speed of consumption.* If consumed rapidly, even relatively few drinks will result in a large concentration gradient that will lead to high blood alcohol concentration.
- *Presence of food.* Food can compete with alcohol for absorption into the bloodstream, slowing the absorption of alcohol. When alcohol absorption is slowed, the alcohol already in the bloodstream can be removed. Slow absorption favors better control of blood alcohol concentration.
- *Body chemistry.* Each person has an individual pattern of physiological functioning that may affect the ability to process alcohol. For example, in some conditions, such as that marked by "dumping syndrome," the stomach empties more rapidly than is normal, and alcohol seems to be absorbed more quickly. The emptying time may be either slowed or quickened by anger, fear, stress, nausea, and the condition of the stomach tissues.

Key Terms

absorption the passage of nutrients or alcohol through the walls of the stomach or intestinal tract into the bloodstream.

• *Gender.* Women produce much less alcohol dehydrogenase than men do.[7] This enzyme is responsible for breaking down alcohol in the stomach. As a result, women absorb about 30% more alcohol into the bloodstream than men, despite an identical number of drinks and equal body weight.

Three other reasons help explain why women tend to absorb alcohol more quickly than men of the same body weight: (1) Women have proportionately more body fat than men. Since alcohol is not stored easily in fat, it enters the bloodstream relatively quickly. (2) Women's bodies have proportionately less water than men's bodies of equal weight. Thus alcohol consumed does not become as diluted as in men. (3) Alcohol absorption is influenced by a woman's menstrual cycle. Alcohol is more quickly absorbed during the premenstrual phase of a woman's cycle. Also, there is evidence that women using birth control pills absorb alcohol faster than usual.[7]

With the exception of a person's body chemistry and gender, all factors that influence absorption can be moderated by the alcohol user.

Blood Alcohol Concentration

A person's **blood alcohol concentration (BAC)** rises when alcohol is consumed faster than it can be removed (oxidized) by the liver.[8] As outlined in Figure 8-3, a fairly predictable sequence of events takes place when a person drinks alcohol at a rate faster than one drink every hour. When the BAC reaches 0.05%, initial measurable changes in mood and behavior take place. Inhibitions and everyday tensions appear to be released, while judgment and critical thinking are somewhat impaired. This BAC would be achieved by a 160-pound person consuming about two drinks in an hour.

At a level of 0.10% (one part alcohol to 1000 parts blood), the drinker typically loses significant motor coordination. Voluntary motor function becomes quite clumsy. At this BAC, most states consider a drinker legally intoxicated and thus incapable of safely operating a vehi-

cle. Although physiological changes associated with this BAC do occur, certain users do not feel intoxicated or do not outwardly appear to be impaired.

As the BAC rises from 0.20% to 0.50%, the health risk of acute alcohol intoxication increases rapidly. A BAC of 0.20% is characterized by the loud, boisterous, obnoxious drunk person who staggers. A 0.30% BAC produces further depression and stuporous behavior, and the drinker becomes so confused that he or she may not be capable of understanding anything. The 0.40% or 0.50% BAC produces unconsciousness. At this level, a person can die, since the brain centers that control body temperature, heartbeat, and breathing may be virtually shut down.

An important factor influencing the BAC is the individual's blood volume. The larger the person, the greater the amount of blood into which alcohol can be distributed. Conversely, the smaller person has less blood into which alcohol can be distributed, and as a result, a higher BAC will develop.

Sobering Up

Alcohol is removed from the bloodstream principally through the process of **oxidation.** Oxidation occurs at a constant rate (about ¼ to ⅓ ounce of pure alcohol per hour) that cannot be appreciably altered. Since each typical drink of beer, wine, or distilled spirits contains about ½ ounce of pure alcohol, it takes about 2 hours for the body to fully oxidize one typical alcoholic drink.[9]

Although people may try to sober up by drinking hot coffee, taking cold showers, or exercising, the oxidation rate of alcohol is unaffected by these measures. Thus far the FDA has not approved any commercial product that can help people achieve sobriety. Passage of time remains the only effective remedy for diminishing alcohol's effects.

First Aid for Acute Alcohol Intoxication

Not everyone who goes to sleep, passes out, or becomes unconscious after drinking has a high BAC. People who are

---

Key Terms
blood alcohol concentration (BAC) the percentage of alcohol in a measured quantity of blood; BACs can be determined directly through the analysis of a blood sample or indirectly through the analysis of exhaled air.
oxidation the process that removes alcohol from the bloodstream.

Figure 8-3

Number of drinks consumed in two hours	Alcohol in blood (percentage)	Typical effects
2	0.05	Judgment, thought, and restraint weakened; tension released, giving carefree sensation
3	0.08	Tensions of everyday life lessened; cheerfulness
4	0.10	Voluntary motor action affected, making hand and arm movements, walk, and speech clumsy
7	0.20	Severe impairment—staggering, loud, incoherent, emotionally unstable, 100 times greater traffic risk; exuberance and aggressive inclinations magnified
9	0.30	Deeper areas of brain affected, with stimulus-response and understanding confused; stuporous; blurred vision
12	0.40	Incapable of voluntary action; sleepy, difficult to arouse; equivalent of surgical anesthesia
15	0.50	Comatose; centers controlling breathing and heartbeat anesthetized; death increasingly probable

Note: A drink refers to a typical 12-ounce bottle of beer, a 1.5-ounce shot of hard liquor, or a 5-ounce glass of wine.

already sleepy, have not eaten well, are sick, or are bored may drink a little alcohol and quickly fall asleep. However, people who drink heavily in a rather short time may be setting themselves up for an extremely unpleasant, toxic, potentially life-threatening experience because of their high BAC.

Although responsible drinking would prevent **acute alcohol intoxication** (poisoning), it will never be a reality for everyone. As a caring adult, what should you know about this health emergency that may help you save a life—perhaps even a friend's life?

The first real danger signs to recognize are the typical signs of **shock.** By the time these signs are evident, a drinker will already be unconscious. He or she will not be able to be aroused from a deep stupor. The person will probably have a weak, rapid pulse (over 100 beats per minute). The skin will be cool and damp, and breathing will be increased to once every 3 or 4 seconds. These breaths may be shallow or deep but will certainly occur in

Key Terms

acute alcohol intoxication a potentially fatal elevation of the BAC, often resulting from heavy, rapid consumption of alcohol.

shock profound collapse of many vital body functions; evident during acute alcohol intoxication and other health emergencies.

Are You Ready for an Alcohol-Related Emergency?

How can I recognize and cope with an acute alcohol emergency?

When you find a person who has been drinking heavily, look for these signs:

- Cannot be aroused
- Has a weak, rapid pulse
- Has an unusual or irregular breathing pattern
- Has cool (possibly damp), pale, or bluish skin

Immediately call for emergency help (call 911). Follow their directions. Position the unconscious person on his or her side to avoid choking in case vomiting occurs.

an irregular pattern. Skin will be pale or bluish. (In the case of a person with dark skin, these color changes will be more evident in the fingernail beds or in the mucous membranes inside the mouth or under the eyelids.) Whenever any of these signs are present, seek emergency medical help immediately (see the Changing for the Better box above for a summary of these signs).

Involuntary regurgitation (vomiting) can be another potentially life-threatening emergency for a person who has drunk too much alcohol. When a drinker has consumed more alcohol than the liver can oxidize, the pyloric valve at the base of the stomach tends to close. Additional alcohol remains in the stomach. This alcohol irritates the lining of the stomach so much that involuntary muscle contractions force the stomach contents to flow back through the esophagus. By removing alcohol from the stomach, vomiting may be a life-saving mechanism for conscious drinkers.

An unconscious drinker who vomits may be lying in such a position that the airway becomes obstructed by the vomitus. This person is at great risk of dying from **asphyxiation.** As a first-aid measure, unconscious drinkers should always be rolled onto their sides to minimize the chance of airway obstruction. If you are with someone who is vomiting, make certain that his or her head is positioned lower than the rest of the body. This position minimizes the chance that vomitus will obstruct the air passages.

It is also important to keep a close watch on anyone who passes out from heavy drinking. Party-goers sometimes make the mistake of carrying these people to bed and then forgetting about them. Monitoring the physical condition of anyone who becomes unconscious from heavy drinking is crucial because of the risk of death. Observe the person at regular intervals until he or she appears to be clearly out of danger. This may mean an evening of interrupted sleep for you, but you

could save a friend's life. Are you aware of any recent alcohol-related deaths among U.S. college students?

Alcohol-Related Health Problems

The relationship of chronic alcohol use to the structure and function of the body is reasonably well understood. Heavy alcohol use causes a variety of changes to the body that lead to an increase in morbidity and mortality. Figure 8-4 on page 218 describes these changes.

Research shows that chronic alcohol use also damages the immune system and the nervous system. Thus chronic users are at high risk for a variety of infections and neurological complications.[1] Additionally, many alcoholics suffer from malnutrition, in part because they do not consume a variety of foods. With the deterioration of the liver, stomach, and pancreas, chronic heavy drinkers also have poor absorption and metabolism of many nutrients.

Fetal Alcohol Syndrome and Fetal Alcohol Effects

A growing body of scientific evidence indicates that alcohol use by pregnant women can result in birth defects in unborn children. When alcohol crosses the **placenta,** it enters the fetal bloodstream in a concentration equal to that in the mother's bloodstream. Because of the underdeveloped nature of the fetal liver, this alcohol is oxidized much more slowly than the alcohol in the mother. During this time of slow detoxification, the developing fetus is certain to be overexposed to the toxic effects of alcohol. Mental retardation frequently develops.

This exposure has additional disastrous consequences for the developing fetus. Low birth weight, facial abnormalities (e.g., small head, widely spaced eyes), and heart problems are often seen in such infants (Figure 8-5). This combination of effects is called **fetal alcohol syndrome.** Recent estimates indicate that the full expression of this syndrome occurs at a rate of between 1 and 3 per 1000

Key Terms

asphyxiation death resulting from lack of oxygen to the brain.

placenta the structure through which nutrients, metabolic wastes, and drugs (including alcohol) pass from the bloodstream of the mother into the bloodstream of the developing fetus.

fetal alcohol syndrome characteristic birth defects noted in the children of some women who consume alcohol during their pregnancies.

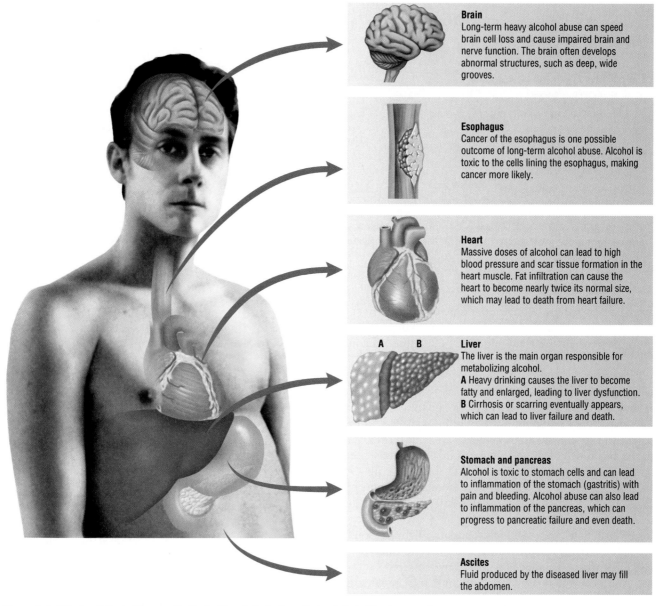

Figure 8-4 Effects of Alcohol Use on the Body. The mind-altering effects of alcohol begin soon after it enters the bloodstream. Within minutes, alcohol numbs nerve cells in the brain. The heart muscle strains to cope with alcohol's depressive action. If drinking continues, the rising BAC causes impaired speech, vision, balance, and judgment. With an extremely high BAC, respiratory failure is possible. Over time, alcohol abuse increases the risk for certain forms of heart disease and cancer and makes liver and pancreas failure more likely.

births. Partial expression (fetal alcohol effects [FAE]) can be seen in 3 to 9 per 1000 live births. In addition, it is likely that many cases of FAE go undetected.[10]

Is there a safe limit to the number of drinks a woman can consume during pregnancy? Since no one can accurately predict the effect of drinking even small amounts of alcohol during pregnancy, the wisest plan is to avoid alcohol altogether.

Because of the critical growth and development that occur during the first months of fetal life, women who have any reason to suspect they are pregnant should stop

all alcohol consumption. Furthermore, women who are planning to become pregnant and women who are not practicing effective contraception must also consider keeping their alcohol use to a minimum.

Alcohol-Related Social Problems

Alcohol abuse is related to a variety of social problems. These problems affect the quality of interpersonal relationships, employment stability, and the financial security

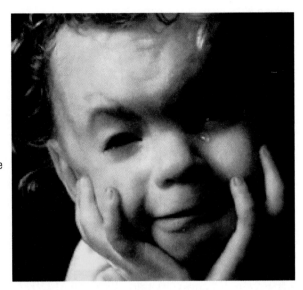

Figure 8-5 Fetal Alcohol Syndrome. The facial features shown are characteristic of affected children. Additional abnormalities in the brain and other internal organs accompany fetal alcohol syndrome but are not obvious in the child's appearance.

of both the individual and the family. Clearly, alcohol's negative social consequences lower our quality of life. In financial terms the annual cost of alcohol abuse and dependence has been estimated at more than $185 billion.[11]

Accidents

The four leading causes of accidental deaths in the United States (motor vehicle collsions, falls, drownings, and fires and burns) have significant statistical connections to alcohol use.

Motor Vehicle Collisions

Data from the National Highway Traffic Safety Administration (NHTSA) indicate that in 2001 over 17,000 alcohol-related vehicular crash deaths occurred. This figure represented 41% of the total traffic fatalities for 2001. Although 17,000 remains an unacceptably high figure, this total represented a 13% reduction from the nearly 20,000 alcohol-related fatalities reported in 1991.[12]

Presently in the United States, an alcohol-related car crash fatality occurs every 30 minutes. Every 2 minutes, an alcohol-related car crash injury happens. An estimated 275,000 people were injured in such crashes in 2001. In 2000, the NHTSA reported that approximately 1.5 million drivers were arrested for drunk driving, reflecting an arrest rate of 1 for every 130 licensed drivers in the United States.[12]

One response to drunk driving has been for all states to raise the minimum legal drinking age to 21 years. This

On August 4, 2000, 23-year-old Casey Ray Beaver was driving with two friends along U.S. Highway 71 near Goodman, Missouri, when an oncoming vehicle crossed the center line and collided with his car. Casey, a recent graduate of the University of Kansas, was pronounced dead at the scene, as was the driver of the other vehicle. The offender, who had seven prior convictions of driving under the influence and whose driver's license had been revoked seven years earlier, had a BAC above .10%. Casey was due to begin classes at the Illinois College of Optometry 10 days after the accident occurred.

Figure 8-6 For most states, a BAC of .08% constitutes legal intoxication. However, lower BACs can impair functioning enough to cause a serious accident.

Number of drinks in a 2-hour period
(1½-oz 86-proof liquor or 12-oz beer)

Body weight (lbs.)									
100	1	2	3	4	5	6	7	8	9
120	1	2	3	4	5	6	7	8	9
140	1	2	3	4	5	6	7	8	9
160	1	2	3	4	5	6	7	8	9
180	1	2	3	4	5	6	7	8	9
200	1	2	3	4	5	6	7	8	9

Could impair driving (BAC to .05%)

Driving significantly impaired (BAC .05% to .09%)

Driving seriously impaired (BAC .10% and up)

was accomplished in the mid-1980s. Another response was a federal law that President Clinton signed in October 2000. This law required all states to lower their drunk driving standard to .08% BAC by October 1, 2003 or the states would risk losing federal highway funds. Do you know if your state has enacted a .08% law? You can search the MADD website at **www.madd.org** to find out current .08% BAC law information (see Figure 8-6).[13]

Other programs and policies are being implemented that are designed to prevent intoxicated people from driving. Many states have enacted **zero tolerance laws** to help prevent underage drinking and driving. Also included have been efforts to educate bartenders to recognize intoxicated customers, to use off-duty police officers as observers in bars, to place police roadblocks, to develop mechanical devices that prevent intoxicated drivers from starting their cars, and to encourage people to use designated drivers.

The use of designated drivers has received some of the credit for the significant reduction in drunk driving deaths mentioned earlier. However, there may be a down side to this solution. Some health professionals are concerned that the use of designated drivers allows the nondrivers to drink more heavily than they might otherwise. In effect, designated drivers "enable" drinkers to be less responsible for their own behavior. The concern is that this freedom from responsibility might eventually lead to further problems for the drinkers. What do you think?

Falls

Many people are surprised to learn that falls are the second leading cause of accidental death in the United States. Alcohol use increases the risk for falls. Various studies suggest that alcohol is involved in between 21% and 77% of deadly falls and between 18% and 53% of nonfatal falls.[14]

Drownings

Drownings are the third leading cause of accidental death in the United States. Studies have shown that alcohol use is implicated in 21% to 47% of these deaths.[14] High percentages of recreational boaters have been found to drink alcohol while boating.[15]

Fires and Burns

Fires and burns are responsible for an estimated 5000 deaths each year in the United States, the fourth leading cause of accidental death. This cause is also connected to alcohol use: studies indicate that half of burn victims have BACs above the legal limit.[14]

Crime and Violence

Have you noticed that most of the violent behavior and vandalism on your campus is related to alcohol use? The connection of alcohol to crime has a long history. Prison populations have large percentages of alcohol abusers and alcoholics: People who commit crimes are more likely to have alcohol problems than are people in the general population. This is especially true for young criminals. Furthermore, alcohol use has been reported in 53% to 66% of all homicides, with the victim, the perpetrator, or both found to have been drinking. In rape situations, rapists are intoxicated 50% of the time and victims 30% of the time.[6]

Because of research methodological problems, pinpointing alcohol's connection to family violence is

Key Terms

zero tolerance laws laws that severely restrict the right to operate motor vehicles for underage drinkers who have been convicted of driving under any influence.

Partying 101: How to Party Responsibly

My friends and I are planning a big holiday party. We want to have fun, but we also want to be responsible about alcohol. What guidelines should we follow?

- Provide other social activities as a primary focus when alcohol is served.
- Respect an individual's decision about alcohol if that decision is either to abstain or to drink responsibly.
- Recognize the decision not to drink and the respect it warrants by providing equally attractive and accessible nonalcohol drinks when alcohol is served.
- Recognize that drunkenness is neither healthy nor safe. One should not excuse otherwise unacceptable behavior solely because of "too much to drink."
- Provide food when alcohol is served.
- Serve diluted drinks, and do not urge that glasses be constantly full.

- Keep the cocktail hour before dinner to a reasonable time and consumption limit.
- Recognize your responsibility for the health, safety, and pleasure of both the drinker and the nondrinker by avoiding intoxication and helping others do the same.
- Make contingency plans for intoxication. If it occurs in spite of efforts to prevent it, assume responsibility for the health and safety of guests—for example, by providing transportation home or overnight accommodations.
- Serve or use alcohol only in environments conducive to pleasant and relaxing behavior.
- Discard unattended drinks immediately. This reduces the possibility of someone consuming a drink containing Rohypnol, GHB, ketamine, (see Chapter 7) or other powerful intoxicants.

difficult.[16] However, it seems clear that among a large number of families, alcohol is associated with violence and other harmful behavior, including physical abuse, child abuse, psychological abuse, and abandonment.[6] The Focus On article on page 230 explores the link between alcohol and violence.

Suicide

Alcohol use has been related to large percentages of suicides. Alcoholism plays a large role in 30% of completed suicides.[17] Also, alcohol use is associated with impulsive suicides rather than with premeditated ones. Drinking is also connected with more violent and lethal means of suicide, such as the use of firearms.[6]

For many of these social problems, alcohol use impairs critical judgment and allows a person's behavior to quickly become reckless, antisocial, and deadly. Because most of us wish to minimize problems associated with alcohol use, acting responsibly when we host a party is a first step in this direction.

Hosting a Responsible Party

Some people might say that no party is totally safe when alcohol is served. These people are probably right, considering the possibility of unexpected **drug synergism**, overconsumption, and the consequences of released inhibitions. Fortunately, an awareness of the value of responsible party hosting seems to be growing among college communities. The impetus for this awareness has come from various sources, including respect for an individual's right to choose not to drink alcohol, the growing recognition that many automobile accidents are alcohol-related, and the legal threats posed by **host negligence.**

Responsibly hosting parties at which alcohol is served is becoming a trend, especially among college-educated young adults. The Education Commission of the States' Task Force on Responsible Decisions about Alcohol has generated a list of guidelines for hosting a social event at which alcoholic beverages are served. The list includes the recommendations shown in the Changing for the Better box above.

In addition, using a **designated driver** is an important component of responsible alcohol use. By planning

---

Key Terms

drug synergism (sin er jism) enhancement of a drug's effect as a result of the presence of additional drugs within the system.

host negligence a legal term that reflects the failure of a host to provide reasonable care and safety for people visiting the host's residence or business.

designated driver a person who abstains from or carefully limits alcohol consumption to be able to safely transport other people who have been drinking.

to abstain from alcohol or to carefully limit their own alcohol consumption, designated drivers are able to safely transport friends who have been drinking.

TALKING POINTS Have you noticed an increased use of designated drivers in your community? Would you be willing to be a designated driver?

Organizations That Support Responsible Drinking

The serious consequences of the irresponsible use of alcohol have led to the formation of a number of concerned-citizen groups. Although each organization has a unique approach, all attempt to deal objectively with two indisputable facts: Alcohol use is part of our society, and irresponsible alcohol use can be deadly.

Mothers Against Drunk Driving

Mothers Against Drunk Driving (MADD) is a national network of over 600 local chapters in the United States and Canada. This organization attempts to educate people about alcohol's effects on driving and to influence legislation and enforcement of laws related to drunk drivers. For more information about MADD, visit its website at **www.madd.org**.[13]

Students Against Destructive Decisions

Many students have known the acronym *SADD* to stand for the youth group Students Against Driving Drunk or Students Against Destructive Decisions. Recently, the group has restructured itself to expand beyond drunk driving to include other high-risk activities that are detrimental to youth, such as underage drinking, drug use, drugged driving, and failure to use seat belts. Founded in 1981, this organization now has millions of members in thousands of chapters throughout the country. Remain-

ing central to the drunk driving aspect of SADD is the "Contract for Life," a pact that encourages students and parents to provide safe transportation for each other if either is unable to drive safely after consuming alcohol. This contract also stipulates that no discussions about the incident are to be started until both can talk in a calm and caring manner. For more information about SADD, visit its website at **www.saddonline.com**.[18]

TALKING POINTS How would you approach asking your parents or friends to join you in signing a "Contract for Life"?

BACCHUS and GAMMA Peer Education Network

BACCHUS (Boost Alcohol Consciousness Concerning the Health of University Students) began in 1975 as an alcohol-awareness organization at the University of Florida. Run by student volunteers, this organization promoted responsible drinking among college students who chose to drink. It was not an anti-alcohol group, but a "harm reduction" group. Over the years, hundreds of chapters were formed on campuses across the country.

When supporters of BACCHUS realized that many students interested in alcohol awareness were from fraternities and sororities, they developed GAMMA (Greeks Advocating Mature Management of Alcohol) to join BACCHUS to form a peer education network. Campuses are now able to choose BACCHUS, GAMMA, or any other acronym or name for their groups.

With the broadening of the original BACCHUS organization has come an expansion of the health issues this group addresses. Originally, the focus was on alcohol abuse and prevention. Now the BACCHUS and GAMMA Peer Education Network confronts a variety of student health and safety issues. For additional information about this organization, check out its website at **www.bacchusgamma.org**.[19]

Other Approaches

Other responsible approaches to alcohol use are surfacing nearly every day. Even among college fraternity organizations, attitudes toward the indiscriminate use of alcohol are changing. Many fraternity rush functions are now conducted without the use of alcohol, and growing numbers of fraternities are alcohol-free.

Another encouraging sign on college campuses is the increasing number of alcohol use task forces. Although each of these groups has its own focus and title, many are meeting to discuss alcohol-related concerns on their particular campus. These task forces often try to formulate detailed, comprehensive policies for alcohol use across the entire campus community. Membership on these committees often includes students (on-campus and off-campus, graduate and undergraduate), faculty and staff members, academic administrators, residence hall advisors, university police, health center personnel, alumni, and local citizens. Does your college have such a committee?

Problem Drinking and Alcoholism

Problem Drinking

At times the line separating **problem drinking** from alcoholism is difficult to distinguish (see the accompanying Star Box). There may be no true line, with the exception that an alcoholic is unable to stop drinking. Problem drinking is a pattern of alcohol use in which a drinker's behavior creates personal difficulties or difficulties for other people. What are some of these behaviors? Examples might be drinking to avoid life stressors, going to work intoxicated, drinking and driving, becoming injured or injuring others while drinking, solitary drinking, morning drinking, an occasional **blackout,** high-risk sexual activity, and being told by others that you drink too much. For college students, two clear indications of problem drinking are missing classes and lowered academic performance caused by alcohol involvement. The Changing for the Better box on page 224 offers suggestions that can help you keep drinking under control.

Problem drinkers are not always heavy drinkers; they might not be daily or even weekly drinkers. Unlike alcoholics, problem drinkers do not need to drink to maintain "normal" body functions. However, when they do drink, they (and others around them) experience problems— sometimes with tragic consequences. It's not surprising that problem drinkers are more likely than other drinkers to eventually develop alcoholism.

 TALKING POINTS Are there people around you who show signs of problem drinking?

Alcoholism

In the early 1990s a revised definition of **alcoholism** was established by a joint committee of experts on alcohol dependence.[20] This committee defined alcoholism as follows:

> Alcoholism is a primary, chronic disease with genetic, psychosocial, and environmental factors influencing its development and manifestations. The disease is often progressive and fatal. It is characterized by impaired control over drinking, preoccupation with the drug alcohol, use of alcohol despite adverse consequences, and distortions in thinking, most notably denial. Each of these symptoms may be continuous or periodic.

Progressive Stages of Alcohol Dependence

Early
- Escape drinking
- Binge drinking
- Guilt feelings
- Sneaking drinks
- Difficulty stopping once drinking has begun
- Increased tolerance
- Preoccupation with drinking
- Occasional blackouts

Middle
- Loss of control
- Self-hate
- Impaired social relationships
- Changes in drinking patterns (more frequent binge drinking)
- Temporary sobriety
- Morning drinking
- Dietary neglect
- Increased blackouts

Late
- Prolonged binges
- Alcohol used to control withdrawal symptoms
- Alcohol psychosis
- Nutritional disease
- Frequent blackouts

This definition incorporates much of the knowledge gained from addiction research during the last two decades. It is well recognized that alcoholics do not drink for the pleasurable effects of alcohol but to escape being sober. For alcoholics, being sober is stressful.

Key Terms

problem drinking an alcohol use pattern in which a drinker's behavior creates personal difficulties or difficulties for other people.

blackout a temporary state of amnesia experienced by a drinker; an inability to remember events that occurred during a period of alcohol use.

alcoholism a primary, chronic disease with genetic, psychosocial, and environmental factors influencing its development and manifestations.

Unlike problem drinking, alcoholism involves a physical addiction to alcohol. For the true alcoholic, when the body is deprived of alcohol, physical and mental withdrawal symptoms become evident. These withdrawal symptoms can be life threatening.

Uncontrollable shaking can progress to nausea, vomiting, hallucinations, shock, and cardiac and pulmonary arrest. Uncontrollable shaking combined with irrational hallucinations is called *delirium tremens* (DT), an occasional manifestation of alcohol withdrawal.[21]

The complex reasons for the physical and emotional dependence of alcoholism have not been fully explained. Why, when more than 100 million adults use alcohol without becoming dependent on it, are 10 million or more others unable to control its use?

Could alcoholism be an inherited disease? Studies in humans and animals have provided strong evidence that genetics plays a role in some cases of alcoholism. Two forms of alcoholism are thought to be inherited: type 1 and type 2. Type 1 is thought to take years to develop and may not surface until midlife. Type 2 is a more severe form and appears to be passed primarily from fathers to sons. This form of alcoholism frequently begins earlier in a person's life and may even start in adolescence.

Genetics may also help protect some Asians from developing alcoholism. About half of all Far East Asians produce low levels of an important enzyme that helps metabolize alcohol. These people cannot tolerate even small amounts of alcohol. Genetic factors pertaining to the absorption rates of alcohol in the intestinal tract have been hypothesized to predispose some Native Americans to alcoholism. It is likely that more research will be undertaken concerning the role of genetic factors in all forms of chemical dependence.

The role of personality traits as conditioning factors in the development of alcoholism has received considerable attention. Factors ranging from unusually low self-esteem to an antisocial personality have been implicated. Additional factors making people susceptible to alcoholism may include excessive reliance on denial, hypervigilance, compulsiveness, and chronic levels of anxiety. Always complicating the study of personality traits is the uncertainty of whether the personality profile is a predisposing factor (perhaps from inheritance) or is caused by alcoholism.

Codependence

Within the last decade, a new term has been used to describe the relationship between drug-dependent people and those around them— **codependence** This term implies a kind of dual addiction. The alcoholic and the person close to the alcoholic are both addicted, one to alcohol and the other to the alcoholic. People who are codependent often find themselves denying the addiction and enabling the alcohol-dependent person.

Unfortunately, this kind of behavior damages both the alcoholic and the codependent. The alcoholic's intervention and treatment may be delayed for a considerable time. Codependent people often pay a heavy price as well. They often become drug- or alcohol-dependent themselves, or they may suffer a variety of psychological consequences related to guilt, loss of self-esteem, depression, and anxiety. Codependents may be at increased risk for physical and sexual abuse.

Researchers continue to explore this dimension of alcoholism. Many students have found some of the resources identified in this chapter to be especially helpful.

Denial and Enabling

Problem drinkers and alcoholics frequently use the psychological defense mechanism of *denial* to maintain their

Key Terms

codependence an unhealthy relationship in which one person is addicted to alcohol or another drug and a person close to him or her is "addicted" to the alcoholic or drug user.

drinking behavior. By convincing themselves that their lives are not affected by their drinking, problem drinkers and alcoholics are able to maintain their drinking patterns. A person's denial is an unconscious process that is apparent only to rational observers.

Formerly, it was up to alcoholics to admit that their denial was no longer effective before they could be admitted to a treatment program. This is not the case today. Currently, family members, friends, or coworkers of alcohol-dependent people are encouraged to intervene and force an alcohol-dependent person into treatment.

TALKING POINTS One of your professors is a known alcoholic. You wonder why no one has persuaded her to seek treatment. Would you intervene in any way to make that happen? If so, how?

During treatment, it is important for chemically dependent people to break through the security of denial and admit that alcohol controls their lives. This process is demanding and often time-consuming, but it is necessary for recovery.

For family and friends of chemically dependent people, denial is part of a process known as **enabling.** In this process, people close to the problem drinker or alcoholic inadvertently support drinking behavior by denying that a problem really exists. Enablers unconsciously make excuses for the drinker, try to keep the drinker's work and family life intact, and in effect make the continued abuse of alcohol possible. For example, college students enable problem drinkers when they clean up a drinker's messy room, lie to professors about a student's class absences, and provide class notes or other assistance to a drinker who can't keep up academically.

Alcohol counselors contend that enablers are an alcoholic's worst enemy because they can significantly delay the onset of effective therapy. Do you know of a situation in which you or others have enabled a person with an alcohol problem?

Alcoholism and the Family

Considerable disruption occurs in the families of alcoholics, not only from the consequences of the drinking behavior (such as violence, illness, and unemployment), but also because of the uncertainty of the family's role in causing and prolonging the situation. Family members often begin to adopt a variety of new roles that will allow them to cope with the presence of the alcoholic in the family. Among the more commonly seen roles are the family hero, the lost child, the family mascot, and the scapegoat.[6] Unless family members receive appropriate counseling, these roles may remain intact for a lifetime.

Once an alcoholic's therapy has begun, family members are encouraged to participate in many aspects of the recovery. This participation will also help them understand how they are affected by alcoholism. If therapy and aftercare include participation in Alcoholics Anonymous (AA), family members will be encouraged to become affiliated with related support groups.

Helping the Alcoholic: Rehabilitation and Recovery

Once an alcoholic realizes that alcoholism is not a form of moral weakness but rather a clearly defined illness, the chances for recovery are remarkably good. It is estimated that as many as two-thirds of alcoholics can recover. Recovery is especially enhanced when the addicted person has a good emotional support system, including concerned family members, friends, and employer.

> **Key Terms**
>
> **enabling** inadvertently supporting a drinker's behavior by denying that a problem exists.

When this support system is not well established, the alcoholic's chances for recovery are considerably lower.

AA is a voluntary support group of recovering alcoholics who meet regularly to help each other get and stay sober. Over 100,000 groups exist in 150 countries worldwide.[22] AA encourages alcoholics to admit their lack of power over alcohol and to turn their lives over to a higher power (although the organization is nonsectarian). Members of AA are encouraged not to be judgmental about the behavior of other members. They support anyone with a problem caused by alcohol.

Al-Anon and Alateen are parallel organizations that give support to people who live with alcoholics. Al-Anon is geared toward spouses and other relatives, and Alateen focuses on children of alcoholics. There are 28,000 Al-Anon groups and 3000 Alateen groups worldwide. Both organizations help members realize that they are not alone and that successful adjustments can be made to nearly every alcoholic-related situation. AA, Al-Anon, and Alateen chapter organizations are usually listed in the telephone book or in the classified sections of local newspapers. You can locate Al-Anon and Alateen on the Web at **www.al-anon.alateen.org**.[23]

For people who feel uncomfortable with the concept that their lives are controlled by a higher power, *secular recovery programs* are becoming popular. These programs maintain that sobriety comes from within the alcoholic. Secular programs strongly emphasize self-reliance, self-determination, and rational thinking about one's drinking. Secular Organizations for Sobriety (SOS) and Rational Recovery are examples of secular recovery programs.

Drugs to Treat Alcoholism

Could there be a medical cure for alcoholism? For nearly 50 years, the only prescription drug physicians could use to help drinkers stop drinking was disulfiram (Antabuse). Antabuse would cause drinkers to become extremely nauseated whenever they used alcohol.

In 1995 the Food and Drug Administration approved the drug naltrexone (ReVia) that works by reducing the craving for alcohol and the pleasurable sensations felt when drinking. Combining naltrexone with conventional behavior modification has shown promising results. Additionally, the use of antidepressants by some alcoholics has been especially helpful during treatment.[1]

Current Alcohol Concerns

Adult Children of Alcoholic Parents

In recent years a new dimension of alcoholism has been identified—the unusually high prevalence of alcoholism

Common Traits of Adult Children of Alcoholics

Adult children of alcoholics may:

- Have difficulty identifying normal behavior
- Have difficulty following a project from beginning to end
- Lie when it would be just as easy to tell the truth
- Judge themselves without mercy
- Have difficulty having fun
- Take themselves very seriously
- Have difficulty with intimate relationships
- Overreact to changes over which they have no control
- Constantly seek approval and affirmation
- Feel that they are different from other people
- Be super-responsible or super-irresponsible
- Be extremely loyal, even in the face of evidence that the loyalty is undeserved
- Tend to lock themselves into a course of action without considering the consequences*

Experts agree that adult children of alcoholics who believe they have come to terms with their feelings can sometimes face lingering problems. Support groups to contact include Al-Anon (**www.al-anon.alateen.org**), Adult Children of Alcohollics (**www.adultchildren.org**), and Children of Alcoholics Foundation (**www.coaf.org**).

*Woititz JG. *Adult children of alcoholics.* Health Communications, Inc., 1990.

among adult children of alcoholics (ACOAs). It is estimated that these children are about four times more likely to develop alcoholism than children whose parents are not alcoholics. Even the ACOAs who do not become alcoholics may have a difficult time adjusting to everyday living. Janet Geringer Woititz, author of the best-selling book *Adult Children of Alcoholics*,[24] describes thirteen traits that most ACOAs exhibit to some degree (see the Star box above).

In response to this concern, support groups have been formed to help prevent the adult sons and daughters of alcoholics from developing the condition that afflicted their parents (see the Star box above). If a stronger link for an inherited genetic predisposition to alcoholism is found, these groups may play an even greater role in the prevention of alcoholism.

Women and Alcohol

For decades, women have consumed less alcohol and had fewer alcohol-related problems than men. At present, evidence is mounting that a greater percentage of women are choosing to drink and that some subgroups of women,

Learning from Our Diversity

Staying Sober: New Pathways for Women

Since 1935, when it was founded by two white American male alcoholics, Alcoholics Anonymous has expanded to encompass millions of members in virtually every region of the world who strive to achieve and maintain sobriety by adhering to AA's well-known 12-step program of recovery. With its strong spiritual orientation emphasizing the acknowledgment of a "higher power," AA offers safety, comfort, and structure to people of all ages and backgrounds, and both sexes. For decades, women as well as men have made AA the cornerstone of their efforts to get sober and stay sober.

Not all women, however, are comfortable with AA's focus on Christian spirituality and the perceived masculine orientation of its chief text, Alcoholics Anonymous (familiarly known as the "Big Book"), and other program literature. These women place an equally high value on sober living as do AA adherents, but they prefer to pursue that goal in other settings. In recent years, alternatives to AA have emerged that offer peer group acceptance and support for recovering alcoholic women, but do so in a nonspiritual, nonsexist context.

One such group, Women for Sobriety, is a mutual aid organization for women with alcohol problems that was founded in 1975 by Dr. Jean Kirkpatrick. The WFS program focuses on improving self-esteem; members achieve sobriety by taking responsibility for their actions and by learning not to dwell on negative thoughts. Another alternative, Rational Recovery, is open to both men and women. RR, which is based on the

theories of psychologist Albert Ellis's Rational Emotive Therapy, also uses a cognitive, nonspiritual approach that fosters cohesiveness and provides the emotional support sought by people who seek to gain and maintain sobriety.

Particularly for "marginalized" alcoholic women such as lesbians, racial and ethnic minorities, and those of non-Christian religious backgrounds, alcoholism treatment professionals increasingly are being encouraged to present the full range of support-group options, including but not emphasizing the approach of Alcoholics Anonymous.

If you were seeking help to achieve and maintain sobriety, would you be more inclined to attend a program based on spirituality, or one that offers a rational, cognitive approach? Why?

Galanter M and others: Rational Recovery: alternative to AA for addiction? *American Journal of Drug and Alcohol Abuse*, 1993, vol. 19, p. 499.

Hall J: Lesbians' participation in Alcoholics Anonymous: experience of social, personal, and political tensions. *Contemporary Drug Problems*, Spring 1996, vol. 23, no. 1, p. 113.

Kaskutas L: A road less traveled: choosing the "Women for Sobriety" program. *Journal of Drug Issues*, Winter 1996, vol. 26, no. 1, p. 77.

Women for Sobriety, Inc. **www.womenforsobriety.org/** accessed 19 June 2003.

especially young women, are drinking more heavily. An increased number of admissions of women to treatment centers may also reflect that alcohol consumption among women is on the rise.[6] Special approaches for women to use for staying sober are discussed in the Learning from Our Diversity box above.

Studies indicate that currently there are almost as many female as male alcoholics. However, there appear to be differences between men and women when it comes to alcohol abuse: (1) More women than men can point to a specific triggering event (such as a divorce, death of a spouse, a career change, or children leaving home) that started them drinking heavily. (2) Alcoholism among women often starts later and progresses more quickly than alcoholism among men. (3) Women tend to be prescribed more mood-altering drugs than men. So women face greater risk of drug interaction or cross-tolerance. (4) Nonalcoholic men tend to divorce their alcoholic spouses nine times more often than nonalcoholic women divorce their alcoholic spouses. Thus alcoholic women are not as likely to have a family support system to aid them in their recovery attempts. (5) Female alcoholics do not tend to receive as much social support as men in their

treatment and recovery. (6) Unmarried, divorced, or single-parent women tend to have significant economic problems that may make entry into a treatment program especially difficult. (7) Women seem to be more susceptible than men to medical complications resulting from heavy drinking.[7] In light of the generally recognized educational, occupational, and social gains made by women during the last two decades, it will be interesting to see whether these male-female differences continue. What's your best guess?

Alcohol Advertising

Every few years, careful observers can see subtle changes in the ways the alcoholic beverage industry markets its products. Recently, the marketing push appears to be directed toward minorities (through advertisements for malt liquor and fortified wines), women (through wine and wine cooler ads), and youth (through trendy, young adult-oriented commercials), and spiffy websites.

On the college campus, aggressive alcohol campaigns have used rock stars, beach party scenes, athletic event sponsorships, and colorful newspaper supplements as vehicles to encourage the purchase of alcohol. Critics claim that most of the collegiate advertising is directed at the "below age 21" crowd and that the prevention messages are not strong enough to offset the potential health damage to this population. How do you feel about alcohol advertising on your campus? If you're a nontraditional-age student, do you find the advertising campaigns amusing or potentially dangerous?

Taking Charge of Your Health

- Determine whether you are affected by someone's drinking by doing the Personal Assessment on page 233.
- Prepare for a possible alcohol-related emergency by reviewing the signs listed in the Changing for the Better box on page 217.
- Assess your level of social responsibility by using the Changing for the Better box on page 221.
- If you think that you are a problem drinker or an alcoholic, join a support group to get help.

- Enter into a "Contract for Life" with your parents or closest friends, a pact that says that you will provide safe transportation for each other if either of you is unable to drive safely after consuming alcohol.
- Make a commitment to responsible alcohol use by joining a campus group that works toward this goal.

Summary

- Alcohol is the drug of choice among college students and the rest of American society.
- Many factors affect the rate of absorption of alcohol into the bloodstream.
- As BAC rises, predictable depressant effects take place.
- People with acute alcohol intoxication must receive first-aid care immediately.
- The health effects of chronic alcohol abuse are quite serious.
- Problem drinking reflects an alcohol use pattern in which a drinker's behavior creates personal difficulties or problems for others.

- Alcoholism is a primary, chronic disease with a variety of possible causes and characteristics.
- Denial, enabling, codependence, ACOAs, and alcohol advertising are current issues related to alcohol abuse in the United States.
- Recovery and rehabilitation programs can be effective in helping alcoholics become sober.
- Antabuse, naltrexone, and antidepressants are drugs prescribed by physicians to help alcoholics in treatment.
- Federal legislation has pushed states to lower the legal BAC standard to .08%.

Review Questions

1. What percentage of American adults consume alcohol? Approximately what percentage of adults are classified as abstainers? What percentage of college students drink?
2. What is binge drinking?
3. What is meant by the term *proof*?
4. What is the nutritional value of alcohol? How do "lite" and low-alcohol beverages compare?
5. Identify and explain the various factors that influence the absorption of alcohol. Why is it important to be aware of these factors?
6. What is BAC? Describe the general sequence of physiological events that takes place when a person drinks alcohol at a rate faster than the liver can oxidize it.

7. What are the signs and symptoms of acute alcohol intoxication? What are the first-aid steps you should take to help a person with this problem?
8. Describe the characteristics of fetal alcohol syndrome and fetal alcohol effects.
9. Explain the differences between problem drinking and alcoholism.
10. What is codependence? What roles do denial and enabling play in alcoholism?
11. What are some common traits of ACOAs?
12. What unique alcohol-related problems exist for women?
13. Describe the activities undertaken by SADD, MADD, BACCHUS, and GAMMA and by AA, Al-Anon, and Alateen.

References

1. U.S. Department of Health and Human Services: *Alcohol and health: tenth special report to the U.S. Congress,* NIH Pub No 00-1583, 2000, U.S. Government Printing Office.
2. U.S. Bureau of the Census: *Statistical abstract of the United States, 1999,* 199th ed. Washington, D.C.: U.S. Government Printing Office, 1999.
3. Dufour M. What is Moderate Drinking? Defining "Drinks" and Drinking Levels. *Alcohol Research and Health,* 23(1), 5–14. 1999.
4. Brown SA, Tapert SF, Granholm E, et al. Neurocognitive functioning of adolescents: effects of protracted alcohol use. *Alcoholism, Clinical and Experimental Research,* 24(2), 164–171. 2000.
5. Zest for Life. Alcohol and ethanol information page (online). Available: **www.anyvitamins.com/alcohol-ethanol-info.htm** accessed 16 June 2003.
6. Kinney J. *Loosening the grip: a handbook of alcohol information,* 7th ed. McGraw-Hill, 2003.
7. Be Responsible About Drinking. Women and Alcohol (online). Available: **www.brad21.org/alcohol_and_women.html** accessed 16 June 2003.
8. Pinger RR, et al. *Drugs: issues for today,* 3rd ed. McGraw-Hill, 1998.
9. Ray O, Ksir C. *Drugs, society and human behavior,* 8th ed. McGraw-Hill, 1999.
10. ADA: Division of Drug and Alcohol Abuse. As a Matter of Fact . . . Fetal Alcohol Syndrome. **www.well.com/user/woa/fsfas.htm** accessed 16 June 2003.
11. National Institute on Alcohol Abuse and Alcoholism. *10th Special Report to the U.S. Congress on Alcohol and Health,* Chapter 6. NIH Publication No. 00-1583. Rockville, MD: U.S. Department of Health and Human Services. 2000.
12. Traffic Safety Facts 2001: Alcohol. U.S. Department of Transportation National Highway Traffic Safety Administration.
13. About Us. Mothers Against Drunk Driving. **www.madd.org** accessed 18 June 2003.
14. Alcohol and Unintentional Injury: A Brief Review of the Literature. The Trauma Foundation. **www.tf.org/tf/alcohol/ariv/reviews/injurev5.html** accessed 16 June 2003.
15. Training Guide for USLA Safety Tips: General Information on Drowning. USLA Lifeguards for Life. **www.usla.org/PublicInfo/Safety_guide.shtml** accessed 16 June 2003.
16. Vaughn C. Children of Alcoholics: At risk for family violence. U.S. Department of Health and Human Services and SAMHSA's National Clearinghouse for Alcohol and Drug Information. 10 February 2003.
17. Facts about Suicide. CDC Prevention, National Center for Health Statistics, 1998.
18. SADD History. Students Against Drunk Driving. **www.saddonline.com** accessed 18 June 2003.
19. Organization History and Mission. The Bacchus & Gamma Peer Education Network. **www.bacchusgamma.org/** accessed 18 June 2003.
20. Morse RM, et al. The definition of alcoholism. *JAMA* 1992; 268(8): 1012–1014.
21. Gossman W. Delirium Tremens *emedicine.com,* Inc. 24 April 2001.
22. AA At a Glance. Alcoholics Anonymous. **www.alcoholics-anonymous.org** accessed 18 June 2003.
23. Website information. Al-Anon/Alateen. **www.al-anon.alateen.org/** accessed 19 June 2003.
24. Woititz JG. *Adult children of alcoholics.* Health Communications, Inc., 1990.

As We Go to Press

During the 2003–2004 academic year, Ball State University suffered the tragic deaths of two students in alcohol-related incidents. In November 2003, a student was fatally shot by a university police officer after a night of excessive drinking. The student allegedly lunged at the officer while he was investigating a reported break-in at a home near the campus. In March 2004, another student was robbed of two dollars and fatally shot after driving some local youths home from an off-campus party.

As we go to press, Ball State University has just launched an anti-alcohol campaign called "Police Yourself." This campaign will highlight the consequences of violating laws related to alcohol use and possible university consequences such as probation, suspension, or expulsion.

Alcohol misuse and abuse continues to be a major issue on most college campuses across the country. Many colleges and universities are using a variety of approaches to curb alcohol abuse on campus. What is your college doing make your students more responsible in this area?

alcohol and violence: a dangerous link

In recent years, there has been an increase in public service messages to raise awareness about driving under the influence of alcohol. In fact, the massive campaign against drinking and driving has been quite successful in reducing the number of drunk-driving accidents and fatalities. However, people may think that as long as a person doesn't get behind the wheel, it's okay to drink. But there are other potential dangers to the abuse of alcohol. One particular problem that perhaps has not been stressed enough in the media is the link between alcohol use and violence.

Obviously, not everyone who drinks becomes violent, but in many violent crimes at least one person involved has been drinking. It has been estimated that alcohol involvement is a factor in 63% of violent crimes.[1]

Alcohol and Types of Violent Crimes

The risk of a person becoming violent is higher among heavy drinkers than light drinkers. Heavy drinkers are also at higher risk of being victims of violent crime and are also more likely to inflict and to receive violent injuries. An environment where alcohol is prevalent is also a risk factor associated with gun injuries, particularly deaths among youths.[1] Alcohol plays a significant role in various types of violent crime. Substantial numbers of sexual-assault victims and offenders were drinking before their crime occurred. Spousal abuse by intoxicated men against women is the leading cause of nonfatal injury to women in the United States.[2]

Marital violence by husbands is common among men who abuse alcohol. Some researchers argue that spousal violence is the result of alcohol interfering with male power needs. Various consequences result from spousal violence that include miscarriage, depression, posttraumatic stress, substance abuse, and spousal homicide.[2] Spousal violence incurs societal costs including mental and physical health care, criminal justice interventions, child welfare, social services, and lost productivity at work.[3] A recent study suggests that in order to reduce marital violence, substance abuse needs to be a focal point during treatment for domestic violence.[2]

Campus Crime and the Effects of Alcohol

Of particular interest to college students are the data linking campus crimes to alcohol use. The CORE Institute conducted a 2001 survey of 54,444 undergraduate students which suggests that when under the influence of alcohol or other drugs the students experienced the following violent consequences:

- Argument or fight · 31.8%
- Been hurt or injured · 16.5%
- Threats of physical violence · 58.8%
- Ethnic harassment · 17.9%
- Actual physical violence · 68.3%
- Forced sexual touching · 76.0%
- Unwanted sexual intercourse · 82.6%
- Theft involving force or threat of force · 54.4%

Other violent consequences the students experienced include damaged property, driving under the influence, DWI/DUI arrests, and taking advantage of another person sexually. This survey reported that 85.3% of the students used alcohol within the last year and 74.4% used alcohol within the 30 days prior to taking the survey. This survey suggests that alcohol and other drugs play a large role in violent acts among college age students.[4] College students tend to drink more heavily than the general population and therefore are at an increased risk of experiencing violence. When sexual assaults and rapes were reported, typically both the perpetrator and the victim had been drinking.[1]

Impact of Alcohol and Violent Behavior

So why is alcohol a contributing factor in violent crime? Alcohol acts as a depressant, which can reduce reaction time, impair cognition, and cloud judgment. Such impairment could decrease the chances of avoiding personal injury once a physical altercation begins. Alcohol also decreases inhibitions and may increase aggressive behavior. It may increase the likelihood of inflicting or receiving a severe injury during a violent act and has been shown to increase the severity of injuries obtained in violent acts. Alcohol use interferes with attention and inhibits communication, both of which can drive aggressive behavior.

What Can You Do?

Although alcohol alone may not cause violence, when alcohol is introduced into a situation that has the potential to become violent, it can increase the chances that violence will occur. As the number of drunk drivers on the road has decreased, so has the number of drunk-driving accidents and fatalities. It seems logical to assume that if alcohol is kept out of the hands of people who are predisposed to violence, the number of alcohol-related crimes may also decrease.

You can choose to use good common sense when you are drinking or if you are with people who are drinking. Try to avoid potentially violent situations, and avoid people drinking around you who are acting in a reckless or violent manner. Drink in moderation, and help your friends recognize when they have had too much. Perhaps you or one of your friends can remain sober (a "designated thinker") to help avoid potentially dangerous situations and stay safe while partying. Finally, you can plan ahead by thinking carefully about an upcoming event before it happens. By "thinking before you drink," you can anticipate problems before they materialize and have solution strategies ready if they are needed.

For Discussion . . .

Have you ever encountered an angry drinker? Is there a safe way to handle a person who is drunk and intending to do harm to someone? If you have ever been drunk, do you feel that you could have controlled your actions in a confrontation while you were drunk?

References

1. Quigley BM, Corbett AB, and Tedeschi JT. Desired Image of Power, Alcohol Expectancies, and Alcohol-Related Agression. *Psychology of Addictive Behaviors,* 16(4), 318–324. 2002.
2. Smart GL, Moore TM, Kahler CW, and Ramsey SE. Substance Abuse and Relationship Violence Among Men Court-Referred to Batterers' Intervention Programs. *Substance Abuse,* 24(2), 107–122. 2003.
3. Schumacher JA, Fals-Stewart W, and Leonard KE. Domestic violence treatment referrals for men seeking alcohol treatment. *Journal of Substance Abuse Treatment,* 24, 279–283. 2003.
4. Core Institute: 2001 Statistics on Alcohol and Other Drug Use on American College Campuses (online). Available: **www.siu.edu/ departments/coreinst/public_html/ recent.html** accessed 16 June 2003.

personal assessment

are you troubled by someone's drinking?

The following questions are designed to help you decide whether you are affected by someone's drinking and could benefit from a program such as Al-Anon. Record your number of yes and no responses in the boxes at the end of the questionnaire.

	Yes	No
1. Do you worry about how much someone else drinks?	____	____
2. Do you have money problems because of someone else's drinking?	____	____
3. Do you tell lies to cover up for someone else's drinking?	____	____
4. Do you feel that if the drinker loved you, he or she would stop drinking to please you?	____	____
5. Do you blame the drinker's behavior on his or her companions?	____	____
6. Are plans frequently upset or meals delayed because of the drinker?	____	____
7. Do you make threats, such as: "If you don't stop drinking, I'll leave you"?	____	____
8. Do you secretly try to smell the drinker's breath?	____	____
9. Are you afraid to upset someone for fear it will set off a drinking bout?	____	____
10. Have you been hurt or embarrassed by a drinker's behavior?	____	____
11. Are holidays and gatherings spoiled because of the drinking?	____	____
12. Have you considered calling the police for help in fear of abuse?	____	____
13. Do you search for hidden alcohol?	____	____
14. Do you often ride in a car with a driver who has been drinking?	____	____
15. Have you refused social invitations out of fear or anxiety that the drinker will cause a scene?	____	____

	Yes	No
16. Do you sometimes feel like a failure when you think of the lengths to which you have gone to control the drinker?	____	____
17. Do you think that if the drinker stopped drinking, your other problems would be solved?	____	____
18. Do you ever threaten to hurt yourself to scare the drinker?	____	____
19. Do you feel angry, confused, or depressed most of the time?	____	____
20. Do you feel there is no one who understands your problems?	____	____
TOTAL	____	____

Interpretation

If you answered yes to three or more of these questions, Al-Anon or Alateen may be able to help. You can contact Al-Anon or Alateen by looking in your local telephone directory or by writing to Al-Anon Family Group Headquarters, Inc., 1600 Corporate Landing Parkway, Virginia Beach, VA 23454-5617, or you may call (888) 4AL-ANON.

To Carry This Further . . .

Sometimes the decision to seek help from a support group is a difficult one. If you answered yes to any of the questions above, spend a few moments reflecting on your responses. How long have you been experiencing problems because of someone else's drinking? How would sharing your feelings with others—people who have dealt with very similar problems—help you cope with your own situation? Knowing you're not alone can often be a great relief; it's up to you to take the first step.

chapter nine

rejecting tobacco use

Online Learning Center Resources

www.mhhe.com/hahn7e

Log on to our Online Learning Center (OLC) for access to these additional resources:

- Chapter key terms and definitions
- Learning objectives
- Student interactive question-and-answer sites

- Self-scoring chapter quiz
- Online assessments
- Key term flash cards

Talking It Over

Supporting a Smoker Who Wants to Quit

My roommate is trying to quit smoking, and I want to help. How can I do that without seeming judgmental?

- Help your friend get through stressful periods by being available for nonsmoking activities, such as walking or playing a sport.
- Establish an award system for "nonsmoking days completed," and participate in the "funding" of the rewards.
- Suggest going to places where nonsmoking is the norm, such as restaurants or coffee houses that are smoke-free.

- Continue being supportive even if your friend fails in her current attempt to stop smoking. Most persons are not successful in their first attempt. Just "being there" often communicates support and understanding better than words do.

CommunicationLinks

www.cancer.org/tobacco/index.html
www.lungusa.org/tobacco/index.html

Eye on the Media

Tobacco Industry Denies Ads Target Kids

On various occasions during the past 5 years, the tobacco industry has run television commercials intended to "educate" the public about the fundamental changes that the tobacco industry has undertaken in terms of marketing, particularly in light of charges that the industry previously targeted children in an attempt to develop a new generation of smokers. In these commercials several changes were described, all of which were attributed to the 1998 settlement (formally signed in 1999) reached between the tobacco industry and the states' attorneys general stemming from a massive class action suit to recoup Medicaid money. There was no mention in the commercials that the original agreement reached between the states and the tobacco industry in June of 1997 was much more restrictive and closely reflective of the intent of the court in curbing the marketing activities of the tobacco industry. The more permissive 1998 settlement, known as the Master Settlement Agreement (MSA), arose when the tobacco industry promised to vigorously fight the 1997 agreement in court. Thus, compromises favoring the tobacco industry were made by the states to save time and resources that would otherwise be lost to additional litigation.

The accompanying chart shows selected examples of the differences between the 1997 agreement and the final 1999 settlement. Because of the tobacco industry's ability to afford media exposure, the American public will continue to be led to believe that the tobacco industry complied completely with the intent of the courts.

Master Settlement Agreement (MSA)

Restriction	1997 Agreement	1999 (MSA)
Outdoor and Transit Ads	Bans all outdoor and transit ads	Allows signs of up to 14 sq feet on any building or property where tobacco products are sold, including those near schools and playgrounds. Bans other billboards and transit ads.
Cartoons and Human Images	Banned	Allows human images, such as the Marlboro man. Bans cartoons.
Brand Name Sponsorships	Banned	Each company allowed one brand name sponsorship of an event or series of events. Prohibits events in which contestants are under 18 years of age.
Free Samples	Banned	Free samples allowed in adult-only facilities.

In yet a more current example of the tobacco industry's relationship to media exposure, RJR withdrew its corporate sponsorship of NASCAR's premier racing series, the Winston Cup Series.[1] By finally complying with the 1999 Master Settlement Agreement RJR can redirect hundreds of millions of dollars once spent on NASCAR into other areas of media exposure, such as advertisements in magazines popular with teens (such as *Sports Illustrated* and *Hot Rod*) and point-of-purchase displays in convenience stores and drug stores.[2] In spite of RJR's absence, the name "Winston" will most likely remain in NASCAR fans' minds for years to come.

Tobacco Use in American Society

If you were to visit certain businesses, entertainment spots, or sporting events in your community, you might leave convinced that virtually every adult is a tobacco user. Certainly, for some segments of society, tobacco use is the rule rather than the exception. You may be quite surprised to find out that the great majority of adults do not use tobacco products. Figure 9-1 shows the states with the highest and lowest smoking rates.[3]

Following the Surgeon General's 1964 report (the first official statement of concern by the federal government regarding the dangers of smoking),[4] the prevalence of smoking began a decline that lasted until 1991, when a leveling off was noted that lasted for the next three years. Since 1994 the percentage of the population who smoke

has declined slowly but progressively. Current statistics reveal that 22.5% of American adults smoke cigarettes on a daily or near-daily basis. Men are more likely to smoke (25.2%) than are women (20.0%).[5] When subsegments of the population, based on race and ethnicity, were studied it

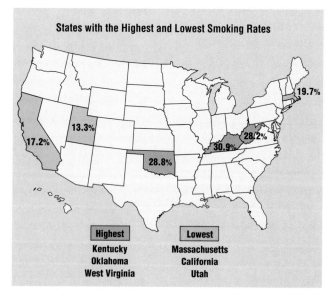

States with the Highest and Lowest Smoking Rates

Highest	Lowest
Kentucky	Massachusetts
Oklahoma	California
West Virginia	Utah

Figure 9-1 Kentucky has the highest smoking rate in the nation. Do you know what the rate is in your state?

Source: Prevalence of current cigarette smoking among adults and changes in prevalence of current and some day smoking—2001. *MMWR.* 52(14). April 2003.

Table 9.1 Patterns of Cigarette Smoking

Prevalence by Sex		
Total	**Men**	**Women**
(+)22.5	(+)25.2	(+)20.0

Note: Subjects have smoked more than one hundred cigarettes and reported smoking every day or some days.

Percentage by Ethnicity and Race					
Total	**White**	**Black**	**Hispanic**	**American Indian or Alaska Native**	**Asian or Pacific Islander**
(+)22.5	(+)24.1	(+)22.5	(+)15.9	(0)40.0	(0)13.7

Note: Subjects have smoked more than 100 cigarettes and smoked at the time of the survey.
(+) = [6]
(0) = [7]

was found that whites and blacks were essentially smoking with the same prevalence (24.1% and 22.5%).[6] At the same time, Hispanics were considerably less likely to smoke, while American Indians and Alaska Natives (40.0%) were more likely to smoke. Persons of Asian or Pacific Island descent were the Americans least likely to smoke (13.7%) (see Table 9.1).[6]

Cigarette Smoking Among College Students

Until very recently, the rate of cigarette smoking among college graduates was lower than that reported for the population as a whole, and it was significantly lower than the rate for persons with very little formal education. In fact, the prevalence of smoking among college students decreased progressively from 21% in 1964 to 14% in 1995.[7] However, an upward trend in cigarette use by college students has been noted, with a recent study suggesting an incidence approaching 36% smoking within the past month.[8] In contrast, a downward trend in smoking by twelfth graders was reported in 2002.[9] Knowing that a segment of those twelfth graders (1998) are now undergraduates on college and university campuses, it is possible that the 35.8% prevalence of cigarette smoking among college students, as reported in 2000, is now experiencing a decline. This is, in fact, probable since among the 2002 twelfth graders with college aspirations, only 15.1% were cigarette smokers.[9]

 TALKING POINTS Your 13-year-old brother inadvertently leaves a tin of smokeless tobacco on the desk in his room and you see it. Would you say anything to him about it? If so, what?

When a college community is viewed as a whole regarding which segments of the student body are most likely to smoke, there appears to be a direct relationship between the level of alcohol consumption and cigarette smoking, and between the importance that students assign to "partying" versus other aspects of the college experience.[10]

The historically predictable relationship between higher levels of completed education and the lessened likelihood of smoking remains clearly evident even today. For example, when comparing the percentage of heavy smokers (a pack or more per day) on the basis of education completed, the influence of education is evident—less than high school (37.5m/31.3f), high school graduate (22.0m/26.2f), some college (25.4m/21.9f), and college graduate (11.0m/10.7f).[11] Unfortunately, the most recently reported incidence of smoking among college students (2002) seems to indicate that the next college graduating classes of 1998–2002 were much closer to the high school dropout rate of cigarette smoking.

The most disturbing aspect of the increase in reported smoking among college students, beyond the eventual influence it will have on health and life expectancy, is its negation of the traditional belief that the college and university experience "protected" this segment of the society from making some ill-informed choices. As recently as the mid-1990s it was still possible to believe that the college population was "too well informed" and "too future oriented" to engage widely in an addictive behavior that fosters dependence, compromises health, and eventually shortens life. Today that proposition seems to lack some of its former validity, but, hopefully, the corner is being turned.

Other Demographic Factors Influencing Tobacco Use

In addition to gender, race, ethnicity, and education level, other demographic facts appear to influence the extent to which smoking occurs. Included among these factors are the age groups into which persons fall, the region of the country in which they live, the size of their communities, and their employment status.

If age grouping is begun with 18- to 25-year-olds and progresses to 65 years of age and older, the general trend is for the percentage of persons smoking (during the past month) within each group to go down. For example, among the younger group (18–25), 28.5m/25.1f% report having smoked during the past month, while in the 26- to 34-year-olds, 29.0m/22.5f% smoked during the past month, and in the 65-plus group, only 10.2m/9.3f% did so.[5] Most likely over the course of time, both quitting and premature death serve to reduce the percentage of smokers.

A Simple Dependency Test Regarding Your Relationships with Cigarettes

To nonsmokers it must seem that smokers would realize the existence of their dependency on cigarettes, however such might not be the case. The Hooked On Nicotine Checklist (HONC) appearing below is a simple way to determine whether a cigarette-based dependency exists. If you are a smoker, answer each question asked by the HONC in an honest manner. When completed, give careful consideration to your findings. If you are a nonsmoker, ask a smoker to complete the HONC and share responses to each item with you. In the latter case, a good discussion could ensue.

Nicotine Addiction's 10 Warning Signs

HONC—Hooked On Nicotine Checklist

1.	Have you ever tried to quit but couldn't?
2.	Do you smoke now because it is really hard to quit?
3.	Have you ever felt like you were addicted to tobacco?
4.	Do you ever have strong cravings to smoke?
5.	Have you ever felt like you really needed a cigarette?
6.	Is it hard to keep from smoking in places where you are not supposed to, like school?

In answering the last four questions, when you tried to stop smoking, or when you have not used tobacco for a while . . .

7.	Did you find it hard to concentrate?
8.	Did you feel more irritable?
9.	Did you feel a strong need or urge to smoke?
10.	Did you feel nervous, restless or anxious because you couldn't smoke?

Answering "yes" to any one of the above ten questions indicates that you may already be hooked on nicotine and are chemically dependent. Think about it! Your "yes" answer is your own honest self assessment that you have already lost the freedom and ability to simply and effortlessly walk away. Two-thirds of all teens who you see smoking regularly will spend their entire life as slaves to nicotine. If you HONC we'll help - www.WhyQuit.com

Source: HONC—(Hooked on Nicotine Checklist), Tobacco Control, Sept. 2002
Dr. JR Difranza, Development of symptoms of tobacco dependency in youths.
Reliability study of HONC factors—July 2002
Created by www.WhyQuit.com—Join us for motivation, education and support!

Comparing smoking during the past month among people in different regions of the country reveals that persons living in the north central portion of the country are the most likely to smoke (26%). In contrast, persons living in the West are least likely to have smoked during the past month (20.0%). People in the South (25.4%) and the Northeast (23.9%) fall in between.[11] In terms of population density, one might be surprised to learn that persons living outside of metropolitan areas are more likely to have smoked during the past month (30.5%), while persons living in small metropolitan areas (27.2%) and large metropolitan areas (26.5%) are less likely to have smoked during the same period.[12]

Employment status too impacts on the likelihood of regular smoking. Persons who are employed part-time are more likely to have smoked during the past month (31.2%) than are people who are employed full-time (25.5%)—most likely reflecting the greater opportunity of the former group to smoke, since today's work place is increasingly a smoke-free environment. In stark contrast to those who have some degree of employment, the unemployed are by far the most likely to have smoked during the past month (50.1%).[12] This may reflect not only the lower level of education found among this group, but also the immediate gratification that smoking brings to persons who may have little opportunity to seriously pursue long-range goals and the postponed gratification that striving for such goals can often require.

Marketing of Tobacco Products

Shredded plant material, wrapped in paper or leaf, ignited with a flame, and then placed on or near the delicate tissues of the mouth . . . what other human behavior does this resemble? If you answered *None!* to this question, then you appreciate that smoking is unique, and, therefore, that it must be learned. How it is learned is currently a less than fully understood process that most likely requires a variety of stimuli ranging from modeling to actual experimentation. The role of advertising as a source of models has long been suspected and intensely debated. Today, as in the past, controversy surrounds the intent of the tobacco industry's advertising. Are the familiar logos seen in a variety of media intended to challenge the brand loyalty of those who have already decided to smoke, as the industry claims? Or are the ads intended to entice new smokers, older children and young adolescents, in sufficient numbers to replace the 3,000 smokers who die each day from the consequences of tobacco use? This latter objective is now known, by admission of the tobacco industry, to have been pursued for decades. Its effectiveness has also been documented. The cartoon character Joe Camel was an especially successful tool for enticing children and teens to begin smoking.

Over the years the tobacco industry has used all aspects of mass media advertising, including radio, television, print, billboards, and sponsorship of televised athletic events and concerts, to sell its products. In addition, it has often distributed free samples and sold merchandise bearing the company or product logo.

Today the tobacco industry has been denied access to television and radio, and it can no longer distribute free samples to minors, but the industry continues to be active and innovative in other aspects of the media to which it has access. For example, Philip Morris has introduced an upscale lifestyle magazine called *Unlimited: Action, Adventure, Good Times,* to be provided free to over 1 million smokers. Interestingly, the magazine features articles about healthful activities that many longtime smokers would be unable to engage in because of the effects of smoking.

In the 9 months following the 1999 Master Settlement Agreement, the tobacco industry increased their magazine advertising budget by 30% over presettlement levels in magazines with 15% or more youth (under 18 years of age) readership, even though they had agreed to discontinue advertising in youth-oriented publications.[13] Most recently, increased tobacco advertising has been noted in magazines that appeal specifically to younger women, working women, and women of color.

The development of nonmarket brands of cigarettes for free distribution to patrons of bars and restaurants who are attempting to "bum" cigarettes represents a second form of "advertising." This "premarketing" introduction of a prototype brand technically does not violate the law regarding the distribution of samples. To date, several hundred establishments in several major cities have participated.

A final current example of the tobacco industry's subtle but effective presence in the mind of the public is that of tobacco use in motion pictures. In spite of a 1990 tobacco industry policy and the 1999 Master Settlement Agreement, both of which prohibit "brand placement" of tobacco products in films, cigarette and cigar smoking continue to be disproportionately represented in current films. Unfortunately, children and adolescents can easily identify with these characters (and their smoking), since they are generally depicted in a positive light. As an example, in a recent survey, two-thirds of the 43 movie stars most frequently named by 10- to 19-year-olds were seen smoking in their most recent films.[14]

Pipe and Cigar Smoking

Many people believe that pipe or cigar smoking is a safe alternative to cigarette smoking. Unfortunately, this is not the case. All forms of tobacco present users with a series of health threats (see the Star box on page 240 and Table 9.3 on page 249).

When compared with cigarette smokers, pipe and cigar smokers have cancer of the mouth, throat, larynx (voice box), and esophagus at the same frequency. Cigarette

Thanks, But No Cigar

If one were to judge on the basis of the number of newly opened cigar stores and clubs catering to cigar smokers, as well as the highly visible magazine *Cigar Aficionado,* one could conclude that cigar smoking was the hottest trend in tobacco use. To a degree this contention is true when one considers that in 1991 only 2.2% of the adult population smoked cigars on a regular basis,[15] while by 1998 the size of the cigar-smoking population had risen to 5.2%.[16] This said, however, a 2000 report demonstrates a decline to 4.5%, suggesting that the appeal of cigars has begun to wane.[17] However, for those cigar smokers who will apparently continue, and for those of you who might be increasingly interested in this form of tobacco use, the following information from the American Lung Association should be considered:

- *Secondhand (sidestream) cigar smoke is more poisonous than secondhand cigarette smoke.* The smoke from one cigar equals that of three cigarettes. Carbon monoxide emissions from one cigar are 30 times higher than for one cigarette.

- *Cigar smoking can cause cancer of the larynx (voice box), mouth, esophagus, and lungs.* Cancer death rates for cigar smokers are 34% higher than for nonsmokers.

- *Ninety-nine percent of cigar smokers have atypical cells found in the larynx.* These cells are the first step toward malignancy (cancer).

- *Cigar smokers are three to five times more likely to die of lung cancer than are nonsmokers.*

- *Cigar smokers have five times the risk of emphysema compared to nonsmokers.*

- *Nicotine does not have to be inhaled to damage the heart and blood vessels.* It is absorbed into the bloodstream through the mucous membranes of the mouth. Nicotine increases the heart rate and constricts the blood vessels, which reduces blood flow to the heart.

---

smokers are more likely than pipe and cigar smokers to have lung cancer, cancer of the larynx, chronic obstructive lung disease (COLD), also called chronic obstructive pulmonary disease (COPD), and heart disease. The cancer risk of death to smokers is four times greater from lung cancer and ten times greater from laryngeal cancer than for nonsmokers.[18]

In comparison to cigarette smokers, pipe and cigar smokers are considerably fewer in number. Interestingly, cigar smoking enjoyed a resurgence through much of the 1990s. However, during 1998–1999 a substantial decline in sales of premium cigars occurred. Whether this downturn represents an emerging dissatisfaction with cigars as an enjoyable use of tobacco or simply reflects adjustments in the import market remains uncertain. In 1995 cigars generated sales of $1 billion, mainly to younger adults, including a very small but growing percentage of women.

Perhaps because of the increase in cigar smoking noted above, the National Cancer Institute commissioned the first extensive study of regular cigar smoking. That report confirmed and expanded upon the health risks identified in earlier smaller studies.[19] A subsequent study reported that cigar smokers are nearly twice as likely as nonsmokers to develop oral, throat, and lung cancer, as well as heart disease and chronic obstructive pulmonary disease.[20] These rates are somewhat lower than those of cigarette smokers.

In response to the recognition of these risks, the FTC now requires that cigar manufacturers must disclose the tobacco content and additives in their products. Most recently the FTC announced its intention of requiring five rotating health warnings to appear on cigars, including two that have been currently agreed upon by the FTC and major cigar manufacturers: *Cigars*

Are Not a Safe Alternative to Cigarettes and *Cigar Smoking Can Cause Cancer of the Mouth and Throat, Even If You Don't Inhale.*

The use of smokeless tobacco, a third alternative to cigarette smoking, is discussed later in the chapter.

Tobacco Use and the Development of Dependence

Although not true for every tobacco user (see the discussion of "chippers" later in this section), the vast majority of users, particularly cigarette smokers, will develop a dependency relationship with the nicotine contained in tobacco. This state of **dependence** causes users to consume greater quantities of nicotine over extended periods of time, further endangering their health.

Dependence can imply both a physical and psychological relationship. Particularly with cigarettes, *physical dependence* or *addiction,* with its associated *tolerance, withdrawal,* and **titration,** is strongly developed by 40 percent of all smokers. The development of addiction

---

Key Terms

dependence a physical and/or psychological need to continue the use of a drug.

titration (tie **tray** shun) the particular level of a drug within the body; adjusting the level of nicotine by adjusting the rate of smoking.

reflects a strong genetic predisposition to physical dependence.[21] Most of the remaining population of smokers will experience lesser degrees of physical dependence. Psychological *dependence* or *habituation,* with its accompanying psychological components of *compulsion* and *indulgence,* is almost universally seen.

Compulsion is a strong emotional desire to continue tobacco use despite restrictions on smoking and the awareness of health risks. Very likely, users are "compelled" to engage in continual tobacco use in fear of the unpleasant physical, emotional, and social effects that result from discontinuing use. In comparison to compulsion, indulgence is seen as "rewarding" oneself for aligning with a particular behavior pattern—in this case, smoking. Indulgence is made possible by the existence of various reward systems built around the use of tobacco, including a perceived image, group affiliation, and even appetite suppression intended to foster weight control.

Much to the benefit of the tobacco industry, dependence on tobacco is easily established. Many experts believe that physical dependence on tobacco is far more easily established than is physical dependence on alcohol, cocaine (other than crack), or heroin. Of all people who experiment with cigarettes, 85% develop various aspects of a dependence relationship.

A small percentage of smokers, known as "chippers," can smoke on occasion without becoming dependent. Most likely, chippers respond differently to environmental cues than do more dependent smokers,[22] thus smoking less frequently. They may be truly "social smokers" in that they smoke with only a few selected friends or in a very limited number of places. Unfortunately, many inexperienced smokers feel that they too are only social smokers; however, a few months, or even a few days, of this type of occasional smoking could be a transitional period into a dependence pattern of tobacco use.

Sandwiched between regular smokers and chippers is a newly emerging group of smokers—part-time smokers. Today these smokers constitute about 23% of all smokers. The practice most likely reflects the reality of the high cost of cigarettes and restrictions in the workplace. The health effects of this form of smoking appear to be the same as for regular smokers.[3]

Theories of Nicotine Addiction

The establishment and maintenance of physical dependence or addiction is less than fully understood. Most experts, however, believe that for a specific individual, addiction has a multifaceted etiology, or cause, with increasing attention being directed toward a genetic basis for addiction. Accordingly, several theories have been proposed to explain the development of dependence. We will present a

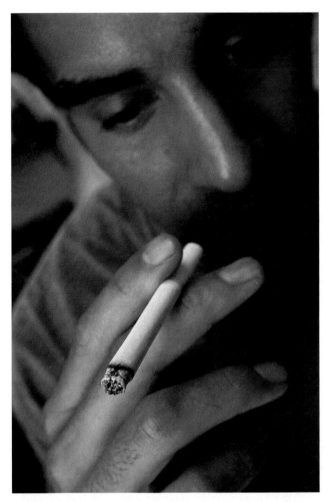

A smoker inhales about 70,000 times during the first year of smoking, resulting in a nicotine addiction that often lasts a lifetime.

brief account of some of these theories. Readers are reminded that many of these theories are technically sophisticated and only a most basic description can be provided in a personal health textbook. The more emotional aspects of dependence formation will be discussed later in the chapter.

Genetic Influences

Although the specific genetic pathways that influence both the initiation and maintenance of smoking (or other forms of tobacco use) are less than fully understood, a role for genetic influence is evident. Applying new statistical techniques to earlier studies of smoking patterns in families and between identical twins, it is now believed that initiation and maintenance of initial smoking is 60% driven by genetic influences. Of course, the smoking of the first few cigarettes is a choice made by beginning smokers. The remaining influence needed for initiation and maintenance of initial smoking is 20% environmental and 20% the unique needs of individuals.[23]

Once the brief period of initial exposure is passed, the role of genetic influences may be even more powerful—providing 70% of the stimulus required over decades of smoking. Environmental and personality factors subside accordingly.[23]

Bolus Theory

In the **bolus theory** of nicotine addiction, one of the oldest and most general theories of addiction, each inhalation of smoke releases into the blood a concentrated quantity of nicotine (a ball or bolus) that reaches the brain and results in a period of neurohormonal excitement. The smoker perceives this period of stimulation as pleasurable but, unfortunately, short lived. Accordingly, the smoker attempts to reestablish this pleasurable feeling by again inhaling and sending another bolus of nicotine on its way to the brain. The 70,000 or more inhalations during the first year of smoking serve to condition the novice smoker, resulting in a lifelong pattern of cigarette dependence. The level needed for arousal is different for each individual smoker, depending on the length of addiction, the level of tolerance, genetic predisposition, and environmental and personal stimuli.

Recognition of two types of smokers emerges from an understanding of the bolus theory of smoking. *Peak smokers* are those smokers who become dependent on the arousal of pleasure centers in the brain (see page 243) that are stimulated by the rapid increase of nicotine levels following inhalation and distribution of nicotine within the CNS. In contrast, the *trough maintenance smokers* maintain an even consistently higher level of nicotine titration in order to avoid the negative consequences of withdrawal.[24] These feelings are experienced as unpleasant, and thus to be avoided.

Adrenocorticotropic Hormone (ACTH) Theory

Yet another theory of dependence suggests that nicotine stimulates the release of adrenocorticotropic hormone (ACTH) from the anterior pituitary, or "master gland" of the endocrine system (see Chapter 3) causing the release of **beta endorphins** (naturally occurring opiate-like chemicals) that produce mild feelings of euphoria. Perhaps this stresslike response mechanism involving ACTH accounts for the increased energy expenditure seen in smokers and thus their tendency to maintain a lower body weight. Others, however, have questioned the ability of nicotine to stimulate endorphin release.[25]

When these physiological responses are viewed collectively, nicotine may be seen as biochemically influencing brain activity by enhancing the extent and strength of various forms of "communication" between different brain areas and even glands of the endocrine system. If this is the case, it is apparent why, once addicted, the functioning of the smoker's control systems is much altered in comparison with that of nonsmokers.

Self-Medication Theory

Another explanation of the addiction to smoking, called self-medication, suggests that nicotine, through the effects of mood-enhancing dopamine, may allow smokers to "treat" feelings of tiredness, lack of motivation, or even depression.[26] In other words, a smoke lifts the spirits, if only briefly. Eventually, however, smokers become dependent on tobacco as a "medication" to make themselves feel better. Thus, because tobacco is a legal drug that is readily available, it becomes preferred to prescription medications and illegal drugs, such as cocaine and the stimulants, that elevate mood.

Regardless of the mechanism involved, as tolerance to nicotine develops, smoking behavior is adjusted to either maintain arousal or prevent the occurrence of withdrawal symptoms. At some point, however, the desire for constant arousal is probably superseded by the smoker's desire not to experience withdrawal.

The importance of nicotine as the primary factor in establishing dependence on tobacco is supported by research that demonstrates that smokers will not select a nontobacco cigarette if a tobacco cigarette is available. Even tobacco cigarettes with a very low level of nicotine seem to be unacceptable to most smokers, as do cigarettes with very low nicotine but with high tar content. Interestingly, users of low-nicotine cigarettes tend to inhale more frequently and deeply to obtain as much nicotine as possible.

Even more impressive (and alarming) regarding nicotine's dependency-producing power is seen in conjunction with the small amount of time needed to become dependent. Using the HONC instruments described in the Star box on page 238, it is now established that beginning smokers (recall that most smokers begin during adolescence) become dependent on cigarettes within 3 weeks to 3 months of smoking on as little as two cigarettes per day. Males are more likely to be a bit more resistant to dependency, taking a month or 2, while females can become dependent in a matter of a very few days of initial experimentation.[27]

Key Terms

bolus theory a theory of nicotine addiction based on the body's response to the bolus (ball) of nicotine delivered to the brain with each inhalation of cigarette smoke.

beta endorphins mood-enhancing, pain-reducing, opiate-like chemicals produced within the smoker's body in response to the presence of nicotine.

Learning from Our Diversity

World No-Tobacco Day Seeks Support from Athletes and Artists

Sports and smoking seem to make strange bedfellows—but not in the world of advertising. For decades, cigarette manufacturers have worked hand-in-glove with professional athletes and teams, exchanging huge sums of money for endorsements of tobacco products or for the promotion and sponsorship of major sporting events. Although cigarette advertising has been banned from American television for over 30 years, the cozy connections continue, with perhaps the most notable example being the women's tennis tournament initially sponsored by Virginia Slims cigarettes (whose slogan, "You've come a long way, baby," resonated with women of a generation ago but is increasingly quoted in tones ranging from irony to contempt).

A step in the opposite direction is World No-Tobacco Day, promoted annually since 1988 by the World Health Organization (WHO), an autonomous unit of the United Nations whose headquarters are in Switzerland. On a designated day each year, WHO urges tobacco users to abstain for at least that day—and, ideally, for good. WHO says the annual observance of World No-Tobacco Day "is a unique opportunity to mobilize athletes, artists, and the media, as well as the public in general, in support of the objective of promoting a society and a way of life where tobacco use is no longer an accepted norm."

In sponsoring World No-Tobacco Day, WHO has focused on smoking in public places, on public transportation, in the workplace, and in medical facilities. A recent campaign escalated the stop-smoking effort with a theme of "United Nations and Specialized Agencies Against Tobacco," with the aim of sharply reducing tobacco use worldwide.

As noted earlier, tobacco interests continue to promote many sporting events, as well as some cultural events. As far as sports are concerned, however, WHO officials see reason for encouragement in the recent smoke-free history of the Olympic Games. Beginning with the 1988 Winter Games in Calgary, all Olympic Games—both summer and winter—have been smoke-free.

While a major cigarette manufacturer congratulates its (female) customers on having "come a long way, baby," the World Health Organization is strongly conveying the message that you'll go a lot farther if you don't smoke.

Which tactic do you think is most likely to reduce the rate of tobacco use worldwide: legal bans and restrictions, campaigns of persuasion like World No-Tobacco Day, or a combination of these two approaches?

TALKING POINTS A smoker says that she does not consider smoking to be a form of drug use. She becomes angry at the suggestion that cigarettes are part of a drug delivery system. How would you respond to her position?

Acute Effects of Nicotine on Nervous System Function

In comparison with the more chronic effects of nicotine on the central nervous system (CNS) that may eventually result in physical dependence or addiction, nicotine also produces changes of short duration. In the CNS, nicotine activates receptors within the nucleus accumbens (a reward center) and the locus caeruleus (a cortical activating center) of the brain. Stimulation of the brain is seen by changes in electroencephalogram (EEG) patterns, reflecting an increase in the frequency of electrical activity. This is part of a general arousal pattern signaled by the release of the neurotransmitters **norepinephrine,** dopamine, acetylcholine, and serotonin. Heavy use of tobacco products, resulting in high levels of nicotine in the bloodstream, eventually produces a blocking effect as more and more receptor sites for these neurotransmitters are filled. The result is a generalized depression of the CNS.

The level of plasma nicotine associated with normal levels of heavy smoking (one to two packs per day) would not likely produce the depressive effect just described. However, in chain smokers (four to eight packs per day), plasma nicotine levels would be sufficient to have a depressive influence on nervous system function. In fact, it has been suggested that chain smoking is driven by the fruitless effort to counter the depressive influence of chronically excessively high levels of nicotine.

In carefully controlled studies involving both animals and humans, nicotine increased the ability of subjects to concentrate on a task. It must be noted, however, that the duration of this improvement was limited. Most would agree that this brief benefit is not enough to justify the health risks associated with chronic tobacco use.

Key Terms

norepinephrine (nor epp in **eff** rin) an adrenalinlike chemical produced within the nervous system.

Non–Nervous System Acute Effects of Nicotine

Outside the CNS, nicotine affects the transmission of nerve signals at the point where nerves innervate muscle tissue (called the *neuromuscular junction*) by mimicking the action of the neurotransmitter acetylcholine. Nicotine occupies receptor sites at the junction and prevents the transmission of nerve impulses from nerve cell to muscle cell.

Nicotine also causes the release of epinephrine from the adrenal medulla (see Chapter 3), which results in an increase in respiration rate, heart rate, blood pressure, and coronary blood flow. These changes are accompanied by the constriction of the blood vessels beneath the skin, a reduction in the motility in the bowel, loss of appetite, and changes in sleep patterns.

Although a lethal dose of nicotine could be obtained through the ingestion of a nicotine-containing insecticide, to "smoke oneself to death" in a single intense period of cigarette use would be highly improbable. In humans, 40 to 60 mg (.06–.09 mg/kg) is a lethal dose.[28] A typical cigarette supplies .05 to 2.5 mg of nicotine, and that nicotine is relatively quickly broken down for removal from the body.

Psychosocial Factors Related to Dependence

You will recall that a psychological aspect of dependence (habituation) exists and is important in maintaining the smoker's need for nicotine. Both research and general observation support many of the powerful influences this aspect of dependence possesses, especially for beginning smokers, prior to the onset of physical addiction. Consequently, in the remainder of this section, we will explore factors that may contribute to the development of this aspect of dependence.

Modeling

Because tobacco use is a learned behavior, it is reasonable to accept that modeling acts as a stimulus to experimental smoking. Modeling suggests that susceptible people smoke to emulate, or model their behavior after, smokers whom they admire or with whom they share other types of social or emotional bonds. Particularly for young adolescents (ages 14 to 17), smoking behavior correlates with the smoking behavior of slightly older peers and very young adults (ages 18 to 22), older siblings, and, most importantly, parents.[29]

Negative parental influences on cigarette smoking by their own children include their own smoking in combination with their failure to clearly state their disapproval of smoking by children.[30] Further, for parents who smoke, it is important that they cease smoking before their children turn 8 years of age if they wish to maximize an anti-smoking message.

Modeling is particularly evident when smoking is a central factor in peer group formation and peer group association and can lead to a shared behavioral pattern that differentiates the group from others and from adults. Further, when risk-taking behavior and disregard for authority are common to the group, smoking becomes the behavioral pattern that most consistently identifies and bonds the group. Particularly for those young people who lack self-directedness or the ability to resist peer pressure, initial membership in a tobacco-using peer group may become inescapable. The ability to counter peer pressure is a salient component of successful anti-smoking programs for use with older children and younger adolescents.[31]

In addition, when adolescents have lower levels of self-esteem and are searching for an avenue to improve self-image, a role model who smokes is often seen as tough, sociable, and sexually attractive. These three traits have been played up by the tobacco industry in their carefully crafted advertisements. In fact, teens from any background may see the very young and attractive models used in tobacco (and beer) advertisements as being more peer-like in age than they really are. FCC regulations require that models for both products be 21 years of age or older, regardless of how youthful they might (and the advertisers hope they do) appear to older children and young adolescents. See the Learning from Our Diversity box on page 243 for a counterapproach to the acceptance of tobacco.

Manipulation

In addition to modeling as a psychosocial link with tobacco use, cigarette use may meet the beginning smoker's need to manipulate something and at the same time provide the manipulative "tool" necessary to offset boredom, feelings of depression, or social immaturity. Clearly the availability of affordable smoking paraphernalia provides smokers with ways to reward themselves. A new cigarette lighter, a status brand of tobacco, or a beach towel with a cigarette's logo are all reinforcements to some smokers. Fortunately, the latter will become increasingly harder to find as logos can no longer be placed on items such as beach towels. For others, the ability to take out a cigarette or fill a pipe adds a measure of structure and control to situations in which they might otherwise feel somewhat ill at ease. The cigarette becomes a readily available and dependable "friend" to turn to during stressful moments.

Susceptibility to Advertising

The images of the smoker's world portrayed by the media can be particularly attractive. For adolescents, women, minorities, and other carefully targeted groups of adults, the tobacco industry has paired suggestions of a better life with the use of its products. To these users and potential users, the self-reward of power, liberation, affluence, sophistication, or adult status is achieved by using the products that they are told are associated with these desired states. Thus the self-rewarding use of tobacco products becomes a means of achievement.

With this multiplicity of forces at work, it is possible to understand why so many who experiment with tobacco use find that they quickly become dependent on tobacco. Human needs, both physiological and psychosocial, are many and complex. Tobacco use meets the needs on a short-term basis, whereas dependence, once established, replaces these needs with a different, more immediate set of needs.

Despite the satisfaction of the dependency that continued smoking brings, approximately 80% of adult smokers have, on at least one occasion, expressed a desire to quit, and the majority of these have actually attempted to become nonsmokers. Today, with the over-the-counter availability of transdermal nicotine patches, nicotine-containing gum, prescription medications such as antidepressants, and nicotine inhalers, the number of smokers making concerted and repeated attempts to stop smoking is up considerably over that seen in the past. It therefore seems apparent that tobacco use is a source of **dissonance.** This dissonance stems from the need to deal emotionally with a behavior that is both highly enjoyable and highly dangerous but known to be difficult to stop. The degree to which this dissonance exists probably varies from user to user.

Preventing Teen Smoking

Even before the 1997 release of tobacco industry documents confirming the targeting of young adolescents, the federal government stated its intention to curb these cigarette advertisements. In August 1995 the FDA described the specific actions that it hoped it would be given authority to implement. Collectively, the restrictions described in the following list were intended to discourage cigarette smoking among America's teens, resulting in 50% fewer adolescents beginning smoking in the year 2002 than in 1995.

1. Limit tobacco advertising in publications that appeal to teens and restrict billboards with tobacco-related content to no closer than 1,000 feet of schools and playgrounds. (An August 1995 study in California found that stores near schools displayed significantly more tobacco-related advertisements than those farther from schools.)
2. Restrict the use of logo and other tobacco-related images on nontobacco-related products, such as towels, T-shirts, and caps.
3. Bar certain sources of access to tobacco products, such as mail order sales, the distribution of free samples, and vending machines.

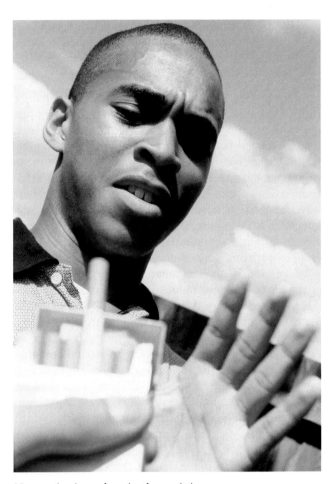

Not starting is much easier than quitting.

4. Halt sponsorship of high-visibility events, such as auto racing and athletic contests in which brand names appear on highly televised surfaces, including hoods, fenders, uniforms, and arena sign boards. (It is estimated that the Marlboro logo is seen 5,933 times during the course of a 90-minute televised Winston Cup auto race.)
5. Require merchants to obtain proof of age when selling tobacco products to adolescents. (This particular component of the initial plan became law in 1997. Merchants are required to validate the age of people whom they suspect to be younger

---

Key Terms

dissonance (**dis** son ince) a feeling of uncertainty that occurs when a person believes two equally attractive but opposite ideas.

than 27 years of age before selling cigarettes to those 18 years of age and older. If found in violation, both the salesperson and the store owner will be fined $500.)

By mid-1998 the federal government's desire to reduce youth smoking through implementation of the steps just described was mired in a larger package of tobacco-related policies being debated in Congress. This undertaking was related to the class action suit filed by all 50 (46 as a single large class and 4 as a smaller class) states against the tobacco industry in an attempt to recoup Medicaid expenditures for treating tobacco-related illnesses. As Congress attempted to construct a settlement that would be acceptable to all parties, the impasse fragmented attempts to reduce youth smoking. Unfortunately, this outcome diluted some restrictions on tobacco advertisements, as well as the FDA's ability to reduce smoking by defining cigarettes as drug delivery systems. In fact, in 2000 the United States Supreme Court ruled that the FDA lacked the regulatory authority to bring tobacco products under its control, unless Congress was willing to rescind laws that currently define tobacco as an agricultural product that can be freely marketed to persons 18 years of age or older. (If defined as a drug delivery system, cigarettes would be obtainable only with a physician's prescription, which would essentially prevent, or greatly limit, children's access to them.)

As noted earlier in the chapter, the Master Settlement Agreement of 1999, that required the tobacco industry to pay the states 246 billion dollars was able to restrict some forms of youth-oriented advertising and funds antismoking education, which may accomplish some of the changes initially proposed. Unfortunately, during the economic downturn some states have used these funds to meet taxation shortfalls.

Tobacco: The Source of Physiologically Active Compounds

When burned, the tobacco in cigarettes, cigars, and pipe mixtures is the source of an array of physiologically active chemicals, many of which are closely linked to significant changes in normal body structure and function. At the burning tip of the cigarette, the 900° C (1,652° F) heat oxidizes tobacco (as well as paper, wrapper, filter, and additives). With each puff of smoke, the body is exposed to approximately 4,700 chemical compounds, hundreds of which are known to be physiologically active, toxic, and carcinogenic (see Table 9.2 for a partial listing).[32] These chemicals have their origin in the tobacco or the over 1,450 additives, including pesticides and other agricultural chemicals. An annual 70,000 puffs taken in by the one-pack-a-day cigarette smoker results in an environment that makes the most polluted urban environment seem clean by comparison.

Particulate Phase

Cigarette, cigar, and pipe smoke can be described on the basis of two phases. These phases include a particulate phase and a gaseous phase. The **particulate phase** includes **nicotine,** water, and a variety of powerful chemicals known collectively as tar. **Tar** includes phenol, cresol, pyrene, DDT, and a benzene-ring group of compounds that includes benzo[a]pyrene. Most of the carcinogenic compounds are found within the tar. A person who smokes one pack of cigarettes per day will collect four ounces of tar in his or her lungs in a year. Only the gases and the smallest particles reach the small sacs of the lungs, called the *alveoli,* where oxygen exchange occurs. The carcinogen-rich particles from the particulate phase are deposited somewhere along the air passage leading to the lungs.

Gaseous Phase

The **gaseous phase** of tobacco smoke, like the particulate phase, is composed of a variety of physiologically active compounds, including carbon monoxide, carbon dioxide, ammonia, hydrogen cyanide, isopyrene, acetaldehyde, and acetone. At least sixty of these compounds have been determined to be **carcinogens** or co-carcinogenic promoters, thus capable of stimulating the development of cancer. Carbon monoxide is, however, the most damaging compound found in this component of tobacco smoke. Its impact is discussed next.

Key Terms

particulate phase portion of the tobacco smoke composed of small suspended particles.

nicotine physiologically active, dependence-producing drug found in tobacco.

tar a chemically rich, syrupy, blackish-brown material obtained from the particulate matter within cigarette smoke when nicotine and water are removed.

gaseous phase portion of the tobacco smoke containing carbon monoxide and many other physiologically active gaseous compounds.

carcinogens environmental agents, including chemical compounds within cigarette smoke, that stimulate the development of cancerous changes within cells.

Table 9.2 A Partial Listing of Toxic and Carcinogenic Components of Cigarette Smoke Including Vapor (Gaseous)-Phase and Particulate-Phase Components

Agent	Toxic	Ciliotoxic	Carcinogenic
Carbon Monoxide	x		
Nitrogen Oxides (NO$_x$)	x		
Hydrogen Cyanide	x	x	
Formaldehyde		x	x
Acrolein		x	
Acetaldehyde		x	
Ammonia	x		
Hydrazine			x
Vinyl Chloride			x
Urethane			x
2-Nitropropane			x
Quinoline			x
Benzo[a]pyrene			x
Dibenz[a,h]anthracene			x
Benzo[b]fluoranthene			x
Benzo[j]fluoranthene			x
Dibenzo[a,h]pyrene			x
Dibenzo[a,i]pyrene			x
Dibenz[a,j]acridine			x
Indeno[1,2,3-cd]pyrene			x
Benz[a]anthracene			x
Benzo[e]pyrene			x
Chrysene			x
Methylchrysene			x
Methylfluoranthene			x
Dibenz[a,c]anthracene			x
Dibenz[a,h]acridine			x
Dibenzo[c,g]carbazole			x
Nitrosodimethylamine			x
Nitrosoethymethylamine			x
Nitrosodiethylamine			x
Nitrosodi-n-propylamine			x
Nitrosodi-n-butylamine			x
Nitrosopyrrolidine			x
Nitrosopiperidine			x
Nitrosomorpholine			x
N'-Nitrosonornicotine			x
4-(methylnitrosamino)-1-(3-pyridyl)-1-butanone			x
N'-Nitrosoanabasine			x
N'-Nitrosoanatabine			x
Aromatic Amines			x
Aromatic Nitrohydrocarbons			x
Polonium-210			x
Nickel			x
Arsenic			x
Cadmium			x

Source: Mulcahy S. *The toxicology of cigarette smoke and environmental tobacco smoke.* A Review of Cigarette Smoke and Its Toxicological Effects. **http://www.csn.ul.ie/-stephen/reports/bc4927.html**

Carbon Monoxide

Like every inefficient engine, a cigarette, cigar, or pipe burns (oxidizes) its fuel with less than complete conversion into carbon dioxide, water, and heat. As a result of this incomplete oxidation, burning tobacco forms **carbon monoxide (CO)** gas. Carbon monoxide is one of the most harmful components of tobacco smoke.

Carbon monoxide is a colorless, odorless, tasteless gas that possesses a very strong physiological attraction for hemoglobin, the oxygen-carrying pigment on each red blood cell. When CO is inhaled, it quickly bonds with hemoglobin and forms a new compound, carboxyhemoglobin. In this form, hemoglobin is unable to transport oxygen to the tissues and cells where it is needed.

Although it is true that normal body metabolism always keeps an irreducible minimum of CO in our blood (0.5% to 1%), the blood of smokers may have levels of 5% to 10% CO saturation.[33] We are exposed to additional CO from environmental sources such as automobiles and buses and other combustion of fossil fuels. By combining a smoker's CO with environmental CO, it is little wonder that smokers more easily become out of breath than nonsmokers. The half-life of CO combined with hemoglobin is approximately 4 to 6 hours.[34] Most smokers replenish their level of CO saturation at far shorter intervals than this.

As mentioned, the presence of excessive levels of carboxyhemoglobin in the blood of smokers leads to shortness of breath and lowered endurance. Because an adequate oxygen supply to all body tissues is critical for normal functioning, any oxygen reduction can have a serious impact on health. Brain function may be eventually reduced, reactions and judgment are dulled, and of course, cardiovascular function is impaired. Fetuses are especially at risk for this oxygen deprivation (hypoxia) because fetal development is so critically dependent on a sufficient oxygen supply from the mother.

Illness, Premature Death, and Tobacco Use

For people who begin tobacco use as adolescents or young adults, smoke heavily, and continue to smoke, the likelihood of premature death is virtually ensured. Two-pack-a-day cigarette smokers can expect to die 7 to 8 years earlier than their nonsmoking counterparts. (Only nonsmoking-related deaths that can afflict smokers and nonsmokers alike keep the difference at this level rather than much higher.) Not only will these people die sooner, but they will also probably be plagued with painful, debilitating illnesses for an extended time. Smoking is responsible for nearly 440,000 premature deaths each year.[35] An overview of illnesses known to be caused or worsened by tobacco use is presented in Table 9.3.[36]

Cardiovascular Disease

Cardiovascular disease is the leading cause of death among all adults, accounting for 945,836 deaths in the United States in 2000.[37] Tobacco use, and cigarette smoking in particular, is clearly one of the major factors contributing to this cause of death. Although overall progress is being made in reducing the incidence of cardiovascular-related deaths, tobacco use impedes these efforts. So important is tobacco use as a contributing factor in deaths from cardiovascular disease that the cigarette smoker more than doubles the risk of experiencing a **myocardial infarction,** the leading cause of death from cardiovascular disease. Smokers also increase their risk of **sudden cardiac death** by two to four times. Fully one-third of all cardiovascular disease can be traced to cigarette smoking.

The relationship between tobacco use and cardiovascular disease is centered on two major components of tobacco smoke: nicotine and carbon monoxide.

Nicotine and Cardiovascular Disease

The influence of nicotine on the cardiovascular system occurs when it stimulates the nervous system to release norepinephrine. This powerful stimulant increases the heart rate. In turn, an elevated heart rate increases cardiac output, thus increasing blood pressure. The extent to which this is dangerous depends in part on the coronary circulation's ability to supply blood to the rapidly contracting heart muscle. The development of **angina pectoris** and the possibility of sudden heart attack are heightened by this sustained elevation of heart rate, particularly in those individuals with existing coronary artery disease (see Chapter 10).

Key Terms

carbon monoxide (CO) chemical compound that can "inactivate" red blood cells.

myocardial infarction heart attack; the death of heart muscle as a result of a blockage in one of the coronary arteries.

sudden cardiac death immediate death resulting from a sudden change in the rhythm of the heart.

angina pectoris (an **jie** nuh **peck** tor is) chest pain that results from impaired blood supply to the heart muscle.

Table 9.3 Selected Established and Suspected Health Effects of Cigarette Smoking

Category of Condition	Established and Suspected Effects
1 Lung Disease	lung cancer, chronic obstructive lung disease; increased severity of asthma; increased risk of developing various respiratory infections
2 Cancer Risk	esophageal, laryngeal, oral, bladder, kidney, stomach, pancreatic, vulvar, cervical, and colorectal cancers
3 Heart Disease	coronary heart disease; angina pectoris; heart attack; repeat heart attack; arrhythmia; aortic aneurysm; cardiomyopathy
4 Peripheral Vascular Disease	pain and discomfort in the legs and feet resulting from restricted blood flow into the extremities
5 Skin Changes	wrinkling; fingernail discoloration; psoriasis; palmoplantar pustulosis
6 Surgical Risk	need for more anesthesia; increased risk of postsurgical respiratory infection; increased need for supplemental oxygen following surgery; delayed wound healing
7 Orthopedic Problems	disc degeneration; less successful back surgery; musculoskeletal injury; delayed fracture healing
8 Rheumatologic Conditions	osteoporosis and osteoarthritis
9 Environmental Tobacco Smoke and Pediatric Illnesses	infections of the lower respiratory tract; more severe asthma; middle ear infections; Crohn's disease and ulcerative colitis; sudden infant death syndrome; impaired delivery of oxygen to body tissues
10 Complications in Obstetrics and Gynecology	infertility; miscarriage; fetal growth retardation; prematurity; stillbirth; transmission of HIV to the fetus from the infected biological mother; birth defects; intellectual impairment of offspring; sudden infant death syndrome; earlier menopause
11 Male Infertility and Sexuality Dysfunctions	decreased sperm motility; decreased sperm density; impotence
12 Neurological Disorders	transient ischemic attack; stroke; worsened multiple sclerosis
13 Brain and Behavior	depression
14 Abnormalities of the Ears, Nose, and Throat	snoring and hearing loss
15 Eyes	cataracts; complications from Graves' disease; macular degeneration; optic neuropathy
16 Oral Health	periodontal disease
17 Endocrine System	increased metabolic rate; blood-sugar abnormalities; increased waist-to-hip ratio; redistribution of body fat
18 Gastrointestinal Diseases	stomach and duodenal ulcers; Crohn's disease
19 Immune System	impaired humoral and cell-mediated immunity
20 Emergency Medicine	injuries from fires; occupational injuries

Source: Kapier KN, et al. *Cigarettes: What the warning label doesn't tell you.* American Council on Science and Health, 1997.

Nicotine is also a powerful vasoconstrictor of the peripheral blood vessels. As these vessels are constricted by the influence of nicotine, the pressure against their walls increases. Recent research shows that irreversible atherosclerotic damage to major arteries also occurs with smoking.

Nicotine also increases blood **platelet adhesiveness.**[38] As the platelets become more and more likely to "clump," a person will be more likely to develop a blood clot. In people already prone to cardiovascular disease, more rapidly clotting blood is an unwelcome liability. Heart attacks occur when clots form within the coronary arteries or are transported to the heart from other areas of the body.

In addition to other influences on the cardiovascular system, nicotine possesses the ability to decrease the proportion of high-density lipoproteins (HDLs) and to increase the proportion of low-density lipoproteins (LDLs) and very-low-density lipoproteins that constitute the body's serum cholesterol. Low-density lipoproteins appear to support the development of atherosclerosis and are clearly increased in the bloodstreams of smokers. (See Chapter 10 for further information about cholesterol's role in cardiovascular disease.)

Key Terms

platelet adhesiveness tendency of platelets to clump together, thus enhancing the speed at which the blood clots.

A healthy lung (right) vs. the lung of a smoker (left).

 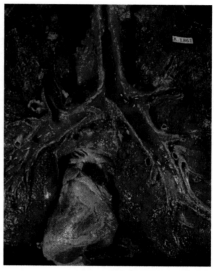

Carbon Monoxide and Cardiovascular Disease

A second substance contributed by tobacco influences the type and extent of cardiovascular disease found among tobacco users. Carbon monoxide interferes with oxygen transport within the circulatory system.

As described earlier in the chapter, carbon monoxide is a component of the gaseous phase of tobacco smoke and readily joins with the hemoglobin of the red blood cells. Carbon monoxide has an affinity for hemoglobin 206 times that of oxygen. Once the hemoglobin of a red cell has accepted carbon monoxide molecules, the hemoglobin is transformed into carboxyhemoglobin. Thereafter, the carboxyhemoglobin permanently weakens the red blood cell's ability to transport oxygen. So long as smoking continues, these red blood cells remain relatively useless during the remainder of their 120-day lives. Levels of carboxyhemoglobin in heavy smokers are associated with significant increases in the incidence of myocardial infarction.

When a person has impaired oxygen-transporting abilities, physical exertion becomes increasingly demanding on both the heart and the lungs. The cardiovascular system will attempt to respond to the body's demand for oxygen, but these responses are themselves impaired as a result of the influence of nicotine on the cardiovascular system. If tobacco does create the good life, as advertisers claim, it also unfortunately lessens the ability to participate actively in that life.

Cancer

Over the past 60 years, research from the most reputable institutions in this country and abroad has consistently concluded that tobacco use is a significant factor in the development of virtually all forms of cancer and the most significant factor in cancers involving the respiratory system.

In describing cancer development, the currently used reference is 20 pack-years, or an amount of smoking equal to smoking one pack of cigarettes a day for 20 years. Thus the two-pack-a-day smoker can anticipate cancer-related tissue changes in as few as 10 years, while the half-pack-a-day smoker may have 40 years to wait. Regardless, the opportunity is there for all smokers to confirm these data by developing cancer as predicted. It is hoped that most people will think twice before disregarding this evidence.

Data supplied by the American Cancer Society (ACS) indicate that during 2003 an estimated 1,334,000 Americans developed cancer.* These cases were nearly equally divided between the sexes and resulted in approximately 556,500 deaths.[35] In the opinion of the ACS, 30% of all cancer cases are heavily influenced by tobacco use.[35] Lung cancer alone accounted for about 171,900 of the new cancer cases and 157,200 deaths in 2003. Fully 87% of men with lung cancer were cigarette smokers.[35] A genetic "missing link" between smoking and lung cancer was established, when mutations to an important tumor suppressor gene were identified. If it was necessary to have a final "proof" that smoking causes lung cancer, that proof appears to be in hand.[39]

Cancer of the entire respiratory system, including lung cancer and cancers of the mouth and throat, accounted for about 185,200 new cases of cancer and 163,700 deaths.[35] Despite these high figures, not all smokers develop cancer.

Respiratory Tract Cancer

Recall that tobacco smoke produces both a gaseous and a particulate phase. As noted, the particulate phase contains the tar fragment of tobacco smoke. This rich chemical

---

*Excluding cases of nonmelanoma skin cancer.

Figure 9-2 Tissue changes associated with bronchogenic carcinoma (lung cancer).

environment contains more than four thousand known chemical compounds, hundreds of which are known to be carcinogens.

In the normally functioning respiratory system, particulate matter suspended in the inhaled air settles on the tissues lining the airways and is trapped in **mucus** produced by specialized *goblet cells*. This mucus, with its trapped impurities, is continuously swept upward by the beating action of hairlike **cilia** of the ciliated columnar epithelial cells lining the air passages (Figure 9-2). On reaching the throat, this mucus is swallowed and eventually removed through the digestive system.

When tobacco smoke is drawn into the respiratory system, however, its rapidly dropping temperature allows the particulate matter to accumulate. This brown, sticky tar contains compounds known to harm the ciliated cells, goblet cells, and the basal cells of the respiratory lining. As the damage from smoking increases, the cilia become less effective in sweeping mucus upward to the throat. When cilia can no longer clean the airway, tar accumulates on the surfaces and brings carcinogenic compounds into direct contact with the tissues of the airway.

At the same time that the sweeping action of the lining cells is being slowed, substances in the tar are stimulating the goblet cells to increase the amount of mucus they normally produce. The "smoker's cough" is the body's attempt to remove this excess mucus.

With prolonged exposure to the carcinogenic materials in tar, predictable changes will begin to occur within the respiratory system's basal cell layer (Figure 9-2). The basal cells begin to display changes characteristic of all cancer cells. In addition, an abnormal accumulation of cells occurs. When a person stops smoking, preinvasive lesions do not repair themselves as quickly as once thought.[41]

By the time lung cancer is usually diagnosed, its development is so advanced that the chance for recovery is very poor. Still today, only 15% of all lung cancer victims survive for 5 years or more after diagnosis.[35] Most die in a very uncomfortable, painful way.

Cancerous activity in other areas of the respiratory system, including the larynx, and within the oral cavity (mouth) follows a similar course. In the case of oral cavity cancer, carcinogens found within the smoke and within the saliva are involved in the cancerous changes. Tobacco users, such as pipe smokers, cigar smokers, and users of smokeless tobacco, have a higher (4 to 10 times) rate of cancer of the mouth, tongue, and voice box.

Key Terms

mucus clear, sticky material produced by specialized cells within the mucous membranes of the body; mucus traps much of the suspended particulate matter within tobacco smoke.

cilia (**sill** ee uh) small, hairlike structures that extend from cells that line the air passages.

In addition to drawing smoke into the lungs, tobacco users swallow saliva that contains an array of chemical compounds from tobacco. As this saliva is swallowed, carcinogens are absorbed into the circulatory system and transported to all areas of the body. The filtering of the blood by the liver, kidneys, and bladder may account for the higher-than-normal levels of cancer in these organs among smokers.

As reported earlier in the chapter, documents released in 1997 from within the tobacco industry clearly show that the major tobacco companies were aware of tobacco's role in the development of cancer and had made a concerted effort to deprive the American public access to such knowledge.

Chronic Obstructive Lung Disease

Chronic obstructive lung disease (COLD), also known as chronic obstructive pulmonary disease (COPD), is a disorder in which the amount of air that flows in and out of the lungs becomes progressively limited. COLD is a disease state that is made up of two separate but related diseases: **chronic bronchitis** and **pulmonary emphysema.**

With chronic bronchitis, excess mucus is produced in response to the effects of smoking on airway tissue, and the walls of the bronchi become inflamed and infected. This produces a characteristic narrowing of the air passages. Breathing becomes difficult, and activity can be severely restricted. With cessation of smoking, chronic bronchitis is reversible.

Emphysema causes irreversible damage to the tiny air sacs of the lungs, the **alveoli.** Chest pressure builds when air becomes trapped by narrowed air passages (chronic bronchitis) and the thin-walled sacs rupture. Emphysema patients lose the ability to ventilate fully. They feel as though they are suffocating. You may have seen people with this condition in malls and other locations as they walk slowly by, carrying or pulling their portable oxygen tanks.

More than 10 million Americans suffer from COLD. It is responsible for a greater limitation of physical activity than any other disease, including heart disease. COLD patients tend to die a very unpleasant, prolonged death, often from a general collapse of normal cardiorespiratory function that results in congestive heart failure (see Chapter 10).

Additional Health Concerns

In addition to the serious health problems stemming from tobacco use already described, other health-related changes are routinely seen. These include a generally poor state of nutrition, the gradual loss of the sense of smell, and premature wrinkling of the skin. Tobacco users are also more likely to experience strokes (a potentially fatal condition), lose bone mass leading to osteoporosis, experience more back pain and muscle injury, and find that fractures heal more slowly. Further, smokers who have surgery spend more time in the recovery room. Although not perceived as a health problem by people who continue smoking in order to control weight, smoking does appear to minimize weight gain. In studies using identical twins, twins who smoked were six to eight pounds lighter than their nonsmoking siblings. Current understanding about why smoking results in lower body weight is less than complete. One factor may be an increase in Basal Metabolic Rate (BMR) (see Chapter 6) brought about by the influence of nicotine on sympathetic nervous system function. Additionally, smokers have a fourfold greater risk of developing serious gum (periodontal) disease. Also, smokers may need supplementation for two important water-soluble vitamins, vitamin C and vitamin B.

Smoking and Reproduction

In all of its dimensions, the reproductive process is impaired by the use of tobacco, particularly cigarette smoking. Problems can be found in association with infertility, problem pregnancy, breastfeeding, and the health of the newborn. So broadly based are reproductive problems and smoking that the term *fetal tobacco syndrome* or *fetal smoking syndrome*[41] is regularly used in clinical medicine. Some physicians even define a fetus being carried by a smoker as a "smoker" and, upon birth, as a "former smoker."

Infertility

Recent research indicates that cigarette smoking by both men and women can reduce levels of fertility. Among men, smoking adversely affects blood flow to erectile tissue, reduces sperm motility, and alters sperm shape, and it

---

Key Terms

chronic bronchitis persistent inflammation and infection of the smaller airways within the lungs.

pulmonary emphysema an irreversible disease process in which the alveoli are destroyed.

alveoli (al **vee** oh lie) thin, saclike terminal ends of the airways; the site at which gases are exchanged between the blood and inhaled air.

causes an overall decrease in the number of viable sperm. Among women, the effects of smoking are seen in terms of abnormal ovum formation, including a lessened ability on the part of the egg to prevent polyspermia, or the fertilization by multiple sperm.[36] Smoking also negatively influences estrogen levels, resulting in underdevelopment of the uterine wall and ineffective implantation of the fertilized ovum. Lower levels of estrogen may also influence the rate of transit of the fertilized egg through the fallopian tube, making it arrive in the uterus too early for successful implantation or, in some cases, restricting movement to the point that an *ectopic,* or *tubal,* pregnancy may develop. Also, the early onset of menopause is associated with smoking.[36]

Problem Pregnancy

The harmful effects of tobacco smoke on the course of pregnancy are principally the result of the carbon monoxide and nicotine to which the mother and her fetus are exposed. Carbon monoxide from the incomplete oxidation of tobacco is carried in the maternal blood to the placenta, where it diffuses across the placental barrier and enters the fetal circulation. Once in the fetal blood, the carbon monoxide bonds with the fetal hemoglobin to form fetal carboxyhemoglobin. As a result of this exposure to carbon monoxide, the fetus is progressively deprived of normal oxygen transport and eventually becomes compromised by chronic **hypoxia.** [41]

Nicotine also exerts its influence on the developing fetus. Thermographs of the placenta and fetus show signs of marked vasoconstriction within a few seconds after inhalation by the mother. This constriction further reduces the oxygen supply, resulting in hypoxia. In addition, nicotine stimulates the mother's stress response, placing the mother and fetus under the potentially harmful influence of elevated epinephrine and corticoid levels (see Chapter 3). Any fetus exposed to all of these agents is more likely to be miscarried, stillborn, or born prematurely.[36] Even when carried to term, children born to mothers who smoked during pregnancy have lower birth weights and may show other signs of a stressful intrauterine life.[41]

Breastfeeding

For women who decide to breastfeed their infants, smoking during this period will continue to expose their children to the harmful effects of tobacco smoke. It is well recognized that nicotine appears in breast milk and thus is capable of exerting its vasoconstricting and stress-response influences on nursing infants. Mothers who stop smoking during pregnancy should be encouraged to continue to refrain from smoking while they are breastfeeding.

Pregnant women and those around them should refrain from smoking to protect the health of the developing fetus.

Neonatal Health Problems

Babies born to women who smoked during pregnancy will, on average, be shorter and have a lower birth weight than children born to nonsmoking mothers. During the earliest months of life, babies born to mothers who smoke experience an elevated rate of death caused by sudden infant death syndrome.[42] Statistics also show that infants are more likely to develop chronic respiratory problems, be hospitalized, and have poorer overall health during their early years of life. Problems such as those just mentioned may also be seen in children of nonsmoking mothers,

---

Key Terms

hypoxia oxygenation deprivation at the cellular level.

when they were exposed prenatally to environmental tobacco smoke. In addition, environmental tobacco smoke exposure extending beyond the home and into the workplace may increase the probability of problem pregnancies and neonatal health problems.[43] Most recently, the interest in the effects of tobacco smoke on pregnancy has been extended to include behavioral differences seen in infants born to women who smoked during pregnancy.[44]

Parenting, in the sense of assuming responsibility for the well-being of children, does not begin at birth, but during the prenatal period. In the case of smoking, this is especially true. Pregnant women who continue smoking are disregarding the well-being of the children they are carrying. Other family members, friends, and coworkers who subject pregnant women to cigarette, pipe, or cigar smoke are, in a sense, exhibiting their own disregard for the health of the next generation.

Oral Contraceptives and Tobacco Use

Women who smoke and use oral contraceptives, particularly after age 35, are placing themselves at a much greater risk of experiencing a fatal cardiovascular accident (heart attack, stroke, or **embolism**) than oral contraceptive users who do not smoke. This risk of cardiovascular complications increases further for oral contraceptive users 40 years of age or older. Women who both smoke and use oral contraceptives are four times more likely to die from myocardial infarction (heart attack) than are women who only smoke. Because of this adverse relationship, *it is strongly recommended that women who smoke should not use oral contraceptives.*

Smokeless Tobacco Use

As the term implies, smokeless tobacco, such as Skoal and Copenhagen, is not burned; rather, it is placed into the mouth. Once in place, the physiologically active nicotine and other soluble compounds are absorbed through the mucous membranes and into the blood. Within a few minutes, chewing tobacco and snuff generate blood levels of nicotine in amounts equivalent to those seen in cigarette smokers.

Chewing tobacco is taken from its foil pouch, formed into a small ball (called a "wad," "chaw," or "chew"), and placed into the mouth. Once in place, the bolus of tobacco is sucked and occasionally chewed, but not swallowed.

Snuff, a more finely shredded smokeless tobacco product, is marketed in small round cans. Snuff is formed into a small mass (or "quid") for dipping or used in prepackaged pouches. The quid or pouch is placed between the jaw and the cheek; the user sucks the quid or pouch, then spits out the brown liquid. Snuff, as once used, was actually a powdered form of tobacco that was inhaled through the nose.

Although smokeless tobacco would seem to free the tobacco user from many of the risks associated with smoking, chewing and dipping are not without their own substantial risks. The presence of *leukoplakia* (white spots) and *erythroplakia* (red spots) on the tissues of the mouth indicate precancerous changes. In addition, an increase in **periodontal disease** (with the pulling away of the gums from the teeth, resulting in later tooth loss), the abrasive damage to the enamel of the teeth, and the high concentration of sugar in processed tobacco all contribute to dental problems among users of smokeless tobacco. In those who develop oral cancer, the risk is dramatically heightened if the cancer metastasizes from the site of origin in the mouth to the brain. Clearly, it is important that users be aware of any signs of damage being done by their use of smokeless tobacco (see the Changing for the Better box on page 255). The validity of this warning was made clear in 1998 when 59% of smokeless tobacco-using major league baseball players were found to have tobacco-related lesions when oral examinations were performed by team physicians on the first day of spring training.

In addition to the damage done to the tissues of the mouth, the need to process the inadvertently swallowed saliva that contains dissolved carcinogens places both the digestive and urinary systems at risk of cancer.

In the opinion of health experts, the use of smokeless tobacco and its potential for life-threatening disease is very real and should not be disregarded. Consequently, television advertisements have been banned, and the following warnings have been placed in rotation on all smokeless tobacco products:

> WARNING: THIS PRODUCT MAY CAUSE MOUTH CANCER

> WARNING: THIS PRODUCT MAY CAUSE GUM DISEASE AND TOOTH LOSS

> WARNING: THIS PRODUCT IS NOT A SAFE ALTERNATIVE TO CIGARETTE SMOKING

Key Terms

embolism a potentially fatal condition in which a circulating blood clot lodges in a smaller vessel.

periodontal disease destruction of soft tissue and bone that surround the teeth.

Clearly, smokeless tobacco is a dangerous product, and little doubt exists that continued use of tobacco in this form is a serious problem to health in all of its dimensions.

The Risks of Involuntary (Passive) Smoking

The smoke generated by the burning of tobacco can be classified as either **mainstream smoke** (the smoke inhaled and then exhaled by the smoker) or **sidestream smoke** (the smoke that comes from the burning end of the cigarette, pipe, or cigar that simply disperses into the air without being inhaled by the smoker). When either form of tobacco smoke is diluted and stays within a common source of air, it can eventually be referred to as **environmental tobacco smoke.** All three forms of tobacco smoke lead to involuntary or passive smoking and can present health problems for both nonsmokers and smokers (see the Discovering Your Spirituality box on page 256).

Surprisingly, mainstream smoke makes up only 15% of our exposure to the harmful substances associated with involuntary smoking. Sidestream smoke is responsible for 85% of the harmful substances associated with second-hand smoke exposure. Because it is not filtered by the tobacco, the filter, or the smoker's body, sidestream smoke contains more free nicotine and produces higher yields of carbon dioxide and carbon monoxide. Much to the detriment of nonsmokers, sidestream smoke has a much higher quantity of highly carcinogenic compounds, called *N-nitrosamines,* than mainstream smoke has.

Current scientific opinion suggests that smokers and nonsmokers are exposed to very much the same smoke when tobacco is used within a common airspace. The important difference is the quantity of smoke inhaled by smokers and nonsmokers. It is likely that for each pack of cigarettes smoked by a smoker, nonsmokers who must share a common air supply with the smokers will involuntarily smoke the equivalent of three to five cigarettes per day. Even today, because of the small size of the particles produced by burning tobacco, environmental tobacco smoke cannot be completely removed from a workplace, restaurant, or shopping mall by the most effective ventilation system.

Recently reported research indicates that involuntary smoke exposure may be responsible for 35,000 to 40,000 premature deaths per year from heart disease among nonsmokers in the United States.[35] Other estimates range upward to 53,000 premature deaths when lung cancer and COPD are included. In addition, large numbers of people exposed to involuntary smoke develop eye irritation, nasal symptoms, headaches, and a cough. Furthermore, most nonsmokers dislike the odor of tobacco smoke.

For these reasons, state, local, and private-sector initiatives to restrict smoking have been introduced. Most

Key Terms

mainstream smoke smoke inhaled and then exhaled by a smoker.

sidestream smoke smoke that comes from the burning end of a cigarette, pipe, or cigar.

environmental tobacco smoke tobacco smoke, regardless of its source, that stays within a common source of air.

The Hidden Price Tag of Smoking

"I started to hug him but felt myself drawing back. It was almost like a reflex action." Those are the words of a young woman after greeting her brother when he returned home from his first semester at college. The young man had recently become a smoker, and his sister was reacting to the strong smell of smoke on his clothes and hair.

Dramatic as it may sound, smoking does set up barriers between people. First, there's the health issue. Some nonsmokers are adamant about not wanting people they care about to smoke. They also want to protect their children from this danger. And they certainly don't want to breathe in smoke themselves. So, at a family gathering, a smoker may want to have a cigarette after dinner, in the living room with everyone else. But the nonsmokers say no—go outside if you want to smoke. In the process, a birthday dinner or a special holiday is marred by this disagreement.

Whether the person is a family member or a friend, it's difficult to feel close to someone who's doing something you disapprove of— such as smoking. But, from the smoker's point of view, it's hard to feel good about someone who acts superior and doesn't accept you as you are. What do children think about all this? Does a "good" aunt or uncle smoke? If smoking is bad, as a little girl constantly hears at school and at home, why does her favorite uncle smoke?

The physical toll that smoking takes is apparent when the smoker finds himself sitting on the sidelines. A young man wants to play basketball with his buddies, but the last time he tried, he had a coughing fit—very embarrassing. A young woman meets some new people, and they ask her to join them for an "easy hike." Well, easy for them. She needs a break after only 10 minutes and sees what looks like pity in her friends' eyes.

On the job, smoking has gone the way of the three-martini lunch. It's just not politically correct. In fact, many companies have a no-smoking policy, or smoking is allowed in designated areas only. Ever drive by a big factory or office building and see a group of people standing outside, perhaps huddled under umbrellas? They're not organizing a strike—they're having a smoke (and being reminded of their high school days). Once again, the smoker feels isolated. Just as in the family group, the smoker feels the judgment of others—only now it's her boss or secretary who's frowning.

The price of smoking is hard to measure. The damage to the smoker's health is beyond dispute. But the spiritual and psychological costs are also real. How does it feel to always be the outsider? The unaccepted? Why does the smoker have to take the chance of missing an exciting play in the stadium to go smoke a cigarette? Or feel the resentment of others at work because he leaves to take a smoking break every hour? It's easy for nonsmokers to say: "Just quit." Smokers know it's not that simple. Many who have stopped smoking—often after several attempts—say that they thought about more than their health in deciding to quit. They thought about many situations—involving family, outdoor activities, and work—before they threw away the pack and said: "That was my last cigarette."

---

buildings in which people work, study, play, reside, eat, or shop now have some smoking restrictions. Some have complete smoking bans. Nowhere is smoking more noticeably prohibited than in the U.S. airline industry. Currently, smoking is banned on all domestic plane flights of less than 6 hours, and most American airlines have extended the ban on smoking to selected international flights as well.

Involuntary smoking poses major threats to nonsmokers within residential settings. Spouses and children of smokers are at greatest risk for involuntary smoking. Scientific studies suggest that nonsmokers married to smokers are three times more likely to experience heart attacks than nonsmoking spouses of nonsmokers, and the former have a 30% greater risk of lung cancer than do the latter. It should be noted, however, that a recent study of 35,561 nonsmoking spouses of smoking partners failed to show significantly higher death rates from heart disease, lung cancer, and COPD than did nonsmoking spouses in nonsmoking relationships.[45]

In spite of what may or may not be the effects of passive smoking on the nonsmoking partners of smokers, the effects of environmental tobacco smoke on the health of children seems well established. The children of parents who smoke are twice as likely as children of nonsmoking parents to experience bronchitis or pneumonia during the first year of life. In addition, throughout childhood these children will experience more wheezing, coughing, and sputum production than will children whose parents do not smoke. Otitis media (middle ear infection), one of the most frequently seen conditions in pediatric medicine, is also significantly more common in children under age 3 who reside with one or more adults who smoke.

In July 1998, the tobacco industry challenged in court the salient 1993 EPA report that was the basis for restricting smoking in a wide array of public places and work sites. The federal judge who heard the case concluded that the principal study used in the report was flawed in its methodology and that its conclusions therefore were of questionable validity. Since this decision, the scientific community has documented to a very substantial degree the inherent dangers of passive or environmental tobacco smoke to the health of nonsmokers and smokers alike. Accordingly, restrictions on public smoking have been large scale and continue to be imposed. The states, cities, and work sites mentioned represent only a partial list of either smoking bans already imposed or bans on tobacco use being considered. Included in this list are statewide bans, including restrictions on all indoor smoking in Delaware; smoking in bars and restaurants in California, Indiana, New York, and Maine; smoking in cars with children under 4 in Georgia; all smoking on school properties in Pennsylvania; and the possession of tobacco products by all teens in Missouri. On a local level, Los Angeles may ban smoking in parks, Purdue University has banned smoking within 25 feet of all residence halls, while the Hartford, Connecticut, Police Department will no longer hire officers who smoke. Perhaps the most encompassing restriction was the March, 2004, banning of smoking in all public buildings in Ireland, including pubs.

Nontobacco Sources of Nicotine

Regardless of whether they are intended as aids to smoking cessation or only supplemental forms of nicotine for use when smoking is not permitted, numerous new forms of nicotine delivery systems have appeared in the marketplace in recent years. An area of growing concerns is, of course, that these nontobacco delivery sources of nicotine could provide introductory exposure to nicotine, at a tragically early age, for the next generation of nicotine-dependent youth. Included among these nontobacco sources of nicotine are multiple flavors of nicotine suckers, nicotine-flavored gum, nicotine straws, nicotine-enhanced water (Nico Water), inhalers, sprays, drops, lozenges, and transdermal patches. To date, only Nico Water has been formally addressed by the Food and Drug Administration, other than those that came into the marketplace as prescription-only or approved OTC products.

Stopping What You Started

Experts in health behavior contend that before people will discontinue harmful health behaviors, such as tobacco use, they must appreciate fully what they are expecting of themselves. This understanding grows in relationship to the following:

1. *Knowledge* about the health risks associated with tobacco use
2. *Recognition* that these health risks are applicable to all tobacco users
3. *Familiarity* with steps that can be taken to eliminate or reduce these risks
4. *Belief* that the benefits to be gained by no longer using tobacco will outweigh the pleasures gained through the use of tobacco
5. *Certainty* that one can start and maintain the behaviors required to stop or reduce the use of tobacco

On closer examination it is evident that these steps combine both knowledge and desire (or motivation). Being knowledgeable about risks, however, will not always stop behaviors that involve varying degrees of psychological and physical dependence. The 75% failure rate thought to be common among tobacco cessation programs suggests that the motivation is not easy to achieve or maintain. In fact, on the basis of information reported by the Hazelden Foundation, for persons who are successful in quitting, approximately 18.6 years elapse between the first attempt to stop and the actual time of quitting. The many health benefits of quitting smoking are shown in Figure 9-3.

A variety of smoking cessation programs exist, including those using highly organized formats, with or without the use of prescription or OTC nicotine replacement systems. In past years, most of the 1.3 million people who managed to quit smoking each year did so by throwing away their cigarettes (going cold turkey) and paying the physical and emotional price of waiting for their bodies to adjust to life without nicotine. Today, however, the use of nicotine replacement products in combination with external smoking cessation approaches, such as those described later in this chapter, or the use of prescription medication, such as antidepressants, is more common. The Changing for the Better box on page 259 provides a plan for smoking cessation that incorporates nicotine replacement products. For those who are concerned

Health on the Web

Behavior Change Activities

Exploring the Benefits of Quitting Smoking

If you or someone you know has been smoking for a long time, you may think it's too late to benefit from quitting. Not so. For encouraging news about quitting smoking, go to **www.wellnessweb.com/smoking/SMOKIQ.HTM** and check your smoking I.Q. While this website is aimed at older smokers, you'll learn why quitting while you're young is better.

Quitting Smoking

There's an old saying that goes, "It's easy to quit smoking—I've done it a hundred times." Quitting smoking is not easy. Few people succeed on their first try. If you'd like some help in making it through this difficult process, go to **www.quitnet.org/.** The site offers quitting tools, e-mail support, and help in finding a local stop-smoking program. Finally, enter your quit date and smoking frequency in the Q Gadget, and the site will keep a running total of how much money you've saved and how much longer you might expect to live as a result of having quit smoking.

Your first year as a nonsmoker

Immediately
- The air around you is no longer dangerous to children and adults

20 Minutes
- Blood pressure improves
- Pulse rate decreases
- Temperature of hands and feet increases to more normal levels

12 Hours
- Body's carbon monoxide level starts to decrease

1 Year
- Risk of early heart disease falls by 50%

24 Hours
- Chance of heart attack decreases

1 to 9 Months
- Fewer coughs, colds, and flu episodes
- Fatigue and shortness of breath decrease
- Lungs increase their ability to remove impurities and reduce infection

Your future years
- Within 10 to 15 years life expectancy comparable to people who never smoked

36 Hours
- Carbon monoxide in blood decreases to healthier levels
- Oxygen in blood increases to healthier levels

2 to 12 Weeks
- Circulation improves
- Lung function improves

48 Hours
- Nerve endings start to regrow
- Exercise gets easier
- Senses of smell and taste improve

Figure 9-3 The health benefits of quitting smoking begin immediately and become more significant the longer you stay smoke-free.

about weight gain following smoking cessation, the Changing for the Better box on page 260 offers some helpful weight management tips.

Programs to help people stop their tobacco use are available in a variety of formats, including educational programs, behavior modification, aversive conditioning, hypnosis, acupuncture, and various combinations of these approaches. Programs are offered in both individual and group settings and are operated by hospitals, universities, health departments, voluntary health agencies, churches, and private practitioners. The better programs will have limited success rates—20% to 50% as measured over one year (with self-reporting), whereas the remainder will have even poorer results. If results are monitored using the assessment of nicotine breakdown products in the blood, the effectiveness rate of these programs falls even lower, as some "successful" self-reporters are not completely honest in their reporting of cessation.

Two methods for weaning smokers from cigarettes to a nontobacco source of nicotine are nicotine-containing chewing gum (Nicorette) and transdermal patches, in either prescription or OTC versions (Nicoderm, Nicotrol, Habitrol, Prostep), using either single-strength or step-

down formulas. A brief description of both gum and the transdermal patch is provided next, although subtle variations exist between prescription and OTC formulations and between brands.

Nicotine-Containing Chewing Gum Correct use of nicotine-containing chewing gum requires an immediate cessation of smoking, an initial determination of dosage (4 mg or 2 mg of nicotine per piece), knowledge of the appropriate manner of chewing each piece of gum, the appropriate time to chew each piece, the maximum number of pieces to be chewed each day, and time to begin withdrawal from the therapy. When used in combination with physician guidance or program support provided by the manufacturer, cessation using nicotine-containing gum may have a success rate of 40% or more, based on blood evaluation. Nicotine-containing chewing gum therapy ranges in cost from an initial $50 kit to weekly refills of approximately $30.

Transdermal Nicotine Patches The more recently developed transdermal (through the skin) nicotine patches appear to be less effective (25%) than the gum just described, but in many ways the patches are more easily used. If a step-down version (21 mg, 14 mg, 7 mg) is employed, determinations must be made as to the appropriate initial dosage (based on number of cigarettes smoked per day and body weight), the length of time at the initial dosage before stepping down, and the manner of withdrawal after a usual 8- to 12-week treatment period. The single-dose (15 mg) version, of course, eliminates the step-down component. Costs associated with transdermal nicotine replacement therapy are similar to those for the gum-based program.

In addition to the nicotine-replacement products already described, a nicotine inhaler and spray has been approved by the FDA. Because of the large surface area of the lungs and rapid absorption into the blood, inhalation-based delivery of nicotine should become a very attractive alternative to transdermal and oral routes of replacement.

In all delivery forms and formulations, nicotine replacement therapy can be associated with contraindications and adverse reactions, including skin irritation, redness, and irregular heart rates.

A recently developed prescription medication, mecamylamine, used in combination with the transdermal nicotine patch improves the latter's effectiveness rate to somewhat above the 40% (perhaps approaching 50%)

level reported for nicotine-containing chewing gum, according to a blood-based assessment. The drug affects receptors in the CNS, reducing the pleasurable effects of nicotine and thus decreasing dependency. An even more recently "discovered" prescription medication for smoking cessation is methoxsalen. Although intended for the treatment of psoriasis, a skin condition, this medication has been found to constructively alter the breakdown of nicotine in persons who have a particular genetic mutation that lessens their need for frequent cigarettes.[46] The most recently approved drug for use in smoking cessation is varenicline. On the basis of clinical trials, it is reported that

How methods of smoking cessation stack up
Of the nation's estimated 48 million smokers, 70% want to quit, and 46% try each year. Only 1 in 40 succeeds. Federal guidelines, based on published studies, estimate varied success rates for a number of medications designed to help smokers quit.

Medications	Nicotine gum	Nicotine inhaler	Buproprion SR (Zyban)	Nicotine spray	Nicotine patch	Combination
Number of studies	13	4	2	3	27	3
Five-month quit rate	23.7%	22.8%	30.5%	30.5%	17.7%	28.6%
Advantage	Can be used to offset cravings	Mimics smoking	Non-nicotine, an antidepressant	Higher nicotine levels	Private, one/day	Combines benefits
Disadvantage	Poor taste	Low nicotine levels	Must screen for seizures	Irritation, sneezing	Skin irritation	Not FDA-approved
Over the counter (OTC) or prescription (Rx)	OTC	Rx	Rx	Rx	Both	Both

Figure 9-4 How methods of smoking cessation stack up.

Source: Treating tobacco use and dependence. U.S Public Health Service: John Hughes, University of Vermont.

nearly one-half of all persons receiving the drug were able to cease smoking.[47] Should this efficacy carry over into long-term trials, this medication would equal or most likely exceed the most effective approaches now available.

Several additional nicotine-free prescription medications to aid smoking cessation have now been approved or are nearing approval. These agents can be used alone or with nicotine replacement therapy. Zyban and Wellbutrin are antidepressant drugs that increase the production of dopamine, a neurotransmitter. Production of dopamine declines when a smoker quits, creating the craving to smoke. Prozac, the serotonin-reuptake inhibitor antidepressant approved for the treatment of depression, bulimia nervosa, PMS, and obsessive-compulsive disorder, has also shown promise as an adjunct to smoking cessation. See Figure 9-4 for a comparison of various cessation approaches.

Those who are concerned that nicotine-replacement therapies are simply a "trade-off" of addictions (from cigarettes to gum or patches) should remember that while using the therapy the former smoker is no longer being exposed to carbon monoxide and carcinogens, while the step-down feature allows for a gradual return to a totally nicotine-free lifestyle. Therefore a short period of cross-addiction should be seen as simply a cost of recovery for those persons who will be successful.

In a recent meta-analysis of smoking cessation program success involving African Americans, it was found that there is no statistically significant difference between the success of this racial group and others. Of interest, however, was a finding that church-based programs might be more successful for smoking cessation than previously recognized.[48]

OnSITE/InSIGHT

Learning to Go: Health

Is smoking a part of your everyday life? Click on Learning to Go: Health on the Online Learning Center at **www.mhhe.com/ Hahn7e** to find more information about tobacco in these lessons:

Lesson 28: Adopt a no-smoking rule.

Lesson 29: Keep your lungs healthy.

Taking Charge of Your Health

- Commit yourself to establishing a smoke-free environment in the places where you live, work, study, and recreate.
- Support friends and acquaintances who are trying to become smoke-free.
- Support legislative efforts, at all levels of government, to reduce your exposure to environmental tobacco smoke.

- Be civil toward tobacco users in public spaces, but respond assertively if they infringe on smoke-free spaces.
- Support agencies and organizations committed to reducing tobacco use among young people through education and intervention.

Summary

- The percentage of American adults who smoke is continuing to decline.
- In spite of a reversal on the part of more recent college graduates, cigarette smoking has traditionally been inversely related to the level of formal education.
- A number of demographical variables influence the incidence of tobacco use.
- The tobacco industry continues to aggressively market its products to potential smokers.
- Multiple theories regarding nicotine's role in dependence have been advanced, including a better understanding of the proportional influences of genetics, environment, and personality.
- Nicotine exerts acute effects both within the central nervous system and on a variety of other tissues and organs.
- Tobacco smoke can be divided into gaseous and particulate phases. Each phase has its unique chemical composition.
- Thousands of chemical components and hundreds of carcinogenic agents are found in tobacco smoke.

- Nicotine and carbon monoxide have predictable effects on the function of the cardiovascular system.
- The development of nearly one-third of all cancers can be attributed to tobacco use, and virtually every form of cancer is found more frequently in smokers than in nonsmokers.
- Chronic obstructive lung disease (COLD), also called chronic obstructive pulmonary disease (COPD), is a likely consequence of long-term cigarette smoking, with early symptoms appearing shortly after beginning regular smoking.
- Smoking alters normal structure and function of the body, as seen in a wide variety of noncardiovascular and noncancerous conditions, such as infertility, problem pregnancy, and neonatal health concerns.

- Additional health concerns include the diminished ability to smell, periodontal disease, vitamin inadequacies, and bone loss leading to osteoporosis.
- The use of smokeless tobacco carries its own health risks, including oral cancer.
- The presence of secondhand smoke results in involuntary (or passive) smoking by those who must share a common air source with smokers. This secondhand smoke threatens the health of the spouse, children, and coworkers of the smoker.
- Stopping smoking can be undertaken in any one of several ways, including within a group setting or on an individual basis. A variety of supportive medications are also available.

Review Questions

1. What percentage of the American adult population smoke? In what direction has change been occurring?
2. What is the current direction that adolescent smoking is taking?
3. What was the outcome of the class action suit brought by the forty-six states, and what was the effect of the Master Settlement Agreement (1999) on the ability of the tobacco industry to market its products?
4. In comparison to cigarettes, what health risks are associated with pipe and cigar smoking?
5. What are the two principal dimensions of nicotine dependence? What are specific aspects seen within physical dependence? To which dimension does compulsion belong?
6. What percentage of smokers appear to be strongly addicted to nicotine?
7. Identify each of the theories of nicotine dependence discussed in the chapter.
8. How do modeling and manipulation explain the development of emotional dependence on tobacco?

9. In the amount consumed by the typical smoker, what is the effect of nicotine on central nervous system function? How does this differ in chain smokers?
10. What effects does nicotine have on the body outside of the central nervous system? How does the influence of nicotine resemble that associated with the stress response?
11. What is the principal effect of carbon monoxide on cardiac function?
12. What influences does passive smoking have on non-smoking adult partners of smokers? On their children?
13. How is the federal government attempting to limit the exposure that children and adolescents currently have to tobacco products and tobacco advertisements?
14. What prescription and OTC products are now available to assist smokers in quitting?
15. What percentage of smokers are able to quit, and how many attempts to quit are generally required?

References

1. *Nextel to take wheel at NASCAR*. CNNMoney, June 18, 2003 (online service).
2. Wakefield MA, et al. Tobacco industry marketing of point of purchase after the 1999 MSA billboard ban. *AJPH* 9, No. 6, June 2002.
3. Prevalence of current cigarette smoking among adults and changes in prevalence of current and some day smoking—2001. *MMWR* 52(14), April 2003.
4. Smoking and Health: Report of the Advisory Committee to the Surgeon General of the Public Health Service. U.S. Department of Health and Human Services. Public Health Service. 1964.
5. U.S. National Center for Health Statistics: *Health, United States, 2002: Early release of selected estimates based on data from the 2002 National Health Interview Survey*, 2002.

6. *Cigarette smoking among adults—United States 1998.* Tobacco Information and Prevention Sources (TIPS).

7. National Center for Health Statistics: *Health, United States, 1998, with socioeconomic status and health chartbook.* NCHS, 1998.

8. *2000 Statistics on Alcohol and Other Drug Uses on College Campuses.* The Core Institute. Southern Illinois University. 2000 http://www.siu/edu/departments/coreinst/public_html/2000.html

9. Johnston LD, O'Malley PM, Bachman JG. *Cigarettes: trends in thirty-day prevalence of use by subgroups for eighth and tenth graders.* Monitoring the Future Study–2002. The University of Michigan, 2003.

10. Rigotti NA, Lee JE, Weschler H. U.S. college use of tobacco products: results of a national survey. *JAMA* 284(6):699–705, 2000.

11. Schoenborn CA, Jackline VL, Barnes PM. *Cigarette smoking behavior of adults: United States, 1998.* Advanced Data from Vital and Health Statistics, No. 331. Division of Interview Statistics, National Center for Vital Statistics, February 2003.

12. *National household survey on drug abuse main findings 1998* (H-11). Substance Abuse and Mental Health Services. Department of Health and Human Services. March 2000.

13. Massachusetts Department of Health, as reported in *USA Today,* 8 May 2000.

14. Tickle JJ, et al. Favourite movie stars, their tobacco use in contemporary movies, and its association with adolescent smoking. *Tob Control* 10(1):16–22, March 2001.

15. Surveillance for selected tobacco-use behaviors— U.S. 1990–1994. *MMWR* 43(SS-3): 1–43, 1995.

16. State-specific prevalence of current cigarette smoking and cigar smoking among adults—United States, 1998. *MMWR* 48(45):1034–1039, 1999.

17. U.S. Substance Abuse and Mental Health Services. *Summary of findings from the 2000 National Household Survey on Drug Abuse,* 2001.

18. Shapiro JA, Jacobs EJ, Thun MJ. Cigar smoking in men and the risk of death from tobacco-related cancers. *J Natl Cancer Inst* 92(4):333–337, 2000.

19. Burns DM, ed. *Cigars: health effects and trends.* Cancer Monograph Series (No. 9) National Cancer Institute, 1998.

20. Iribarren C, et al. Evidence of cigar smoking on the risk of cardiovascular disease, chronic obstructive pulmonary disease, and cancer in men. *N Engl J Med* 340(23):1173–1180, 1999.

21. Zickler P. Evidence builds that genes influence cigarette smoking. *NIDA Notes* 15(3)1–15, 2000.

22. Sayette MA, et al. A multi-dimensional analysis of cue-elicited craving in heavy smokers and tobacco chippers. *Addiction* 96(10):1419–1432, 2001.

23. Sullivan PK, Kendler KS. The genetic epidemiology of smoking. *Nicotine Tob Res, Suppl.* 2:S51–7, 1999.

24. Longnecker GL. *How drugs work: drug abuse and the human body.* Ziff-Davis Press. 1994.

25. Olive MF, et al. Stimulation of endorphin neuro-transmission in the nucleus accumbens by ethanol, cocaine, and amphetamine. *J of Neurosci* 21(23):RC 184, December 2001.

26. Balfour DJ, Ridley DL. The effects of nicotine on neural pathways implicated in depression. *Pharmacol Biochem Behav* 66(1):79–85, 2000.

27. DiFranza JR, et al. Development of symptoms of tobacco dependence in youth: 30-month follow-up from the DANDY study. *Tob Control* 11(3):228–235, 2002.

28. *17. Tobacco.* School of Veterinary Medicine. Purdue University. http://www.vet.purdue/edu/depts/addl/toxic/plant17.htm

29. Simons-Morton BG. Prospective analysis of peer and parental influences on smoking initiation among early adolescents. *Prev Sci* 3(4):275–283, December 2002.

30. Bricker JB, et al. Nine-year prospective relationship between parental smoking cessation and children's daily smoking. *Addiction* 98(5):585–593, May 2003.

31. Pechmann C, Reibling RT. Anti-smoking advertising campaigns targeting youth: case studies from USA and Canada. *Tob Control* 9 Suppl. :118–131, 2000.

32. Mulcahy S. *The toxicology of cigarette smoke and environmental tobacco smoke.* A Review of Cigarette Smoke and Its Toxicological Effects. http://www.csn.ul.ie/-stephen/reports/bc4927.html

33. Saladin KS. *Anatomy and physiology: the unit of form and function.* 3rd ed. McGraw-Hill, 2004.

34. Hecht MI. Smoking cessation: pre-operative. *University of Wisconsin anesthesia topics.* November 1998.

35. *Cancer facts & figures—2003.* Atlanta: Cancer Society, 2002.

36. Kapier KN, et al. *Cigarettes: What the warning label doesn't tell you.* American Council on Science and Health, 1997.

37. American Heart Association. *Heart disease and stroke Statistics—2003 update.* 2002.

38. Lilienberg G, Venge P. Platelet adhesion in patients prone to arterial and venous thrombosis: the impact of gender, smoking and heredity. *Scand J Clin Lab Invest* 58(4):279–284. 1998.

39. Campling B, EI-Deiry W. Clinical implications of p53 mutation in lung cancer. *Mol Biotechnol* 24(2):141–156, June 2003.

40. Lam S, et al. Sex-related differences in bronchial epithelial changes associated with tobacco smoking. *J Natl Cancer Inst* 91(8):691–696 April, 1999.

41. Habek D, et al. Fetal tobacco syndrome and perinatal outcome. *Fetal Diagn Ther* 17(6):367–371, November–December 2002.

42. Fleming PJ, et al. Sudden infant death syndrome and social deprivation: assessing epidemiological factors after post-matching for deprivation. *Paediatr Perinat Epidemiol* 17(3):272–280. July 2003.

43. Misra DP, Nguyen RH. Environmental tobacco smoke and low birth weight: a hazard in the workplace? *Enviro Health Perspect* 107 (suppl) (6):897–904. 1999.

44. Keknabson IA, et al. Maternal smoking during pregnancy and behavioral characteristics in 2–4-month infants. *Klin Padiatr* 214(6):359–364. 2002.

45. Enstrom JE, Kabat GC. Environmental tobacco smoke- and tobacco-related mortality in a prospective study of Californians, 1660–1998. *BMJ.* 326(7398):1048–1049, May 2003.

46. Sellers EM, Kaplan HL, Tyndale RF. Inhibition of cytochrome P450 2A6 increases nicotine's oral bioavailability and decreases smoking. *Clin Pharmacol Ther* 68(1):35–43. 2000.

47. Pfizer unveils anti-smoking drug. *CNN Money,* June 17, 2003. http://www.money.cnn.com/2003/06/17/news/companies/pfizer/index.htm

48. Pederson LL, et al. Smoking cessation among African Americans: what we know and do not know about interventions and self-quitting. *Prev Med* 31(1):23–38. 2000.

As We Go to Press

On pages 255–257 your textbook discusses the growing displeasure with smoking that results from the inclusion of environmental tobacco smoke in the lives of nonsmokers. Two recent events lend further credence to the continuing efforts to ban all public smoking.

The first report stems from an initial follow-up study of a small group of New York City bar and restaurant workers three months following the introduction (July 2004) of laws prohibiting smoking in virtually all of the city's public buildings, including their places of employment. Using as a baseline the blood levels of a nicotine breakdown product, cotinine, taken just before the ban went into effect, the researchers found that by the end of three months an 85% decrease in cotinine levels had occurred. On the basis of this significant drop in cotinine in such a relatively short period of time, a clearer picture of the negative influences associated with environmental tobacco smoke exposure can be more fully appreciated.

A second aspect of the ongoing movement to protect nonsmokers from the harmful effects of environmental tobacco smoke is the recent recommendation of the state of Maine's Health and Human Services Committee to ban smoking in the homes and cars of foster parents when foster children are present. If approved by the state's House and Senate and signed into law by the governor, this ban will most likely serve as a model for other states who hold concerns for the well-being of foster children—whose care is paid for through state funds.

focus on

hypnotism: a solution for smokers?

On at least one occasion each year a "professional" hypnotist visits the community in which we (the authors) live. A large advertisement appears in the local paper a day or two before his visit to identify his location (usually a motel conference room) and the problems (obesity and smoking) that his brand of hypnosis will prove effective against. The cost of a one-time session generally ranges between $30 (for one condition) and $50 (for both conditions), with a discount for groups of two or more preregistered persons. Effective rates are generally stated to be 97.5 percent for weight reduction and 98 percent for smoking abatement. The term "effective" is, of course, never defined.

In terms of smoking abatement, what about the services of a clinically trained and hospital-based psychologist who specializes in the use of hypnosis? Does hypnosis of this type have efficacy in smoking abatement—either as a sole treatment modality or in combination with other therapies?

In an attempt to answer this question, a Med-Line search using the key word "hypnosis" was conducted with the following results. In the time period between January and August 2000, sixty-eight studies addressing the clinical application of hypnosis were published in the medical literature. Of these, three studies were related to the use of hypnosis in smoking abatement. Two of the three studies reported involved the meta-analysis of 59 and 9 earlier studies, respectively. On the basis of 59 earlier studies, the authors of the largest of the current studies concluded that "hypnosis cannot be considered a specific and efficacious treatment for smoking cessation." They did acknowledge that hypnosis is "possibly efficacious," but only when cognitive/behavioral and educational intervention that often accompanies hypnosis is included in the study.[1] The authors of the second and smallest (9 earlier studies) of the current studies concluded that they were unable to show "that hypnotherapy

has a greater effect on six month quit rates than other interventions or no treatment."[2]

Searches involving the websites of The National Center for Complementary and Alternative Medicine and American Psychological Association failed to identify studies related to hypnosis and smoking cessation. In all three searches, however, ample evidence was found related to the efficacy of hypnosis in the treatment of inflammatory bowel disease, inflammatory conditions of the oral cavity, temporal-mandibular joint dysfunction, tension headaches, radiological procedures involving the injection of contrast mediums, and an array of other conditions in both adults and children.

1. Green JD, Lynn SJ. Hypnosis and suggestion-based approaches to smoking cessation: an examination of the evidence. *Int J Clin Hypn.* 48(2): 195–224. 2000.

2. Abbot NC, et al. Hypnotherapy for smoking cessation. *Cochrane Data Base Syst Rev.* 2000.

personal assessment

how much do you know about cigarette smoking?

Are the following assumptions about smoking true or false?
Take your best guess, and then read the answer to the right of
each statement.

Assumption

1. There are now safe cigarettes on the market.

2. A small number of cigarettes can be smoked without risk.

3. Most early changes in the body resulting from cigarette smoking are temporary.

4. Filters provide a measure of safety to cigarette smokers.

5. Low-tar, low-nicotine cigarettes are safer than high-tar, high-nicotine brands.

6. Mentholated cigarettes are better for the smoker than are nonmentholated brands.

7. It has been scientifically proven that cigarette smoking causes cancer.

8. No specific agent capable of causing cancer has ever been identified in the tobacco used in smokeless tobacco.

9. The cure rate for lung cancer is so good that no one should fear developing this form of cancer.

10. Smoking is not harmful as long as the smoke is not inhaled.

11. The "smoker's cough" reflects underlying damage to the tissue of the airways.

12. Cigarette smoking does not appear to be associated with damage to the heart and blood vessels.

13. Because of the design of the placenta, smoking does not present a major risk to the developing fetus.

14. Women who smoke cigarettes and use an oral contraceptive should decide which they wish to continue because there is a risk in using both.

15. Air pollution is a greater risk to our respiratory health than is cigarette smoking.

16. Addiction, in the sense of physical addiction, is found in conjunction with cigarette smoking.

Discussion

F   Depending on the brand, some cigarettes contain less tar and nicotine; none are safe, however.

F   Even a low level of smoking exposes the body to harmful substances in tobacco smoke.

T   Some changes, however, cannot be reversed—particularly changes associated with emphysema.

T   However, the protection is far from adequate.

T   Many people, however, smoke low-tar, low-nicotine cigarettes in a manner that makes them just as dangerous as stronger cigarettes.

F   Menthol simply makes cigarette smoke feel cooler. The smoke contains all of the harmful agents found in the smoke from regular cigarettes.

T   Particularly lung cancer and cancers of the larynx, esophagus, oral cavity, and urinary bladder.

F   Unfortunately, smokeless tobacco is no safer than the tobacco that is burned. The user of smokeless tobacco swallows much of what the smoker inhales.

F   Approximately 14% of people who have lung cancer will live the 5 years required to meet the medical definition of "cured."

F   Because of the toxic material in smoke, even its contact with the tissue of the oral cavity introduces a measure of risk in this form of cigarette use.

T   The cough occurs in response to an inability to clear the airway of mucus as a result of changes in the cells that normally keep the air passages clear.

F   Cigarette smoking is in fact the single most important risk factor in the development of cardiovascular disease.

F   Children born to women who smoked during pregnancy show a variety of health impairments, including smaller birth size, premature birth, and more illnesses during the first year of life. Smoking women also have more stillbirths than do nonsmokers.

T   Women over 35 years of age, in particular, are at risk of experiencing serious heart disease should they continue using both cigarettes and an oral contraceptive.

F   Although air pollution does expose the body to potentially serious problems, the risk is considerably less than that associated with smoking.

T   Dependence, including true physical addiction, is widely recognized in cigarette smokers.

1. #1
2. blood
3. a, h, g, r
4. heart
5. CVD
6. < 120/80
7. 200 or less
8. CHF
9. ♂ for women
10. Art. plaque
11. Aspirin
12. (long one)
13. aneurysm
14. diabetes
15. children

chapter ten

reducing your risk of cardiovascular disease

Chapter Objectives

After reading this chapter, you should be able to:

▌ describe the prevalence of cardiovascular disease compared to other diseases.

▌ list the cardiovascular disease risk factors and distinguish between those that can vs. cannot be modified.

▌ explain how each of the modifiable cardiovascular disease risk factors can be changed.

▌ explain the signs of a heart attack and the recommended action that should be taken.

▌ explain how coronary heart disease is diagnosed and treated.

▌ explain the recommendations for prevention and treatment of hypertension.

▌ distinguish between the different types of stroke.

Online Learning Center Resources

www.mhhe.com/hahn7e

Log on to our Online Learning Center (OLC) for access to these additional resources:

- Chapter key terms and definitions
- Learning objectives
- Student interactive question-and-answer sites

- Self-scoring chapter quiz
- Online assessments
- Key term flash cards

Talking It Over

Encouraging Children to Be Active

You understand the value of being physically active. The challenge is to communicate this message to your kids—kids who are avalanched by video games, fast foods, rented movies, big screen TV, and hundreds of television channels!

- *Be a positive role model.* By your actions, show children that physical activity is fun.
- *Play with your kids.* Ask if they want to shoot baskets or teach you dance steps.
- *Don't preach.* Lectures just aren't as interesting as TV.

- *Support efforts at physical activity.* Praise kids when they're active. Help them get involved in activities they enjoy and help them be successful at them.
- *Limit passive activities.* Set time limits on TV watching and video-game playing.

CommunicationLinks

www.a1.com/ncppa
www.kidshealth.org
www.fantasyfit.com

Eye on the Media

How Credible Are Online Health Sites?

If you're looking for accurate health information on the Internet, make the site's credibility your first priority. Since just about anyone can post information on the web (within legal limits), what you find there ranges from opinion to balanced, carefully researched information. Your challenge is to distinguish between reliable and dubious information.

According to health professionals Kotecki and Chamness,[1] certain key information can help you determine a health information website's credibility. They suggest using the following six criteria: (1) scope, (2) accuracy, (3) authority,

If you're a traditional-age college student, you may have a difficult time realizing the importance of **cardiovascular** health. Unless you were born with a heart problem, it's easy to think that cardiovascular damage will not occur until you reach your 50s or 60s. During your young adult years, you're much more likely to be concerned about cancer and sexually transmitted diseases.

Yet autopsy reports on teenagers and young adults who have died in accidents are now showing that relatively high percentages of young people have developed changes consistent with coronary artery disease; that is, fatty deposits have already formed in their coronary arteries. (See the Learning from Our Diversity box on page 272 to discover why these changes have occurred.) Since the foundation for future heart problems starts early in life, cardiovascular health is a very important topic for all college students.

Heart disease continues to be the number one killer of Americans; between 1990 and 2000 the death rates from cardiovascular disease (CVD) declined 17%.[2] The

American Heart Association, in its 2004 *Heart and Stroke Statistical Update,* credits this reduction to a combination of changing American lifestyles and medical advances in the diagnosis and treatment of CVD.[2]

This chapter explains how the heart works. It also will help you identify your CVD risk factors and suggest ways you can alter certain lifestyle behaviors to reduce your risk of developing heart disease.

Prevalence of Cardiovascular Disease

Cardiovascular diseases were directly related to 38.5% of deaths in the United States in 2001 and indirectly related to a large percentage of additional deaths.[2] Heart disease, stroke, and related blood vessel disorders combined to kill nearly 1 million Americans in 2001 (Figure 10-1).[2] This figure represents more deaths than were caused by cancer, accidents, pneumonia, influenza, lung diseases, diabetes, and AIDS combined. CVD causes one out of every 2.6 deaths in the United States.[2] Indeed, cardiovascular disease is our nation's number one "killer" (see Table 10.1).

Normal Cardiovascular Function

The cardiovascular or circulatory system uses a muscular pump to send a complex fluid on a continuous trip

Table 10.1 Estimated Prevalence of Major Cardiovascular Diseases*

Coronary heart disease	12,900,000
Hypertension	58,000,000
Stroke	4,700,000
Congenital heart disease	1,000,000
Rheumatic heart disease	1,800,000
Congestive heart failure	4,900,000
TOTAL[†]	83,300,000

*61,800,000 people total.
[†]The sum of the individual estimates exceeds 61,800,000 because many people have more than one cardiovascular disorder. For example, many people with coronary heart disease also have hypertension.

Key Terms

cardiovascular pertaining to the heart (cardio) and blood vessels (vascular).

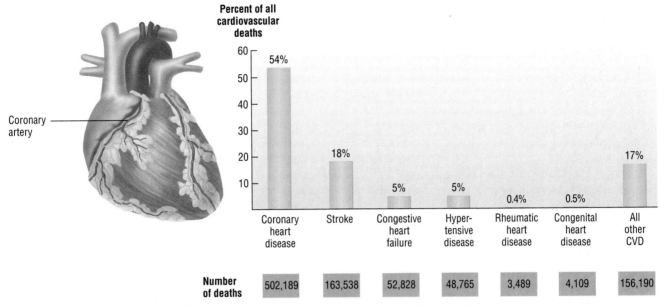

Figure 10-1 Of the 931,108 deaths in the United States in 2001* resulting from cardiovascular diseases, half were attributable to heart attack.[2] (**The most recent year for which statistics are available.*)

through a closed system of tubes. The pump is the heart, the fluid is blood, and the closed system of tubes is the network of blood vessels.

The Vascular System

The term *vascular system* refers to the body's blood vessels. Although we might be familiar with the arteries (vessels that carry blood away from the heart) and the veins (vessels that carry blood toward the heart), arterioles, capillaries, and venules are also included in the vascular system.

Arterioles are the farther, small-diameter extensions of arteries. These arterioles lead eventually to capillaries, the smallest extensions of the vascular system. At the capillary level, exchanges of oxygen, food, and waste occur between cells and the blood.

Once the blood leaves the capillaries and begins its return to the heart, it drains into small veins, or venules. The blood in the venules flows into increasingly larger vessels called *veins*. Blood pressure is highest in arteries and lowest in veins, especially the largest veins, which empty into the right atrium of the heart.

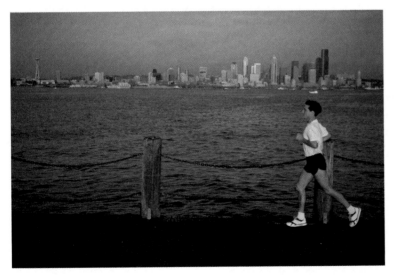

Regular exercise helps strengthen the heart muscle and increase HDL cholesterol.

The Heart

The heart is a four-chambered pump designed to create the pressure required to circulate blood throughout the body. Usually considered to be about the size of a person's clenched fist, this organ lies slightly tilted between the lungs in the central portion of the **thorax.** The heart does not lie completely in the center of the chest. Approximately two-thirds of the heart is to the left of the body midline, and one third is to the right.

Two upper chambers, called *atria,* and two lower chambers, called *ventricles,* form the heart.[3] The thin-walled atrial chambers are considered collecting chambers, and the thick-walled muscular ventricles are considered the pumping chambers. The right and left sides of the heart are divided by a partition called the *septum.* Use Figure 10-2 to follow the flow of blood through the heart's four chambers.

For the heart muscle to function well, it must be supplied with adequate amounts of oxygen. The two main **coronary arteries** (and their numerous branches) accomplish this. These arteries are located outside the heart (see Figure 10-1). If the coronary arteries are diseased, a heart attack (myocardial infarction) is possible.

Heart Stimulation

The heart contracts and relaxes through the delicate interplay of **cardiac muscle** tissue and cardiac electrical centers called *nodes.* Nodal tissue generates the electrical impulses necessary to contract heart muscle.[4] The heart's electrical activity is measured by an instrument called an *electrocardiograph* (ECG or EKG), which provides a printout called an electrocardiogram, which can be evaluated to determine cardiac electrical functioning.

Blood

The average-sized adult has approximately 5 quarts of blood in his or her circulatory system. The functions of blood, which are performed continuously, are similar to the overall functions of the circulatory system and include the following:

- Transportation of nutrients, oxygen, wastes, hormones, and enzymes
- Regulation of water content of body cells and fluids
- Buffering to help maintain appropriate pH balance of body fluids

Key Terms

thorax the chest; portion of the torso above the diaphragm and within the rib cage.

coronary arteries vessels that supply oxygenated blood to heart muscle tissues.

cardiac muscle specialized muscle tissue that forms the middle (muscular) layer of the heart wall.

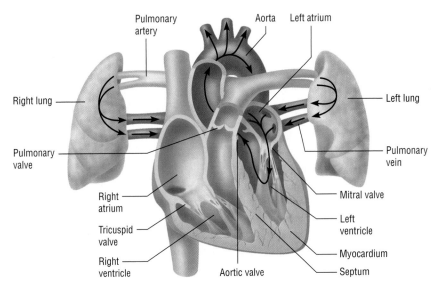

Pulmonary artery

Aorta

Left atrium

Right lung

Left lung

Pulmonary valve

Pulmonary vein

Right atrium

Mitral valve

Tricuspid valve

Left ventricle

Right ventricle

Myocardium

Aortic valve

Septum

Figure 10-2 The heart functions like a complex double pump. The right side of the heart pumps deoxygenated blood to the lungs. The left side of the heart pumps oxygenated blood through the aorta to all parts of the body. Note the thickness of the walls of the ventricles. These are the primary pumping chambers.

- Regulation of body temperature; the water component in the blood absorbs heat and transfers it
- Prevention of blood loss; by coagulating or clotting, the blood can alter its form to prevent blood loss through injured vessels
- Protection against toxins and microorganisms, accomplished by chemical substances called *antibodies* and specialized cellular elements circulating in the bloodstream

Cardiovascular Disease Risk Factors

As you have just read, the heart and blood vessels are among the most important structures in the human body. By protecting your cardiovascular system, you lay the groundwork for an exciting, productive, and energetic life. The best time to start protecting and improving your cardiovascular system is early in life, when lifestyle patterns are developed and reinforced (see Learning from Our Diversity, page 272). Of course, it's difficult to move backward through time, so the second best time to start protecting your heart is today. Improvements in certain lifestyle activities can pay significant dividends as your life unfolds. Complete the Personal Assessment on page 291 to determine your risk for heart disease.

The American Heart Association encourages people to protect and enhance their heart health by examining the ten cardiovascular risk factors related to various forms of heart disease.[5] A *cardiovascular risk factor* is an attribute that a person has or is exposed to that increases the likelihood that he or she will develop some form of heart disease. The first three risk factors are ones you will be unable to change. An additional six risk factors are ones you can change. One final risk factor is one that is thought to be a contributing factor to heart disease.

Risk Factors That Cannot Be Changed

The three risk factors that you cannot change are increasing age, male gender, and heredity.[5] However, your knowledge that they might be an influence in your life should encourage you to make a more serious commitment to the risk factors you can change.

Increasing Age

Heart diseases tend to develop gradually over the course of one's life. Although we may know of a few people who experienced a heart attack in their twenties or thirties, most of the serious consequences of heart disease are evident in older ages. For example, approximately 84% of people who die from heart diseases are age 65 and older.[2]

Male Gender

Women have lower rates of heart disease than men prior to age 55. Yet when women move through menopause (typically in their fifties), their rates of heart disease are similar to those of men (see the Star box on page 274). It is thought that women are somewhat more protected from heart disease than men because of their natural production of the hormone estrogen during their fertile years.

Heredity

Like increasing age and male gender, heredity cannot be changed. By the luck of the draw, some people are born into families in which heart disease has never been a serious problem; others are born into families in which heart disease is quite prevalent. In this latter case, children

Women and Heart Disease

Is heart disease mainly a problem for men? According to the American Heart Association, the answer is a resounding NO. In fact, data indicate that 53% of all cardiovascular disease deaths occur in women. Cardiovascular disease is the leading cause of death for American women and kills nearly twice as many women as do all forms of cancer combined. Presently, one in five women has some sort of heart or blood vessel disease. Over 60% of stroke deaths occur in women. Also 38% of women who have heart attacks will die within a year, compared with 25% of men. From age 55, higher percentages of women than men have high blood pressure.[1]

For many years, it was thought that men were at much greater risk than women for the development of cardiovascular problems. Today it is known that young men are more prone to heart disease than young women, but once women reach menopause (usually in their early to middle 50s), their rates of heart-related problems quickly equal those of men.

The protective mechanism for young women seems to be the female hormone estrogen. Estrogen appears to help women maintain a beneficial profile of blood fats. When the production of estrogen is severely reduced at menopause, this protective factor no longer exists. Prescribing estrogen replacement therapy (ERT) was a common practice by many physicians in treating a number of factors in postmenopausal women. One of the benefits of ERT was considered to be prevention of cardiovascular diseases. However, in 2002 a major clinical research trial was stopped due to the finding that more women on ERT were experiencing heart attacks and strokes. Thus, the American Heart Association now recommends that ERT should not be used for the purpose of preventing cardiovascular diseases. Certainly, ERT may still be utilized for other purposes (i.e., relief of menopausal symptoms or osteoporosis prevention).[2] Women who are prescribed ERT need to be aware of the increased risk for cardiovascular disease in evaluating its value. Certainly, much more research is underway that may influence the use of ERT in the future. Women should discuss the risks and benefits of ERT with their physicians.

Young women should not rely solely on naturally produced estrogen to prevent heart disease. The general recommendations for maintaining heart health—good diet, adequate physical activity, monitoring blood pressure and cholesterol levels, controlling weight, avoiding smoking, and managing stress—will benefit women at every stage of life.

1. American Heart Association: **www.americanheart. org/Heart and Stroke A Z Guide/womens/,** September 1, 2001.
2. American Heart Association: **http://www.americanheart.org/presenter.jhtml?identifier=4536,** July 21, 2003.

are said to have a genetic predisposition (tendency) to develop heart disease as they grow and develop throughout their lives. These people have every reason to be highly motivated to reduce the risk factors they can control.

Race is also a consideration related to heart disease. African Americans have moderately high blood pressure at rates twice that of whites and severe hypertension at rates three times higher than whites (for a detailed discussion of this topic, see the Focus On article on page 288). Hypertension significantly increases the risk of both heart disease and stroke; however, it can be controlled through a variety of methods. It is especially important for African Americans to take advantage of every opportunity to have their blood pressure measured so that preventive actions can be started immediately if necessary.

Risk Factors That Can Be Changed

There are six cardiovascular risk factors that are influenced largely by our lifestyle choices. These risk factors are cigarette and tobacco smoke, physical inactivity, high blood cholesterol level, high blood pressure, diabetes mellitus, and obesity and overweight.[4] Healthful behavior changes you make for these "big six" risk factors can help you protect and enhance your cardiovascular system.

Tobacco Smoke

Smokers have a heart attack risk that is 2–4 times that of nonsmokers. Smoking cigarettes is the major risk factor associated with sudden cardiac death. In fact, smokers have two to four times the risk of dying from sudden cardiac arrest than nonsmokers.

Cigarette or tobacco smoke also adversely affects nonsmokers who are exposed to environmental tobacco smoke. Studies suggest that the risk of death caused by heart disease is increased about 30% in people exposed to secondhand smoke in the home. Because of the health threat to nonsmokers, restrictions on indoor smoking in public areas and business settings are increasing tremendously in every part of the country.

For years, it was believed that if you had smoked for many years, it was pointless to try to quit; the damage to one's health could never be reversed. However, the American Heart Association now indicates that by quitting smoking, regardless of how long or how much you have smoked, your risk of heart disease declines rapidly. For people who have smoked a pack or less of cigarettes per day, within 3 years after quitting smoking, their heart disease risk is virtually the same as those who never smoked.

This news is exciting and should encourage people to quit smoking, regardless of how long they have smoked. Of course, if you have started to smoke recently, the healthy approach would be to quit now—before the nicotine controls your life and leads to heart disease or damages your lungs or causes lung cancer. (For additional information about the health effects of tobacco, see Chapter 9.)

 TALKING POINTS A friend complains of not being able to quit smoking after several serious attempts. How could you direct this person toward a new approach?

Physical Inactivity

Lack of regular physical activity is a significant risk factor for heart disease. Regular aerobic exercise (discussed in Chapter 4) helps strengthen the heart muscle, maintain healthy blood vessels, and improve the ability of the vascular system to transfer blood and oxygen to all parts of the body. Additionally, physical activity helps lower overall blood cholesterol levels for most people, encourages weight loss and retention of lean muscle mass, and allows people to moderate the stress in their lives.

With all the benefits of physical activity, it amazes health professionals that so many Americans refuse to become regularly active. Some people feel that they don't have enough time or that they must work out strenuously. However, you'll recall from Chapter 4 that only 20 to 60 minutes of moderate aerobic activity three to five times each week can decrease your risk of heart disease. This is not a large price to pay for a lifetime of cardiovascular health. Find a partner and get started! Discovering Your Spirituality (page 276) discusses how the benefits of physical activity extend into the spiritual dimension of your life.

If you are middle-aged or older and have been inactive, consult with a physician before starting an exercise program. Also, if you have any known health condition that could be aggravated by physical activity, check with a physician first.

 TALKING POINTS You've started exercising many times by yourself, but you can't seem to stick to it. How would you convince a new friend that you can help each other get started on regular physical activity and keep it up?

High Blood Cholesterol Level

The third controllable risk factor for heart disease is high blood cholesterol level. Generally speaking, the higher the blood cholesterol level, the greater the risk for heart disease. When high blood cholesterol levels are combined with other important risk factors, the risks become much greater.

Fortunately, blood cholesterol levels are relatively easy to measure. Many campus health, fitness, and wellness centers provide cholesterol screenings for employees and students. These screenings help identify people whose

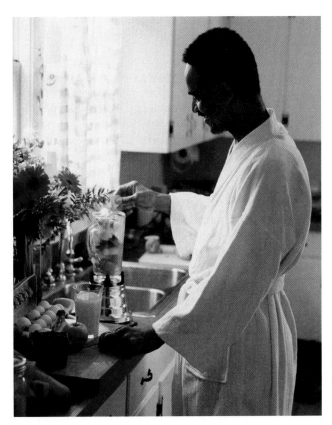

People who have high cholesterol should follow a heart-healthy diet based on the Food Guide Pyramid (see Chapter 5).

cholesterol levels (or profiles) may be potentially dangerous. Medical professionals have been able to determine the link between a person's diet and his or her cholesterol levels. People with high blood cholesterol levels are encouraged to consume a heart-healthy diet (see Chapter 5) and to become physically active. In recent years a variety of cholesterol-lowering drugs have also been developed that are very effective. Cholesterol will be discussed further later in this chapter.

Health on the Web

Behavior Change Activities

Reducing Your Cholesterol Level

Too much cholesterol in the blood can lead to cardiovascular disease. Even though we can make many lifestyle changes to lower our cholesterol and protect ourselves, half of all Americans have levels that are too high. Go to **www.americanheart.org/cholesterol/do.jsp** and learn how to reduce your blood cholesterol—and cut your risk of heart disease and stroke.

High Blood Pressure

The fourth of the "big six" cardiovascular risk factors is high blood pressure, or *hypertension*. You will soon be reading more about hypertension, but for now, suffice it to say that high blood pressure can seriously damage a person's heart and blood vessels. High blood pressure causes the heart to work much harder, eventually causing the heart to enlarge and weaken. It increases the chances for stroke, heart attack, congestive heart failure, and kidney disease.

When high blood pressure is present along with other risk factors, the risk for stroke or heart attack is increased tremendously. Yet this "silent killer" is easy to monitor and can be effectively controlled using a variety of approaches. This is the positive message about high blood pressure.

Diabetes Mellitus

Diabetes mellitus (discussed in detail on page 317) is a debilitating chronic disease that has a significant effect on the human body. In addition to increasing the risk of developing kidney disease, blindness, and nerve damage, diabetes increases the likelihood of developing heart and blood vessel diseases. Over 65% of people with diabetes die of some type of heart or blood vessel disease. The cardiovascular damage is thought to occur due to the abnormal levels of cholesterol and blood fat found in individuals with diabetes. With weight management, exercise, dietary changes, and drug therapy, diabetes can be relatively well controlled in most people. Even with careful management of this disease, diabetic patients are susceptible to eventual heart and blood vessel damage.

TALKING POINTS How would you show support for a friend who is struggling with the dietary requirements of diabetes?

Obesity and Overweight

Even if they have no other risk factors, obese people are more likely than nonobese people to develop heart disease and stroke. Obesity, particularly if located primarily around the abdomen, places considerable strain on the heart, and it tends to influence both blood pressure and blood cholesterol levels. Also, obesity tends to trigger diabetes in predisposed people. The importance of maintaining body weight within a desirable range minimizes the chance of obesity ever happening. To accomplish this, maintain an active lifestyle and follow the dietary guidelines in Chapter 5.

TALKING POINTS How could you tactfully bring up a friend's weight problem to show concern for his or her health?

Contributing Risk Factors

The American Heart Association identifies other risk factors that may contribute to CVD. These include *individual response to stress, sex hormones, birth control pills,* and *drinking too much alcohol.* Unresolved stress can encourage negative health dependencies (for example, smoking, poor dietary practices, underactivity) that lead to changes in blood fat profiles, blood pressure, and heart workload. Female sex hormones tend to protect women from CVD until they reach menopause, but male hormones do the opposite. Birth control pills (see Chapter 14) can increase the risk of blood clots and heart attack, although the risk is small unless the woman also smokes and is over age 35. The consumption of too much alcohol can cause elevated blood pressure, heart failure, and lead to stroke, although moderate drinking (no more than one drink per day for women and two drinks per day for men) is associated with lower risk of heart disease.[2]

Forms of Cardiovascular Disease

The American Heart Association describes the six major forms of CVD as coronary heart disease, hypertension, stroke, congenital heart disease, rheumatic heart disease, and congestive heart failure. A person may have just one of these diseases or a combination of them at the same time. Each form exists in varying degrees of severity. All are capable of causing secondary damage to other body organs and systems.

Coronary Heart Disease

This form of CVD, also known as *coronary artery disease,* involves damage to the vessels that supply blood to the heart muscle. The bulk of this blood is supplied by the coronary arteries. Any damage to these important vessels can cause a reduction of blood (and its vital oxygen and nutrients) to specific areas of heart muscle. The ultimate result of inadequate blood supply is a heart attack.

Atherosclerosis

The principal cause for the development of coronary heart disease is atherosclerosis (Figure 10-3). **Atherosclerosis** produces a narrowing of the coronary arteries. This narrowing stems from the long-term buildup of fatty deposits, called *plaque,* on the inner walls of the arteries. This buildup reduces the blood supply to specific portions of the heart. Some arteries of the heart can become so blocked (occluded) that all blood supply is stopped. Heart muscle tissue begins to die when it is deprived of oxygen and nutrients. This damage is known as **myocardial infarction.** In lay

Figure 10-3 Progression of atherosclerosis. This diagram shows how plaque deposits gradually accumulate to narrow the lumen (interior space) of an artery. Although enlarged here, coronary arteries are only as wide as a pencil lead.

terms, this event is called a *heart attack.* The Changing for the Better box on page 278 explains how to recognize the signs of a heart attack and what to do next.

Cholesterol and Lipoproteins For many years, scientists have known that atherosclerosis is a complicated disease that has many causes. Some of these causes are not well understood, but others are clearly understood. *Cholesterol,* a soft, fatlike material, is manufactured in the liver and small intestine and is necessary in the formation of sex hormones, cell membranes, bile salts, and nerve fibers. Elevated levels of serum cholesterol (200 mg/dl or more for adults age 20 and older, and 170 mg/dl or more for young people below age 20) are associated with an increased risk for developing atherosclerosis[2] (see the Changing for the Better box on page 279).

About half of American adults age 20 and older exceed the "borderline high" 200 mg/dl cholesterol level. It

---

Key Terms

atherosclerosis buildup of plaque on the inner walls of arteries.

myocardial infarction heart attack; the death of part of the heart muscle as a result of a blockage in one of the coronary arteries.

is estimated that nearly 40% of American youth age 19 and below have "borderline high" cholesterol levels of 170 mg/dl and above. About one out of five American adults has a "high" blood cholesterol level, that is, 240 mg/dl or greater.

Initially, most people can help lower their serum cholesterol level by adopting three dietary changes: lowering their intake of saturated fats, lowering their intake of dietary cholesterol, and lowering their caloric intake to a level that does not exceed body requirements. The aim is to reduce excess fat, cholesterol, and calories in the diet while promoting sound nutrition. By carefully following such a diet plan, people with high serum cholesterol levels may be able to reduce their cholesterol levels by 30 to 55 mg/dl. However, dietary changes do not affect people equally; some will experience greater reductions than others. Some will not respond at all to dietary changes and may need to take cholesterol-lowering medications and increase their physical activity.

Cholesterol is attached to structures called lipoproteins. Lipoproteins are particles that circulate in the blood and transport lipids (including cholesterol).[5] Two major classes of lipoproteins exist: **low-density lipoproteins (LDLs)** and **high-density lipoproteins (HDLs).** A person's total cholesterol level is chiefly determined by the amount of the LDLs and HDLs in a measured sample of blood. For example, a person's total cholesterol level of 200 mg/dl could be represented by an LDL level of 130 and an HDL level of 40, or an LDL level of 120 and an HDL level of 60. (Note that other lipoproteins do exist and carry some of the cholesterol in the blood.)

After much scientific study, it has been determined that high levels of LDL are a significant promoter of atherosclerosis. This makes sense because LDLs carry the greatest percentage of cholesterol in the bloodstream. LDLs are more likely to deposit excess cholesterol into the artery walls. This contributes to plaque formation.

Key Terms

low-density lipoprotein (LDL) the type of lipoprotein that transports the largest amount of cholesterol in the bloodstream; high levels of LDL are related to heart disease.

high-density lipoprotein (HDL) the type of lipoprotein that transports cholesterol from the bloodstream to the liver, where it is eventually removed from the body; high levels of HDL are related to a reduction in heart disease.

For this reason, LDLs are often called the "bad cholesterol." High LDL levels are determined partially by inheritance, but they are also clearly associated with smoking, poor dietary patterns, obesity, and lack of exercise.

On the other hand, high levels of HDLs are related to a decrease in the development of atherosclerosis. HDLs are thought to transport cholesterol out of the bloodstream. Thus HDLs have been called the "good cholesterol." Certain lifestyle alterations, such as quitting smoking, reducing obesity, increasing physical activity, and replacing saturated fats with monosaturated fats, help many people increase their level of HDLs.

Reducing total serum cholesterol levels is a significant step in reducing the risk of death from coronary heart disease. For people with elevated cholesterol levels, a 1% reduction in serum cholesterol level yields about a 2% reduction in the risk of death from heart disease. Thus a 10% to 15% cholesterol reduction can reduce risk by 20% to 30%.[6] See Table 10.2 for cholesterol classifications and current recommended follow-up.

Angina Pectoris When coronary arteries become narrowed, chest pain, or *angina pectoris,* is often felt. This pain results from a reduced supply of oxygen to heart muscle tissue. Usually, angina is felt when the coronary artery disease patient becomes stressed or exercises too strenuously. Angina reportedly can range from a feeling of mild indigestion to a severe viselike pressure in the chest. The pain may extend from the center of the chest to the arms and even up to the jaw. Generally, the more severe the blockage, the more pain is felt.

Some cardiac patients relieve angina with the drug *nitroglycerin,* a powerful blood vessel dilator. This prescription drug, available in slow-release transdermal (through the skin) patches or small pills that are placed under the

Changing for the Better

Monitoring Your Cholesterol Level

The last time I had a physical exam, I was embarrassed to ask what the cholesterol numbers meant. I thought if there was a problem, the doctor would have notified me. Now I think I should have asked for more information. What should I do next time?

The next time you get your blood cholesterol level checked, try to find out more than just your total cholesterol level. Ask for the following three measurements, and compare them with the desirable measurements for adults, listed below.

Readings for	Your measurement	Desirable measurement
HDL level:	_____	Above 40 mg/dl
LDL level:	_____	Below 130 mg/dl
Total level:	_____	Below 200 mg/dl
Triglycerides level:	_____	Below 150 mg/dl

How do your measurements compare with the desirable measurements? If they are not satisfactory, refer to Table 10.2 and the discussion to improve your levels.

patient's tongue, causes a major reduction in the workload of the heart muscle. Other cardiac patients may be prescribed drugs such as **calcium channel blockers** or **beta blockers.**

Emergency Response to Heart Crises

Heart attacks need not be fatal. The consequences of any heart attack depend on the location of the damage to the heart, the extent to which heart muscle is damaged, and the speed with which adequate circulation is restored. Injury to the ventricles may very well prove fatal unless medical countermeasures are immediately undertaken.

Table 10.2 Classification and Recommended Follow-up Based on LDL Cholesterol Level

LDL Cholesterol Level	Classification	Initiate Therapeutic Lifestyle Changes (TLC)
<100	Optimal	—
100–129	Near Optimal/ Above Optimal	If CHD or diabetes is present
130–159	Borderline High	If you have 2 or more risk factors
160–189	High	Yes, and see physician
≥190	Very High	Yes, and see physician

Note: The National Cholesterol Education Program (NCEP) now recommends that all adults have their LDL-cholesterol measured. See: http://nhlbi.nih.gov/about/ncep/index.htm

Key Terms

calcium channel blockers drugs that prevent arterial spasms; used in the control of blood pressure and the long-term management of angina pectoris.

beta blockers drugs that prevent overactivity of the heart, which results in angina pectoris and helps control blood pressure.

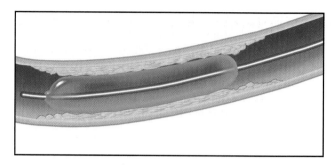

A   **B**

Figure 10-4 Angioplasty. A, A "balloon" is surgically inserted into the narrowed coronary artery. **B,** The balloon is inflated, compressing plaque and fatty deposits against the artery walls.

The recognition of a heart attack is critically important (see the Changing for the Better box on page 278).

Cardiopulmonary resuscitation (CPR) is one of the most important immediate countermeasures that trained people can use when confronted with a victim of heart attack. Programs sponsored by the American Red Cross and the American Heart Association teach people how to recognize, evaluate, and manage heart attack emergencies. CPR trainees are taught how to restore breathing and circulation in persons requiring emergency care. Frequently, colleges offer CPR training through courses in various departments. With revised CPR procedures in place in 2001, we encourage students to take a new course and become certified. Additionally, members of the public are encouraged to obtain training in the use of automated external defibrillators (AED). These devices are now found in most public buildings and can markedly improve the chances of resuscitating a victim.

Diagnosis and Coronary Repair

Once a person's vital signs have stabilized, further diagnostic examinations can reveal the type and extent of damage to heart muscle. Initially an ECG might be taken, which may be able to identify if areas of ischemia (insufficient blood flow) or damage has occurred to the heart muscle. Another test which may be used is echocardiography. This procedure can also detect ischemia. The diagnostic ability of both of these tests is improved if used in conjunction with exercise (i.e., stress ECG or stress echocardiography). This test analyzes the electrical activity of the heart. *Heart catheterization,* also called *coronary arteriography,* is a minor surgical procedure that starts with placement of a thin plastic tube into an arm or leg artery. This tube, called a *catheter,* is guided through the artery until it reaches the coronary circulation, where a *radiopaque dye* is then released. X-ray films called *angiograms* record the progress of the dye through the coronary arteries so that areas of blockage can be easily identified.

Once the extent of damage is identified, a physician or team of physicians can decide on a medical course of action. Currently popular is an extensive form of surgery called **coronary artery bypass surgery.** An estimated 516,000 patients had bypass surgeries in 2001.[2] The purpose of such surgery is to detour (bypass) areas of coronary artery obstruction by usually using a section of an artery from the patient's chest (the internal mammary artery) and grafting it from the aorta to a location just beyond the area of obstruction. Multiple areas of obstruction result in double, triple, or quadruple bypasses.

Angioplasty Angioplasty, an alternative to bypass surgery, involves the surgical insertion of a doughnut-shaped "balloon" directly into the narrowed coronary artery (Figure 10-4). When the balloon is inflated, plaque and fatty deposits are compressed against the artery walls, widening the space through which blood flows. The balloon usually remains in the artery for less than 1 minute. Renarrowing of the artery will occur in about one quarter of angioplasty patients. Balloon angioplasty can be used for blockages in the heart, kidneys, arms, and legs. The decision whether to have angioplasty or bypass surgery can be a difficult one to make. Nearly 1,050,000 angioplasty procedures were performed in 2001.[2]

The FDA approved a device for clearing heart and leg arteries. This device is called a *motorized scraper.* Inserted through a leg artery and held in place by a tiny inflated balloon, this motor-driven cutter shaves off plaque deposits from inside the artery. A nose cone in the scraper unit stores the plaque until the device is removed.

The use of laser beams to dissolve plaque that blocks arteries has been slowly evolving. The FDA has approved three laser devices for use in clogged leg arteries. In 1992 the FDA approved the use of an excimer laser for use in coronary arteries.

Aspirin Studies released a decade ago highlighted the role of aspirin in reducing the risk of heart attack in men with no history of previous attacks. Specifically, the studies concluded that for men with hypertension, elevated cholesterol levels, or both, taking one aspirin per day was a significant factor in reducing their risk of heart attack. Aspirin works by making the blood less able to clot. This reduces the likelihood of blood vessel blockages. Presently, there is differing opinion regarding the age at which this preventive action should begin. The safest advice is to check with your physician before starting aspirin therapy. Recent research now indicates that aspirin therapy is also beneficial for women.[7]

Alcohol For years, scientists have been uncertain about the extent to which alcohol consumption is related to a reduced risk for heart disease. The current thinking is that moderate drinking (defined as no more than two drinks per day for men and one drink per day for women) is related to a lower heart disease risk. However, the benefit is much smaller than proven risk reduction behaviors such as stopping smoking, reducing cholesterol level, lowering blood pressure, and increasing physical activity. Experts caution that heavy drinking increases cardiovascular risks and that nondrinkers should not start to drink just to reduce heart disease risk.

Heart Transplants and Artificial Hearts For approximately 30 years, surgeons have been able to surgically replace a person's damaged heart with that of another human being. Although very risky, these transplant operations have added years to the lives of a number of patients who otherwise would have lived only a short time. In 2001, 2,202 heart transplants were performed in the United States.[2]

Artificial hearts have also been developed and implanted in humans. These hearts have extended the lives of many patients, but they have kept them unpleasantly tethered with tubes and wires to large power source machines. However, a major medical breakthrough took place in July 2001, when the world's first self-contained artificial heart was successfully implanted into a 59-year-old patient.

Hypertension

Just as your car's water pump recirculates water and maintains water pressure, your heart recirculates blood and maintains blood pressure. When the heart contracts, blood is forced through your arteries and veins. Your blood pressure is a measure of the force that your circulating blood exerts against the interior walls of your arteries and veins.

Blood pressure is measured with a *sphygmomanometer*. This instrument is attached to an arm-cuff device that can be inflated to stop the flow of blood temporarily in the brachial artery. This artery is a major supplier of blood to the lower arm. It is located on the inside of the upper arm, between the biceps and triceps muscles.

A health professional using a stethoscope will listen for blood flow while the pressure in the cuff is released. Two pressure measurements will be recorded: the **systolic pressure** is the highest blood pressure against the vessel walls during the heart contraction, and the **diastolic pressure** is the lowest blood pressure against the vessel walls when the heart relaxes (between heartbeats). Expressed in units of millimeters of mercury displaced on the sphygmomanometer, blood pressure is recorded as the systolic pressure over the diastolic pressure, for example, 115/82.

Key Terms

systolic pressure blood pressure against blood vessel walls when the heart contracts.

diastolic pressure blood pressure against blood vessel walls when the heart relaxes.

Although a blood pressure of less than 120/80 is considered "normal" for an adult, lower values do not necessarily indicate a medical problem. In fact, many young college women of average weight will indicate blood pressures that seem to be relatively low (100/60, for example), yet these lowered blood pressures are quite "normal" for them.

 TALKING POINTS You're having a regular physical examination, and your doctor remarks that your blood pressure puts you in the category of "borderline hypertension." What questions would you ask about managing this condition?

Hypertension refers to a consistently elevated blood pressure. Generally, concern about a young adult's high blood pressure begins when he or she has a systolic reading of 140 or above or a diastolic reading of 90 or above. Now those with prehypertension are advised to seek lifestyle measures to prevent any further elevation in their blood pressure. Approximately 58 million American adults and children have hypertension. The American Heart Association reports that African Americans, Hispanic Americans, and American Indians have higher rates of high blood pressure than white Americans.[2,5] In contrast, Asian/Pacific Islanders have significantly lower rates of hypertension.[2]

Although the reasons for 90% to 95% of the cases of hypertension are not known, the health risks produced by uncontrolled hypertension are clearly understood. Throughout the body, long-term hypertension makes arteries and arterioles become less elastic and thus incapable of dilating under a heavy workload. Brittle, calcified blood vessels can burst unexpectedly and produce serious strokes (brain accidents), kidney failure (renal accidents), or eye damage **(retinal hemorrhage)**. Furthermore, it appears that blood clots are more easily formed and dislodged in a vascular system affected by hypertension. Thus hypertension can be a cause of heart attacks. Clearly, hypertension is a potential killer.

Ironically, despite its deadly nature, hypertension is referred to as "the silent killer" because people with hypertension often are not aware that they have the condition. They cannot feel the sensation of high blood pressure. The condition does not produce dizziness, headaches, or memory loss unless one is experiencing a medical crisis. It is estimated that approximately 30% of the people who have hypertension do not realize they have it.[8] Many who are aware of their hypertension do little to control it. Only a small percentage (34%) of people who have hypertension control it adequately, generally through dietary control, regular exercise, relaxation training, and drug therapy.

Hypertension is not thought of as a curable disease; rather, it is a controllable disease. Once therapy is stopped,

the condition returns. As a responsible adult, use every opportunity you can to measure your blood pressure on a regular basis.

Prevention and Treatment

Weight reduction, physical activity, moderation in alcohol use, and sodium restriction are often used to reduce hypertension. For overweight or obese people, a reduction in body weight may produce a significant drop in blood pressure. Physical activity helps lower blood pressure by expending calories (which may lead to weight loss in those who are overweight or obese) and through other physiological changes that affect the circulation. Moderation in alcohol consumption (no more than 1–2 drinks daily) helps reduce blood pressure in some people.

The restriction of sodium (salt) in the diet also helps some people reduce hypertension. Interestingly, this strategy is effective only for those who are **salt sensitive** — estimated to be about 25% of the population. Reducing salt intake would have little effect on the blood pressure of the rest of the population. Nevertheless, since our daily intake of salt vastly exceeds our need for salt, the general recommendation to curb salt intake still makes good sense.

Many of the stress reduction activities discussed in Chapter 3 are receiving increased attention in the struggle to reduce hypertension. In recent years, behavioral scientists have reported the success of meditation, biofeedback, controlled breathing, and muscle relaxation exercises in reducing hypertension. Look for further research findings in these areas in the years to come.

Key Terms

retinal hemorrhage uncontrolled bleeding from arteries within the eye's retina.

salt sensitive term used to describe people whose bodies overreact to the presence of sodium by retaining fluid and thus experience an increase in blood pressure.

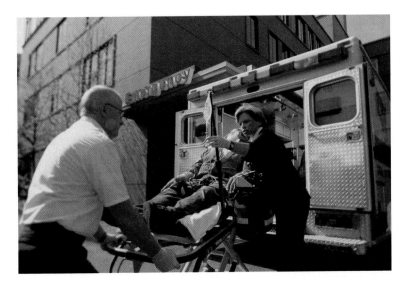

Emergency response teams help keep cardiac patients alive during transit to a medical facility.

There are literally dozens of drugs available for use by people with hypertension. Unfortunately, many patients refuse to take their medication on a consistent basis, probably because of the mistaken notion that "you must feel sick to be sick." Nutritional supplements, such as calcium, magnesium, potassium, and fish oil, have not been proven to be effective in lowering blood pressure.

Stroke

Stroke is a general term for a wide variety of crises (sometimes called *cerebrovascular accidents* [CVAs] or brain attacks) that result from blood vessel damage in the brain. African Americans have a much greater risk of stroke than white Americans do, probably because African Americans have a greater likelihood of having hypertension than white Americans. Data for 2001 indicate that 163,538 deaths and half a million new cases of stroke occurred.[2] Just as the heart muscle needs an adequate blood supply, so does the brain. Any disturbance in the proper supply of oxygen and nutrients to the brain can pose a threat.

Perhaps the most common form of stroke results from the blockage of a cerebral (brain) artery. Similar to coronary occlusions, **cerebrovascular occlusions** can be started by a clot that forms within an artery, called a *thrombus,* or by a clot that travels from another part of the body to the brain, called an *embolus* (Figure 10-5, *A* and *B*). The resultant accidents (cerebral thrombosis or cerebral embolism) cause more than 60% of all strokes. The portion of the brain deprived of oxygen and nutrients can literally die.

A third type of stroke can result from an artery that bursts to produce a crisis called *cerebral hemorrhage* (Figure 10-5, *C*). Damaged, brittle arteries can be especially susceptible to bursting when a person has hypertension.

A fourth form of stroke is a *cerebral aneurysm.* An aneurysm is a ballooning or outpouching on a weakened area of an artery (Figure 10-5, *D*). Aneurysms may occur in various locations of the body and are not always life-threatening. The development of aneurysms is not fully understood, although there seems to be a relationship between aneurysms and hypertension. It is quite possible that many aneurysms are congenital defects. In any case, when a cerebral aneurysm bursts, a stroke results. See the Changing for the Better box on page 284 to learn the warning signs of stroke.

A person who reports any warning signs of stroke or any mini stroke, called a **transient ischemic attack (TIA),** will undergo a battery of diagnostic tests, which could include a physical examination, a search for possible brain tumors, tests to identify areas of the brain affected, use of the electroencephalogram, cerebral arteriography, and the use of the **CT** (computed tomography) **scan** or **MRI** (magnetic resonance imaging) **scan.** Many additional tests are also available.

> ### Key Terms
>
> **cerebrovascular occlusion** blockages to arteries supplying blood to the cerebral cortex of the brain; strokes.
>
> **transient ischemic attack (TIA)** strokelike symptoms caused by temporary spasm of cerebral blood vessels.
>
> **CT scan** computed tomography scan; an x-ray procedure that is designed to visualize structures within the body that would not normally be seen through conventional x-ray procedures.

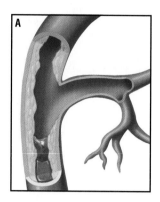

Thrombus
A clot that forms within a narrowed section of a blood vessel and remains at its place of origin.

Embolus
A clot that moves through the circulatory system and becomes lodged at a narrowed point within a vessel.

Hemorrhage
The sudden bursting of a blood vessel.

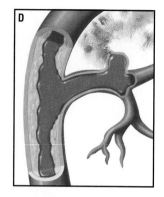

Aneurysm
A sac formed when a section of a blood vessel thins and balloons; the weakened wall of the sac can burst, or rupture, as shown here.

Figure 10-5 Causes of stroke.

Treatment of stroke patients depends on the nature and extent of the damage. Some patients require surgery (to repair vessels and relieve pressure) and acute care in the hospital. Others undergo drug treatment, especially the use of anticoagulant drugs, including aspirin and TPA (tissue plasminogen activators; the "clot buster" drug).

The advancements made in the rehabilitation of stroke patients are amazing. Although some severely affected patients have little hope of improvement, our increasing advancements in the application of computer technology to such disciplines as speech and physical therapy offer encouraging signs for stroke patients and their families.

Congenital Heart Disease

A congenital defect is one that is present at birth. The American Heart Association estimates that each year about 40,000 babies are born with a congenital heart defect. In 2001, 4,109 children (mostly infants) died of congenital heart disease.[2]

A variety of abnormalities may be produced by congenital heart disease, including valve damage, holes in the walls of the septum, blood vessel transposition, and an underdevelopment of the left side of the heart. All of these problems ultimately prevent a newborn from adequately oxygenating tissues throughout the body. A bluish skin color (cyanosis) is seen in some infants with such congenital heart defects. These infants are sometimes referred to as *blue babies.*

The cause of congenital heart defects is not clearly understood, although one cause, *rubella,* has been identified. The fetuses of mothers who contract the rubella

Key Terms

MRI scan magnetic resonance imaging scan; an imaging procedure that uses a giant magnet to generate images of body tissues.

★ **Risk Factors for Congenital and Rheumatic Heart Disease**

Risk Factors for Congenital Heart Disease

Fetal exposure to rubella, other viral infections, pollutants, alcohol, or tobacco smoke during pregnancy

Risk Factors for Rheumatic Heart Disease

Streptococcal infection

Common Symptoms of Strep Throat

Sudden onset of sore throat, particularly with pain when swallowing
Fever
Swollen, tender glands under the angle of the jaw
Headache
Nausea and vomiting
Tonsils covered with a yellow or white pus or discharge

virus during the first 3 months of pregnancy are at great risk of developing *congenital rubella syndrome (CRS)*, a catch-all term for a wide variety of congenital defects, including heart defects, deafness, cataracts, and mental retardation. Other hypotheses about the development of congenital heart disease implicate environmental pollutants; maternal use of drugs, including alcohol, during pregnancy; and unknown genetic factors (see the Star box above).

Treatment of congenital defects usually requires surgery, although some conditions may respond well to drug therapy. Defective blood vessels and certain malformations of the heart can be surgically repaired. This surgery is so successful that many children respond quite quickly to the increased circulation and oxygenation. Many are able to lead normal, active lives.

Rheumatic Heart Disease

Rheumatic heart disease is the final stage in a series of complications started by a streptococcal infection of the throat (strep throat). The Star box above lists symptoms of strep throat. This bacterial infection, if untreated, can result in an inflammatory disease called *rheumatic fever* (and a related condition, scarlet fever). Rheumatic fever is a whole-body (systemic) reaction that can produce fever, joint pain, skin rashes, and possible brain and heart damage. A person who has had rheumatic fever is more susceptible to subsequent attacks. Rheumatic fever tends to run in families. Over 3,400 Americans died from rheumatic fever and rheumatic heart disease in 2001.[2]

Damage from rheumatic fever centers on the heart's valves. For some reason the bacteria tend to proliferate in the heart valves. Defective heart valves may fail either to open fully *(stenosis)* or to close fully *(insufficiency)*. Diagnosis of valve damage might initially come when a physician hears a backwashing or backflow of blood (a **murmur**). Further tests—including chest X rays, cardiac catheterization, and echocardiography—can reveal the extent of valve damage. Once identified, a faulty valve can be replaced surgically with a metal or plastic artificial valve or a valve taken from an animal's heart.

Congestive Heart Failure

Congestive heart failure is a condition in which the heart lacks the strength to continue to circulate blood normally throughout the body. In 2001, 52,828 people died from congestive heart failure. During congestive heart failure, the heart continues to work, but it cannot function well enough to maintain appropriate circulation. Venous blood flow starts to "back up." Swelling occurs, especially in the legs and ankles. Fluid can collect in the lungs and cause breathing difficulties and shortness of breath, and kidney function may be damaged.[2]

Congestive heart failure can result from heart damage caused by congenital heart defects, lung disease, rheumatic fever, heart attack, atherosclerosis, or high blood pressure. Generally, congestive heart failure is treatable through a combined program of rest, proper diet, modified daily activities, and the use of appropriate drugs. Without medical care, congestive heart failure can be fatal.

Additional Conditions

Besides the cardiovascular diseases already discussed, the heart and blood vessels are also subject to other pathological

---

Key Terms

rheumatic heart disease chronic damage to the heart (especially heart valves) resulting from a streptococcal infection within the heart; a complication associated with rheumatic fever.

murmur an atypical heart sound that suggests a backwashing of blood into a chamber of the heart from which it has just left.

congestive heart failure inability of the heart to pump out all the blood that returns to it; can lead to dangerous fluid accumulations in veins, lungs, and kidneys.

conditions. Tumors of the heart, although rare, occur. Infectious conditions involving the pericardial sac that surrounds the heart *(pericarditis)* and the innermost layer of the heart *(endocarditis)* are more commonly seen. In addition, inflammation of the veins *(phlebitis)* is troublesome to some people.

Peripheral Artery Disease **Peripheral artery disease (PAD)**, also called *peripheral vascular disease (PVD)*, is a blood vessel disease characterized by pathological changes to the arteries and arterioles in the extremities (primarily the legs and feet but sometimes the hands). These changes result from years of damage to the peripheral blood vessels. Important causes of PAD are cigarette smoking, a high-fat diet, obesity, and sedentary occupations. In some cases, PAD is aggravated by blood vessel changes resulting from diabetes.

PAD severely restricts blood flow to the extremities. The reduction in blood flow is responsible for leg pain or cramping during exercise, numbness, tingling, coldness, and loss of hair in the affected limb. The most serious consequence of PAD is the increased likelihood of developing ulcerations and tissue death. These conditions can lead to gangrene and may eventually necessitate amputation.

The treatment of PAD consists of multiple approaches and may include efforts to improve blood lipid levels (through diet, exercise, or drug therapy), reduce hypertension, reduce body weight, and eliminate smoking. Blood vessel surgery is also a possible treatment approach.

Key Terms

peripheral artery disease (PAD) damage resulting from restricted blood flow to the extremities, especially the legs and feet.

Taking Charge of Your Health

- Complete the Personal Assessment on page 291 to determine your risk for heart attack and stroke.
- Review the Food Guide Pyramid in Chapter 5 (page 115), and make changes to your diet so that it is more "heart healthy."
- Begin or continue an aerobic exercise program that is appropriate for your current fitness level.
- If you are a smoker, resolve to quit smoking. Visit your physician to talk about safe and effective approaches. Begin putting your plan into action.

- Develop a plan to lower your dietary intake of fat to keep your blood cholesterol level low.
- Have your blood pressure checked, and review your weight, physical activity, alcohol intake, and salt intake to determine whether you can make changes in any of these areas.
- If you are overweight or obese, develop a plan to combine dietary changes and increased physical activity to lose weight gradually but steadily.

Summary

- Cardiovascular disorders are responsible for more disabilities and deaths than any other disease.
- The cardiovascular system consists of the heart, blood, and blood vessels. This system performs many functions.
- Our overall health depends on the health of the cardiovascular system.
- A cardiovascular risk factor is an attribute that a person has or is exposed to that increases the likelihood of heart disease.
- The "big six" risk factors are tobacco smoke, physical inactivity, high blood cholesterol level, high blood

pressure, diabetes mellitus, and obesity and overweight. These are controllable risk factors.
- Increasing age, male gender, and heredity are risk factors that cannot be controlled.
- Four contributing risk factors to heart disease are individual response to stress, sex hormones, birth control pills, and drinking too much alcohol.
- The major forms of cardiovascular disease include coronary artery disease, hypertension, stroke, congenital heart disease, rheumatic heart disease, and congestive heart failure. Each disease develops in a specific way and may require a highly specialized form of treatment.

Review Questions

1. Identify the principal components of the cardiovascular system. Trace the path of blood through the heart and cardiovascular system.
2. How much blood does the average adult have? What are some of the important functions of blood?
3. Define cardiovascular risk factor. What relationship do risk factors have to cardiovascular disease?
4. Identify those risk factors for cardiovascular disease that cannot be changed. Identify those risk factors that can be changed. Identify the risk factors that can be contributing factors.
5. What are the six major forms of cardiovascular disease? For each of these diseases, describe what the disease is, its cause (if known), and its treatment.
6. Describe how high-density lipoproteins differ from low-density lipoproteins.
7. What problems does atherosclerosis produce?
8. Why is hypertension referred to as "the silent killer"?
9. What are the warning signals of stroke?
10. What is peripheral artery disease?

References

1. Kotecki JE, Chamness BE. A valuable tool for evaluating health-related www sites, *Journal of Health Education* 30:1, January/February 1999, 56–58.
2. American Heart Association. *2004 Heart and stroke statistical update*, 2004.
3. Seeley RR, Stephens TD, Tate P. *Essentials of anatomy and physiology*, ed 3, 1999, McGraw-Hill.
4. Brubaker PH, Kaminsky LA, Whaley MH. *Coronary Artery Disease*, Human Kinetics, 2002.
5. American Heart Association. **www.americanheart.org/ Heart_and_Stroke_A_Z_Guide/** July 19, 2003.
6. Cholesterol: up with the good, *Harvard Heart Letter* 5:11, July 1995, 3–4.
7. Aspirin for coronary disease: beneficial in women, too, *Harvard Heart Letter* 7:7, March 1997, 8.
8. National Heart Lung and Blood Institute. **www.nhlbi.nih.gov/guidelines/hypertension/ index.htm** July 21, 2003.

As We Go to Press

The American College of Sports Medicine[1] recently released a new Position Stand on *Exercise and Hypertension*. Among the notable statements in this report are that "Exercise remains a cornerstone therapy for the prevention, treatment, and control of hypertension."

[1]American College of Sports Medicine. Exercise & Hypertension Position Stand. *Medicine and Science in Sports and Exercise.* 36:533–553, 2004.

As noted in Table 10.1 (page 270), hypertension is a condition that exists in 58 million Americans. Thus, lifestyle measures, which include exercise, can play a significant role in both preventing people from developing this condition and in the treatment of those that have hypertension.

hypertension in african americans: targeting prevention

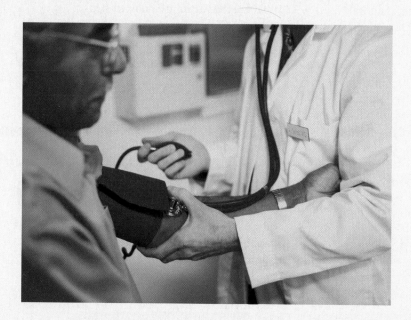

Development of disease is an area in which each societal group is disadvantaged in one way or another. Practically every group has a tendency to develop one or more afflictions at a higher rate than the general population. For the African American community, one particular problem is hypertension.

The existing data show that hypertension is more common in African Americans[1,2] and is more aggressive and less well managed in African Americans than in whites. African Americans also have higher rates of morbidity and mortality from diseases related to high blood pressure, such as stroke and renal failure. The natural nocturnal fall in blood pressure is less pronounced in African Americans, and their systolic blood pressure while awake is higher than in people of other races.[1]

The exact causes of these differences have not been pinpointed, but research seems to be focused in two general areas.

Some research suggests that certain physical and genetic factors contribute to increased incidence of hypertension in African Americans, whereas other studies have shown that hypertension in African Americans is related to environmental stress. This debate involves not just medical data but socioeconomic factors as well. In short, it is a nature vs. nurture debate, and there are supporting data for both arguments.

Nature vs. Nurture

Studies have shown that environmental stress may contribute to increased hypertension in African Americans. A study conducted by Dr. Norman Anderson of Duke University[3] shows that chronic stress may lead to an increase in the release of the hormone norepinephrine to the bloodstream. Norepinephrine reduces the amount of salt eliminated from the kidneys, and the resulting increase in

blood salt content can lead to increased blood pressure. This chain reaction has been shown to occur in animal studies. The high rate of chronic exposure to stress in many African American communities has been well documented.[3] If these studies hold true for humans, it would lend credence to the idea that certain stressful factors found in some African American communities could cause hypertension. Stressors such as poverty, unemployment, the threat of violence, and racial discrimination could be shown to cause kidneys to reduce elimination of salt and thus may also increase the risk of hypertension.[3]

Anger in response to racism may be a significant contributing factor in increased hypertension in African Americans. A study conducted jointly at the University of Tennessee and Saint Louis University showed that blood pressure in African Americans increased significantly when they were shown film clips of racially motivated violence.[4] The responses of African Americans to these scenes of racial discrimination were more pronounced than their responses to viewing scenes that were anger-provoking but had no racial component. The increases in blood pressure were not into the hypertension range, but researchers believe that over time, such continued elevation of blood pressure could become dangerous.

Such conclusions seem to suggest that socioeconomic factors are the main cause of hypertension among African Americans. A study performed on twenty-six African American women on strict low-fat diets seems to support this. The data showed that women of higher socioeconomic status had more excretion of salt than those of lower status.[3] Since proportionately more

African Americans are in lower socioeconomic classes than whites, increased stress from lower status could be the main factor behind the inflated rate of hypertension among the African American population.

But is it all due to environment? Perhaps not. Other groups of traditionally lower socioeconomic status, such as Hispanics, Asians, and Native Americans, have been found to have the same incidence of hypertension as whites.[1] African American children have been found to have higher blood pressure in general than white children;[1] it is not known whether stress plays a significant role in affecting the blood pressure of these children so early in life.

There is also evidence that African Americans may be predisposed to hypertension at the cellular level. Microscopic studies of blood vessels in African Americans with severe hypertension revealed that renal arterioles were thickened and had reduced flow. This thickening, not found in the renal arterioles of hypertensive whites, was caused by hypertrophy (excess growth) of smooth muscle cells in the muscle walls of the arterioles. This thickening reduced the size of the lumen (inside opening) of the vessels, and the resulting reduced blood flow may have caused increased blood pressure. The smooth muscle cells were thought to be responding abnormally to growth factors, which caused the hypertrophy to occur.[2] The reason behind this abnormal reaction was not determined, however.

The best explanation of why African Americans are more prone to develop hypertension may not involve environment or genetics alone, but a combination of the two. Stress factors unique to the African American community may serve to aggravate or intensify an existing physical predisposition toward hypertension. It has already been shown that the tendency toward developing hypertension can be passed from parents to their children. Add several unique stress factors to a population already predisposed to high blood pressure, and the potential exists for high numbers of people to develop hypertension. Commenting on the UT-SLU study, Dr. Elijah Saunders agreed that "racism and Black rage are emotional stressors that could worsen a physiological tendency toward hypertension."[4]

Treatment for Hypertension in African Americans

The good news is that African Americans respond to medical treatment in a similar manner to whites. The treatment regimen for African Americans may have to be altered somewhat, however, since they do not respond as well to some hypertension medications as people of other races. For unknown reasons, drugs such as beta-blockers and ACE (angiotensin converting enzyme) inhibitors do not work as well in African Americans and may need to be supplemented by other medications, such as diuretics.[1]

Lifestyle changes may also be needed and may be a more effective tool in lowering blood pressure in African Americans than in people of other races.[1] Effort should be made to exercise and lose weight if needed, since excess weight can be a contributing factor in hypertension. Hypertensive African Americans tend to have lower intakes of potassium and calcium, so diet changes should be made that ensure that these minerals are in adequate supply. A reduction in sodium may also be desirable, since research suggests that African Americans may be more sensitive to the effects of sodium on the cardiovascular system.[1]

Although African Americans are more likely to develop high blood pressure, prevention and treatment can help keep hypertension from becoming a deadly affliction. Proper diagnosis is essential, so people at risk should see their doctors to determine whether they have hypertension or are at risk for developing it. Through recommending lifestyle modifications, prescribing medications, or both, a physician can help manage this condition or help prevent its onset.[5]

For Discussion . . .

Do you feel that people in lower (or higher) socioeconomic groups suffer more from everyday stress? Do you believe physiological or genetic differences may exist between different ethnic or racial groups?

References

1. Kaplan NM. Ethnic aspects of hypertension, *Lancet* 344(8920), 1994.
2. Dustan HP. Growth factors and racial differences in severity of hypertension and renal diseases, *Lancet* 339(8805), 1992.
3. Haywood RL. Why Black Americans suffer with more high blood pressure than Whites, *Jet* Dec 5, 1994, 87(5).
4. Study reveals anger over racism causes high blood pressure in Blacks, *Jet* May 14, 1990, 78(5).
5. Too little attention paid to high blood pressure, *Tufts University Health and Nutrition Letter,* (15:11), January 1998, p. 1.

personal assessment

what is your risk for heart disease?

Cholesterol

Your serum cholesterol level is:

0	190 or below
+ 2	191 to 230
+ 6	231 to 289
+12	290 to 319
+16	Over 320

Your HDL cholesterol is:

− 2	Over 60
0	45 to 60
+ 2	35 to 44
+ 6	29 to 34
+12	23 to 28
+16	Below 23

Smoking

You smoke now or have in the past:

0	Never smoked, or quit more than 5 years ago
+ 1	Quit 2 to 4 years ago
+ 3	Quit about 1 year ago
+ 6	Quit during the past year

You now smoke:

+ 9	½ to 1 pack a day
+12	1 to 2 packs a day
+15	More than 2 packs a day

The quality of the air you breathe is:

0	Unpolluted by smoke, exhaust, or industry at home and at work
+ 2	Live or work with smokers in unpolluted area
+ 4	Live and work with smokers in unpolluted area
+ 6	Live or work with smokers **and** live or work in air-polluted area
+ 8	Live **and** work with smokers **and** live and work in air-polluted area

Blood Pressure

Your blood pressure is:

0	120/75 or below
+ 2	120/75 to 140/85
+ 6	140/85 to 150/90
+ 8	150/90 to 175/100
+10	175/100 to 190/110
+12	190/110 or above

Exercise

Your exercise habits are:

0	Exercise vigorously 4 or 5 times a week
+ 2	Exercise moderately 4 or 5 times a week
+ 4	Exercise only on weekends
+ 6	Exercise occasionally
+ 8	Little or no exercise

Weight

Your weight is:

0	Always at or near ideal weight
+ 1	Now 10% overweight
+ 2	Now 20% overweight
+ 3	Now 30% or more overweight
+ 4	Now 20% or more overweight and have been since before age 30

Stress

You feel overstressed:

0	Rarely at work or at home
+ 3	Somewhat at home but not at work
+ 5	Somewhat at work but not at home
+ 7	Somewhat at work **and** at home
+ 9	Usually at work **or** at home
+12	Usually at work **and** at home

Diabetes

Your diabetic history is:

0	Blood sugar always normal
+ 2	Blood glucose slightly high (prediabetic) or slightly low (hypoglycemic)
+ 4	Diabetic beginning after age 40 requiring strict dietary or insulin control
+ 5	Diabetic beginning before age 30 requiring strict dietary or insulin control

Alcohol

You drink alcoholic beverages:

0	Never or only socially, about once or twice a month, or only one 5-ounce glass of wine or 12-ounce glass of beer or 1½ ounces of hard liquor about 5 times a week
+ 2	Two to three 5-ounces glasses of wine or 12-ounce glasses of beer or 1½ ounce cocktails about 5 times a week
+ 4	More than three 1½-ounce cocktails or more than three 5-ounce glasses of wine or 12-ounce glasses of beer almost every day

Interpretation

Add all sources and check next page.

0 to 20:   **Low risk.** Excellent family history and lifestyle habits.

21 to 50:   **Moderate risk.** Family history or lifestyle habits put you at some risk. You might lower your risks and minimize your genetic predisposition if you change any poor habits.

51 to 74:   **High risk.** Habits and family history indicate high risk of heart disease. Change your habits now.

Above 75:   **Very high risk.** Family history and a lifetime of poor habits put you at very high risk of heart disease. Eliminate as many of the risk factors as you can.

To Carry This Further . . .

Were you surprised with your score on this assessment? What were your most significant risk factors? Do you plan to make any changes in your lifestyle to reduce your cardiovascular risks? Why or why not?

chapter eleven

living with cancer and other chronic conditions

Chapter Objectives

Upon completing this chapter, you will be able to:

▌ describe cancer statistics and identify groups who are at high risk for developing particular forms of cancer.

▌ explain the role of cell regulation in the development of cancer, and discuss the relationship of genetic mutations, viral infections, and carcinogens to the loss of cell regulation.

▌ name specific steps that individuals can take to aid in early detection of specific cancers.

▌ explain and discuss the role of self-examination in detecting certain cancers, including breast cancer, melanoma, and testicular cancer.

▌ discuss the importance of medical screening for specific cancers, and identify several procedures used to screen for particular forms of cancer.

▌ offer several lifestyle changes that effectively reduce your cancer risk.

▌ summarize the status of our current "War on Cancer."

▌ explain what an autoimmune disorder is.

▌ describe the genetic causes and the symptoms of several inherited conditions.

▌ discuss treatment options for a number of chronic conditions.

▌ explain the difference between Type 1 and Type 2 diabetes, and discuss the importance of physical activity and diet in remaining glucose tolerant as we get older.

Online Learning Center Resources

www.mhhe.com/hahn7e

Log on to our Online Learning Center (OLC) for access to these additional resources:

- Chapter key terms and definitions
- Learning objectives
- Student interactive question-and-answer sites
- Self-scoring chapter quiz
- Online assessments
- Key term flash cards

Talking It Over

Telling Coworkers About Your Cancer

When you decide it's time to tell your boss and coworkers that you have cancer, you'll have many things to consider—how much information to give, how this news will affect other people's perception of you, and how your condition will affect your ability to do your job.

- Tell people what they need to know.
- Ask for help when you need it, but remember that your coworkers have their own responsibilities.

- Consider how you want to present yourself—as a victim or a fighter—because your coworkers are likely to reinforce your attitude.

CommunicationLinks

Living With It www.livingwithit.org
Prostate Info www.prostateinfo.com

Eye on the Media

Support Is Just a Click Away

Support groups are composed of people who come together to help each other through the demands of a chronic health condition. These groups have traditionally been organized by institutions in the local health care community, such as hospitals, by the local affiliates of national organizations, such as the American Cancer Society, or by citizens who have the same chronic condition. Increasingly common today, however, we find support groups whose members are connected, not by physical proximity, but by the Internet.

Health self-help groups on the Internet develop in one of two ways. The first occurs when a brick-and-mortar organization, such as a national agency or health care institution, develops a support group for its homepage. The second way is for a person with the condition (or a family member of that person) to organize an online group.

You can find a health support group simply by surfing the net. Or you can be referred to a site by a health care professional, friend, family member, colleague, or someone with a similar condition. You can also go to the

Most people can attest to the disruptive influence an illness can have on their ability to participate in day-to-day activities. When we are ill, school, employment, and leisure activities are replaced by periods of lessened activity and even periods of bed rest or hospitalization. When an illness is chronic, the effect of being ill may extend over long periods, perhaps even an entire lifetime. People with chronic illness must eventually find a balance between day-to-day function and the continuous presence of their condition. Cancer is usually a chronic illness.

In spite of our understanding of its relationship to human health and our ceaseless attempts to prevent and cure it, progress in "the war on cancer" has been relatively limited. In this regard, cancer is clearly an "expensive" condition, both in terms of its human consequences and its monetary costs. It is estimated that 1,334,100 people developed cancer in 2003 and that, since 1990, nearly 17 million new cases of cancer have developed in this country. Once diagnosed, approximately 62% (adjusted for other causes of death) of this group will be alive 5 years later.[1] The 5-year period that defines *relative survivability* encompasses "persons who are living 5 years after diagnosis, whether disease free, in remission, or under treatment with evidence of cancer."[1] Understandably, the use of the term *cured* is guarded since an initially diagnosed case of cancer can impact on survivability beyond the end of the 5-year time period. Regardless of survivability, for those who develop cancer, the physical, emotional, and social costs will be substantial.

No single explanation can be given for why progress in eliminating cancer has been so limited. It is a combination of factors, including the aging of the population, continued use of tobacco, the high-fat American diet, the continuing urbanization and pollution of our environment, the lack of health insurance for an estimated 41.2 million Americans to pay for early diagnosis and proper treatment,[2] or simply our recognition of cancer's true role

in deaths once ascribed to other causes. Regardless, we continue to be challenged to control this array of abnormal conditions that we collectively call cancer. There is, however, increasing optimism that with new pharmacological agents and the completion of the Human Genome Project real progress will finally be made.

 TALKING POINTS A close friend justifies her high cancer–risk lifestyle by saying that "Everyone will die of something." How would you counter this point?

Cancer: A Problem of Cell Regulation

Just as a corporation depends on individuals to staff its various departments, the body depends on its basic units of function, the cells. Cells band together as tissues, such as muscle tissue, to perform a prescribed function. Tissues in turn join to form organs, such as the heart, and organs are assembled into the body's several organ systems, such as the cardiovascular system. Such is the "corporate structure" of the body.

If individuals and cells are the basic units of function for their respective organizations, the failure of either to perform in a prescribed, dependable manner can erode the overall organization to the extent that it might not be able to continue. Cancer, the second leading cause of death among adults, is a condition reflecting cell dysfunction in its most extreme form. In cancer, the normal behavior of cells ceases.

Cell Regulation

Most of the body's tissues lose cells over time. This continual loss requires that replacement cells come from areas of young and less specialized cells. The process of specialization required to turn the less specialized cells into mature cells is controlled by genes within the cells. On becoming specialized, these newest cells copy, or replicate, themselves. These two processes are carefully monitored by the cells' **regulatory genes.** Failure to regulate specialization and replication results in abnormal, or potentially cancerous, cells.

In addition to genes that regulate specialization and replication, cells also have genes designed to repair mistakes in the copying of genetic material (the basis of replication) and genes to suppress the growth of abnormal cells should it occur. Thus, repair genes and tumor suppressor genes, such as the *p53* gene (altered or missing in half of all cancers), can also be considered regulatory genes in place to prevent the development of abnormal cells. Should these genes fail to function properly, resulting in the development of malignant (cancerous) cells, the immune system (see Chapter 12) will ideally recognize their presence and remove them before a clinical (diagnosable) case of cancer can develop.

Because specialization, replication, repair, and suppressor genes can become cancer-causing genes, or **oncogenes,** when not working properly, these four types of genes could also be referred to as **proto-oncogenes,** or potential oncogenes.[3] How proto-oncogenes become oncogenes is a question that cannot be completely answered at this time. Regardless, abnormal cells produce abnormal proteins, and the absence of normal proteins alters the body's ability to function appropriately, from the molecular to the organ system level.

Oncogene Formation

Recognizing that all cells have proto-oncogenes, what events alter otherwise normal regulatory genes so that they become cancer-causing genes? Three mechanisms, genetic mutations, viral infections, and carcinogens, have received much attention.

Genetic mutations develop when dividing cells miscopy genetic information. If the gene that is miscopied is a gene that controls specialization, replication, repair, or tumor suppression (a proto-oncogene), the oncogene that results will allow the formation of cancerous cells. A variety of factors, including aging, free radical formation, and radiation, are associated with the miscopying of the complex genetic information that comprises the genes found within the cell, including those intended to prevent cancer.

In both animals and humans, cancer-producing viruses, such as the feline leukemia virus in cats and the human immunodeficiency virus (HIV) and multiple forms of the human papilloma virus (HPV) in humans (see Chapter 12) have been identified. These viruses seek out cells of a particular type, such as cells of the immune system, or the lining of the cervix, and substitute some of their genetic material for some of the cells' thus converting them into virus-producing cells. In so doing, however, they change the makeup of the specialization, replication, repair, or suppressor genes, converting the proto-oncogenes into oncogenes. Once converted into oncogenes, the altered genes are passed on through cell division.

A third possible explanation for the conversion of proto-oncogenes into oncogenes involves the presence of environmental agents known as *carcinogens.* Over an extended period, carcinogens, such as chemicals found in tobacco smoke, polluted air and water, toxic wastes, and even high-fat foods, may convert proto-oncogenes into oncogenes. These carcinogens may work alone or in combination with co-carcinogenic promoters (see Chapter 9, Table 9.2) to alter the genetic material, including regulatory genes, within cells. Thus people might develop lung cancer only if they are exposed to the right combination of carcinogens over an extended period.

You may already see that some of the specific risk factors in each area—such as radiation in the development of mutations, sexually transmitted viruses in cancers of the reproductive tract, and smoking introduced carcinogens in the development of lung cancer—can be moderated by adopting health-promoting behaviors.

In light of the complexity of cancer, some in the scientific community believe that cancer can never be truly prevented. Rather, they feel that the ability to stop and then reverse cancerous changes at an early stage of their development is more likely than prevention of this complex disease process. However, this text will address the concepts of prevention in the belief that prevention-based practices reflect our personal contribution to the "war on cancer."[4]

The Cancerous Cell

Compared with noncancerous cells, cancer cells function in similar and dissimilar ways. It is the dissimilar aspects that often make them unpredictable and difficult to manage.

Key Terms

regulatory genes genes that control cell specialization, replication, DNA repair, and tumor suppression.

oncogenes faulty regulatory genes that are believed to activate the development of cancer.

proto-oncogenes (pro toe **on** co genes) normal regulatory genes that may become oncogenes.

Perhaps the most unusual aspect of cancerous cells is their infinite life expectancy. Specifically, it appears that cancerous cells can produce an enzyme, *telomerase*, that blocks the cellular biological clock that informs normal cells that it is time to die.[5] In spite of this ability to live forever, cancer cells do not necessarily divide more quickly than normal cells. In fact, they can divide at the same rate or even on occasion at a slower rate.

In addition, cancerous cells do not possess the *contact inhibition*[6] (a mechanism that influences the number of cells that can occupy a particular space at a particular time) of normal cells. In the absence of this property, cancer cells accumulate, altering the functional capacity of the tissue or organ they occupy. Further, the absence of *cellular cohesiveness*[6] (a property seen in normal cells that "keeps them at home") allows cancer cells to spread through the circulatory or lymphatic system to distant points via **metastasis** (Figure 11-1). Interest-ingly, once migrating cancer cells arrive at a new area of the body, they "rediscover" their cellular cohesive capabilities. A final unique characteristic of cancerous cells is their ability to command the circulatory system to send them additional blood supply to meet their metabolic needs and to provide additional routes for metastasis. This *angiogenesis*[6] capability of cancer cells makes them extremely hardy compared with noncancerous cells.

Benign Tumors

Noncancerous, or **benign,** tumors can also form in the body. These **tumors** are usually enclosed by a membrane and do not spread from their point of origin. Benign tumors can be dangerous when they crowd out normal tissue within a confined space.

Types of Cancer

Cancers are named according to the types of cells or tissues from which they originate. Although physicians routinely use these labels, another set, to be described later, is more familar to laypersons:

carcinoma—Found most frequently in the skin, nose, mouth, throat, stomach, intestinal tract, glands, nerves, breasts, urinary and genital structures, lungs, kidneys, and liver; approximately 85% of all malignant tumors are classified as carcinomas

sarcoma—Formed in the connective tissues of the body; bone, cartilage, and tendons are the sites of sarcoma development; only 2% of all malignancies are of this type

melanoma—Arises from the melanin-containing cells of skin; found most often in people who have had extensive sun exposure, particularly a deep, penetrating sunburn; although once rare, the amount of this cancer has increased markedly in recent years; remains among the most deadly forms of cancer

neuroblastoma—Originates in the immature cells found within the central nervous system; neuroblastomas are rare; usually found in children

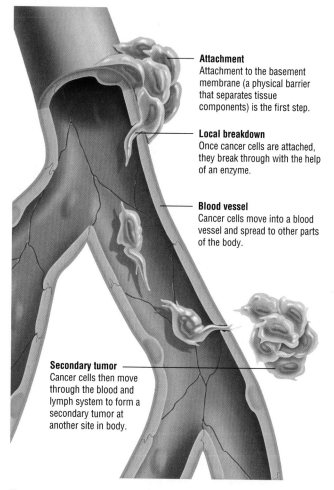

Attachment
Attachment to the basement membrane (a physical barrier that separates tissue components) is the first step.

Local breakdown
Once cancer cells are attached, they break through with the help of an enzyme.

Blood vessel
Cancer cells move into a blood vessel and spread to other parts of the body.

Secondary tumor
Cancer cells then move through the blood and lymph system to form a secondary tumor at another site in body.

Figure 11-1 How cancer spreads. Locomotion (movement) is essential to the process of metastasis (spread of cancer). Scientists have identified a protein that causes cancer cells to grow arms, or pseudopodia, enabling them to move to other parts of the body.

Key Terms

metastasis (muh **tas** ta sis) the spread of cancerous cells from their site of origin to other areas of the body.

benign noncancerous; tumors that do not spread.

tumor mass of cells; may be cancerous (malignant) or noncancerous (benign).

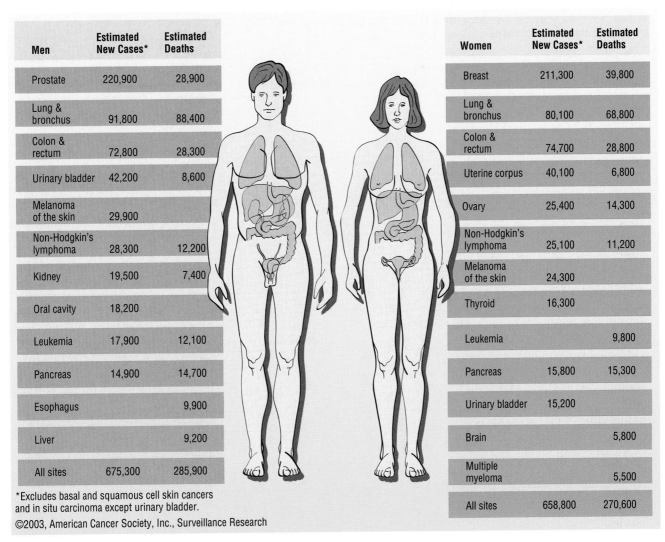

Men	Estimated New Cases*	Estimated Deaths
Prostate	220,900	28,900
Lung & bronchus	91,800	88,400
Colon & rectum	72,800	28,300
Urinary bladder	42,200	8,600
Melanoma of the skin	29,900	
Non-Hodgkin's lymphoma	28,300	12,200
Kidney	19,500	7,400
Oral cavity	18,200	
Leukemia	17,900	12,100
Pancreas	14,900	14,700
Esophagus		9,900
Liver		9,200
All sites	675,300	285,900

*Excludes basal and squamous cell skin cancers and in situ carcinoma except urinary bladder.

©2003, American Cancer Society, Inc., Surveillance Research

Women	Estimated New Cases*	Estimated Deaths
Breast	211,300	39,800
Lung & bronchus	80,100	68,800
Colon & rectum	74,700	28,800
Uterine corpus	40,100	6,800
Ovary	25,400	14,300
Non-Hodgkin's lymphoma	25,100	11,200
Melanoma of the skin	24,300	
Thyroid	16,300	
Leukemia		9,800
Pancreas	15,800	15,300
Urinary bladder	15,200	
Brain		5,800
Multiple myeloma		5,500
All sites	658,800	270,600

Figure 11-2 These 2003 estimates of new cases of cancer and deaths from cancer revealed some significant similarities between men and women. Note that lung cancer is the leading cause of cancer deaths for both genders.

adenocarcinoma—Derived from cells of the endocrine glands

hepatoma—Originates in cells of the liver; although not thought to be directly caused by alcohol use, seen more frequently in people who have experienced **sclerotic changes** in the liver

leukemia—Found in cells of the blood and blood-forming tissues; characterized by abnormal, immature white blood cell formation; several forms are found in children and adults

lymphoma—Arises in cells of the lymphatic tissues or other immune system tissues; includes lymphosarcomas and Hodgkin's disease; characterized by abnormal white cell production and decreased resistance

Figure 11-2 presents information about the estimated new cases of cancer and deaths from cancer at various sites in both men and women.[1] Table 11.1 shows that cancer incidence and mortality rates vary among different racial and ethnic groups.

> **Key Terms**
>
> **sclerotic changes** (skluh **rot** ick) thickening or hardening of tissues.

Table 11.1 Incidence and Mortality Rates* by Site, Race, and Ethnicity, United States, 1992–1999

Incidence	White	African American	Asian/ Pacific Islander	American Indian/ Alaskan Native	Hispanic[†]
All Sites					
Males	568.2	703.6	408.9	277.7	393.1
Females	424.4	404.8	306.5	224.2	290.5
Total	480.4	526.6	348.6	244.6	329.6
Breast (female)	137.0	120.7	93.4	59.4	82.6
Colon & rectum					
Males	64.4	70.7	58.7	40.7	43.9
Females	46.1	55.8	39.5	30.8	29.7
Total	53.9	61.9	47.9	35.2	35.7
Lung & bronchus					
Males	82.9	124.1	63.8	51.4	44.1
Females	51.1	53.2	28.5	23.3	22.8
Total	64.3	82.6	44.0	35.4	31.5
Prostate	172.9	275.3	107.2	60.7	127.6

Mortality	White	African American	Asian/ Pacific Islander	American Indian/ Alaskan Native	Hispanic[†]
All Sites					
Males	258.1	369.0	160.6	154.4	163.7
Females	171.2	204.5	104.4	110.4	105.7
Total	205.1	267.3	128.6	128.6	129.2
Breast (female)	29.3	37.3	13.1	14.8	17.5
Colon & rectum					
Males	26.7	34.8	16.5	14.6	16.6
Females	18.4	25.4	11.6	11.3	10.6
Total	21.9	29.1	13.7	12.8	13.2
Lung & bronchus					
Males	81.7	113.0	42.3	49.3	38.2
Females	41.1	39.6	19.3	24.9	13.8
Total	57.9	68.9	29.3	35.5	24.1
Prostate	32.9	75.1	15.1	18.8	22.6

* Per 100,000, age-adjusted to the 2000 US standard population. Incidence rates obtained from SEER registries covering 10%–15% of the US population. Mortality data are from all states.

[†] Hispanics are not mutually exclusive from whites, African Americans, Asian/Pacific Islanders, and American Indian/Alaskan Natives

Source: Surveillance, Epidemiology, and End Results Program, 1973–99, Division of Cancer Control and Population Sciences, National Cancer Institute. Bethesda, MD, 2002.

American Cancer Society, Surveillance Research, 2003

Cancer at Selected Sites in the Body

A second and more familiar way to describe cancer is on the basis of the organ site at which it occurs. The following discussion relates to some of these more familiar sites. A lack of space, in combination with the wide array of human cancers, limits the number of specific malignancies that can be described. Remember, also, that regular screening procedures can lead to early identification of cancer at these sites (see the Changing for the Better box on page 300).

Lung Cancer

Lung cancer is one of the most lethal and frequently diagnosed forms of cancer. Primarily because of the advanced stage of the disease at the time symptoms first appear, only 15% of all people with lung cancer (all stages) survive 5 years beyond diagnosis.[1] By the time a person is sufficiently concerned about having a persistent cough, blood-streaked sputum, and chest pain, it is often too late for treatment to be effective. This failure to be able to diagnose lung cancer in its earlier stages could, however, begin to change. Currently the National Cancer Institute is studying the efficacy of *spiral CT scans* in detecting lung tumors earlier than can be done by conventional chest x-rays. However, an initial assessment of the technology questions its cost-effectiveness and potential for excessive false-positive findings.[8]

Risk Factors

Today it is known that a genetic predisposition is important in the development of lung cancer. Perhaps, in fact, the majority of people who develop this form of cancer have an inherited "head start." When people who are genetically at risk also smoke, their level of risk for developing lung cancer is significantly greater than it is for nonsmokers. Of particular interest at this time are multiple genes on chromosome 3. Damage to three tumor suppressors on this chromosome is found in virtually every case of small-cell lung cancer and 90% of nonsmall-cell lung cancer.[9] Most of the remaining lung cancer cases appear in people who smoke but are not genetically predisposed.

Cigarette smoking is unquestionably the single most important behavioral factor in the development of lung cancer. For men who smoke, the rate of lung cancer is twenty-three times higher than for men who do not smoke. For women who smoke, the rate is eleven times higher than for women who do not smoke. Smokers account for the vast majority of all reported cases of lung cancer, and lung cancer itself produces at least 30% of all cancer-caused deaths.[1]

Since 1987, lung cancer has exceeded breast cancer as the leading cause of cancer deaths in women. The incidence of lung cancer has shown an encouraging decline in men that parallels their declining use of tobacco products, although it remains the leading cause of cancer deaths in men as well. Environmental agents, such as radon, asbestos, and air pollutants, make a smaller contribution to the development of lung cancer. Radon alone may be the principal causative agent in most lung cancer found in nonsmokers.

Prevention

The preceding information clearly suggests that not smoking or quitting smoking (see page 258) and avoidance of environmental tobacco smoke (see page 255) are the most important factors in the prevention of lung cancer. In addition, place of residence, particularly as it relates to air pollution, is a long-suspected risk factor for lung cancer.[10] Nonsmokers who are considering living with a smoker or working in a confined area where environmental tobacco smoke is prevalent should carefully consider the risk of developing lung cancer. A recent study does, however, lessen concern over moderate alcohol use and the risk of developing lung cancer.[11]

Treatment

The prognosis for surviving lung cancer remains extremely guarded. Depending on the type of lung cancer, its extent, and factors related to the patient's overall health, various combinations of surgery, radiation, and chemotherapy remain the physicians' primary approach to treatment. Today, for persons with early stage lung cancer, chemotherapy, following surgery, has increased survivability slightly.[12] Additionally, new medications that primarily shrink tumors are also available. Although these newer therapies have improved short-term survival, full recovery remains unlikely in all but a small percentages of cases.

Breast Cancer

Surpassed only by lung cancer, breast cancer is the second leading cause of death from cancer in women. It is the third leading cause of cancer deaths overall. Nearly one in eight women will develop breast cancer in her lifetime, resulting in an estimated 211,300 new invasive cases and 40,200 deaths in 2003.[1] In men, an estimated 1,300 new cases and 400 deaths occurred in 2003[1] (see the Learning from Our Diversity box on page 302). As they age, women's risk of developing breast cancer increases. Early detection is the key to complete recovery. Ninety-seven percent of women who discover their breast cancer before it has spread (metastasized) will survive more than 5 years.[1]

Screening Guidelines

For the Early Detection of Cancer in Asymptomatic People

Site	Recommendation
Breast	Women 40 and older should have an annual mammogram, an annual clinical breast examination (CBE) by a health care professional, and should perform monthly breast self-examinations (BSE). Ideally the CBE should occur before the scheduled mammogram. Women ages 20–39 should have a CBE by a health care professional every three years and should perform BSE monthly.
Colon & rectum	Beginning at age 50, men and women should follow one of the examination schedules below: • A fecal occult blood test (FOBT) every year • A flexible sigmoidoscopy (FSIG) every five years • Annual fecal occult blood test and flexible sigmoidoscopy every five years* • A double-contrast barium enema every five years • A colonoscopy every 10 years *Combined testing is preferred over either annual FOBT, or FSIG every 5 years, alone. People who are at moderate or high risk for colorectal cancer should talk with a doctor about a different testing schedule.
Prostate	The PSA test and the digital rectal examination should be offered annually, beginning at age 50, to men who have a life expectancy of at least 10 years. Men at high risk (African American men and men with a strong family history of one or more first-degree relatives diagnosed with prostate cancer at an early age) should begin testing at age 45. For both men at average risk and high risk, information should be provided about what is known and what is uncertain about the benefits and limitations of early detection and treatment of prostate cancer so that they can make an informed decision about testing.
Uterus	**Cervix:** Screening should begin approximately three years after a woman begins having vaginal intercourse, but no later than 21 years of age. Screening should be done every year with regular Pap tests or every two years using liquid-based tests. At or after age 30, women who have had three normal test results in a row may get screened every 2–3 years. However, doctors may suggest a woman get screened more often if she has certain risk factors, such as HIV infection or a weak immune system. Women 70 years and older who have had three or more consecutive normal Pap tests in the last 10 years may choose to stop cervical cancer screening. Screening after total hysterectomy (with removal of the cervix) is not necessary unless the surgery was done as a treatment for cervical cancer. **Endometrium:** The American Cancer Society recommends that all women should be informed about the risks and symptoms of endometrial cancer, and strongly encouraged to report any unexpected bleeding or spotting to their physicians. Annual screening for endometrial cancer with endometrial biopsy beginning at age 35 should be offered to women with or at risk for hereditary nonpolyposis colon cancer (HNPCC).
Cancer-related checkup	For individuals undergoing periodic health examinations, a cancer-related checkup should include health counseling, and depending on a person's age, might include examinations for cancers of the thyroid, oral cavity, skin, lymph nodes, testes, and ovaries, as well as for some nonmalignant diseases.

American Cancer Society guidelines for early cancer detection are assessed annually in order to identify whether there is new scientific evidence sufficient to warrant a re-evaluation of current recommendations. If evidence is sufficiently compelling to consider a change or clarification in a current guideline or the development of a new guideline, a formal procedure is initiated. Guidelines are formally evaluated every 5 years regardless of whether new evidence suggests a change in the existing recommendations. There are nine steps in this procedure, and these "guidelines for guideline development" were formally established to provide a specific methodology for science and expert judgment to form the underpinnings of specific statements and recommendations from the Society. These procedures constitute a deliberate process to insure that all Society recommendations have the same methodological and evidence-based process at their core. This process also employs a system for rating strength and consistency of evidence that is similar to that employed by the Agency for Health Care Research and Quality (AHCRQ) and the US Preventive Services Task Force (USPSTP).

Source: American Cancer Society, Cancer Facts & Figures 2003.

Risk Factors

Although all women and men are at some risk of developing breast cancer, the following groups of women have a higher risk.

• Women whose menstrual periods began at an early age, or whose menopause occurred late (although the former may be more powerful than the latter)[13]

Chemotherapy is a treatment for many types of cancer.

- Women who had no children, had their first child later in life, or did not nurse[14]
- Women who have used hormone replacement therapy[15]
- Women whose diets are high in saturated fats, those who are sedentary, and those with excessive central body cavity fat[16] (see Chapter 6)
- Women with a family history of breast cancer

As presented in the bulleted list, significant concerns exist regarding the long-term use of hormone replacement therapy and the development of breast cancer in post-menopausal women. In fact, in a government-sponsored study (Women's Health Initiative Study) the link appeared so strongly and early that the study was terminated much earlier than had been planned. Researchers found that tumor development in women taking HRT versus those on a placebo was more common, that tumors were larger at diagnosis, and that tumors were more often invasive.[15] Physicians are now advising that HRT be used only on a very short-term basis to relieve the symptoms of menopause, rather than the much longer period of time previously deemed appropriate.

The effects of environmental pollutants and regional influences have also been investigated as causative factors in the development of breast cancer.[17] Environmental pollutants vary from region to region and are influenced by a number of factors, including the type of industrial and agricultural activity in a particular area. A wide array of regional factors may be involved, including genetic background of people in a given area and lifestyle differences involving diet, alcohol consumption, and exercise patterns.

The role of genetic predisposition in the development of breast cancer has also received considerable attention.

For example, a small percentage (perhaps 5%) of women with breast cancer have inherited or developed mutations in one or both of two tumor suppressor genes (proto-oncogenes), *BRCA1* and *BRCA2*. Discovered in 1994 and 1995, respectively, and currently the focus of extensive research, more than two hundred mutations in these genes have been identified. In a recent study involving 5,000 Ashkenazi Jews (Jews of Central and Eastern European descent) living in the Washington, D.C., area, mutation in the *BRCA1* gene resulted in a 56% greater chance of developing breast cancer by age 70 (versus a 13% greater risk for people without a mutated version of the gene).[18] A more recent study suggests a role not only for mutations to *BRCA1* but to genetic material nearby on the same chromosome.[19] A mutation in the *BRCA2* gene has

OnSITE/InSIGHT

Learning to Go: Health

Are you concerned about developing cancer? Want to know how to live with a chronic condition? Click on Learning to Go: Health on the Online Learning Center at **www.mhhe.com/hahn7e** and check out the following lessons:

Lesson 30: Guard against breast cancer.

Lesson 31: Protect your skin from the sun.

Lesson 32: Reduce your risk of cancer.

Lesson 34: Learn to live with diabetes.

Lesson 35: Control your chronic pain.

Lesson 36: Learn how to manage your asthma.

been found to be less likely to foster the development of breast cancer than the *BRCA1* mutation.[18] Both of these genes are also associated with increased risk of developing ovarian cancer (see page 306) and, perhaps, prostate cancer in men.

Other genetic links to breast cancer have been identified. For example, one involves an increased risk for breast cancer development in black women.[20] The gene in question is *BPI*, a gene that, if shut off, allows cancer cells to establish cellular immortality. Factors that influence this gene to become dysfunctional have not been identified. The Personal Assessment on page 327 may be helpful in determining your relative level of risk for developing breast cancer.

Prevention

As already discussed, a variety of risk factors are thought to be important in the development of most cases of breast cancer. Accordingly, some degree of prevention is possible when factors such as diet; alcohol use; physical activity level; decisions about contraception, pregnancy, and breastfeeding; occupational exposure to toxins; and even place of residence are considered.

For women who have a primary family history of breast cancer (sisters, mother, or grandmothers with the disease) and who have been found to carry one or both of the mutated suppressor genes discussed, an extreme form of prevention is also possible— **prophylactic mastectomy.** In this surgical procedure, both noncancerous breasts are re- moved, in an attempt to eliminate the possibility of future cancer development. When carefully planned, breast reconstruction surgery can be undertaken immediately, with satisfactory results. A high level of satisfaction was found among women who had undergone this procedure.

At the present time pharmacological prevention represents the newest approach to reducing the incidence of breast cancer. Two medications, Evista, or raloxifene (a drug developed for use in osteoporosis prevention), and tamoxifen (an estrogen-receptor blocker developed for use in the treatment of cancer) have been found to be effective in lowering the risk of cancer in high-risk women. However, a warning (August 2000) from the FDA reminds physicians that tamoxifen can have serious side effects, including the development of uterine cancer and potentially fatal blood clots.[21]

Early Detection: Breast Self-Examination

For several decades a fundamental component of early detection of breast cancer has been breast self-examination

Key Terms
prophylactic mastectomy surgical removal of the breasts to prevent breast cancer in women who are at high risk of developing the disease.

I've never felt confident about doing a breast self-exam. What is the proper technique?

The following explains how to do a breast self-examination:

1. In the shower: Examine your breasts during a bath or shower; hands glide more easily over wet skin. With your fingers flat, move gently over every part of each breast. Use right hand to examine left breast, left hand for right breast. Check for any lump, hard knot, or thickening. This self-examination should be done monthly, preferably a day or two after the end of the menstrual period.

2. Before a mirror: Inspect your breasts with arms at your sides. Next, raise your arms high overhead. Look for any changes in contour of each breast, a swelling, dimpling of skin, changes in the nipple. Then rest palms on hips, and press down firmly to flex your chest muscles. Left and right breast will not exactly match—few women's breasts do.

3. Lying down: To examine your right breast, put a pillow or folded towel under your right shoulder. Place right hand behind your head—this distributes breast tissue more evenly on the chest. With left hand, fingers flat, press gently in small circular motions around an imaginary clock face. Begin at outermost top of your right breast for 12 o'clock, then move to 1 o'clock, and so on around the circle back to 12 o'clock. A ridge of firm tissue in the lower curve of each breast is normal. Then move in an inch toward the nipple; keep circling to examine every part of your breast, including the nipple. This requires at least three more circles. Now slowly repeat the procedure on your left breast with a pillow under your left shoulder and left hand behind head. Notice how your breast structure feels. Finally, squeeze the nipple of each breast gently between thumb and index finger. Any discharge, clear or bloody, should be reported to your doctor immediately.

Breast cancer can occur in men too. Therefore this examination should be performed monthly by men. Regular inspection shows what is normal for you and will give you confidence in your examination.

InfoLinks

www.mskcc.org

(BSE). Generally recommended for women 20 years of age and older, the procedure was to be performed during the menstrual period or during the day immediately following the end of the menstrual period, when estrogen levels are at their lowest and cystic activity in breast tissue is minimal (or on the same day of each month by postmenopausal women). The proper technique is illustrated in the Changing for the Better box above. Although breast self-examination is an easily learned technique, today its value is being strongly challenged by researchers in both this country and in China.[22] It has, in fact, become the contention of some that teaching BSE to another generation of women is a misuse of time and money that could be better spent on other screening techniques. Others, however, feel that women who know the technique should not be discouraged from using BSE, but they also should be regularly reminded of its significant limitations in finding tumors. In 2003, the American Cancer Society revised its recommendation for breast cancer screening to better address the doubts regarding BSE's limitations. Specific to BSE the following statement summarizes the ACS's current position.[23]

Previously, the guidelines (for BSE) recommended women perform breast self-exam every month. Now, (we) recommend that, beginning in their 20s, women should be told about the benefits and limitations of BSE, and that it is acceptable for women to choose not to do BSE, or to do it occasionally. The importance of promptly reporting changes to a physician is emphasized.

The reason for this change is that research has shown that BSE plays a very small role in detecting breast cancer compared with self-awareness.

Regardless, monthly BSE can be viewed as an adjunct to regularly scheduled breast examination conducted by a physician and to the routine use of mammography.

Early Detection: Mammography

Although researchers once disagreed about the age at which women should begin routine mammography and the extent to which mammography is effective in finding masses in dense breast tissue, today mammograms are physicians' best tool for the early detection of breast cancer. Accordingly, the American Cancer Society recommends that mammography begin at age 40.

Whether women begin routine mammography at 40, as advised by the ACS, or as early as 35 years of age, particularly for women with earlier symptoms or a family history of breast disease, women should continue these examinations on an annual basis. Recommendations regarding mammography for older women (65+) are, however, a bit more individually determined and should be discussed annually with physicians. For older women, overall health status and expectations for reaching a normal life expectancy will be weighed relative to the lowering cost-effectiveness of mammography.

Because of the important role routine mammography plays in the early identification of breast lesions, the Mammography Quality Standards Act (MQSA), formulated by the FDA (April 1998), is a valuable step toward ensuring that mammography is performed by experienced technicians, using correctly calibrated equipment, and interpreted by skilled radiologists. Every woman should be certain that her mammography is being performed in a MQSA-certified facility.

Treatment

Regardless of the method of detection, if a lump is found, a breast biopsy can determine whether the lump is cancerous. If the lump is cancerous but localized, treatment is highly effective, with cure rates at nearly 100 percent. The most frequently used treatments are **lumpectomy** combined with radiation, lumpectomy without radiation, and mastectomy. The use of chemotherapy following surgery is strongly advocated as well.[24]

When drug therapy is deemed desirable in treating breast cancer, oncologists may consider two drugs that have recently become available or whose earlier protocols have been redefined. The first, tamoxifen, discussed earlier in terms of breast cancer prevention, is a hormonelike drug that prevents estrogen from stimulating cancer cell growth. The use of tamoxifen has proven highly effective in women who have the type of breast cancer stimulated by the presence of estrogen.

The second drug, herceptin, is an antibodylike agent used in combination with other chemotherapeutic drugs in highly advanced breast cancer. This newly approved drug interferes with the activity of a protein produced by the HER-2 oncogene that normally fosters tumor cell division.

Cervical Cancer

In 2003 an estimated 12,200 new cases of cancer of the cervix (the anatomical neck of the uterus) occurred in the United States.[1] Fortunately, the death rate from cervical cancer has dropped greatly since 1950, largely because of the **Pap test.** This test screens for precancerous cellular changes (called *cervical intraepithelial neoplasia,* or *CIN*) and malignant cells. If malignant cells are found, it is hoped that they represent only cancer in situ (at the site of origin), rather than a more advanced invasive stage of the disease. Unfortunately, this simple and relatively inexpensive screening test is still underused, particularly in women over age 60, the group in which cervical cancer is most frequently found.

Key Terms

lumpectomy a surgical treatment for breast cancer in which a minimal amount of breast tissue is removed; when appropriate, this procedure is an alternative to mastectomy, in which the entire breast and underlying tissue are removed.

Pap test a cancer screening procedure in which cells are removed from the cervix and examined for precancerous changes.

Risk Factors

Because of the clear association between sexually transmitted infections and cervical cancer, risk factors for this form of cancer include early age of first intercourse, large number of sexual partners, history of infertility (which may indicate chronic pelvic inflammatory disease), and clinical evidence of *human papillomavirus* infections (see page 351 in Chapter 12). For patients with previous HPV infections or whose sexual history suggests a higher risk for HPV, a ThinPrep Pap test has been shown effective in detecting the DNA from four HPVs that are known to be cancer causing, while being as easy to use as the more widely used Pap smear. Today the test is only approved for identifying HPV infection, but it is also capable of detecting both chlamydia and gonorrhea. At the time of writing, human trials (Stage 1) are underway on a vaccine designed to protect against some HPV infections. Initial human studies have been highly effective in preventing infections from the most virulent of the HPVs, type 16.[25] Cigarette smoking and socioeconomic factors are also risk factors for cervical cancer. The latter most likely relates to less frequent medical assessment, including infrequent Pap tests. The Personal Assessment on page 327 will help women evaluate their risk of developing cervical cancer.

 TALKING POINTS Three risk factors are associated with HPV-induced cervical cancer: early age of first sexual intercourse, higher-than-average number of partners, and lack of protection against sexually transmitted diseases (e.g., condoms). How would you introduce this topic to a teenage daughter, sister, or niece?

Prevention

Sexual abstinence would be the most effective way of reducing the risk of developing cervical cancer (for example, Catholic nuns have extremely low rates of cervical cancer). However, since this is unlikely to be the choice for most women, other alternatives include fewer sexual partners, more careful selection of partners to minimize those at high risk, the use of condoms, and the use of spermicides. In addition, of course, regular medical assessment, including annual Pap tests (and the ThinPrep Pap test), represents prevention through early detection. Of course, when widely available, the HPV vaccine will further increase prevention.

Early Detection

At this time, the importance of women having Pap tests for cervical cancer performed on a regular basis cannot be overemphasized. However, the specific scheduling of cervical screening is undergoing adjustment. For young sexually active women, initial screening using the Pap smear (preferably in combination with the ThinPrep) should be undertaken within 3 years of first exposure. For young women not sexually at risk, or for women who have had a hysterectomy, the initial screening with the Pap smear can be determined in consultation with health care providers. Once initiated, however, following three consecutive annual negative tests, the interval between tests may be increased upon discussion with health care providers. The American Cancer Society estimates that cervical cancer claimed the lives of 4,100 women in 2002.

The Pap test is not perfect, however. When tests are read in laboratories highly experienced in interpreting Pap slides, about 7% will be false negatives, resulting in a 93% accuracy rate. In less-experienced laboratories, false negatives may be as high as 20%. (The Star box below explains what the possible Pap smear results mean.) In addition, not all women whose test results are accurately assessed as abnormal receive adequate follow-up care, nor do they have subsequent Pap tests regularly enough.

In addition to changes discovered by a Pap test, symptoms that suggest potential cervical cancer include abnormal vaginal bleeding between periods and frequent spotting.

What Pap Smear Results Mean

Pap smear results and their meanings can include:

- **Normal.** The cervical cells are healthy.
- **Unsatisfactory for evaluation.** The slide can't be read. Causes include douching, bleeding, infection, or not enough cells on the slide. The test should probably be repeated in 2–3 months.
- **Benign.** The Pap smear showed infection, irritation, or normal cell repair. If you have an infection, you might need medication.
- **Ascus.** The Pap smear showed some abnormal changes in the cells, but the cause is not clear. Infection is a common cause.
- **Low-grade changes.** You might have been infected with the human papilloma virus (HPV). Some types of the virus are associated with an increased risk for cancer of the cervix. Your health care provider will recommend specific follow-up. This might include another Pap smear or a colposcopy—a look at the cervix with a high-power microscope.
- **High-grade changes.** The cells of the cervix can progress toward cancer, but they aren't cancer yet. Fewer than half of the women with this test will develop cancer. Colposcopy is needed. Biopsy and treatment might be necessary.

Treatment

Should precancerous cellular changes (CIN) be identified, treatment can include one of several alternatives. Physicians can destroy areas of abnormal cellular change using cryotherapy (freezing), electrocoagulation, laser destruction, or surgical removal of abnormal tissue. More advanced (invasive) cancer of the cervix can be treated with a hysterectomy combined with other established cancer therapies. A combination of radiation and chemotherapy is the most effective treatment for cervical cancer.

Uterine (Endometrial) Cancer

The American Cancer Society estimates that in 2003, 40,100 cases of uterine cancer (cancer within the inner wall of the body of the uterus, rather than within the cervix or neck of the uterus) were diagnosed in American women. In addition, 6,600 women died of the disease.[1] Although African Americans have a lower incidence of uterine cancer than white women, their death rate is nearly twice as high.[1]

Risk Factors

Unlike cervical cancer, in which a strong viral link has been identified, the principal risk factor related to the development of endometrial cancer is a high estrogen level. Accordingly, the following factors are related to higher levels of estrogen and, thus, to the development of endometrial cancer:

- Early menarche (early onset of menstruation)
- Late menopause
- Lack of ovulation
- Never having given birth
- Estrogen replacement therapy (ERT not moderated with progesterone)
- Use of tamoxifen (a drug used in breast cancer therapy)

To some degree, endometrial cancer is seen more frequently in people who are diabetic, obese, or hypertensive or who have gallbladder disease,[1] or a family history of colon cancer.

Prevention

The risk factors associated with high levels of estrogen are areas in which prevention might be targeted. In addition, the need for regular gynecological care that includes pelvic examination is a principal factor in minimizing the risk of uterine cancer. Pregnancy and the use of oral contraceptives both provide some protection from endometrial cancer.[1]

Early Detection

Compared with cervical cancer, which is routinely identified through Pap tests, endometrial cancer is much more likely to be suspected on the basis of symptoms (irregular or postmenopausal bleeding) and confirmed by biopsy. Although more invasive, biopsy is a more effective method than ultrasound to diagnose uterine cancer.

Treatment

The treatment for early or localized endometrial cancer is generally surgical removal of the uterus (hysterectomy). Other therapies, such as radiation, chemotherapy, and hormonal therapy, may then be added to the treatment regimen. However, in terms of hormone replacement therapy (HRT), in which estrogen is combined with a synthetic progesterone, the FDA, The National Institute on Aging, and various medical associations now advise that no women 65 or older should take HRT due to several concerns, including an increased risk for endometrial cancer. For women who are undergoing menopause and experiencing troublesome symptoms such as night sweats and hot flashes, HRT should be used in the smallest doses that provide relief and for the shortest duration of time possible.

Ovarian Cancer

Since the death in 1989 of actress Gilda Radner, a star in the early years of *Saturday Night Live,* public awareness of ovarian cancer has increased in the United States. The American Cancer Society estimates that in 2003, there were 25,400 new cases diagnosed and 14,300 women died of the disease.[1] Most cases develop in women over age 40 who have not had children or began menstruation at an early age. The highest rate is in women over age 60. Today ovarian cancer causes more deaths than any other form of female reproductive system cancer.

For a relatively small percentage of all women (10%), the inheritance of either the *BRCA1* or *BRCA2* suppressor gene mutation (see page 301) significantly increases the risk of developing both breast and ovarian cancer. Today it is estimated that about 20% of all cases of ovarian cancer stem from these genetic mutations.

Beyond the 20% of cases attributed to genetic mutations, what might account for the majority of ovarian cancers? Today accumulated evidence points to the several decades during which millions of menopausal and postmenopausal women were placed on estrogen replacement therapy (ERT), often for years to counter the symptoms of menopause, maintain bone mass, and continue hormonal protection from cardiovascular disease.[26] As mentioned in conjunction with endometrial cancer, today hormone replacement therapy (HRT) is used, and then for only the briefest period of time.

Prevention

Methods of preventing or lowering the risk of developing ovarian cancer are very similar to those recommended for breast cancer. These include using oral contraceptives, giving birth and breastfeeding (for at least three months), reducing dietary fat intake, abstaining from alcohol use, and performing regular physical activity.

For the small group of women with a strong family history of ovarian cancer, a **prophylactic oophorectomy** should be seriously considered. In this surgical procedure, both ovaries are removed. Carefully monitored hormone replacement therapy is then used to provide the protective advantages of estrogen in maintaining cardiovascular health and bone density.

Early Detection

Because of its vague symptoms, ovarian cancer has been referred to as a *silent cancer*. Women in whom ovarian cancer has been diagnosed often report that the only symptoms of their cancer's presence were digestive disturbances, gas, and stomach distention. For this reason, annual pelvic examinations are important.

For women with a strong family history of ovarian cancer (four primary family members who have had breast or ovarian cancer, with two or more cases occurring before age 50) or women of Ashkenazi Jewish descent (see page 301), genetic screening and transvaginal ultrasound screening are likely to be recommended. These women may also be referred for participation in one of several prevention trials now under way.

Treatment

At this time, treatment of ovarian cancer requires surgical removal of the ovary, followed by aggressive use of chemotherapy. Use of the chemotherapeutic drug Taxol, obtained from the bark and needles of the Pacific yew tree, results in a 50% survival rate 19 months after the completion of therapy. Most recently, use of an experimental three-drug combination has resulted in a 70% survival rate 22 months after chemotherapy.

Prostate Cancer

If the names Bob Dole, General Norman Schwarzkopf, Colin Powell, and Rudy Giuliani are familiar, then you know four older men who have been diagnosed with and treated for prostate cancer. In fact, prostate cancer is so common that in 2003 an estimated 220,900 new cases were diagnosed and 28,900 men died of the disease.[1] Prostate cancer is the second leading cause of cancer deaths in American men, exceeded only by lung cancer deaths. Cancer of the prostate is the third most common form of cancer in men and a leading cause of death from cancer in older men.

The prostate gland is a walnut-size gland located near the base of the penis. It surrounds the neck of the bladder and the urethra. The prostate secretes a number of components of semen, such as nutrients used to fuel sperm motility.

Risk Factors

Compared with other cancers, the risk factors for prostate cancer are less clearly defined. The most predictable risk factor is age. Nearly 80% of all prostate cancer cases are diagnosed in men over 65 years of age, while cases in men under age 50 are infrequent. African American men and men with a family history of prostate cancer are at greater risk of developing this form of cancer. A link between prostate cancer and dietary fat intake, including excessive red meat and dairy product consumption, has also been suggested. With the discovery of the *BRCA1* and *BRCA2* genes related to breast and ovarian cancer, a genetic link with prostate cancer was also established. Men with one of these genetic mutations have an increased risk of developing prostate cancer.

Prevention

Although the American Cancer Society does not specifically address prevention of prostate cancer, prevention is not an unrealistic goal. Clearly, moderation of dietary fat intake is a preventive step.[27] Increased dietary intake levels of vitamin E and the micronutrient selenium have been shown to play a preventive role in prostate cancer.[28] In addition, effective treatment of benign prostatic hyperplasia (BPH) (prostate enlargement) with the drug Proscar (finasteride) has proven effective in preventing low-grade tumors in clinical trials.[29]

Early Detection

The symptoms of prostate disease, including prostate cancer, are listed in the Star box on page 308. A physician should be consulted if any of these symptoms appear, particularly in men aged 50 or older. Screening for prostate cancer should begin by age 40. This screening consists of an annual rectal examination performed by a physician and a blood test, the **prostate-specific antigen (PSA) test,** administered every 2 years. Another version of the PSA test has also been developed. This test can identify the "free"

Key Terms

prophylactic oophorectomy surgical removal of the ovaries to prevent ovarian cancer in women at high risk of developing the disease.

prostate-specific antigen (PSA) test a blood test used to identify prostate-specific antigen, an early indicator that the immune system has recognized and mounted a defense against prostate cancer.

- Difficulty urinating
- Frequent urination, particularly at night
- Continued wetness for a short time after urination
- Blood in the urine
- Low back pain
- Ache in the upper thighs

antigen most closely associated with the more aggressive forms of prostate cancer, thus cutting down on the false positives and extensive use of biopsies. In addition, an ultrasound rectal examination is used in men whose PSA scores are abnormally high. In spite of the important contribution made by the PSA test, there is some concern about the possibility of overtreating 30% of men in the 60 to 84 age group, particularly in light of the side effects of treatment described below.[30]

Treatment

Today prostate cancer is treated surgically, or through the use of external radiation or the implantation of radioactive seeds (brachytherapy) into the gland. Of course, each form of treatment carries the potential for side effects, including an 80% chance of impotence over a 10-year period;[30] incontinence with surgery; diarrhea and tiredness with external radiation; and some anal discomfort in association with the implantation of radioactive seeds into the prostate with internal radiation. The latter form of radiation therapy is highly effective for early-stage disease. One form of prostate cancer grows so slowly that men whose cancer is of this type, whose tumors are very localized, and whose life expectancy is less than 10 years at the time of diagnosis will not receive treatment but rather will be closely monitored for any progression of the cancer. For men who have the more aggressive form of the cancer, or whose tumor is no longer localized, physicians can employ a range of therapies, including surgery, radiation, chemotherapy, and hormonal therapy. In addition, an experimental vaccine has recently been tested on humans.

Testicular Cancer

Cancer of the testicle is among the least common forms of cancer; however, it is the most common solid tumor in men ages 15 to 34. Awareness of this type of cancer was raised in 1996 and 1997, when five-time winner of the tour de France Lance Armstrong and champion figure skater Scott Hamilton were diagnosed with testicular can-

cer. In both men, chronic fatigue and abdominal discomfort were the first symptoms of the disease. The American Cancer Society estimates that in 2003 testicular cancer was diagnosed in 7,600 men and caused the deaths of 400.[1]

Risk Factors

Risk factors for testicular cancer are variable, ranging from family history to environmental factors. The disease is more frequently seen in African Americans and in men whose testicles were undescended during childhood. Additional risk factors, such as difficulty during the mother's pregnancy, elevated temperature in the groin, and mumps during childhood, have been reported. The incidence of this cancer has been increasing in recent decades, while a corresponding drop in sperm levels has also been observed. Although no single explanation can be given for these changes, environmental factors such as agricultural pesticide toxicity may be involved. Once pesticides are concentrated in the tissues of the human body, during pregnancy they mimic estrogen. This, in turn, leads to testicular dysgenesis syndrome, or the failure of the testicles to develop normally.[31]

Testicular cancer is more frequently seen among white-collar workers than among people in blue-collar occupations. The suspicion that testicular cancer is linked to vasectomies appears to be unfounded.

Prevention

Because risk factors for testicular cancer are so variable, prevention is limited to regular self-examination of the testicles. Symptoms such as fatigue, abdominal discomfort, and enlargement of the testicle should be reported to a physician, since these can be associated with other disease processes. A male infant with one or both testicles in the undescended position (resulting in an empty scrotum) should be seen promptly by a physician so that corrective procedures can be undertaken.

Early Detection

In addition to the fatigue and abdominal distress reported by both Armstrong and Hamilton, other symptoms of testicular cancer include a small, painless lump on the side or near the front of the testicle, a swollen or enlarged testicle, and a heaviness or dragging sensation in the groin or scrotum. The importance of testicular self-examination, as well as early diagnosis and prompt treatment, cannot be overemphasized for men in the at-risk age group of 15 to 34 years. The Changing for the Better box on page 309 explains how to perform a testicular self-examination.

Treatment

Depending on the type, stage, and degree of localization of the tumor, surgical intervention generally includes re-

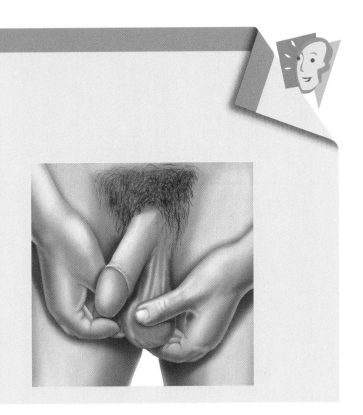

moval of the testicle, spermatic cord, and regional lymph nodes. Chemotherapy and radiation might also be used. Today, treatment is very effective, with 95% of all testicular cancer patients surviving 5 years and 99% surviving 5 years when the cancer was localized at the time of diagnosis. It should be noted, however, that concern exists regarding the development of other forms of cancer, such as leukemia, later in life.[32]

Colorectal Cancer

Cancer of the colon and rectum (colorectal cancer) has a death rate second only to that of lung cancer. In the most general sense, two types of tumors, carcinoma and lymphoma, can be found in both the colon and rectum. However, even within the most common form of colorectal cancer, there may subtle difference in type of tumors (or their origins) which influence the degree of potential spread and, thus, the nature of treatment itself. Fortunately, when diagnosed in a localized state, colorectal cancer has a relatively high survival rate (90% when localized and 65% for all stages).[1]

Risk Factors

Underlying the development of colorectal cancer are at least two potentially important areas of risk: genetic susceptibility and dietary patterns. Genes have recently been discovered that lead to familial colon cancer and familial polyposis (abnormal tissue growth that occurs before the formation of cancer) and are believed to be responsible for the tendency of colorectal cancer to run in families. Dietary risk factors include diets that are high in saturated fat from red meat and low in fruits and vegetables, which contain antioxidant vitamins and fiber. In regard to fiber's ability to prevent colorectal cancer, however, the ability of dietary fiber, when taken in supplement form, is in question. In addition, an association between colorectal polyps and smoking has been identified.[33]

Prevention

Small outpouchings in the lower intestinal tract wall, called *polyps*, are frequently important in the eventual development of colorectal cancer. Prompt removal of polyps has been shown to lower the risk of colorectal cancer. Further, some evidence indicates that the development of colorectal cancer may be prevented or slowed through regular exercise, the regular use of aspirin, an increase in dietary calcium intake, and long-term folic acid supplementation. Additionally, oral contraceptive use may be protective for women.

   Again, routine screening for colorectal cancer should be considered a form of prevention, much as PSA testing is for prostate cancer and mammography is for breast cancer.

Early Detection

Symptoms of colorectal cancer include bleeding from the rectum, blood in the stool, and a change in bowel habits. In addition, a family history of inflammatory bowel disease, polyp formation, or colorectal cancer should make one more alert to symptoms.[1] In people over age 50, any sudden change in bowel habits that lasts 10 days or longer should be evaluated by a physician. The American Cancer Society recommends preventive health care that includes digital (manual) rectal examination after age 40, a stool blood test after age 50, and sigmoidoscopy every 3 to 5 years and **colonoscopy** every 10 years after age 50. At this time some experts are questioning the advisability of using sigmoidoscopy as the routine screening procedure for colorectal cancer in comparison to using colonoscopy, which can more effectively find distal (higher up in the colon) cancerous changes.[34]

Although colonoscopy is currently the "gold standard" in the screening for colorectal cancer, new technologies are on the horizon. Three alternatives include the PreGen-Plus test that identifies cancer-indicating DNA mutations appearing in stool samples; a yet-named blood test capable of identifying "loss of imprinting" (LOI) factor associated with a high risk for colorectal cancer; and the CT colonography (CTC) that uses serial tomography to visualize the colon, thus eliminating the need to scope the colon.

Treatment

When one or more of these screening procedures suggests the possibility of disease within the lower intestinal tract, a careful visual evaluation of the entire length of the colon will be undertaken. During colonoscopy, areas of concern can be biopsied and the presence of a malignancy confirmed. Upon diagnosis, a localized and noninvasive malignancy will be removed surgically. When an invasive tumor is identified, supportive treatment with radiation or chemotherapy is necessary. Metastatic cancer requires chemotherapy.

Pancreatic Cancer

Pancreatic cancer is one of the most lethal forms of cancer, with a survival rate of only 4% 5 years after diagnosis.[1] Because of this gland's important functions in both digestion and metabolic processes related to glucose utilization (see the discussion of diabetes mellitus), its destruction by a malignancy leaves the body in a state incompatible with living.

In 2003 an estimated 30,700 new cases of pancreatic cancer were diagnosed and 30,000 deaths occurred.[1]

Risk Factors

Pancreatic cancer is more common in men than women, occurs more frequently with age, and develops most often in African American men. Smoking is clearly a risk factor for this form of cancer, with smokers more than twice as likely to develop the disease. Other risk factors have been tentatively suggested, such as chronic inflammation of the pancreas (pancreatitis), diabetes mellitus, alcohol-induced liver deterioration (cirrhosis), obesity, and high-fat diets.[1] Relatively little else is known about risk factors and, thus, prevention.

Prevention

Not smoking and abstaining from alcohol use are the most effective steps toward preventing this form of cancer. Further, reducing the risk of type 2 diabetes mellitus, through weight loss and exercise, (see page 317) would also make an important contribution to prevention. Annual medical examinations are, of course, associated with overall cancer prevention.

Early Detection

Early detection of this cancer is difficult because of the absence of symptoms until late in its course. Perhaps for people with a history of chronic pancreatitis, physicians might consider routine ultrasound assessment or computerized axial tomography scans (CAT scans). Once symptoms appear, a biopsy will be performed.

Treatment

At this time there is no effective treatment for pancreatic cancer. Surgical removal of malignant sites within the gland, in addition to radiation and chemotherapy, is usually tried. Certainly, if a particular patient with pancreatic cancer qualifies, enrollment in a clinical trial would be worth consideration.

Lymphatic Cancer

An estimated 61,000 new cases of lymphoma (7,600 cases of Hodgkin's disease and 53,400 cases of non-Hodgkin's lymphoma) were diagnosed in 2003. The number of deaths from both forms of lymphoma was near 31,900. The incidence of Hodgkin's disease has declined over the last 25 years, while the incidence of non-Hodgkin's disease has nearly doubled.[1]

Key Terms

colonoscopy (co lun **os** ko py) examination of the entire length of the colon, using a flexible fiberoptic scope to inspect the structure's inner lining.

Risk Factors

Risk factors for lymphoma are difficult to determine. Some possible factors are a general reduction in immune protection, exposure to toxic environmental chemicals such as pesticides and herbicides, and viral infections.[1] As you will learn in Chapter 12, the virus that causes AIDS (HIV) is a leukemia/lymphoma virus that was initially called HTLV-III (human T-cell leukemia/lymphoma virus-type III). A related leukemia/lymphoma virus, HTLV-I, is also suspected in the development of lymphatic cancer.

Prevention

Beyond limiting exposure to toxic chemicals and sexually transmitted viruses, few recommendations can be made about prevention. Again, early detection and diagnosis can serve as a form of prevention, since early-stage cancer is more survivable than advanced disease.

Early Detection

Unlike other cancers, the early symptoms of lymphoma are diverse and similar to symptoms of other illnesses, most of which are not serious. These symptoms include enlarged lymph nodes (frequently a sign of any infection that the immune system is fighting), fever, itching, weight loss, and anemia.

Treatment

Although surgery (beyond a biopsy) is usually not associated with the treatment of lymphoma, a variety of other therapies are employed. Depending on the stage and type of lymphoma, therapy may involve only radiation treatment of localized lymph nodes, as is seen in non-Hodgkin's lymphoma. Radiation combined with chemotherapy is generally used in the treatment late-stage non-Hodgkin's lymphoma. More recently, other therapies, including more aggressive chemotherapy, monoclonal antibody therapy, and bone marrow and stem cell transplantation, have been employed.

After completion of therapy, one-year survival rates for Hodgkin's disease are near 95% and near 77% for non-Hodgkin's lymphoma. By the end of 5 years, these rates have dropped to 84% and 55%, respectively.[1] Lower rates of survival are seen at 10 years and beyond.

Skin Cancer

Thanks largely to our desire for a fashionable tan, many teens and adults have spent more time in the sun (and in tanning booths) than their skin can tolerate. As a result, skin cancer, once common only among people who had to work in the sun, is occurring with alarming frequency. In 2003, nearly 1.3 million Americans developed basal or squamous cell skin cancer and 54,200 cases of highly dangerous malignant melanoma were diagnosed.[1]

Deaths from skin cancer do occur, with 9,600 estimated in 2002. More than 80% of these deaths were the result of malignant melanoma.

Risk Factors

Severe sunburning during childhood and chronic sun exposure during adolescence and younger adulthood are largely responsible for the "epidemic" of skin cancer being reported. The current emphasis on screening for skin cancer may also be increasing the incidence of early-stage cancer being reported. Occupational exposure to some hydrocarbon compounds can also cause skin cancer.

Prevention

Prevention of skin cancer should be a high priority for people who enjoy the sun or must work outdoors. The use of sunscreen with an a sun protection factor (SPF) of 15 or greater is very important. In addition, parents can help their children prevent skin cancer later in life by restricting their outdoor play from 11:00 A.M. to 2:00 P.M., requiring them to wear hats that shade their faces, and applying a sunscreen with an SPF of 15 on them regardless of skin tone. A recent evaluation of sunscreen effectiveness studies by Sloan-Kettering Cancer Center, however, suggests that sunscreens provide little protection against the deeply penetrating UV-A rays associated with the development of melanoma in susceptible people, and less protection than once thought against the UV-B rays associated with burning and wrinkling of the skin. Practicing dermatologists nonetheless continue to recommend their use. Regardless of the extent to which sunscreens provide protection, users are reminded that the level of protection provided is not doubled by simply doubling the SPF—for example, a sunscreen carrying an SPF of 30 does not provide twice the protection provided by a product with an SPF of 15. Therefore, the compliant use of a SPF-15 product is deemed not only appropriate, but may also save money over the more expensive products with a higher SPF rating.

The Personal Assessment on page 327 will help you determine your own risk of developing this kind of cancer.

Early Detection

Although many doctors do not emphasize this point enough, the key to the successful treatment of skin cancer is early detection. For basal cell or squamous cell cancer, a pale, waxlike, pearly nodule or red, scaly patch may be the first symptom. Other types of skin cancer may be indicated by a gradual change in the appearance of an existing mole. A physician should be consulted if such a change is noted. Melanoma usually begins as a small, molelike growth that increases progressively in size, changes color, ulcerates, and bleeds easily. To help detect melanoma, the American Cancer Society recommends using the guidelines below:

A is for asymmetry.

B is for border irregularity.

C is for color (change).

D is for a diameter greater than 6 mm.

E is for elevation (raised margins).

Figure 11-3 shows a mole that would be considered harmless and one that clearly demonstrates the ABCDE characteristics just described. The Changing for the Better box on page 313 shows how to make a regular inspection of the skin.

Most recently, a relationship between the presence of abnormal moles, called *dysplastic nevi* (flat, irregularly shaped, mottled in color, with irregular edges), and the risk of developing malignant melanoma has been established.[35] By counting these "indicator moles," physicians can judge the relative risk of developing this serious form of skin cancer before it first appears.

Treatment

When nonmelanoma skin cancer is found, an almost 100% cure rate can be expected. Treatment of these skin cancers can involve surgical removal by traditional excising or laser vaporization, destruction by burning or freezing, or destruction using x-ray therapy. When the more serious melanomas are found at an early stage, a high cure rate (95%) is accomplished using the same techniques. However, when malignant melanomas are more advanced, extensive surgery and chemotherapy will be necessary. The 5-year survival rate for regionalized forms of

the disease drops to 60%, and, unfortunately, long-term disease recovery is uncommon (14%).[1]

Status of the "War On Cancer"

It has been nearly 35 years since President Nixon declared a national "War On Cancer" and today the results are both encouraging and discouraging. On the positive side impressive technological advances have been and continue to be made in the diagnosis and treatment of cancer. As mentioned throughout the chapter, new screening procedures as well as treatment protocols seem to appear at a consistent rate. Additionally, the death rates from a variety of cancers have fallen, including a 70% decrease in the rate for Hodgkin's disease and a 14% decline in the death rate for breast cancer. Death rates for cervical, stomach, uterine, colon, bladder, and thyroid cancers have also fallen. Particularly important is a general increase in the public's awareness of cancer prevention and early detection.[36]

On the negative side is the reality that cancer is not only a biological disease, but also a disease (or more than 100 diseases) with strong sociopolitical implications. Central to this area are factors such as the inability of the majority of Americans to make needed changes in lifestyle, as it relates to smoking, alcohol use, exercise, weight management, and dietary practices. Also impeding progress is the absence of health care insurance for 41.4 million Americans that prevents early diagnosis and treatment of cancer. In fact, virtually every cancer in adults is impacted negatively by one or more of these largely modifiable complicating factors. This said, the federal government continues funding research in biological, behavioral, and education aspects of the war on cancer.[37]

A   B

Figure 11-3 A, Normal mole. This type of lesion is often seen in large numbers on the skin of young adults and may affect any body site. Note its symmetrical shape, regular borders, uniform color, and relatively small size (about 6 millimeters). **B,** Malignant melanoma. Note its asymmetrical shape, irregular borders, uneven color, and relatively large size (about 2 centimeters).

Cancer's Seven Warning Signals

Listed below are the seven warning signs of cancer, which the acronym CAUTION will help you remember:

1. **C**hange in bowel or bladder habits
2. **A** sore that does not heal
3. **U**nusual bleeding or discharge
4. **T**hickening or lump in the breast or elsewhere
5. **I**ndigestion or difficulty in swallowing
6. **O**bvious change in a wart or mole
7. **N**agging cough or hoarseness

If you have a warning signal for more than 5 days, see your doctor!

In the final analysis, the "war" remains very challenging: progress is being made, setbacks occur, and the victory remains far from being in hand. The "Big C" remains.[36]

Prevention Through Risk Reduction

Because cancer will probably continue to be the second most common cause of death among adults, it is important that you explore ways to reduce your risk of developing cancer. The following factors, which could make you vulnerable to cancer, can be controlled or at least recognized.

- *Know your family history.* You are the recipient of the genetic strengths and weaknesses of your biological parents and your more distant relatives. If you are able to determine that cancer is prevalent in your family medical history, you cannot afford to disregard this fact. It may be appropriate for you to be screened for certain types of cancer more often or at a young age. The importance of family history was clearly seen in our discussion of the *BRCA1/BRCA2* inheritance pattern and related decisions about prophylactic mastectomy and prophylactic oophorectomy.

- *Select and monitor your occupation carefully.* Because of recently discovered relationships between cancer and occupations that bring employees into contact with carcinogenic agents, you must be aware of the risks posed by certain job selections and assignments. Worksites where you will come into frequent contact with pesticides, strong solvents, volatile hydrocarbons, and airborne fibers could pay well but also shorten your life. The importance of this point is evident in reviewing the current list of environmental carcinogens studies funded by the National Cancer Institute. Included are studies that focus on indoor air pollution (tobacco smoke and cooking oils), dust (cotton, grain, plastic, and wood), organic solvents (benzene, carbon tetrachloride, toluene, xylene, and chlordane), organophosphates (diazinon, dichlorvos, malathion, triazines, and cyaniazine), polybrominated biphenyls, polychlorinated biphenyls, fumigants (ethylene), water pollution (chloride, phosphene, and fluoride), petroleum products (diesel fuel, gasoline, jet fuel), radiation (radon, neutron therapy, and reactor accidents), biological agents (chlamydia, HIV/HPV, helicobacter, hepatitis B and C) and radioisotopes (iodine and radium).

- *Do not use tobacco products.* You may want to review Chapter 9 on the overwhelming evidence linking all forms of tobacco use (including smokeless tobacco) to the development of cancer. Smoking is so detrimental to health that it is considered the number one preventable cause of death.

- *Monitor environmental exposure to carcinogens.* When carcinogenic concerns related to types of employment, residential radon levels, ozone depletion leading to increased exposure to solar radiation, and environmental tobacco smoke are seen in totality, it is apparent that the environment holds great potential as a source of carcinogenic exposure. To the extent to which it is possible to select the environment in which you will reside, work, and recreate, you should add selecting a low-risk environment to your list of cancer-prevention activities.

- *Follow a sound diet.* As mentioned in conjunction with folic acid and colorectal cancer and high-fat diets and prostate cancer, dietary patterns are known to play both a causative and a preventive role in cancer. Review Chapter 5 for information about dietary practices and the incidence of various diseases, including cancer. In that chapter, the role of fruits and vegetables known to be sources of cancer-preventing phytochemicals is introduced. Good sources include a wide variety of fruits and vegetables, particularly the cruciferous vegetables, including cauliflower, broccoli, and brussels sprouts, and fruits high in beta-carotene, vitamin C, and fiber. Should research demonstrate an even clearer role for nutrients, **chemoprevention** may become an even more widely practiced component of cancer prevention. Chemoprevention is not limited to food items and dietary supplements but can also involve pharmaceutical

agents, such as aspirin, estrogen replacement therapy, and hormone replacement therapy.

- *Control your body weight.* For women, obesity is related to a higher incidence of cancer of the uterus, ovary, and breast because obesity correlates with high estrogen levels. Maintaining a desirable body weight could improve overall health and lead to more successful management of cancer should it develop. Additionally, consider carefully whether you want to follow the currently popular high-protein, high-fat diets (Chapter 6), given their recognized carcinogenic potential.

- *Exercise regularly.* Chapter 4 discusses in detail the importance of regular moderate exercise to all aspects of health, including reducing the risk of chronic illnesses. Moderate exercise increases the body's ability to deliver oxygen to its tissues and thus to reduce the formation of cancer-enhancing free radicals formed during incomplete oxidation of nutrients. Moderate exercise also stimulates the production of enzymes that remove free radicals.

- *Limit your exposure to the sun.* It is important to heed this message even if you enjoy many outdoor activities. Particularly for people with light complexions, the radiation received through chronic exposure to the sun may foster the development of skin cancer.

- *Consume alcohol in moderation if at all.* Heavier users of alcohol have an increased prevalence of several types of cancer, including cancer of the oral cavity, larynx, and esophagus. Whether this results directly from the presence of carcinogens in alcohol or is more closely related to the alcohol user's tendency to smoke has not yet been established.

Cancer and Wellness

When you carefully consider the preceding suggestions, it should be obvious that you can do a great deal to prevent or at least minimize the development of cancer. A wellness-oriented lifestyle is the best weapon in your "personal war against cancer." However, all risk factor reduction is

---

Key Terms

chemoprevention cancer prevention using food, food supplements, or medications thought to bolster the immune system or reduce the damage caused by carcinogens.

relative. Observation and experience tell us that life cannot be totally structured around the desire to achieve maximum longevity or reduce morbidity at all costs. Most people need to strike a balance between life that is emotionally, socially, and spiritually satisfying and life that is structured solely for the purpose of living a long time and minimizing exposure to illness. Regardless of our personal lifestyle, however, we can educate others, provide comfort and support to those who are living with cancer, and support the funding of continuing and innovative new cancer research. Resources available for people with cancer and their families are listed in the Star boxes above.

Chronic Health Conditions

In addition to the two most widely recognized chronic health problems of adulthood—cardiovascular disease and cancer—adults can experience an array of other chronic health conditions. What all of these chronic conditions have in common is the ability to cause significant change in the lives of people—both on the part of the affected person and his or her family members and friends (see Discovering Your Spirituality on page 317).

Some of these conditions are seen in early adulthood, such as lupus and Crohn's disease. Others, such as diabetes mellitus type 2, generally do not appear until nearer middle age. However, some chronic diseases seen during adulthood have their origins in childhood, such as diabetes mellitus type 1.

Systemic Lupus Erythematosus

Systemic lupus erythematosus (SLE), or simply *lupus*, is perhaps the most familiar of a class of chronic conditions know as **autoimmune** disorders, or connective tissue diseases. Collectively, these conditions reflect a concentrated and inappropriate attack by the body's immune system on its own tissues, which then serve as *self-antigens* (see Chapter 12 for a discussion of the immune response).

The name *systemic lupus erythematosus* reflects the widespread (systemic, or system-wide) destruction of fibrous connective tissue and other tissues and the appearance in some patients of a reddish rash (erythematosus) that imparts a characteristic "mask" to the face. Lupus is most often seen in women who developed the condition during young adulthood. The course of the condition is gradual, with intermittent periods of inflammation, stiffness, fatigue, pleurisy (chest pain), and discomfort over wide areas of the body, including muscles, joints, and skin. Similar changes may also occur with tissue of the nervous system, kidneys, and heart.[38] Diagnosis is made on the basis of symptoms and several laboratory tests.

Why the immune system turns on the body in such an aggressive manner is not fully understood. It is likely, however, that a combination of genetic predisposition and an earlier viral infection or environmental exposure may be involved. Episodes (called *flares*) of lupus often follow exposure to the sun, periods of fatigue, or an infectious disease; all these should be avoided to the fullest extent possible. Management of the condition generally may involve long-term (and low-dose) use of prednisone (a corticosteroid) or newer medications, such as Plaquenil (hydroxychloroquine), may be employed.

Crohn's Disease

A wide array of chronic conditions that involve the gastrointestinal system are collectively referred to as inflammatory bowel disease (IBD). One type of IBD is Crohn's disease, a deterioration of the inner surface and muscular layer of the intestinal wall that affects nearly 500,000 Americans, many of traditional college age. The disease commonly affects the terminal end of the small intestine and the beginning of the large intestine, or colon. When the disease is active (it frequently has long periods of remission), symptoms include abdominal pain, fever, diarrhea, weight loss, and rectal bleeding that leads to anemia.

Although the cause of Crohn's disease is not fully understood, a genetic predisposition and an autoimmune response are the principal factors. A gene (*NOD*2) with implications for Crohn's was identified.[39] Multiple forms of Crohn's disease are thought to exist, with each reflecting different genetic components.

When a person reports the symptoms just described, the physician quickly suspects some form of IBD, such as Crohn's disease. Accordingly, blood tests and a complete series of gastrointestinal (GI) X rays are undertaken. Additional diagnostic procedures could include a CT scan of the GI tract, endoscopic examination of the GI tract, and a biopsy of the intestinal wall. Positive results of these tests confirm the existence of Crohn's disease.

Today an array of medications is available or in development for use in management of Crohn's disease. Among the most recently introduced of these medications is infliximab (Remicade), an antibody to tumor necrosis factor (TNF) that has proven effective in managing some forms of the disease.

Although Crohn's disease can be well managed, intestinal obstructions can occur as a result of the progressive thickening of the intestinal wall in the areas of inflammation. Surgery may be necessary to remove the obstruction. People with Crohn's disease may encounter further complications, including gallstones, arthritis, and chronic irritation of the skin.

Multiple Sclerosis

For proper nerve conduction to occur in the brain and spinal cord, an insulating sheath of myelin must surround the neurons. In the progressive disease multiple sclerosis (MS), the cells that produce myelin are destroyed and myelin production ceases. Eventually, the vital functions of the body can no longer be carried out. The cause of MS is not fully understood. Research continues to focus on virus-induced autoimmune mechanisms in which T cells attack viral-infected myelin-producing cells.

Usually, MS first appears during the young adult years. It may take one of four forms, depending on the interplay of periods of stabilization (remitting), renewed deterioration (relapsing), continuous deterioration (progressive) or combinations of the above. The initial symptoms are often visual impairment, prickling and burning in the extremities, or an altered **gait.** Deterioration of nervous system function occurs in various forms during the course of MS. In the most advanced stages of MS, movement is greatly impaired, and mental deterioration may be present.

Treatment of MS involves reducing the severity of the symptoms and extending the periods of remission. Today

---

Key Terms

autoimmune an immune response against the tissues of a person's own body.

gait pattern of walking.

a variety of therapies are used, including immune-targeted drugs, steroid drugs, drugs that relieve muscle spasms, injection of nerve blockers, and physical therapy.

The development of immune system–related medications is at the center of today's treatment of MS. Four interferon-based medications, Avonex, Betaserone, Copaxone, and Novantrone, are currently at the forefront of treating MS. Depending on the specific form of MS being addressed, these medications are generally able to slow the progression of the illness, thus delaying the occurrence of the most debilitating symptoms, or to reduce the duration of relapses. In addition to these medications, other interferon-based medications, such as Rebif and Antegren, await full-scale entry into the marketplace. Additional medications are available to address complications of MS, such as spasticity. Also, initial studies involving the implantation of human adult stem cells into MS patients has proven promising in reducing the number of brain lesions,[40] as has the use of statins (cholesterol-lowering drugs) in MS-developing laboratory mice.

In addition to drug therapy, psychotherapy is an important adjunct to the treatment of MS. Profound periods of depression often accompany the initial diagnosis of this condition. Emotional support is helpful in dealing with the progressive impairments associated with most forms of the condition.

Diabetes Mellitus

Diabetes mellitus is not a single condition but rather two metabolic disorders with important similarities and differences.

Non–Insulin-Dependent Diabetes Mellitus (Type 2)

In people who do not have diabetes mellitus the body's need for energy is met through the "burning" of glucose (blood sugar) within the cells. Glucose is absorbed from the digestive tract and carried to the cells by the blood system. Passage of glucose into the cell is achieved through a transport system that moves the glucose molecule across the cell's membrane. Activation of this glucose transport mechanism requires the presence of the hormone insulin. Specific receptor sites for **insulin** can be found on the cell membrane. In addition to its role in the transport of glucose into sensitive cells, insulin is required for the conversion of glucose into glycogen in the

Key Terms
insulin a pancreatic hormone required by the body for the effective metabolism of glucose (blood sugar).

liver and the formation of fatty acids in adipose cells. Insulin is produced in the cells of the islets of Langerhans in the pancreas. The release of insulin from the pancreas corresponds to the changing levels of glucose within the blood.[41]

In adults with a **genetic predisposition** for developing non-insulin-dependent diabetes mellitus, a trigger mechanism (most likely obesity) begins a process through which the body cells become increasingly less sensitive to the presence of insulin, although a normal (or slightly greater than normal) amount of insulin is produced by the pancreas. The growing ineffectiveness of insulin in getting glucose into cells results in the buildup of glucose in the blood. Elevated levels of glucose in the blood lead to *hyperglycemia,* a hallmark symptom of non–insulin-dependent diabetes mellitus.

In response to this buildup, the kidneys begin the process of filtering glucose from the blood. Excess glucose then spills over into the urine. This removal of glucose in the urine demands large amounts of water, a process called *diuresis,* a second important symptom of adult-onset diabetes. Increased thirst, a third symptom of developing diabetes, results in response to the movement of fluid from extracellular spaces into the circulatory system to maintain homeostasis.

For many adults with diabetes, dietary modification (with an emphasis on monitoring total carbohydrate intake, not just sugar) and regular exercise is the only treatment required to maintain an acceptable glucose level. Weight loss will improve the condition by "releasing" more insulin receptors, and exercise increases the actual number of receptor sites. With better insulin recognition, the affected person can better maintain glucose levels.

For people whose condition is more advanced, dietary modification and weight loss are not sufficient, and a hypoglycemia agent must be used. Most recently, Rezulin, a widely used medication that increases the cells' sensitivity to available insulin, was shown to be associated with serious liver damage. However, a similar drug, Avandia, which has fewer harmful effects on the liver, has won FDA approval. For those who require insulin by injection or other delivery methods (e.g., nasal spray or implanted pump), management is much more demanding.

In addition to genetic predisposition and obesity, unresolved stress appears to be involved in the development of hyperglycemic states. Although stress alone probably cannot produce a diabetic condition, it is likely that stress can create a series of endocrine changes that can lead to a state of hyperglycemia.

Diabetes can cause serious damage to several important structures within the body. The rate and extent to which people with diabetes develop these changes can be markedly influenced by the nature of their condition and their compliance with its management requirements. For those who already have diabetes, an understanding of the condition and a commitment to its management are important elements in living with diabetes mellitus.

In 2003 renewed expressions of concern were aroused regarding an alarming increase in the numbers of adults and even children who were seen with either definitive type 2 diabetes mellitus or clear glucose intolerance, also called borderline diabetes mellitus. By mid-2003 it was estimated that 17 million Americans were already diabetic (90% being type 2) and another 16 million were borderline. For this latter group, at least three of the five characteristics of the "metabolic syndrome" were found: abdominal obesity, elevated fasting blood triglycerides, low levels of HDL (the "good" cholesterol), high fasting blood glucose levels, and hypertension (high blood pressure).[42] Underlying these factors and thus exposing millions to future diabetes mellitus and cardiovascular disease are excessive caloric intake and a sedentary lifestyle (see Chapters 4, 7, and 10 for information on reducing these risk factors).

Perhaps the most distressing aspect of the situation described above is the increasing number of young children, most often overweight or obese, accompanied by an equally overweight parent, presenting in pediatric offices across the country. Many of these children already have two or three of the five "metabolic syndrome" risk factors. As these children progress into adulthood, the number of persons with type 2 diabetes mellitus could increase to 50 million by midcentury.[43]

Insulin-Dependent Diabetes Mellitus (Type 1)

A second type of diabetes mellitus is insulin-dependent diabetes mellitus, or type 1 diabetes. The onset of this condition generally occurs before age 35, most often during childhood. In contrast to type 2 diabetes, in which

TALKING POINTS You learn that two young women who are your co-workers have recently been diagnosed with lupus and Crohn's disease, respectively. How can you be supportive of them? What should you say to them about their conditions, particularly on days when it is obvious that they are not feeling well?

Key Terms

genetic predisposition an inherited tendency to develop a disease process if necessary environmental factors exist.

Differences Between Types of Diabetes Mellitus

Insulin-Dependent (Type 1)

(These symptoms usually develop rapidly.)

- Extreme hunger
- Extreme thirst
- Frequent urination
- Extreme weight loss
- Irritability
- Weakness and fatigue
- Nausea and vomiting

Non–Insulin-Dependent (Type 2)

(These symptoms usually develop gradually.)

- Any of the symptoms for insulin-dependent diabetes
- Blurred vision or a change in sight
- Itchy skin
- Tingling or numbness in the limbs

If you notice these symptoms occurring, bring them to the attention of your physician.

Common Complications of Diabetes

- Cataract formation
- Glaucoma
- Blindness
- Dental caries
- Stillbirths/miscarriages
- Neonatal deaths
- Congenital defects
- Cardiovascular disease
- Kidney disease
- Gangrene
- Impotence

insulin is produced but is ineffective because of insensitivity, in type 1 diabetes the body does not produce insulin at all. Destruction of the insulin-producing cells of the pancreas by the person's immune system (possibly in combination with a genetic predisposition) accounts for this sudden and irreversible loss of insulin production.[41]

In most ways the two forms of diabetes are similar, with the important exception that insulin-dependent diabetes mellitus requires the use of insulin from an outside source. Today this insulin is obtained either from animals or through genetically engineered bacteria. It is taken by injection (one to four times per day), through the use of an insulin pump that provides a constant supply of insulin to the body, by transdermal patch, or through nasal inhalation. An insulin pill, now under development, will hopefully be available within the next few years. The use of a glucometer, a highly accurate device for measuring the amount of glucose in the blood, allows for sound management of this condition and a life expectancy that is essentially normal. With both forms of diabetes mellitus, sound dietary practice, weight management, planned activity, and control of stress are important for keeping blood glucose levels within normal ranges. Without good management of diabetes mellitus, several serious problems can result, including blindness, gangrene of the extremities, kidney disease, and heart attack. These and other common complications of diabetes are listed in the

Star box above. People who cannot establish good control are likely to live a shorter life than those who can.

Sickle-Cell Trait and Sickle-Cell Disease

Among the hundreds of human diseases, few are found almost exclusively in a particular racial or ethnic group. Such is the case, however, for the inherited condition *sickle-cell trait/sickle-cell disease.* In the United States, sickle-cell abnormalities are virtually unique to African Americans.

Of all the chemical compounds found in the body, few occur in as many forms as hemoglobin, which helps bind oxygen to red blood cells. Two forms of hemoglobin are associated with sickle-cell trait and sickle-cell disease. African Americans can be the recipients of either form of this abnormal hemoglobin. Those who inherit the trait form do not develop the disease but can transmit the gene for abnormal hemoglobin to their children. In the past, those who inherited the disease form faced a shortened life characterized by periods of pain and impairment. Today, however, with effective screening and new therapeutic approaches to treatment, life expectancy is being extended. Central to this progress has been the implantation of stem cells into young sickle cell victims that have been taken from the bone marrow of compatible donors, particularly siblings.[44] In the future, technological advances will hopefully allow the use of embryonic stem cells, although that is unlikely in this country, and cells taken from unrelated donors. Additionally, a cancer and AIDS chemotherapy agent, hydroxyurea, has been found effective in the management of sickle cell disease.[45]

About 8% of all African Americans have the gene for sickle-cell trait; they experience little impairment, but they can transmit the abnormal gene to their children. For about 1.5% of African Americans, sickle-cell disease is a painful, incapacitating, and life-shortening disease.

In the fully expressed disease form, red blood cells are elongated, crescent-shaped (sickled), and unable to pass through the body's minute capillaries. The body responds to the presence of these abnormal red blood cells by removing them very quickly. This sets the stage for anemia. Thus the condition is often called *sickle-cell anemia*. In addition to anemia, the disease form of the condition can cause many serious medical problems, including impaired lung function, congestive heart failure, gallbladder infections, bone changes, and abnormalities of the eye and skin.

If a key exists for preventing sickle-cell trait and disease, it lies in genetic counseling and testing in preparation for reproduction or in the use of in vitro fertilization followed by genetic testing of the embryo before implantation. At present, both of these preventive approaches are very expensive and limited in availability. However, further research and testing could make these methods more affordable and increase their availability to people who are at high risk.

Alzheimer's Disease

Although it affects less than 2% of the elderly, **Alzheimer's disease** is an incapacitating, emotionally painful, and costly affliction. It is the best known of the dementia disorders, affecting an estimated 4 to 5 million adults. Today, more than ever before, it is *the* disease associated with aging.

The first signs of Alzheimer's disease are often subtle and may be confused with mild depression. Initially, the person might have difficulty answering questions such as "What is today's date?" Over the next several months, greater memory loss, confusion, and *dementia* (or loss of normal thought processes) occur. In the advanced stages, people with Alzheimer's disease become incontinent, show infantile behavior, and finally become incapacitated as brain tissue is destroyed. With advanced Alzheimer's disease, institutionalization becomes necessary.

Alzheimer's disease is difficult to diagnose because its symptoms are similar to those of other types of dementia. It is only after the person's death, if an autopsy is performed, that the characteristic changes in the brain can be used to make a definitive diagnosis. As a practical matter, a probable diagnosis of Alzheimer's disease is made by the process of elimination. Newer medical imaging technologies, such as MRI, have become so refined that it is now almost possible to confirm the diagnosis of Alzheimer's disease before death.

Medications to cure Alzheimer's disease do not exist at this time. However, four currently available drugs

(tacrine, donepezil, rivastigamine, and galantamine) provide temporary improvement in intellectual function during the early stages of the disease by inhibiting the breakdown of acetylcholine, whose diminished availability is the basis of the disease. Of the four drugs, donepezil is most widely used; while galantamine, the newest, influences receptors for three other neurotransmitters, as well as nicotine receptors, all of which play roles in the disease.[46] At least six additional drugs are in various clinical trial phases, including metrifonate and physostigmine.

Several theories have been advanced about the cause of Alzheimer's disease. Increasing evidence indicates that genetic mutations on chromosomes 10, 14, 19, and 21 may encourage the development of the disease. Research into the function of various proteins in fostering the disease's development is also under way. Prevention-oriented trials involving the use of ibuprofen, folic acid, estrogen, and vitamin E are also continuing. Research into a method of stopping and reversing the course of the disease through implantation of stem cells is also under consideration. Additionally, two vaccines intended to block the development of the disease are under development.

Taking Charge of Your Health

- Stay attuned to media reports about chronic conditions so that you can make informed choices.
- Support agencies devoted to the prevention of chronic health conditions.
- Monitor your work, home, and recreational environments to determine whether they are placing you at risk for cancer.
- Perform regular self-examinations for forms of cancer that can be detected through these techniques.
- Undergo the recommended cancer screening procedures for your age and sex.
- If you have a chronic condition, participate actively in your own treatment.

Summary

- More than one and a quarter million people in the United States develop cancer each year.
- Cancer is a condition in which the body is unable to control the specialization, replication, and repair of cells or the suppression of abnormal cell formation.
- Genes that control the replication, specialization, and repair of cells and the suppression of abnormal cellular activity have the potential to become oncogenes and thus can be considered proto-oncogenes.
- A variety of agents, including genetic mutations, viruses, and carcinogens, stimulate the conversion of regulatory genes (proto-oncogenes) into oncogenes.
- Cancer cells demonstrate unique characteristics in comparison to normal cells.
- Cancer can be described on the basis of the type of tissue from which it originates, such as carcinoma, sarcoma, and melanoma.
- Cancer can be described on the basis of its location within the body, such as lung, breast, and prostate cancer.
- Cigarette smoking and genetic predisposition are both related to the development of lung cancer.
- Spiral CT scans may allow for earlier diagnosis of lung cancer.
- Most cases of breast cancer do not demonstrate a clear familial pattern that suggests a genetic predisposition, although some do.
- Long-term exposure to high levels of estrogen is an important risk factor for breast cancer.
- Mammograms are an important component of breast cancer identification. Drugs capable of preventing breast cancer are available; however, their use is being carefully studied.
- Regular use of Pap tests is related to the early detection of cervical cancer. Sexually transmitted viral infections are strongly suspected of causing cervical cancer.
- For women at high risk of HPV infections, screening for infections may be as effective in cervical cancer detection as the Pap test.
- Uterine (endometrial) cancer is more common than cervical cancer. High levels of estrogen are strongly associated with this form of cancer.
- The excessively long use of HRT is a strongly suspected cause of uterine cancer.
- Ovarian cancer is often "silent" in its presentation of symptoms.
- Prostate cancer is the second leading cause of cancer deaths in men.
- The PSA test improves the ability to diagnose prostate cancer. Age, high-fat diets, and inheritance of a mutated suppressor gene are known risk factors.
- Regular self-examination of the testicles leads to early detection of testicular cancer. Environmental factors may be associated with an increasing rate of testicular cancer.
- Colorectal cancer has a strong familial link and is seen in populations that consume diets high in fat and low in fruits and vegetables. Polyp formation is associated with an increased risk of this form of cancer.
- Colonoscopy is the most effective method of detecting polyps and colorectal cancers.
- Pancreatic cancer is very difficult to survive, in part because of the absence of symptoms early in the disease's course.
- Lymphatic cancers display a wide array of initial symptoms that reflect failure of the immune system to function fully. Viral infections and environmental toxins are suspected causative agents.
- Basal cell and squamous cell carcinomas are highly curable forms of skin cancer when detected early. Malignant melanoma is life threatening if not detected early.
- Skin cancer prevention requires protection from excessive sun exposure.
- Early detection based on self-examination and screening is the basis for the identification and successful treatment of many cancers.
- The "War On Cancer" is experiencing both successes and failures.
- Risk reduction, through living a wellness lifestyle remains at the heart of cancer prevention.
- Chronic conditions may be lifelong or they may arise during later adulthood.
- In SLE the body's immune system attacks the body's connective tissues.
- Crohn's disease, a form of IBD, involves an autoimmune deterioration of the gastrointestinal wall.
- Multiple sclerosis is an autoimmune disorder in which the insulation on motor neurons and in the brain is destroyed, leading to a decreasing ability to control muscles.
- Diabetes mellitus type 1 and type 2 both reflect the body's inability to utilize glucose, but have different causes and usually require different forms of treatment.
- Sickle cell trait/disease are inherited conditions appearing in African Americans that result in abnormal hemoglobin.
- Alzheimer's disease reflects a progressive decline in cognitive function, leading eventually to death, and appears primarily in later life.

Review Questions

1. What is the relationship between regulatory genes and tumor suppressor genes in the development of cancer? Why are regulatory genes called both proto-oncogenes and oncogenes?
2. What properties do cancer cells possess that are lacking in normal cells?
3. What are some types of cancer, based on the tissue from which they originate? What are some of the more familiar cancers based on organ of origin?
4. What are the principal factors that contribute to the development of lung cancer? Of breast cancer? What is prophylactic mastectomy and who might consider its use?
5. When should regular use of mammography begin, and which women should begin using it earliest?
6. What important information can be obtained with the use of Pap tests? What innovations are associated with the Thin Prep Pap Test?
7. Why is ovarian cancer described as a "silent" cancer?
8. How does the PSA test contribute to the early detection of prostate cancer?
9. What are the steps for effective self-examination of the breasts and testicles? What is the new status of Breast Self-Examination?
10. What signs indicate the possibility that a skin lesion has become cancerous?
11. Why is pancreatic cancer among the most lethal of all cancers?
12. What are the risk reduction activities identified in this chapter?
13. What are the problems that arise with SLE and how is this autoimmune condition managed?
14. What larger family of conditions is Crohn's disease a part of, and what changes occur in the digestive tract when it is present?
15. What critically important material within the nervous system is eroded by the immune system in conjunction with multiple sclerosis? What are the consequences of losing the ability to continue production of this material?
16. How are type 1 and type 2 diabetes similar and how are they clearly different conditions? What is the "metabolic syndrome" and how does it relate to type 2 diabetes mellitus?
17. What racial group is most susceptible to sickle cell trait/disease? What is sickle cell trait/disease? How could genetic counseling be used in the prevention of this condition?
18. In terms of Alzheimer's disease, what is the cause of its victims' cognitive decline? How effective are current medication used in the treatment of AD?

References

1. American Cancer Society. *Cancer facts & figures 2003.* The Society, 2003.
2. *Number of Americans with and without health insurance rise.* Census Bureau Reports. United States Department of Commerce News. U.S. Census Bureau Public Information Office. 2002. **http://www.census.gov/press-release/www/2002/ cb02-127.html**
3. Clark DP, Russell LD. *Molecular biology made simple and fun.* Cache River Press. 1997.
4. Hoover RN. Cancer—nature, nurture, or both. *N Engl J Med* 343(2):135–136. 2000.
5. Schwab M (ed). *Encyclopedic reference of cancer.* Springer. 2001.
6. Bertino JR (ed). *Encyclopedia of cancer,* 2nd ed. (Vols 1–4). Academic Press. 2002.
7. Hamann B. *Disease: identification, prevention, and control* (2nd ed). McGraw-Hill. 2001.
8. Mahadevia PJ, et al. Lung cancer screening with helical computed tomography in older adult smokers: a decision and cost-effectiveness analysis. *JAMA* 289(3):313–322, 2003.
9. Zabarovsky ER, Lerman MI, Minna JD. Tumor suppressor genes on chromosome 3p involved in the pathogenesis of lung and other cancers. *Oncogene* 21(45):6135–6195, 2003.
10. Pope CA 3rd, et al. Lung cancer, cardiopulmonary mortality, and long-term exposure to fine particulate air pollution. *JAMA* 287(9):1132–1141, 2002.
11. Djousse L, et al. alcohol consumption and risk of lung cancer; the Framingham Study. *J Natl Cancer Inst* 94(24):1877–1882, 2002.
12. Massarelli E, et al. A retrospective analysis of the outcome of patients who have received two prior chemotherapy regimens including platinum and docetaxel for recurrent non-small cell lung cancer. *Lung Cancer* 39(1):55–61, 2003.
13. Hamilton AS, Mack TM. Puberty and genetic susceptibility to breast cancer in a case control study of twins. *N Engl J Med* 348(23):2313–2322, 2003.
14. Collaborative Group on Hormonal Factors in Breast Cancer. Breast cancer and breastfeeding reanalysis of individual data from 47 epidemiological studies in 30 countries, including 50302 women with breast

cancer and 96973 women without the disease. *Lancet* 360(9328):203–210, 2002.

15. Chlebowski RT. Influence of estrogen plus progestin on breast cancer and mammography in healthy postmenopausal women: the Women's Health Initiative Randomized Trial. *JAMA* 289(24):3243–3253, 2003.

16. Folsom AR, et al. Association of general and abdominal obesity with multiple health outcomes in older women: the Iowa Women's Health Study. *Arch Intern Med* 160(14):2117–2128, 2000.

17. Blot WJ, McLaughlin JK. Geographic patterns of breast cancer among American women. *J Natl Cancer Inst* 87(24):1819–1820, 1995.

18. Krainer M, et al. Differential contributions of BRCA1 and BRCA2 to early on-set breast cancer. *N Engl J Med* 336(20):1416–1421, 1997.

19. Thompson JA, et al. BRCA1 susceptibility markers and postmenopausal breat cancer: the Iowa Women's Health Study. *Cancer Epidemiol Biomarkers Prev* 9(5):507–511, 2000.

20. Fu SW, et al. Correlation of expression of BP1, a homeobox gene, with estrogen receptor status in breast cancer. *Breast Cancer Res* 5(4):R82–87, Epub 2003.

21. Freedman AN, et al. Estimates of the number of U.S. women who could benefit from tamoxifen for breast cancer chemoprevention. *J Natl Cancer Inst* 95(7):526–532, 2003.

22. Thomas DB, et al. Randomized trial of breast self-examination in Shanghai: final results. *J Natl Cancer Inst* 94(19):1454–1457. 2002.

23. ACS New Center. *Updated breast cancer screening guidelines released.* American Cancer Society. **http://www.cancer.org/updated_breast_cancer_ screening_guidelines_released.**

24. Du XL. Re: trends in use of adjuvant multi-agent chemotherapy and tamoxifen for breast cancer in the United States: 1975–1999. *J Natl Cancer Inst* 95(9):683, 2003.

25. Crum CP. The beginning of the end of cervical cancer? *N Engl J Med* 347(21):1703–1705, 2002.

26. Lacey JV Jr, et al. Menopausal hormone replacement therapy and risk of ovarian cancer. *JAMA* 288(3):2544, 2002.

27. Kushi L, Giovannucci E. Dietary fat and cancer. *Am J Med* 113 Suppl 9B:63S–70S, 2002.

28. Klein EA, et al. The selenium and vitamin e cancer prevention trial. *World J Urol* 21(1):21–27, 2003.

29. Thompson IM, et al. The influence of finasteride on the development of prostate cancer. *N Engl J Med* 349(3):215–224, 2003.

30. Etzioni R, et al. Overdiagnosis due to prostate-specific antigen screening: lessons from U.S. prostate

cancer incidence trends. *J Natl Cancer Inst* 94(3):981–990. 2002.

31. Skakkebaek NE. Endocrine disrupters and testicular dysgenesis syndrome. *Horm Res* 57 Suppl 2:43, 2002.

32. Travis LB, et al. Treatment-associated leukemia following testicular cancer. *J Natl Cancer Inst* 92(14):1165–1171, 2000.

33. Lieberman DA, et al. Risk factors for advanced colonic neoplasia and hyperpastic polyps in asymptomatic individuals. *JAMA* 290(22):2959–2967, 2003.

34. Lieberman DA, et al: Use of colonoscopy to screen asymptomatic adults for colorectal cancer. Veterans Affairs Cooperative Study 380. *N Engl J Med* 343(3):162–168, 2000.

35. Hussein MR, et al. Identification of novel deletion Loci at 1p36 and 9p22-21 in melanocytic dysplastic nevi and cutaneous malignant melanomas. *Arch Dermatol* 139(6):816–817. 2003.

36. *30 years of war on cancer.* Americans for Medical Progress. **http://www.amprogress.org/files/ files.ctm?=136&c=68**

37. Halpern IM, Waters B. Fiscal year 2003 appropriations essential step forward in war against cancer. *ONS News* 18(4):11. 2003.

38. Braunwald E, et al. *Harrison's principles of internal medicine,* 15ed. McGraw-Hill Professional. 2001.

39. Cho JH. Significant role of genetics in IBD: the NOD2 gene. *Rev Gastroenterol Disord.* 3 Suppl 1:18–22, 2003.

40. Fassas A, et al. Hematopoietic stem cells transplantation for multiple sclerosis. A retrospective multicenter study. *J Neurol* 249(8):1088–1097, 2002.

41. Saladin KS. Anatomy and physiology: the unity of form and function. McGraw-Hill, 2004.

42. Sattar N, et al. Metabolic Syndrome with and without C-Reactive Protein as a predictor of coronary heart disease and diabetes in the West of Scotland Coronary Prevention Study. *Circulation* July 2003. [Epub ahead of print]

43. Boyle JP, et al. Projection of diabetes burden through 2050: impact of changing demography and disease prevalence in the U.S. *Diabetes Care* 24(11):1936–1940, 2001.

44. Vermylen C. Hematopoietic stem cell transplantation in sickle cell disease. *Blood Rev* 17(3):163–166, 2003.

45. Steinberg MH, et al. Effect of hydroyurea on mortality and morbidity in adult sickle cell anemia: risks and benefits up to 9 years of treatment. *JAMA* 289(13):1692–1694, 2003.

46. Reichman WE. Current pharmacologic options for patients with Alzheimer's disease. *Ann Gen Hosp Psychiatry* 2(1):1, 2003.

In the early 1990s a few small studies conducted in this country suggested a link between abortions and an increased risk for the development of breast cancer. In the politically charged atmosphere that generally surrounds the abortion issue, this information was frequently used to substantiate larger claims regarding the need to appeal the 1974 Supreme Court ruling legalizing abortions. However, upon review of these studies, the U.S. National Cancer Institute, in 1995, found the studies too flawed to be considered valid.

The most recent return of the question regarding the link between breast cancer and abortion appeared near the end of March 2004, when 53 separate studies, involving 44,000 women who had abortions and 39,000 women who had been diagnosed with breast cancer, were subjected to a meta-analysis. The new data analysis, conducted by the Collaborative Group on Hormonal Factors in Breast Cancer of Oxford University, found that no link between abortion or miscarriage and the increased risk of developing breast cancer could be found. Findings were reported in *The Lancet*, England's most prestigious medical journal.

focus on

Chronic illness and the demands of Caregiving

In the chapter you have just read, your textbook focused on several representative chronic illnesses. With what you have learned about these conditions, you should be able to imagine that a person whose ability to care for him- or herself has been gravely compromised by the ravages of cancer or Alzheimer's. They would have great difficulty meeting the specific demands of their illness, as well as the activities of daily living that are required for even minimal independence. If they hope to remain in a non-institutional setting, they will, most assuredly, need the assistance of a caregiver at some point, perhaps around the clock.

The need for caregivers is not limited to those suffering from Alzheimer's and Parkinsons. Many victims of stroke, brain and spinal cord injuries require long-term care. Epilepsy, rheumatoid arthritis, chronic obstructive pulmonary disease, asthma, diabetes mellitus, glaucoma, hemophilia, renal failure, cleft lip and palate, and systemic lupus erythematosis are but a few of the other chronic conditions that at some point in their progression will require the afflicted person to receive care from others.[1]

Sixty-five percent of older persons requiring long term care rely on family and friends as caregivers; an additional 30% make use of paid providers in addition to family and friends.[2] The average caregiver is 46 years old and female, and has the added responsibilities of being married and working outside the home.[3] Our nation has come to rely on families, rather than social service agencies, nursing homes, or other health care providers, to provide long term care for the chronically ill. It is estimated that the combined economic value of these unpaid care-givers exceeds $257 billion each year.[4]

It is particularly important to recognize that under the law, few persons other than health care professionals, parents of dependent children, legally defined guardians, and specified public servants are required to meet the needs of the chronically ill. But when it comes to our aging and infirm population, it is most often those who are not required to do so who take care of their elderly parents, other family members, friends and neighbors. More than 22.4 million Americans are informal caregivers who provide some degree of assistance to older persons or persons with some limitations on their ability to care for themselves.[4]

So, the decision to become the primary caregiver for a parent, grandparent, relative or friend who is chronically ill is a personal one. Thus, a person considering becoming a voluntary caregiver of a chronically ill person must carefully consider many issues related to the endeavor. Among the most pressing of these are:

- *What are the present and future needs of the chronically ill person whose care you are assuming?* Are you able to manage their care now? Will you be able to take on more responsibilities and difficulties should their condition worsen?
- *Whose needs are most fundamentally at stake in this venture?* In other words, are you stepping forward in the role of caregiver in order to meet your own unfulfilled needs, or are you genuinely focused on the person whose illness-related needs you are trying to meet?
- *What resources are available to assist you in meeting the needs of this chronically ill person?* Are there private, state or federal programs and/or facilities available that might provide you with assistance? Are you capable of accessing the agencies whose expertise and assistance would be beneficial?
- *Can you remain above feelings of resentment once you have accepted the role of caregiver, knowing that others apparently have been comfortable setting aside the same ethical obligations?* In other words, will you find yourself feeling bitter toward a sibling who did not volunteer to help you care for a parent?[5]

It is crucial that you ask yourself these questions, and honestly deal with your feelings, before taking on the role of caregiver. If you are able to resolve these issues in a healthy manner, then you may be entering into one of the most demanding but rewarding undertakings that a person can experience.

For Discussion

Would you be willing to take on the full-time care of a parent if he or she became chronically ill? Should those in need of assistance be entitled to some level of government-funded at home care? How might employers be able to help workers who are struggling to balance work with the responsibilities of caregiving?

References

1. Chui, D. Occupational therapy in Community Rehabilitation Network. Hong Kong Occupational Association. 2003.
2. U.S Administration on Aging. *America's Families Care: A report on the needs of America's family caregivers.* Fall 2000.
3. National Alliance for Caregiving (1997). *Family Caregiving in the*

United States: Findings from a national survey. **http://www.caregiving.org/finalreport.pdf**

4. The U.S. Department of Health and Human Services, Administration on Aging. *What We Do Makes Difference: Fact Sheet on Family Caregiving.* **http://www.aoa.gov/prof/aoaprog/caregiver/carefam/taking care of others/taking care.asp**

5. Pressing worldwide challenge of long-term care for ill and disabled presents difficult ethical questions. World Health Organization. 2003. **http://www.who.int/mediacentre/notes/2003/np3/en**

personal assessment

are you at risk for skin, breast, or cervical cancer?

Some people may have more than an average risk of developing particular types of cancer. These people can be identified by certain risk factors.

This simple self-testing method is designed by the American Cancer Society to help you assess your risk factors for three common types of cancer. These are the major risk factors but by no means represent the only ones that might be involved.

Check your response to each risk factor. Add the numbers in the parentheses to arrive at a total score for each cancer type. Find out what your score means by reading the information in the "Interpretation" section. You are advised to discuss the information with your physician if you are at a higher risk.

Skin Cancer

1. Frequent work or play in the sun
   A. Yes (10)
   B. No (1)
2. Work in mines, around coal tars, or around radioactivity
   A. Yes (10)
   B. No (1)
3. Complexion—fair skin or light skin
   A. Yes (10)
   B. No (1)

Your total points _____

Explanation

1. Excessive ultraviolet light causes skin cancer. Protect yourself with a sunscreen.
2. These materials can cause skin cancer.
3. Light complexions need more protection than others.

Interpretation

Numerical risks for skin cancer are difficult to state. For instance, a person with a dark complexion can work longer in the sun and be less likely to develop cancer than can a light-complected person. Furthermore, a person wearing a long-sleeved shirt and a wide-brimmed hat may work in the sun and be less at risk than a person who wears a bathing suit and stays in the sun for only a short period. The risk increases greatly with age.

The key here is if you answered "yes" to any question, you need to realize that you have above-average risk.

Breast Cancer

1. Age group
   A. 20–34 (10)
   B. 35–49 (40)
   C. 50 and over (90)
2. Race/nationality
   A. Asian American (5)
   B. African American (20)
   C. White (25)
   D. Mexican American (10)
3. Family history of breast cancer
   A. Mother, sister, or grandmother (30)
   B. None or unknown (10)
4. Your history
   A. No breast disease (10)
   B. Previous noncancerous lumps or cysts (25)
   C. Previous breast cancer (100)
5. Maternity
   A. First pregnancy before age 25 (10)
   B. First pregnancy after age 25 (15)
   C. No pregnancies (20)

Your total points _____

Interpretation

Under 100	Low-risk women should follow the 2003 ACS cancer screening guidelines. Note that the role of BSE has been redefined. Consult your physician for possible modifications to this protocol.
100–199	Moderate-risk women should consult their physicians to determine whether the ACS guideline should be followed as stated or, possibly, be modified in terms of scheduling or procedures employed. Note that the role of BSE has been redefined.
200 or more	High-risk women should consult their physicians to determine whether the ACS guidelines should be followed as stated or, very likely, be modified in terms of scheduling or procedures employed. Note that the role of BSE has been redefined.

Cervical Cancer*

1. Age group
   A. Less than 25 (10)
   B. 25–39 (20)
   C. 40–54 (30)
   D. 55 and over (30)
2. Race/nationality
   A. Asian American (10)
   B. Puerto Rican (20)
   C. African American (20)
   D. White (10)
   E. Mexican American (20)

*Lower portion of uterus. These questions would not apply to a woman who has had a complete hysterectomy.

Cervical Cancer

3. Number of pregnancies
   A. 0 (10)
   B. 1 to 3 (20)
   C. 4 and over (30)
4. Viral infections
   A. Herpes and other viral infections or ulcer formations on the vagina (10)
   B. Never (1)
5. Age at first intercourse
   A. Before 15 (40)
   B. 15–19 (30)
   C. 20–24 (20)
   D. 25 and over (10)
6. Bleeding between periods or after intercourse
   A. Yes (40)
   B. No (1)

Your total points _____

Explanations

1. The highest occurrence is in the 40-and-over age group. The numbers represent the relative rates of cancer for different age groups. A 45-year-old woman has a risk three times higher than that of a 20-year-old.

2. Puerto Ricans, African Americans, and Mexican Americans have higher rates of cervical cancer.
3. Women who have delivered more children have a higher occurrence.
4. Viral infections of the cervix and vagina are associated with cervical cancer.
5. Women with earlier intercourse and with more sexual partners are at a higher risk.
6. Irregular bleeding may be a sign of uterine cancer.

Interpretation/To Carry This Further . . .

40–69	This is a low-risk group. Ask your doctor for a Pap test. You will be advised how often you should be tested after your first test.
70–99	In this moderate-risk group, more frequent Pap tests may be required.
100 or higher	You are in a high-risk group and should have a Pap test (and pelvic examination) as advised by your doctor.

Regardless of score, you should discuss with your physician the desirability of the ThinPrep-Pap test (or one similar to it), as it is designed to identify the presence of DNA from one or more of the HPV strains associated with cervical cancer.

chapter twelve

preventing infectious diseases

Chapter Objectives

Upon completing this chapter, you should be able to:

▌ describe the movement of a cold virus through each link in the chain of infectious disease.

▌ explain why persons with HIV/AIDS do not generally progress beyond the clinical stage of their disease.

▌ develop and then implement a plan to protect (or enhance) your immune system.

▌ assess your own immunizations status, and make arrangements for any additional immunizations such as flu shots.

▌ understand and describe the importance of frequent hand washing, particularly during the cold and flu season.

▌ recognize the importance of testing dead birds found on campus or in your neighborhood for the presence of the West Nile virus.

▌ identify those forms of hepatitis that are potentially sexually transmitted, in comparison to those that are not.

▌ take proper precautions to protect yourself from HIV/AIDS and other sexually transmitted diseases.

Online Learning Center Resources

www.mhhe.com/hahn7e

Log on to our Online Learning Center (OLC) for access to these additional resources:

- Chapter key terms and definitions
- Learning objectives
- Student interactive question-and-answer sites

- Self-scoring chapter quiz
- Online assessments
- Key term flash cards

Talking It Over

Chronic Fatigue Syndrome: Real or Imaginary?

Communication with a friend who has chronic fatigue syndrome can sometimes be strained. You may think that the person is just being lazy. Or, because the person doesn't look sick, you may wonder if he is faking it.

- Show respect for your friend by letting him talk about it—just as you would behave if he had any other illness.
- Acknowledge the fact that your friend has a recognized medical condition. Don't suggest that he can "snap out of it."

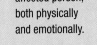

- Do what you can to support the affected person, both physically and emotionally.

CommunicationLinks

www.cdc.gov/ncidod/diseases/cfs/index.htm
www.cfids.org/csn.html
www.chronicfatiguenews.com

Eye on the Media

From Fear to Hope—AIDS in the News

In the early days of news coverage about AIDS, magazines like *Time* and *Newsweek* ran articles called: "The AIDS Epidemic," "Epidemic of Fear," "Plague Mentality," "Fear of Sex," "The Growing Threat," "A Spreading Scourge," "The New Untouchables," "AIDS Spreading Panic Worldwide," "A Grim Race Against the Clock," and "The Lost Generation." The titles reflected fear of the unknown, a new killer disease.

When the case of Kimberley Bergalis broke into the news in 1991, a routine visit to the dentist was suddenly fraught with risk.

Bergalis was the first American to die of AIDS after being infected by her dentist, Dr. David Acer. Four of Acer's other patients became infected with AIDS—all traced back to Acer. The public's reaction was near-hysteria. *Time* ran an article called "Should You Worry About Getting AIDS from Your Dentist?" People started asking their dentists (and other doctors) about their use of sterile precautions and even whether they had been tested for HIV.

Eye on the Media *continued*

By 1996, when the "cocktail" approach to AIDS treatment started showing remarkably good results, Magic Johnson was on the cover of both *Time* and *Newsweek* the same week. After more than 4 years of retirement from pro basketball—and the announcement that he had tested positive for HIV—he was back in the game. The secret to his survival? New drug treatments, a healthy diet, regular exercise, support from family and friends, and a positive attitude.

By the late 1990s, many news articles reflected a more hopeful tone: "Living Longer with AIDS," "Hope with an Asterisk," "Are Some People Immune?" and "What—I'm Gonna Live?" Doctors, too, are feeling more positive about the disease. As one AIDS specialist said: "I go to work feeling like there's something I can do for my patients."

For people with HIV/AIDS in the most highly developed countries the future holds different things. For some, who can't afford or tolerate the new drugs, it's still a matter of waiting to die. Others feel that they've been given a second chance. They can think about having relationships again—something many put on hold when they learned they were HIV positive. They can make plans for what they want to do with the rest of their lives—however long that may be.

Most people with HIV/AIDS are buying time—hoping for the big breakthrough, the cure for AIDS. They're trying new drug treatments, hoping that one treatment won't disqualify them from the next one. They're watching TV news, reading the newspapers, and using the Internet with greater attention. Will protease-inhibiting drugs be the answer? Are the even newer antiviral medications the breakthrough hoped for? Is a vaccine on the horizon?

Today, the media are calling our attention to yet other aspects of the AIDS pandemic. For the more developed countries, the failure of younger gays and bisexuals to protect themselves from exposure to HIV has led to a reversal in the progress made over the last 20 years. In ways all too familiar to public health professionals, a younger generation can too easily forget the progress against disease and premature death made by those who came before, and in doing so, unravel the threads of progress.

Increasingly, media attention has also been focused on the plight of the millions of HIV/AIDS victims in third world countries, particularly in Africa and areas of Asia. Television increasingly exposes the suffering in countries where diagnosis is inadequately undertaken and, once done, virtually no effective treatment exists for those infected. Beyond the suffering and limited hope for those infected, the media has also publicized the plights of the tens of thousands of orphaned children in these areas whose parents have died from AIDS. Our federal government and pharmaceutical industry has been exposed to this suffering as well, and initial responses are being mustered.

Sources: Gayle HD. Curbing the global AIDS epidemic. *N Engl J Med* 348(18):1802–1805. 2003. Klausner RD, et al. Medicine. The need for a global HIV vaccine enterprise. *Science* 300(5628):2036–2039. 2003.

In the nineteenth century, infectious diseases were the leading cause of death. These deaths came after exposure to the organisms that produced such diseases as smallpox, tuberculosis (TB), influenza, whooping cough (pertussis), typhoid, diphtheria, and tetanus. However, since the early 1900s, improvements in public sanitation, the widespread use of antibiotic drugs, and vaccinations have considerably reduced the number of people who die from infectious diseases. People now die more often from chronic disease processes.

Today, however, we have a new respect for infectious diseases. We have learned that AIDS threatens 70 million people in many areas of the world. We are witnessing the resurgence of TB. We recognize the role of pelvic infections in infertility. We also know that failure to fully immunize children has laid the groundwork for a return of whooping cough, polio, and other serious childhood diseases. In fact, some experts suggest that because of HIV/AIDS and the emergence and re-emergence of infectious diseases, today's young adults may have a lower life expectancy than the generation immediately ahead of them.

Several new types of infectious disease have appeared, and new concerns have been raised about the spread of familiar infectious diseases.

Infectious Disease Transmission

Infectious diseases can generally be transmitted from person to person, although the transfer is not always direct. Infectious diseases can be especially dangerous because they can spread to large numbers of people, producing epidemics or pandemics. The following sections explain the process of disease transmission and the stages of infection.

Pathogens

For a disease to be transferred, a person must come into contact with the disease-producing agent, or **pathogen,** such as a virus, bacterium, or fungus. When pathogens enter our bodies, the pathogens can sometimes resist

---

Key Terms

pathogen a disease-causing agent.

Table 12.1 Pathogens and Common Infectious Diseases

Pathogen	Description	Representative Disease Processes
Viruses	Smallest common pathogens; nonliving particles of genetic material (DNA) surrounded by a protein coat	Rubeola, mumps, chickenpox, rubella, influenza, warts, colds, oral and genital herpes, shingles, AIDS, genital warts
Prion	Potentially self-replicating protein, lacking both DNA and RNA, viruslike in size, clinically called TSE (transmissible spongiform encephalopathies)	Creutzfeldt-Jakob disease, Gerstmann-Straussler-Scheinker syndrome, "mad cow" disease
Bacteria	One-celled microorganisms with sturdy, well-defined cell walls; three distinctive forms: spherical (cocci), rod shaped (bacilli), and spiral shaped (spirilla)	Tetanus, strep throat, scarlet fever, gonorrhea, syphilis, chlamydia, toxic shock syndrome, Legionnaires' disease, bacterial pneumonia, meningitis, diphtheria, food poisoning, Lyme disease
Fungi	Plant-like microorganisms; molds and yeasts	Athlete's foot, ringworm, histoplasmosis, San Joaquin Valley fever, candidiasis
Protozoa	Simplest animal form, generally one-celled organisms	Malaria, amebic dysentery, trichomoniasis, vaginitis
Rickettsia	Virus-like organisms that require a host's living cells for growth and replication	Typhus, Rocky Mountain spotted fever, rickettsialpox
Parasitic worms	Many-celled organisms; represented by tapeworms, leeches, and roundworms	Dirofilariasis (dog heartworm), elephantiasis, onchocerciasis

body defense systems, flourish, and produce an illness. We commonly call this an *infection*. Because of their small size, pathogens are sometimes called *microorganisms* or *microbes*. Table 12.1 above describes infectious disease agents and some of the illnesses they produce.[1]

Chain of Infection

The movement of a pathogenic agent through the various links in the chain of infection (Figure 12-1 on page 332) explains how diseases spread.[1] Not every pathogenic agent moves all the way through the chain of infection, because various links in the chain can be broken. Therefore, the presence of a pathogen creates only the potential for causing disease.

Agent

The first link in the chain of infection is the disease-causing **agent.** Whereas some agents are very **virulent** and lead to serious infectious illnesses such as HIV, which causes AIDS, others produce far less serious infections, such as the common cold. Through mutation, some pathogenic agents, particularly viruses, can become more virulent.

Reservoir

Infectious agents require the support and protection of a favorable environment to survive. This environment forms the second link in the chain of infection and is called the *reservoir*. For many of the most common infectious diseases, the reservoirs are the bodies of people who are already infected. Here the agents thrive before being spread to others. These infected people are, accordingly,

the hosts for particular disease agents. In some infectious illnesses a person's reservoir status may be restored after treatment and apparent recovery from the original infection. This is because some pathogens, particularly viruses, can remain sequestered (hidden), emerging later to give rise to another infection. The herpes viruses are often sequestered.

For other infectious diseases, however, the reservoirs are the bodies of animals. Rabies is a well-known animal-reservoir disease. The infected animals are not always sick and do not always show symptoms similar to those seen in infected people.

The third type of reservoir in which disease-causing agents can live is in a nonliving environment, such as the soil. The spores of the tetanus bacterium, for example, can survive in soil for up to fifty years, entering the human body in a puncture wound.

Portal of Exit

For pathogenic agents to cause diseases and illnesses in others, they must leave their reservoirs. Thus the third link in the chain of infection is the portal of exit, or the point at which agents leave their reservoirs.

Key Terms

agent the causal pathogen of a particular disease.

virulent (**veer** yuh lent) capable of causing disease.

Figure 12-1 The six links in the chain of infection. The example above shows a rhinovirus, which causes the common cold, being passed from one person to another. 1. the *agent* (pathogen) is a rhinovirus; 2. the *reservoir* is the infected person; 3. the *portal of exit* is the respiratory system (coughing); 4. the *mode of transmission* is indirect hand contact; 5. the *portal of entry* is the mucous membranes of the uninfected person's eye; 6, the virus now has a *new host.*

The principal portals of exit are familiar—the digestive system, urinary system, respiratory system, reproductive system, and the blood, especially with infectious diseases that infect humans.

Mode of Transmission

The fourth link in the chain of infection is the mode of transmission, or the way in which pathogens move from reservoirs to susceptible hosts. Two principal methods are direct transmission and indirect transmission.

We see three types of direct transmission in human-to-human transmission. These include contact between body surfaces (such as kissing, touching, and sexual intercourse), droplet spread (inhalation of contaminated air droplets), and fecal-oral spread (feces on the host's hands are brought into contact with the new host's mouth), as could occur when changing the diaper of an infected infant.

Indirect transmission between infected and uninfected people occurs when infectious agents travel by means of nonhuman materials. Vehicles of transmission include inanimate objects (known as *fomites*), such as water, food, soil, towels, clothing, and eating utensils.

Infectious agents can also be indirectly transmitted through vectors. The term *vector* describes living things, such as insects, birds, and other animals, that carry

diseases from human to human. An example of a vector is the deer tick, which transmits Lyme disease.

Airborne indirect transmission includes the inhalation of infected particles that have been suspended in an air source for an extended time. Unlike droplet transmission, in which both infected and uninfected people must be in close physical proximity, noninfected people can become infected through airborne transmission by sharing air with infected people who were in the same room hours earlier. Viral infections such as German measles can be spread this way.

Portal of Entry

The fifth link in the chain of infection is the portal of entry. As with the portals of exit, portals of entry have three primary methods that allow pathogenic agents to enter the bodies of uninfected people. These are through the digestive system, respiratory system, and reproductive system. In addition, a break in the skin provides another portal of entry. In most infectious conditions, the portals of entry are the same systems that served as the portals of exit from the infected people. In HIV, however, we see cross-system transmission. Oral and anal sex allow infectious agents to pass between the warm, moist tissues of the reproductive and digestive systems.

The New Host

All people are, in theory, at risk for contracting infectious diseases and thus could be called susceptible hosts. In practice, however, factors such as overall health, acquired immunity, health care services, and health-related behavior can affect susceptibility to infectious diseases.

Stages of Infection

When a pathogenic agent assaults a new host, a reasonably predictable sequence of events begins. That is, the disease moves through five distinctive stages.[1] You may be able to recognize these stages of infection each time you catch a cold.

1. *The incubation stage.* This stage lasts from the time a pathogen enters the body until it multiplies enough to produce signs and symptoms of the disease. The duration of this stage can vary from a few hours to many months, depending on the virulence of the organisms, the concentration of organisms, the host's level of immune responsiveness, and other health problems. This stage has been called a *silent stage.* The pathogen can be transmitted to a new host during this stage, but this is not likely. A host may be infected during this stage but not infectious. HIV infection is an exception to this rule.

2. *The prodromal stage.* After the incubation stage, the host may experience a variety of general signs and symptoms, including watery eyes, runny nose, slight fever, and overall tiredness for a brief time. These symptoms are nonspecific and may not be severe enough to force the host to rest. During this stage the pathogenic agent continues to multiply. Now the host is capable of transferring pathogens to a new host, but this is not yet the most infectious stage of an infectious disease. One should practice self-imposed isolation during this stage to protect others. Again, HIV infection is different in this stage.

3. *The clinical stage.* This stage, also called the *acme* or *acute stage,* is often the most unpleasant stage for the host. At this time the disease reaches its highest point of development. Laboratory tests can identify or analyze all of the clinical (observable) signs and symptoms of the particular disease. The likelihood of transmitting the disease to others is highest during this peak stage; all of our available defense mechanisms are in the process of resisting further damage from the pathogen.

4. *The decline stage.* The first signs of recovery appear during this stage. The infection is ending or, in some cases, falling to a subclinical level. People may suffer a relapse if they overextend themselves.

5. *The recovery stage.* Also called the *convalescence stage,* this stage is characterized by apparent recovery from the invading agent. The disease can be transmitted during this stage, but this is not probable. Until the host's overall health has been strengthened, he or she may be especially susceptible to another (perhaps different) disease pathogen. Fortunately, after the recovery stage, further susceptibility to the pathogenic agent is typically lower because the body has built up immunity. This buildup of immunity is not always permanent; for example, many sexually transmitted diseases can be contracted repeatedly.

Later in the chapter HIV/AIDS will be discussed. However, prior to that time, it may be helpful to state that this critically important pandemic infectious disease does not easily fit into the five-stage model of infectious diseases just presented. In individuals infected with HIV there is an initial asymptomatic *incubation stage,* followed by a *prodromal stage* characterized by generalized signs of immune system inadequacy. However, once the level of specific protective cells of the immune system declines to the point that the body cannot be protected from opportunistic diseases, and the label AIDS is assigned, the five-stage model becomes less easily applied.

Body Defenses: Mechanical and Cellular-Chemical Immune Systems

Much as a series of defensive alignments protect a military installation, so too is the body protected by sets of defenses. These defenses can be classified as either mechanical or cellular-chemical. Mechanical defenses are first-line defenses, because they physically separate the internal body from the external environment. Examples include the skin, the mucous membranes that line the respiratory and gastrointestinal tracts, earwax, the tiny hairs and cilia that filter incoming air, and even tears. These defenses serve primarily as a shield against foreign materials that may contain pathogenic agents. These defenses can, however, be disarmed, such as when tobacco smoke kills the cilia that protect the airway, resulting in chronic bronchitis, or when contact lenses reduce tearing, leading to irritation and eye infection.

The second component of the body's protective defenses is the cellular-chemical system or, more commonly, the **immune system.** The cellular-chemical

---

Key Terms

immune system the system of cellular and chemical elements that protects the body from invading pathogens, foreign protein, and abnormal cells.

component is far more specific than the mechanical defenses. Its primary mission is to eliminate microorganisms, foreign protein, and abnormal cells from the body. A wellness-oriented lifestyle, including sound nutrition, effective stress management, and regular exercise, supports this important division of the immune system. The microorganisms, foreign protein, or abnormal cells that activate this cellular component are collectively called *antigens*.[2]

Divisions of the Immune System

Closer examination of the immune system, or cellular-chemical defenses, reveals two separate but highly cooperative groups of cells. One group of cells originates in the fetal thymus gland and thus has become known as *T cell-mediated immunity*, or simply *cell-mediated immunity*. The second group of cells that makes up cellular immunity are the B cells (bursa of Fabricius), which are the working units of *humoral immunity*.[3] Cellular elements of both cell-mediated and humoral immunity can be found within the bloodstream, the lymphatic tissues of the body, and the fluid that surrounds body cells.

Although we are born with the structural elements of both cell-mediated and humoral immunity, developing an immune response requires that components of these cellular systems encounter and successfully defend against specific antigens. When the immune system has done this once, it is, in most cases, primed to respond quickly and effectively if the same antigens appear again. This confrontation produces a state of **acquired immunity (AI).**[1] Acquired immunity develops in different ways.

- **Naturally acquired immunity (NAI)** develops when the body is exposed to infectious agents. Thus when we catch an infectious disease, we fight the infection and in the process become immune (protected) from developing that illness if we encounter these agents again. Before the advent of immunizations, this was the only way of developing immunity.

- **Artificially acquired immunity (AAI)** occurs when the body is exposed to weakened or killed infectious agents introduced through vaccination or immunization. As in NAI, the body fights the infectious agents and records the method of fighting the agents. Young children, older adults, and adults in high-risk occupations should consult their physicians about immunizations.

- **Passively acquired immunity (PAI),** a third form of immunity, results when extrinsic antibodies are introduced into the body. These antibodies are for a variety of specific infections, and they are produced outside the body (either in animals or by the genetic manipulation of microorganisms). When intro-

Are Americans Too Clean?

Infectious disease specialists are increasingly concerned about the widespread popularity and availability of antimicrobial cleaning products and the contribution they may be making to the development of antibiotic-resistant "super bugs." In fact, it is estimated that approximately 75% of all liquid hand soaps and nearly 30% of all bar soaps contain either triclocarban or triclosan, antibacterial chemicals to which pathogenic agents are already showing resistance.

As concern about our increasing reliance on antimicrobial products grows, we are reminded of the first personal hygiene rule that most Americans were taught as children at home and in school: Wash your hands thoroughly with soap and *hot water!* Even today, microbiologists remind us that nothing is more effective in cleaning our bodies, our homes, and our work places than "old-fashioned" soap and hot water.

duced into the human body, they provide immediate protection until the body can develop a more natural form of immunity. Note that in PAI no actual pathogenic agents are introduced into the body—only the antibodies against various forms of disease-causing agents.

Regardless of how infectious agents are acquired, either through naturally acquired immunity (NAI) or through artificially acquired immunity (AAI), the result is an "arming" of the body's own immune system. This

Key Terms

acquired immunity (AI) the major component of the immune system; forms antibodies and specialized blood cells capable of destroying pathogens.

naturally acquired immunity (NAI) a type of acquired immunity resulting from the body's response to naturally occurring pathogens.

artificially acquired immunity (AAI) a type of acquired immunity resulting from the body's response to pathogens introduced into the body through immunizations.

passively acquired immunity (PAI) a temporary immunity achieved by providing antibodies to a person exposed to a particular pathogen.

process is frequently labeled as *active immunity.* This contrasts to passively acquired immunity (PIA) in which the body "borrows" another's immune elements, without actual involvement of the body's own immune system. This latter case is called *passive immunity.*[4]

In addition to the forms of immunity just described, infants are also provided with a period of short-term immunity via the biological mothers' immune system elements crossing the placental barrier (see Chapter 14) and following birth via breast milk. This *maternal immunity,* however, gradually deteriorates but is concurrently being replaced by the child's own increasingly functional immune system.

Collectively, these forms of immunity can provide important protection against infectious disease.

The Immune Response

Fully understanding the function of the immune system requires a substantial understanding of human biology and is beyond the scope of this text. Figure 12-2 on page 336 presents a simplified view of the immune response.

When antigens (whether microorganisms, foreign substances, or abnormal cells) are discovered within the body, various types of white blood cells confront and destroy some of these antigens. Principal among these blood cells are the *macrophages* (very large white blood cells) that begin ingesting antigens as they are encountered. In conjunction with this "eating" of antigens, macrophages display segments of the antigen's unique protein coat on their outer surface. Now in the form of macrophage/antigen complexes, macrophages transport their captured antigen identifiers to awaiting helper T cells whose recognition of the antigen will initiate the full expression of the cell-mediated immune response. This involves the specialization of "basic" T cells into four specialized forms: helper T cells, killer T cells, suppressor T cells, and memory T cells.

Once helper T cells have been derived from the "parent" T cells by the presence of the macrophage/antigen complex, they notify a second component of cellular immunity, the killer T cells. Killer T cells produce powerful chemical messengers that activate specific white blood cells that destroy antigens through the production of caustic chemicals called cytotoxins, or "cell poisons." In addition to the helper T cells' activation of killer T cells, helper T cells also play a critical role in the activation of B cells, principal players in the expression of humoral immunity.

Activation of the humoral immunity component of the overall immune response involves the helper T cells' ability to construct a working relationship between themselves, the macrophage/antigen complexes (mentioned

earlier), and the small B cells. Once these three elements have been constituted into working units, the B cells are transformed into a new version of themselves called *plasma cells.* Plasma cells then utilize the information about the antigen's identity to produce massive numbers of "locks" called **antibodies.** Upon release from the plasma cells, these antibodies then circulate throughout the body and "lock-up" or capture free antigens in the form of *antigen/antibody complexes.*[4] The "captured" antigens are now highly susceptible to a variety of white blood cells that ingest or chemically destroy these infectious agents.

To assure that the initial response to the presence of the antigen can be appropriately controlled, a third group of T cells, the suppressor T cells, have been formed by the initial activation of parent T cells. These suppressor T cells monitor the outcome of the humoral response (antibody formation) and when comfortable with the number of antibodies produced, turn off further plasma cell activity. The fourth group of specialized T cells, the memory T cells, record this initial recognition-based game plan for fighting the original antigen invasion so that any subsequent similar antigen appearance will be quickly mounted.

An additional group of cells that operate independently from the T cell/B cell interplay just described are the *natural killer* (NK) cells. These immune cells continuously patrol the blood and intracellular fluids looking for abnormal cells, including cancer cells and viral-infected cells. When these are found, the NK cells attack them with destructive cytotoxins in a process called *lysing.*[4]

Clearly, without a normal immune system employing both cellular and humoral elements, we would quickly fall victim to serious and life-shortening infections and malignancies. As you will see later, this is exactly what occurs in many people infected with HIV (see the Learning from Our Diversity box on page 337).

Emerging medical technology holds promise for repairing damaged immune systems. In a current form of treatment, *adult stem cells* are harvested from non-diseased tissues of a person's body or from a biologically related family member and used to replace damaged or diseased cells within the immune system.[5,6] A second form of immune system repair involves harvesting *cord blood (stem) cells* taken from the umbilical cord blood

---

Key Terms

antibodies chemical compounds produced by the body's immune system to destroy antigens and their toxins.

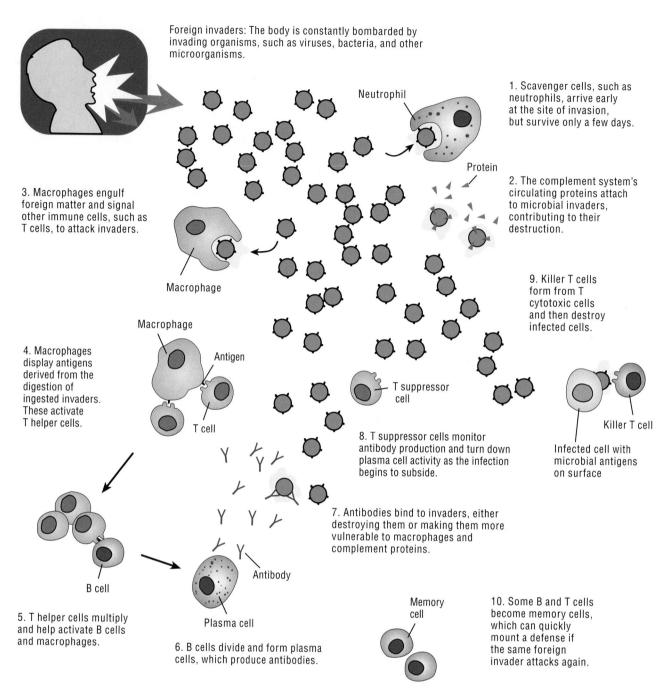

Foreign invaders: The body is constantly bombarded by invading organisms, such as viruses, bacteria, and other microorganisms.

Neutrophil

1. Scavenger cells, such as neutrophils, arrive early at the site of invasion, but survive only a few days.

Protein

2. The complement system's circulating proteins attach to microbial invaders, contributing to their destruction.

3. Macrophages engulf foreign matter and signal other immune cells, such as T cells, to attack invaders.

Macrophage

9. Killer T cells form from T cytotoxic cells and then destroy infected cells.

Macrophage

Antigen

4. Macrophages display antigens derived from the digestion of ingested invaders. These activate T helper cells.

T cell

T suppressor cell

Killer T cell

Infected cell with microbial antigens on surface

8. T suppressor cells monitor antibody production and turn down plasma cell activity as the infection begins to subside.

7. Antibodies bind to invaders, either destroying them or making them more vulnerable to macrophages and complement proteins.

B cell

Antibody

Memory cell

10. Some B and T cells become memory cells, which can quickly mount a defense if the same foreign invader attacks again.

5. T helper cells multiply and help activate B cells and macrophages.

Plasma cell

6. B cells divide and form plasma cells, which produce antibodies.

Figure 12-2 Biological warfare The body commands an army of defenders to reduce the danger of infection and guard against repeat infections. Antigens are the ultimate targets of all immune responses.

collected and "banked" at birth. After careful matching, these cells can be transplanted into a recipient in anticipation that they will specialize into the cell type needed by the damaged or diseased immune system.[7] It is important to note that considerable controversy now surrounds the use of stem cells obtained from embryonic or fetal tissue sources. Even though these are considered to be the "best" stem cells, restrictions by the federal government (and several states) on their collection and use have forced clinicians to use stem cells from the sources mentioned earlier, as well as from cadavers.[8,9]

Immunizations

Although the incidence of several childhood communicable diseases is at or near the lowest level ever, we are risking a resurgence of diseases such as measles, polio,

It's not always easy for young adults in excellent health to recover quickly and completely from some infectious diseases. Later in life the recovery often becomes much more difficult and in some cases impossible. For a variety of reasons older adults do not respond to infectious conditions with the same resiliency as they once did.

Central to this issue is the gradual degradation of the immune system over time. For reasons not fully understood, the immune system loses both its ability to recognize the presence of pathogens that have entered the body and its ability to mount an effective response against them. Particularly important in this regard are the decreased prevalence of active immune system cells and the inability of existing immune cells to respond effectively. Whether this reduced level of immune protection is a "programmed" aspect of aging (all human life does end at some point in time) or whether it reflects a process that is preventable (perhaps through lifestyle modifications) remains hotly debated. Perhaps no group of older adults is at greater risk because of a compromised immune system than are those with AIDS. The nearly eighty thousand persons over age 50 with this immune system–destroying disease have a decreased ability to resist all infectious conditions, even when their HIV levels are suppressed through drug therapy.

In addition to the normal aging of their immune systems, older adults are generally afflicted with a variety of chronic conditions. The presence of multiple chronic illnesses (known as comorbidity) places the body under great stress, which also undermines the immune system. The combined effects of these conditions result in damage to different organ systems of the body—most importantly, the cardiovascular system, the respiratory system, and the renal system. Any time these systems are compromised by the effects of illness, either chronic or acute, the body becomes particularly vulnerable to infectious agents that routinely exist in our environment.

Compounding this situation is the inability of many older adults to understand the potential seriousness of infections at this stage of their lives. They may even have a false sense of confidence that their bodies are just as "good" at warding off infections as they once were. In addition, a lack of social support, isolation from health care facilities, and the inability to afford expensive prescription medication together make important medical care less available at a time when it could be effective.

When these factors are combined, as they are for many older adults, serious and even fatal infectious conditions become a reality. Therefore, anyone who is responsible for the health and well-being of older persons needs to understand their susceptibility to infectious conditions and recognize the fact that timely and competent care is of critical importance.

---

diphtheria, and rubella. This possible increase in childhood infectious illnesses is based on the disturbing finding that fewer than half of American preschoolers are adequately immunized, which is principally due to the failure of many parents to complete their children's immunization programs. Today health professionals are attempting to raise the level of immunization to 90% of all children under the age of 2 years.

Vaccinations against several potentially serious infectious conditions are available and should be given. These include the following:

- *Diphtheria:* A potentially fatal illness that leads to inflammation of the membranes that line the throat, to swollen lymph nodes, and to heart and kidney failure
- *Whooping cough:* A bacterial infection of the airways and lungs that results in deep, noisy breathing and coughing
- *Hepatitis B:* A viral infection that can be transmitted sexually or through the exchange of blood or bodily fluids; seriously damages the liver
- *Haemophilus influenzae type B:* A bacterial infection that can damage the heart and brain, resulting in meningitis, and can produce profound hearing loss

- *Tetanus:* A fatal infection that damages the central nervous system; caused by bacteria found in the soil
- *Rubella (German measles):* A viral infection of the upper respiratory tract that can cause damage to a developing fetus when the mother contracts the infection during the first trimester of pregnancy
- *Measles (red measles):* A highly contagious viral infection leading to a rash, high fever, and upper respiratory tract symptoms
- *Polio:* A viral infection capable of causing paralysis of the large muscles of the extremities
- *Mumps:* A viral infection of the salivary glands
- *Chicken pox:* A varicella zoster virus spread by airborne droplets, leading to a sore throat, rash, and fluid-filled blisters
- *Pneumococcal infection:* A bacterium capable of causing infections, including pneumonia, heart, kidney, and middle ear infections

Parents of newborns should take their infants to their family-care physicians, pediatricians, or well-baby clinics operated by county health departments to begin the immunization schedule. The new chicken pox vaccine, VariVax, is now available. Currently the vaccine is recommended for the child 1 year of age or older who does not have a reliable history of having had chickenpox as determined by the health care provider. For children at high risk for pneumococcal infections of the upper respiratory system (including resultant middle ear infections), a vaccine is now available. For these children, including Native American children, African American children, and children with congenital immunodeficiency, chronic cardiopulmonary disease, immunosuppressive neoplastic disease, chronic renal insufficiency, and those on chemotherapy, immunization with pneumococcal conjugate and pneumococcal polysaccharide vaccines is recommended. Early studies regarding a decrease in middle ear infections (otitis media) in children having received the pneumococcal vaccine was encouraging. More recent reviews of previous studies, however, suggest that the reduction is very small, and should not be viewed as the basis on which this immunization is advised.[10] Researchers are also attempting to develop a single immunization that would combine many individual vaccines now used. In addition, research is being conducted on new delivery systems, including a skin patch, nasal spray, and vaccine-enriched foods, such as potatoes.

 TALKING POINTS Through community service work, you meet a couple that say that they have not had their children immunized and don't see the reason for doing so. How would you explain the importance of having this done?

In recent years concern has arisen regarding the role of childhood immunizations in the development of other serious childhood physical and emotional health problems, such as type 1 diabetes mellitus,[11] asthma,[12] autism,[13] and SIDS.[14] At this time studies investigating the possible relationship between recommended immunizations and conditions mentioned above have found no demonstrable cause-and-effect relationships.

Although immunization is universally viewed as important for infants and children, adults have immunization needs that can be unmet. Accordingly, CDC's National Immunization Program has just released its first immunization schedule for adults which recommends eight immunizations that should be updated or initially received by adults. Adults are particularly underprotected in regard to diphtheria and tetanus.[15]

Causes and Management of Selected Infectious Diseases

This section focuses on some of the common infectious diseases and some diseases that are less common but serious. You can use this information as a basis for judging your own disease susceptibility.

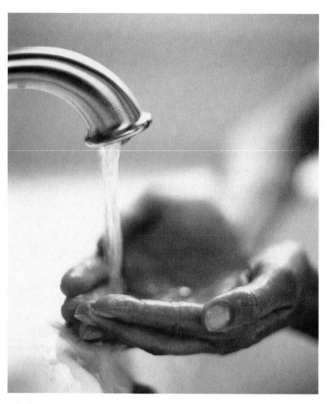

Washing your hands often is the best way to prevent the common cold.

The Common Cold

The common cold, an acute upper-respiratory-tract infection, must reign as humankind's supreme infectious disease. Also known as **acute rhinitis,** this highly contagious viral infection can be caused by any of the nearly 200 known rhinoviruses. Colds are particularly common when people spend time in crowded indoor environments, such as classrooms.

The signs and symptoms of a cold are fairly predictable. Runny nose, watery eyes, general aches and pains, a listless feeling, and a slight fever all may accompany a cold in its early stages. Eventually the nasal passages swell, and the inflammation may spread to the throat. Stuffy nose, sore throat, and coughing may follow (Table 12.2 on page 339). The senses of taste and smell are blocked, and appetite declines.

Key Terms
acute rhinitis the common cold; the sudden onset of nasal inflammation.

Table 12.2 Is It a Cold or the Flu?

	Cold	Flu
Symptoms		
Fever	Rare	Characteristic, high (102°–104°+ F); lasts 3–4 days
Headache	Rare	Prominent
General aches, pains	Slight	Usual; often severe
Fatigue, weakness	Quite mild	Can last up to 2–3 weeks
Extreme exhaustion	Never	Early and prominent
Stuffy nose	Common	Sometimes
Sneezing	Usual	Sometimes
Sore throat	Common	Sometimes
Chest discomfort, cough	Mild to moderate; hacking cough	Common; can become severe
Complications	Sinus congestion, earache	Pneumonia, bronchitis; can be life threatening
Prevention	Avoidance of infected people	Annual vaccination; amantadine or rimantadine (antiviral drugs)
Treatment	OTC products for symptom relief	Amantadine or rimantadine within 24–48 hours after onset of symptoms

Note: The need to consult a physician as the result of complications that might arise during the course of a cold or flu is not unknown. During the course of a cold any of the following should be called to the attention of a physician: (1) when a cold fails to resolve within 5 to 7 days, (2) when an elevated temperature develops (above 103°F), or (3) when a "deep chest" cough develops that produces either a brownish-tinged sputum or does not respond to OTC cough medication. Similar complications can occur in conjunction with the flu and require consultation with a physician. In addition, prolonged vomiting and diarrhea also should be called to the attention of a physician. Upon contracting the flu, children, older adults, pregnant women, and all persons with chronic conditions such as diabetes mellitus, cardiovascular diseases, and malignancies should be carefully monitored and complications should be promptly reported to a physician.

When you notice the onset of symptoms, you should begin managing the cold promptly. After a few days, most of the cold's symptoms subside. In the meantime, you should isolate yourself from others, drink plenty of fluids, eat moderately, and rest.

At this time there is no effective way to prevent colds. In 1999 a medication, pleconaril, appeared to be effective in reducing the extent and duration of colds once initial symptoms had developed. However, in 2002 the FDA denied approval of pleconaril (brand name Picovir) due, in part, to adverse reactions in some women using the drug and oral contraceptives; and the possibility of developing resistance to the drug within the family of viruses for which it is intended.

Some of the many OTC cold remedies can help you manage a cold. These remedies will not cure your cold but may lessen the discomfort associated with it. Nasal decongestants, expectorants, cough syrups, and aspirin or acetaminophen can give some temporary relief. Follow label directions carefully.

If a cold persists, as evidenced by prolonged chills, fever above 103 degrees Fahrenheit, chest heaviness or aches, shortness of breath, coughing up rust-colored mucus, or persistent sore throat or hoarseness, you should contact a physician. Because we now consider colds to be transmitted most readily by hand contact, you should wash your hands frequently.

Influenza

Influenza is also an acute contagious disease caused by viruses. Some influenza outbreaks have killed many people, such as the influenza pandemics of 1889 to 1890, 1918 to 1919, 1957 and 2003/2004. The viral strains that produce this infectious disease have the potential for more severe complications than the viral strains that produce the common cold. The viral strain for a particular form of influenza enters the body through the respiratory tract. After brief incubation and prodromal stages, the host develops signs and symptoms not just in the upper respiratory tract but throughout the entire body. These symptoms include fever, chills, cough, sore throat, headache, gastrointestinal disturbances, and muscular pain (Table 12.2 above).

Antibiotics are generally not prescribed for people with influenza, except when the patient has a possible secondary bacterial infection. Physicians may recommend only aspirin, fluids, and rest. Parents are reminded not to give aspirin to children because of the danger of Reye's syndrome. Reye's syndrome is an aspirin-enhanced complication of influenza in which central nervous system changes can occur, including brain swelling. For a person seeking a quicker resolution to the debilitating symptoms of flu, four antiviral medications are currently available; two are intended for influenza virus type A and two for both virus types A and B. Specific recommendations regarding use of these prescription medications, including age limitations, also exist.[16]

Most young adults can cope with the milder strains of influenza that appear each winter or spring. However, pregnant women and older people—especially older people with additional health complications, such as heart disease, kidney disease, emphysema, and chronic bronchitis—are not as capable of handling this viral attack. People who regularly come into contact with the general public, such as teachers, should also consider annual flu shots.

Today approximately 70 million Americans receive annual "flu shots." In past years, these annual immunizations, tailored to work against the flu viruses anticipated for the coming flu season, were principally received by adults over 50 years of age and others with special needs. During the flu epidemic of 2003/2004, younger adults moved into the recipient population. Today, CDC is extending flu shots recommendations to include all children 6 to 23 months of age and youth between 6 months to 18 years of age who are residing with adults at greatest risk for contracting influenza due to illness or occupational exposure. In June of 2003, the FDA approved the sale of Flumist, a noninvasive nasal spray inhalation delivery system for influenza vaccine. Its use is approved for people ages 5 to 49. Its use is not, at this time, recommended for persons most in need of the highest level of protection.

Tuberculosis

Experts considered TB, a bacterial infection of the lungs resulting in chronic coughing, weight loss, and even death, to be under control in this country until the mid-1980s. The number of cases surged then, however, with a peak of 26,283 cases in 1992. The number has declined since then, with 15,989 cases reported in 2001, a 2% decline from 2000.[17] However, public health officials must continually watch this infectious disease, as people immigrate to the United States from areas of the world in which TB is considerably more common and drug-resistant strains of the bacterium emerge. As an example, it is estimated that 60% of all cases of TB in New York City are among foreign born residents; and that 10 to 15 million U.S. residents have latent tuberculosis, from which 10% will develop an active case of TB.[18]

Tuberculosis thrives in crowded places where infected people are in constant contact with others, since TB is spread by coughing. This includes prisons, hospitals, public housing units, and even college residence halls. In such settings, a single infected person can spread the TB agents to many others.

When healthy people are exposed to TB agents, their immune systems can usually suppress the bacteria enough to prevent symptoms from developing and to reduce the likelihood of infecting others. When the immune system is damaged, however, such as in some older adults, malnourished people, and those who are infected with HIV, the disease can become established and eventually be transmitted to other people at risk.

A new serum-based TB screening test, ELISPOT, has been developed.[19] Similar to the screening test used to detect HIV infection, this test identifies T cells that have been sensitized to an antigen component of the principal tuberculosis bacterium, mycobacterium. This test is more accurate in identifying infected persons than the older and more familiar skin tests.

Pneumonia

Pneumonia is a general term that describes a variety of infectious respiratory conditions. There are bacterial, viral, fungal, rickettsial, mycoplasmal, and parasitic forms of pneumonia. However, bacterial pneumonia is the most common form and is often seen with other illnesses that weaken the body's immune system. In fact, pneumonia is so common in the frail older adult that it is often the specific condition causing death. *Pneumocystis carinii* pneumonia, a parasitic form, is important today because it is a principal opportunistic infection associated with AIDS in HIV-infected people.

Older adults with a history of chronic obstructive lung disease, cardiovascular disease, diabetes, or alcoholism often encounter a potentially serious midwinter form of pneumonia known as *acute (severe) community-acquired pneumonia*.[20] Characteristics of this condition are the sudden onset of chills, chest pain, and a cough producing sputum. In addition, a symptom-free form of pneumonia known as *walking pneumonia* is also commonly seen in adults and can become serious without warning.

As the number of older Americans grows, recommendations regarding immunization against pneumococcal pneumonia have been established and vaccination programs undertaken. Today, these recommendations encourage vaccination beginning at 50 years of age. The cost effectiveness of pneumonia immunizations for older adults, and particularly for minority older adults, is well established.[21]

The first known drug-resistant strains of pneumonia have been identified in this country. As a result, some experts are calling for an even more comprehensive vaccination plan for older adults.

Mononucleosis

College students who contract **mononucleosis ("mono")** can be forced into a long period of bed rest during a semester when they can least afford it. Other common diseases can be managed with minimal disruption, but the overall weakness and fatigue seen in many people with mono sometimes require a month or two of rest and recuperation.

Mono is a viral infection in which the body produces an excess of mononuclear leukocytes (a type of white blood cell). After uncertain, perhaps long, incubation and prodromal stages, the acute symptoms of mono can appear, including weakness, headache, low-grade fever, swollen lymph glands (especially in the neck), and sore throat. Mental fatigue and depression are sometimes reported as side effects of mononucleosis. After the acute symptoms disappear, the weakness and fatigue usually persist—perhaps for a few months.

Mono is diagnosed by its characteristic symptoms. The Monospot blood smear can also be used to identify the prevalence of abnormal white blood cells. In addition, an antibody test can detect activity of the immune system that is characteristic of the illness.

This disease is most often caused by an Epstein-Barr virus, so antibiotic therapy is not recommended. Treatment usually includes bed rest and the use of OTC remedies for fever (aspirin or acetaminophen) and for sore throat lozenges. Corticosteroid drugs can be used in extreme cases. Rupture of the spleen is an occasional, but serious, consequence of the condition, particularly in persons who are too physically active during their recovery.[22] Adequate fluid intake and a well-balanced diet are also important in the recovery stages of mono. Fortunately, the body tends to develop NAI (naturally acquired immunity) to the mono virus, so repeat infections of mono are unusual.

For years, mono has been labeled the "kissing disease"; however, mono is not highly contagious and is known to be spread by direct transmission in ways other than kissing. No vaccine has been developed to confer AAI for mononucleosis. The best preventive measures are the steps that you can take to increase your resistance to most infectious diseases: (1) eat a well-balanced diet, (2) exercise regularly, (3) sleep sufficiently, (4) use health care services appropriately, (5) live in a reasonably healthful environment, and (6) avoid direct contact with infected people.

Chronic Fatigue Syndrome

Chronic fatigue syndrome (CFS) may be the most perplexing "infectious" condition physicians see. First identified in 1985, this mononucleosis-like condition is most often seen in women in their thirties and forties. People with CFS, often busy professional people, report flulike symptoms, including severe exhaustion, fatigue, headaches, muscle aches, fever, inability to concentrate, allergies, intolerance to exercise, and depression. Examinations of the first people with CFS revealed antibodies to the Epstein-Barr virus (EBV). Thus observers assumed CFS to be an infectious viral disease (and initially called it *chronic Epstein-Barr syndrome*).

Since its first appearance, the condition has received a great deal of attention regarding its exact nature. Today, opinions vary widely as to whether the condition is a specific viral infection, a condition involving both viral infections and nonviral components, or some other disorder.[23]

In recent years it has been noted that another chronic condition, fibromyalgia, appears in a manner similar to CFS. As in CFS, the person with fibromyalgia demonstrates fatigue, inefficient sleep patterns, localized areas of tenderness and pain, morning stiffness, and headaches. The onset of this condition, like that of CFS, can follow periods of stress, infectious disease, physical trauma such as falls, thyroid dysfunction, or in conjunction with a connective tissue disorder.[24] Therefore some clinicians believe that the two conditions might be very closely related,[25] drawing on an explanation based on immune system involvement.

Regardless of its cause or causes, CFS is extremely unpleasant for its victims. Certainly, those experiencing the symptoms over an extended time need to be seen by a physician experienced in dealing with CFS.

Bacterial Meningitis

Since approximately 1995, a formerly infrequently seen but potentially fatal infectious disease, meningococcal meningitis, has appeared on college campuses, suggesting that college students are currently at greater risk of contracting the disease than are their noncollege peers. Particularly interesting is the fact that among college students, the risk of contracting this infection on campus is highest for those students living in residence halls, suggesting that close living quarters, as well as sharing cigarettes and beverages, kissing (exchanging infectious oral fluids), and contact with students from

---

Key Terms

mononucleosis ("mono") a viral infection characterized by weakness, fatigue, swollen glands, sore throat, and low-grade fever.

chronic fatigue syndrome (CFS) an illness that causes severe exhaustion, fatigue, aches, and depression; mostly affects women in their thirties and forties.

other areas of the world favor transmission of the bacteria. Since many colleges and universities require that first-year students reside in residence halls, it is in this group that the incidence of meningococcal meningitis is highest.[26] Additionally, this group of students is most likely to be in large section lecture classes and take meals in large dining facilities. Since 1997 the American College Health Association has strongly suggested that parents have incoming students vaccinated against this condition—a $75 investment that could save a life. Annually, about 150 cases of meningococcal meningitis occur on American college campuses, resulting in 15 deaths per year. Understandably, more and more colleges and universities are requiring, as a condition of admission, documentation of immunization against bacterial meningitis. Fortunately, new vaccines, initially used in Canada and Europe, are now available for use in this country.

Meningococcal meningitis is a bacterial infection of the thin membranous coverings of the brain. In its earliest stages, this disease can easily be confused with the flu. Symptoms usually include a high fever, severe headache, stiff neck, nausea with vomiting, extreme tiredness, and the formation of a progressive rash. For about 10% of people who develop this condition, the infection is fatal, often within 24 hours. Therefore the mere presence of the symptoms described above signals the need for immediate medical evaluation. If done promptly, treatment is highly effective.[27]

Lyme Disease

Lyme disease is an infectious disease that is becoming increasingly common in eastern, southeastern, upper midwestern, and West Coast states, with 23,763 cases in 2002. The significant increase in the number of cases of Lyme disease since 1992 (when 9,909 cases were reported) most likely reflects a wider geographical distribution of the disease, a greater awareness of its symptoms by the general public, and more consistent reporting by physicians. This bacterial disease results when infected deer ticks, usually in the nymph (immature) stage, attach to the skin and inject the infectious agent as they feed on a host's blood. Deer ticks become infected by feeding on infected white-tailed deer or white-footed mice.

The symptoms of Lyme disease vary but typically appear within 30 days as small red bumps surrounded by a circular red rash at the site of bites. The red rash, traditionally described as being "bulls eye" in shape, with a whitish center, may also be circular with redness throughout. Flulike symptoms may accompany this phase I stage, including chills, headaches, muscle and joint aches, and low-grade fever. A phase II stage develops in about 20% of infected people. This phase may produce disorders of the nervous system or heart. Those who remain untreated even to this stage can develop a phase III stage, which can include chronic arthritis, lasting up to 2 years. Fortunately, Lyme disease can be treated with antibiotics.[28] Unfortunately, however, no immunity develops, so infection can recur. Because some physicians order tests and begin antibiotic therapy too quickly, however, the basis of concern should be the appearance of phase I symptoms, not simply having been bitten by a tick. Lyme disease may be more difficult to diagnose in children than in adults.

People who live in susceptible areas, including near small urban/suburban wood lots,[29] and participate in outdoor activities can encounter the nearly invisible tick nymphs that have fallen from deer or infected mice into the grass. Thus these people should check themselves frequently to be sure that they are tick-free. They should tuck shirts into pants, tuck pants into socks, and wear gloves and hats when possible. They should also shower after coming inside from outdoors and check clothing for evidence of ticks. Pets can carry infected ticks into the house. If you find ticks, they should be carefully removed from the skin with tweezers and the affected area washed. A vaccine, once available and reasonably effective, has been removed from the marketplace due to declining sales.

Hantavirus Pulmonary Syndrome

Since 1993 a small but rapidly growing number of people have been dying of extreme pulmonary distress caused by the leakage of plasma into the lungs. In the initial cases, the people lived in the Southwest, had been well until they began developing flulike symptoms over one or two days, then quickly experienced difficulty breathing, and died only hours later. Epidemiologists quickly suspected a viral agent such as the hantavirus, known to exist in Asia and, to a lesser degree, in Europe. Exhaustive laboratory work led to the culturing of the virus and confirmed that all of these patients had been infected with an American version of the hantavirus.

Today hantavirus pulmonary syndrome has been reported in areas beyond the Southwest, including most of the western states and some of the eastern states. The common denominator in all these areas is the presence of deer mice. We now know that this common rodent serves as the reservoir for the virus. In fact, so common is the mouse that in 2000 the National Park Service began warning hikers, campers, and off-road bikers that hantavirus probably existed in every national park and that caution should be taken to avoid high-risk sites.

The virus moves from deer mice to humans when people inhale dust contaminated with dried virus-rich rodent urine or saliva-contaminated materials, such as nests. Health experts now warn people who live in areas with deer mouse populations (most of the United States) to be extremely careful when cleaning houses and barns in which deer mouse droppings are likely to be found. If you must remove rodent nests, wear rubber gloves, pour disinfectant or bleach on the nests and soak them thoroughly, and finally, pick up the nests with shovels and burn them or bury them in holes that are several feet deep. These procedures should greatly reduce the airborne spread of the viral particles.

Key Terms

Lyme disease a bacterial infection transmitted by deer ticks.

Because there is no vaccine for hantavirus pulmonary syndrome, people who are likely to be exposed to the infected excrement of deer mice should seek early evaluation of flulike symptoms.

West Nile Virus

First detected in New York City in 1999, the West Nile virus was, by the summer of 2000, identified in six eastern states—New York, Connecticut, New Jersey, Maryland, Rhode Island, and Massachusetts. By the end of 2002 the West Nile virus had spread westward and to include 34 states, with a reported 4,156 cases and 284 deaths. Incomplete data for 2003 (through August) report 1,442 cases and 21 deaths, with anticipated weekly doubling to occur through September 2003. The West Nile virus was found in all but 2 of the 48 contiguous states by the end of 2003.

This vector-borne infectious virus is transmitted from a reservoir, most often birds, by mosquitoes that in turn infect humans.[1] Human to human transmission (via mosquitoes) apparently does not occur. West Nile virus infection involves flulike symptoms, including fever, headache, muscle ache, fatigue, and joint pain. In young children, persons with immune systems weakened by HIV, and older adults, West Nile virus infection may involve encephalitis, a potentially fatal inflammation of the brain that closely resembles St. Louis encephalitis. Physicians recommend that any unusual neurological symptoms be considered as a possible West Nile infection. The West Nile virus deaths that have occurred since the infection's initial appearance in 1999 have been the result of encephalitis.

In an attempt to determine the extent of the West Nile virus range, public health officials throughout the eastern United States have tested mosquitoes, sentinel chickens, crows, other birds, cows, and other animals, including humans. Additionally, mosquito habitats are being treated in an attempt to reduce the vector population. Public service announcements focusing on protection against mosquito bites are routinely made in high-risk areas.

In the period 1999–2003, additional aspects of the disease were reported to CDC; these include transmission of the virus through blood transfusions, a possible case of prenatal transmission, and the presence of the virus in breast milk. Additionally, a new test to accurately screen for infected blood has been developed, as has a new diagnostic test, developed in Australia, that significantly reduced the time needed to obtain confirmation of the West Nile virus.

Toxic Shock Syndrome

Toxic shock syndrome (TSS) made front-page headlines in 1980, when the CDC reported a connection between TSS and the presence of a specific bacterial agent (*Staphylococcus aureus*) in the vagina associated with the use of tampons. In addition to tampon misuse-induced TSS, the condition can be caused in conjunction with nasal packing following surgery, infected burns, and subcutaneous abscesses.

TSS causes the signs and symptoms listed in the Star box on this page. Superabsorbent tampons can irritate the vaginal lining three times more quickly than regular tampons. This vaginal irritation is aggravated when the tampon remains in the vagina for a long time (more than five hours). When this irritation begins, the staphylococcal bacteria (which are usually present in the vagina) have relatively easy access to the bloodstream. When these bacteria proliferate in the circulatory system, their resultant toxins produce toxic shock syndrome. A woman with TSS can die, usually as a result of cardiovascular failure, if left untreated. Fortunately, less than 10% of women diagnosed as having TSS die.

In comparison to other infectious diseases, the extent of TSS is limited. In 1998, the last year for which data are available, 133 cases were reported. More recently only about 10 cases have been reported annually. However, because of a tendency of many physicians to not report this

Signs and Symptoms of Toxic Shock Syndrome

- Fever (102°F or above)
- Headache
- Vomiting
- Sore throat
- Diarrhea
- Muscle aches
- Sunburnlike rash
- Low blood pressure
- Bloodshot eyes
- Disorientation
- Reduced urination
- Peeling of skin on the palms of the hands and soles of the feet

Key Terms

toxic shock syndrome (TSS) a potentially fatal condition caused by the proliferation of certain bacteria in the vagina that enter the general blood circulation.

condition, it may be far more prevalent than recent data suggest. Accordingly, every woman should exercise reasonable caution in the use of tampons. Consider these recommendations: (1) tampons should not be the sole form of sanitary protection used, and (2) tampons should not remain in place for too long. Women should change tampons every few hours and intermittently use sanitary napkins. Tampons should not be used during sleep. Some physicians recommend that tampons not be used at all if a woman wants to be extraordinarily safe from TSS.

 TALKING POINTS As a parent you are preparing yourself to discuss menstruation with your rapidly maturing daughter. What would you say regarding the safe use of tampons?

Hepatitis

Hepatitis is an inflammatory process in the liver that can be caused by several viruses. Types A, B, C (once called non-A and non-B), D, and E have been recognized. Hepatitis can also be caused indirectly from abuse of alcohol and other drugs. General symptoms of hepatitis include fever, nausea, loss of appetite, abdominal pain, fatigue, and jaundice (yellowing of the skin and eyes).[1]

Type A hepatitis is often associated with consuming fecal-contaminated food, such as raw shellfish, or water. Poor sanitation, particularly in the handling of food and diaper-changing activities, has produced outbreaks in child care centers. Experts estimate that up to two hundred thousand people per year experience this infection. This number far exceeds the reported 26,000 to 27,000 cases per year, suggesting that a very large reservoir exists among children, who are routinely asymptomatic prior to 6 years of age. Therefore, it is currently recommended that children living in states with high levels of reported hepatitis A be vaccinated, as well as children with weakened immune systems, and those who will travel outside the United States.[30]

Type B hepatitis (HBV) is spread in various ways, including sexual contact, intravenous drug use, tattooing, body piercing, and even sharing electric razors. On the basis of these modes of transmission, college students should be aware of the potential risk that they too carry for HBV infection. Beyond the risk factors just identified, medical and dental procedures are also a potential means of transmitting the virus, including patient to practitioner, and practitioner to patient transmission. Chronic HBV infection has been associated with liver cirrhosis and is the principal cause of liver cancer. An effective immunization for hepatitis B is now available. Although it is given during childhood, it should be seriously considered for older unvaccinated people and college students. In 2002 the American Academy of Pediatrics recommended that all newborns be immunized prior to leaving the hospital. A new vaccine against both hepatitis A and B is now available. Earlier concerns regarding hepatitis B vaccine and multiple sclerosis have been largely dismissed.[31]

Hepatitis C is contracted in ways similar to hepatitis B (sexual contact, tainted blood, and shared needles). In the absence of immunization, the pool of infected people is in excess of four million and the death rate is expected to climb. Currently a dual-drug therapy for HCV involving multiple forms of interferon in combination with the drug ribavirin is the treatment of choice. It should also be noted that many infected persons remain asymptomatic for decades, and many persons infected with HCV recover from this liver-threatening infection. In a recent study a two-drug combination treatment resulted in a virus-free state for nearly 60% of a large group of infected persons treated for 1 year. In spite of encouraging news such as this, recovery from HCV infection seems less likely the case for infected African Americans, a phenomenon that cannot currently be explained.[32]

The newly identified type D (delta) hepatitis is very difficult to treat and is found almost exclusively in people already suffering from type B hepatitis, since the hepatitis D virus requires the presence of the hepatitis B virus in order to gain full pathogenicity. This virus, like type B hepatitis and HIV, makes unprotected sexual contact, including anal and oral sex, very risky. Hepatitis E, associated with water contamination, is rarely seen in this country other than in people returning from hepatitis E virus-endemic areas of the world.

Sudden Acute Respiratory Syndrome (SARS)

In February 2003, the world became aware of a previously unknown respiratory disease, initially thought to be a form of pneumonia. This disease, characterized by high fever (100.4+°F), chills, headaches and, a few days later a dry cough, was, in fact, a new viral disease, Sudden Acute Respiratory Syndrome (SARS). First reported in Hanoi, then in Singapore, mainland China, and other Asian countries, the disease quickly presented in Europe and North America. In actuality, the disease had first appeared in a rural area of China, during the fall of 2002, but the Chinese government had apparently chosen not to disseminate this information.

With the rapid spread of SARS, the World Health Organization and CDC issued travel advisories against unnecessary travel to several areas and cities of Asia, as well as to Toronto, Canada. At the same time, scientists isolated the virus responsible for the respiratory disease and identified it as a member of the coronavirus family—a viral family with links to upper respiratory infection (colds). This particular virus, however, apparently entered the human germ pool in conjunction with the eating of civet cats—a delicacy in China—again demonstrating that many infectious conditions in humans have their origins in other animals—**zoonosis.**

With news of the SARS outbreak, the international scientific community began a cooperative effort to understand the disease's human-to-human transmission. It was quickly determined that the virus was transmitted by respiratory droplets. It was further determined that the frail, the elderly, and the young were at greatest risk, as well as persons in direct contact with symptomatic persons (family members and hospital staff). Soon thereafter, a diagnostic test was developed and treatment protocols became more focused and effective. These developments, in combination with concerted public health measures regarding the recognition of symptoms and curtailment of transmission opportunities, led to a rapid decline of reported new cases. On June 5, 2003, the World Health Organization declared that SARS had peaked and was subsiding in all infected areas.[33] By the WHO-defined end of the pandemic, August 15, 2003, 33 people in the United States had been infected and none had died, while worldwide 8,422 had been infected and 916 had died.[34] Clearly, in terms of a potentially pandemic disease, the global village had been condensed in size by international travel and commerce.

AIDS

AIDS (acquired immunodeficiency syndrome) has become the most devastating infectious disease in recent history and it is virtually certain to be the most devastating disease in history unless a cure is forthcoming. Setting aside for the present the international scope of the HIV/AIDS epidemic, statistics for the United States alone paint a distressing picture. On the basis of data reported through December 2001, a total of 816,149 Americans have been diagnosed with the AIDS, and 467,910 have died from its effects (or 57.3% of all cases).[35]

Cause of AIDS

AIDS is the disease caused by HIV, a virus that attacks the helper T cells of the immune system (see pages 335–336). When HIV attacks helper T cells, people lose the ability to fight off a variety of infections that would normally be easily controlled. Because these infections develop while people are vulnerable, they are collectively called *opportunistic infections*. HIV-infected (HIV+) patients become increasingly vulnerable to infection by bacteria, protozoa, fungi, and several viruses. A variety of malignancies (see Chapter 11) also develop during this period of immune-system vulnerability.

HIV+ with AIDS was originally diagnosed based on the presence of specific conditions. Among these were *Pneumocystis carinii* pneumonia and Kaposi's sarcoma, a rare but deadly form of skin cancer. Gradually, experts recognized that additional conditions were associated with advancing deterioration of the immune system and thus added them to the list of AIDS conditions. This list now includes almost thirty definitive conditions, with more conditions being added as they become apparent. Among the conditions found on the current version of the list are toxoplasmosis within the brain, cytomegalovirus retinitis with loss of vision, lymphoma involving the brain, recurrent salmonella blood infections, and a wasting syndrome that includes invasive cervical cancer in women, recurrent pneumonia, and recurrent tuberculosis. Today, however, experts tend to assign the label of HIV+ with AIDS to HIV-infected people when their level of helper T cells drops below 250 cells per cubic millimeter of blood, regardless of whether specific conditions are present.

Spread of HIV

HIV cannot be contracted easily in comparison to other infectious conditions such as colds, flu, and some childhood infections that can spread quickly within a classroom or office complex. The chances of contracting HIV through casual contact with HIV-infected people at work, school, or home are extremely low or nonexistent. HIV is known to be spread only by direct sexual contact involving the exchange of bodily fluids (including blood, semen, and vaginal secretions), the sharing of hypodermic needles, transfusion of infected blood or blood products, and perinatal transmission (from an infected mother to a fetus or newborn baby). For HIV to be transmitted, it must enter the bloodstream of the noninfected person, such as through needles or tears in body tissues lining the rectum, mouth, or reproductive system. Current research also indicates that HIV is not transmitted by sweat, saliva, tears, or urine, although the virus may be found in very low concentrations in these fluids. The virus cannot enter the body through the gastrointestinal system because digestive enzymes destroy the virus. An exception to this generalization, however, might exist, as studies conducted in Africa indicate that transmission can occur in conjunction with breast-feeding infants.[36] A second exception involves the transmission of HIV between infected persons and their uninfected sexual partners during episodes of unprotected oral sex when the uninfected persons have evident gingivitis and bleeding gums.[37]

Key Terms

zoonosis the transmission of diseases from animals to humans.

Women are at much greater risk than men of contracting HIV through heterosexual activity because of the higher concentration of lymphocytes in semen (± 10 million lymphocytes/tsp.) than in vaginal secretions (± 1,200 thousand lymphocytes/tsp).[38] This susceptibility is seen in part by the increasing percentage of women with AIDS who were infected through heterosexual contact—from 8% in 1981, to 19% in 1993, and 36% in 2001.[35] Women under age 25 contract the virus principally through heterosexual contact. Figure 12-3 shows the estimated number of new cases of HIV worldwide.

Signs and Symptoms of HIV Infection

Most people infected with HIV initially feel well and have no symptoms (that is, they are asymptomatic). Experts generally consider the *incubation stage* for HIV infection to be 6 months to 10 or more years, with the average approximately 6 years. Despite the long period between infection and the first clinical observation of damage to the immune system, antibodies to HIV may appear within several weeks to three months of contracting the virus. Of course, relatively few people are tested for HIV infection at any time during the incubation period. Thus infected people could remain asymptomatic (currently described as HIV+ without symptoms) and be carriers of HIV for years before they experience signs of illness sufficient to warrant a physical examination.

Without symptoms of immune-system deterioration or AIDS-testing results, sexually active people need to redefine the meaning of monogamy. Couples must now account for the sexual partners they have both had over the past 10 years. Unfortunately, people do this so infrequently that some observers are labeling today's young adults "a generation in jeopardy."

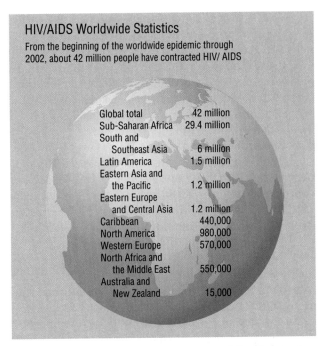

HIV/AIDS Worldwide Statistics

From the beginning of the worldwide epidemic through 2002, about 42 million people have contracted HIV/ AIDS

Global total	42 million
Sub-Saharan Africa	29.4 million
South and Southeast Asia	6 million
Latin America	1.5 million
Eastern Asia and the Pacific	1.2 million
Eastern Europe and Central Asia	1.2 million
Caribbean	440,000
North America	980,000
Western Europe	570,000
North Africa and the Middle East	550,000
Australia and New Zealand	15,000

Figure 12-3 For every person counted in these statistics, there is a face and a story. What are you doing to protect yourself from HIV/AIDS?

Source: UNAIDS and World Health Organization.

Most people infected with HIV, in the absence of early screening and prophylactic drug treatment, eventually develop signs and symptoms of a more advanced stage of the disease. These signs and symptoms include tiredness, fever, loss of appetite and weight, diarrhea, night sweats, and swollen glands (usually in the neck, armpits, and groin). At this point, they are said to be HIV+ with symptoms. (See Table 12.3 below.)

Table 12.3 The Spectrum of HIV Infection

	HIV+ without Symptoms (Asymptomatic)	HIV+ with Symptoms	HIV+ with AIDS
External signs	No symptoms Looks well	Fever Night sweats Swollen lymph glands Weight loss Diarrhea Minor infections Fatigue	Kaposi's sarcoma *Pneumocystis carinii* pneumonia and/or other predetermined illnesses Neurological disorders One or more of an additional 30+ diagnosable conditions or a helper T cell count falls below 250 per cubic milliliter of blood
Incubation	Invasion of virus to 10 years	Several months to 10 or more years	Several months to 10–12 or more years
Internal level of infection	Antibodies are produced Immune system remains intact Positive antibody test	Antibodies are produced Immune system weakened Positive antibody test	Immune system deficient Positive antibody test
Infectious?	Yes	Yes	Yes

Given sufficient time, perhaps as long as 15 years, most infected people without prophylactic drug treatment will move beyond HIV with symptoms into the *acute stage*. At this point, the label HIV+ with AIDS is applied, either on the basis of clinically defined conditions or more likely on the basis of a helper T cell count below 250 per cubic millimeter of blood. A normal helper T cell range is 800 to 1,000. The efficacy of treatment is based in part on improvements in the T cell count over time.

A small percentage of infected people can suppress the infection and have survived for over two decades without developing AIDS, but experts do not fully understand this ability (possibly attributing it to a suppressor compound formed by specific immune system cells).

Diagnosis of HIV Infection

HIV infection is diagnosed through a clinical examination, laboratory tests for accompanying infections, and an initial screening test. Should the initial screening test produce a negative result, persons at risk for infection should be rescreened in 3 to 6 months. For persons reluctant to present themselves for screening in a clinical setting, home screening tests are also available. Regardless, once initial screening has been undertaken, to eliminate the small chance of a false positive having occurred, more sensitive tests can be administered, including the enzyme-linked immunosorbent assay (ELISA) and Western blot test. Although expensive and not completely reliable, even more recently developed tests are now available. One of these tests identifies the existence of viral mutations known to be drug resistant,[39] while another helps determine whether a particular drug will function in suppressing the contracted viral strain. This information helps physicians structure treatment protocols.

Treatment of HIV and AIDS

There is no cure for HIV infection and the resultant AIDS. It is critically important, however, that treatment begin upon diagnosis. Current treatment uses a combination of drugs drawn principally from two distinct groups: the *reverse-transcriptase* inhibitors and the *protease inhibitors*.

The reverse-transcriptase inhibitors block (or inhibit) the action of reverse transcriptase, an enzyme the virus requires to replicate itself within the host's infected T helper cells. Currently a combination of two of the many available reverse-transcriptase inhibitors is used to formulate a portion of the drug "cocktail" employed in treating HIV infection.

Introduction of the protease inhibitors, in combination with the reverse-transcriptase inhibitors, has revolutionized the treatment of HIV infection. These drugs inhibit the ability of the virus to undertake the replication process. In most treatment protocols, one protease inhibitor is combined with two reverse-transcriptase inhibitors to complete the drug cocktail.

Protease inhibitors have revolutionized AIDS care, reducing HIV to undetectable levels in thousands of people. The number of deaths from AIDS has decreased dramatically, from 49,985 in 1995 to 14,499 in 2000.[35] However, people should not consider this improvement to mean that the emergency is over. In fact, when the drug cocktail therapy described above is discontinued, viral loads frequently move back toward pretreatment levels. This suggests the existence of well-protected sequestered (hidden) viruses within other tissues of the body.

In addition to reverse-transcriptase inhibitors and protease inhibitors, three recently introduced types of medications, including two entry inhibitors, two co-receptor inhibitors, and two fusion inhibitors, have been developed to further enhance the battle against HIV/AIDS.[40] Now, newer and even more potent "cocktails" are developed by combining both older and new medication. The treatment is deemed highly active antiretroviral therapy, or *HAART*. HAART has proven highly effective in extending the life of many persons with HIV/AIDS by significantly reducing the level of HIV (viral load) in the body. Decision as to what a given patients' HAART will consist of is determined by factors such as the viral load data and the presence of pre-existing conditions.

In the final analysis, however, as effective as HAART is in improving the length and quality of life for persons with HIV/AIDS, mortality concerns remain, and life expectancy is compromised. The inability of persons with AIDS to move into and through the *decline stage* and on to the *recovery stage* reflects the relationship between the disease and the immune system itself. Although drug cocktails stabilize the downward movement of the helper T cell count for an extended period, the viral load moves rapidly upward when drugs are discontinued. Additionally, drug therapy is demanding on the overall body, opportunistic infections continue to develop, and pre-existing conditions may often worsen, such as incipient cardiovascular disease.[41]

In addition to the antiviral drugs, physicians also have a variety of medications to treat the symptoms associated with various infections and malignancies that make up AIDS. These drugs, of course, cannot reverse HIV status or cure AIDS.

Researchers continue to search for vaccines to prevent HIV infection. One large-scale clinical trial involving a vaccine is now completed. The vaccine, AIDSVAX, that employed two genetically altered AIDS virus types (North American and European strains), did not, however, result in the anticipated level of protection. It did, however, provide a slightly higher level of protection for Blacks and Asian than for whites.[42] The FDA has advised the manufacturer that they will certify the vaccine for sale, if the level of protection can reach 30%.

The reality of HIV/AIDS in Africa and Asia is only now being recognized worldwide. With an estimated 29.4

million infected persons in Sub-Saharan Africa and an additional 6.0 million infected persons in Southeast Asia, the need for a vaccine specific to the viral strains of these areas is growing rapidly.[43] In late 2000, a radically new and relatively inexpensive vaccine using segments of HIV DNA attached to salmonella bacteria underwent its initial human trials in Uganda. Should this innovative approach prove safe and effective, then progress can be made in quelling the potential catastrophe that is taking form on these two continents. Conversely, in the absence of a vaccine (and the inability to effectively treat those currently infected), it is projected that African life expectancy will drop to 29 years and that more than 29 million orphans will need care. Similar consequences would be expected in areas of Asia.

Prevention of HIV Infection

Can HIV infection be prevented? The answer is a definite yes. HIV infection rates on college campuses are considered low (approximately 0.2%), but students can be at risk. Every person can take several steps to reduce the risk of contracting and transmitting HIV. All of these steps require understanding one's behavior and the methods by which HIV can be transmitted. Some appropriate steps for college-aged people are abstinence, safer sex, sobriety, and communication with potential sexual partners. To ensure the greatest protection from HIV, one should abstain from sexual activity. Other than this, the Changing for the Better box lists recommendations for safer sex, sobriety, and the exchange of honest, accurate information about sexual histories.

TALKING POINTS In a job interview with a representative from a large pharmaceutical company, you are asked about your feelings regarding the affordability of HIV/AIDS medications in third world countries. What would your response be?

Changing for the Better

Reducing Your Risk of Contracting HIV

I've had only one partner in the past, but now I'm starting to date others with whom I may become sexually active. What should I do to protect myself from HIV and sexually transmitted diseases?

It is important to keep in mind that sexual partners may not reveal their true sexual history or drug habits. If you are sexually active, you can lower your risk of infection with HIV and STDs by adopting the following safer sex practices.

- Learn the sexual history and HIV status of your sex partner.
- Limit your sexual partners by practicing abstinence or by maintaining long-term monogamous relationships.
- Always use condoms correctly and consistently.
- Avoid contact with body fluids, feces, and semen.
- Curtail use of drugs that impair good judgment.
- Never share hypodermic needles.
- Refrain from sex with known injectable drug abusers.*
- Avoid sex with HIV-infected persons, those with signs and symptoms of AIDS, and the partners of high-risk individuals.*
- Get regular tests for STD infections.
- Do not engage in unprotected anal intercourse.

How easy will it be to adopt these behaviors? How real is your risk of becoming HIV-positive?

*Current studies indicate that the elimination of high-risk people as sexual partners is the single most effective safer sex practice that can be implemented.

InfoLinks

www.caps.ucsf.edu/FSindex.html

Sexually Transmitted Diseases

Sexually transmitted diseases (STDs) were once called venereal diseases (for Venus, the Roman goddess of love). Today the term *venereal disease* has been superseded by the broader terms *sexually transmitted disease* or *sexually transmitted infections*. Table 12.4 shows statistics on reportable STDs by age, gender, and ethnicity. Experts currently emphasize the successful prevention and treatment of STDs rather than the ethics of sexuality. Thus one should consider the following points: (1) By age 25 years approximately one-third of all adults will have contracted a sexually transmitted disease—most often chlamydia, herpes simplex, or human papillomavirus infection; (2) a person can have more than one STD at a time; (3) the symptoms of STDs can vary over time and from person to person; (4) the body develops little immunity for STDs; and (5) STDs can predispose people to additional health problems, including infertility, birth defects in their children, cancer, and long-term disability. In addition, the risk of HIV infection is higher when sexual partners are also infected with STDs.

This section focuses on the STDs most frequently diagnosed among college students (chlamydia, gonorrhea, human papillomavirus infection, herpes simplex, syphilis, and

---

Key Terms

sexually transmitted diseases (STDs) infectious diseases that are spread primarily through intimate sexual contact.

Table 12.4 Selected Sexually Transmitted Diseases by Number of Cases, Sex, Age, Race, and Ethnicity. 2001 (and 1998)

Disease	Male	Females	15–19	20–24	25–29	White	Black	Hispanic	Asian Pacific Islander	American Indian Alaska Native
Chlamydia	141,138	547,247	254,176	252,425	93,776	206,348	319,667	136,617	13,590	13,165
Gonorrhea	117,541	184,217	101,065	116,226	56,084	58,323	271,871	26,190	2,935	2,439
Primary and Secondary Syphilis	4,132	1,968	387	836	876	1,387	3,813	754	55	90
			15–25	**26–39**	**40–64**					
Hepatitis B	5,929	3,887	1,757	4,357	3,117	3,958	855	850	683	80 (1998)
Hepatitis C	2,171	1,272	166	1,101	1,619	1,921	468	392	33	46 (1998)

Note: Similar data on AIDS appears in Table 13.5.

Sources: 2001 data: STD Surveillance 2001. National Center for HIV, STD, and TB Prevention Centers for Disease Control and Prevention. 2001 **http://www.cdc/gov.std/stats/TOC2001.htm** 1998 data: Table 13.8. *Understanding Your Health*, 7ᵗʰ ed. McGraw-Hill, 2002

pubic lice). Complete the Personal Assessment on page 361 to determine your risk of contracting an STD. See the Changing for the Better box on page 349 for safer sex practices.

Chlamydia (Nonspecific Urethritis)

Chlamydia is thought to be the most prevalent STD in the United States today. Chlamydia infections occur an estimated five times more frequently than gonorrhea and up to ten times more frequently than syphilis. Because of its high prevalence in sexually active adolescents, they should be screened for chlamydia twice a year, even in the absence of symptoms. Because chlamydia frequently accompanies gonorrheal infections, a dual therapy is often appropriate when gonorrhea is found. Sexually active people in the 20- to 24-year age range should also be considered for routine screening, particularly if they have a history of multiple sex partners and have not practiced a form of barrier contraception (Figure 12-4).[44]

Chlamydia trachomatis is the bacterial agent that causes the chlamydia infection. Chlamydia is the most common cause of nonspecific urethritis (NSU). NSU describes infections of the **urethra** and surrounding tissues that are not caused by the bacterium responsible for gonorrhea. About 80 percent of men with chlamydia display gonorrhea-like signs and symptoms, including painful urination and a whitish pus discharge from the penis. As in gonorrheal infections and many other STDs, most women report no overt signs or symptoms. A few women might exhibit a mild urethral discharge, painful urination, and swelling of vulval tissues. The recommended treatment for chlamydia is either a single dose of azithromycin (1 g) or doxycycline (100 mg) given orally twice a day for 7 days.

Average Number of Sexual Partners

Women
Men

0: 3% 3%
1: 31% 20%
2-4: 36% 21%
5-10: 20% 23%
10-20: 6% 16%
21 or more: 3% 17%

Figure 12-4 Average number of sexual partners men and women have had since age 18. The fewer the number of partners you've had, the lower your risk of contracting HIV or an STD.

Source: Michael RT, Gagnon JH, Laumann EO, Kolata G: *Sex in America: a definitive study.*

Key Terms

chlamydia the most prevalent sexually transmitted disease; caused by a nongonococcal bacterium.

urethra (yoo **ree** thra) the passageway through which urine leaves the urinary bladder.

The infected person should carefully comply with instructions to abstain from sexual intercourse.[44]

Both sexual partners should receive treatment to avoid the ping-pong effect—the back-and-forth reinfection that occurs among couples when only one partner receives treatment. Furthermore, as with other STDs, having chlamydia once does not effectively confer immunity.

Unresolved chlamydia can lead to the same negative health consequences that result from untreated gonorrheal infections. In men the pathogens can invade and damage the deeper reproductive structures (the prostate gland, seminal vesicles, and Cowper's glands). Sterility can result. The pathogens can spread further and produce joint problems (arthritis) and heart complications (damaged heart valves, blood vessels, and heart muscle tissue).

In women the pathogens enter the body through the urethra or the cervical area. If the invasion is not properly treated, it can reach the deeper pelvic structures, producing a syndrome called **pelvic inflammatory disease (PID).** The infection may attack the inner uterine wall (endometrium), the fallopian tubes, and any surrounding structures to produce this painful syndrome. A variety of further complications can result, including sterility, ectopic pregnancies, and **peritonitis.** Infected women can transmit a chlamydia infection to the eyes and lungs of newborns during a vaginal birth. Detecting chlamydia and other NSUs early is of paramount concern for both men and women.

Human Papillomavirus

The appearance of another STD, **human papillomavirus (HPV),** is unwanted news. Because HPV infections are generally asymptomatic, the exact extent of the disease is unknown. A study of a group of sexually active college women found HPV infection in approximately 20% of the women. HPV-related changes to the cells of the cervix are found in nearly 5% of the Pap smears taken from women under age 30. Researchers currently believe that risk factors for HPV infection in women include: (1) sexual activity before age 20, (2) intercourse with three or more partners before age 35, and (3) intercourse with a partner who has three or more partners. The extent of HPV infection in men is even less clearly known, but it is probably widespread.

HPV infection is alarming because some of the more than fifty forms of the virus are strongly associated with precancerous changes to cells lining the cervix, thus the importance of new viral Pap smears (see Chapter 11). Additionally, visible genital warts (cauliflower-like, raised, pinkish-white lesions) are associated with viral forms 6 or 11, while viral forms 16, 18, 31, 33, and 35 foster changes in other areas[44] (Figure 12-5). Found most commonly on the penis, scrotum, labia, cervix, and around the anus, these lesions represent the most common symptomatic viral STD in this country. Although most genital wart colonies are small, they may become very large and block the anus or birth canal during pregnancy.

Treatment for HPV, including genital warts, may include patient-applied gels or creams or physician-administered cryotherapy, topical medication, or surgery. Regardless of treatment, however, the viral colonies will probably return. One should use condoms to attempt to prevent transmission of HPV.

Key Terms

pelvic inflammatory disease (PID) an acute or chronic infection of the peritoneum or lining of the abdominopelvic cavity and fallopian tubes; associated with a variety of symptoms or none at all and a potential cause of sterility.

peritonitis (pare it ton **eye** tis) inflammation of the peritoneum, or lining of the abdominopelvic cavity.

human papillomavirus (HPV) sexually transmitted viruses, some of which are capable of causing precancerous changes in the cervix; causative agent for genital warts.

Figure 12-5 A human papillomavirus infection (genital warts).

Gonorrhea

Another extremely common (600,000 cases/year estimated and 360,000 cases/year reported) STD, gonorrhea is caused by a bacterium *(N. gonorrhoea)*. The incidence of gonorrhea rose 18% between 1997 and 2001,[45] perhaps, in part, because of decreasing fear of HIV/AIDS brought about by the effectiveness of the protease inhibitors being widely reported at that time. In men this bacterial agent can produce a milky-white discharge from the penis, accompanied by painful urination. About 80% of men who contract gonorrhea report varying degrees of these symptoms. This figure is approximately reversed for women: Only about 20% of women are symptomatic and thus report varying degrees of frequent, painful urination, with a slimy yellow-green discharge from the vagina or urethra. Oral sex with an infected partner can produce a gonorrheal infection of the throat (pharyngeal gonorrhea). Gonorrhea can also be transmitted to the rectal areas of both men and women.

An interesting finding relative to gonorrhea in adolescents appeared in the 28 April 2000 issue of the *Morbidity and Mortality Weekly Report*.[46] In that issue, it was reported that the incidence of gonorrhea within the adolescent population correlated closely with the consumption of beer, suggesting that alcohol consumption fosters a higher level of high-risk sexual behavior, including earlier onset of sexual activity, an increased number of partners, and less selectivity in choosing those partners. With heavy consumption of beer on many college campuses, this finding does not bode well for the highly asymptomatic female population.

Physicians diagnose gonorrhea by culturing the bacteria. Because of the paired occurrence of chlamydia and gonorrhea, dual therapy with doxycycline or azithromycin in combination with ofloxacin is used in susceptible populations, particularly adolescent women. Outside of these groups, recommended treatment for uncomplicated cases involves the use of one of several antimicrobial drugs. Although prevalent in other areas of the world, drug-resistant strains are not extensive in the United States.[43] This said, however, it should be noted that a clear increase in drug-resistant strains has been reported along the west coast, in various Pacific areas, such as Hawaii, other Pacific Islands, and Asia. Infected persons who might have contracted the disease while in these areas should report this information to their physicians.

Testing for gonorrhea is included as a part of prenatal care so that infections in mothers can be treated before they give birth. If the birth canal is infected, newborns can easily contract the infection in the mucous membranes of the eye.

Herpes Simplex

Public health officials think that the sexually transmitted genital herpes virus infection rivals chlamydia as the most prevalent STD. To date about forty-five million Americans have been diagnosed, although the asymptomatic (thus undiagnosed) population could increase this figure substantially. Herpes is really a family of more than fifty viruses, some of which produce recognized diseases in humans (chicken pox, **shingles,** mononucleosis, and others). One subgroup, called herpes simplex 1 virus (HSV-1), produces an infection called labial herpes (oral or lip herpes). Labial herpes produces common fever blisters or cold sores around the lips and oral cavity. Herpes simplex 2 virus (HSV-2) is a different strain that produces similar clumps of blisterlike lesions in the genital region (Figure 12-6). Laypeople call this second type of herpes the STD type, but both types produce identical clinical pictures. About 5 to 30% of cases are caused by HSV-1.[45] Oral-genital sexual practices most likely account for this crossover infection.

Herpes appears as a single sore or as a small cluster of blisterlike sores. These sores burn, itch, and (for some) become very painful. The infected person might also report swollen lymph glands, muscular aches and pains, and fever. Some patients feel weak and sleepy when they have blisters. The lesions may last from a few days to a few weeks. Viral shedding lasts a week on average; then the blisters begin

Key Terms

shingles painful fluid-filled skin eruptions along underlying sensory nerve pathways—due to reactivation of once-sequestered herpes zoster (chicken pox) viruses

Figure 12-6 A severe herpes infection.

scabbing, and new skin is formed. Even when the patient has become asymptomatic, viral transmission is still possible.

Herpes is an interesting virus for several reasons. It can lie dormant for long periods. For reasons not well understood but perhaps related to stress, diet, or overall health, the viral particles can be stimulated to travel along the nerve pathways to the skin and then create an active infection. Thus herpes can be considered a recurrent infection. Fortunately for most people, recurrent infections are less severe than the initial episode and do not last as long. Recommended treatment for an initial outbreak of herpes calls for the use of one of three medications: acyclovir, famciclovir, or valacyclovir. These medications are taken orally, multiple times each day, for seven to ten days. Because herpes may occur at intervals following initial treatment, two choices exist. One is to treat each recurrence as it arises (episodic recurrent treatment), and the second is to attempt to suppress recurrence through continuous use of medication (daily suppressive therapy). The treatment choices described above appear to be equally effective for HSV-1 and HSV-2.[44] Additionally, physicians may recommend other medications for relief of various symptoms. Genital herpes is almost always diagnosed through a clinical examination.

Currently, the best method of preventing herpes infection is to avoid all direct contact with a person who has an ac-

tive infection. Do not kiss someone with a fever blister—or let them kiss you (or your children) if they have an active lesion. Do not share drinking glasses or eating utensils. Check your partner's genitals. Do not have intimate sexual contact with someone who displays the blisterlike clusters or rash. (Condoms are only marginally helpful and cannot protect against lesions on the female vulva or the lower abdominal area of men.) Be careful not to infect yourself by touching a blister and then touching any other part of your body. The Changing for the Better box below gives helpful advice about talking with your partner if you have genital herpes.

Syphilis

Like gonorrhea, syphilis is caused by a bacterium (*Treponema pallidum*) and is transmitted almost exclusively by sexual intercourse. The incidence of syphilis, a CDC-

---

Changing for the Better

Talking with Your Partner about Herpes

My girlfriend told me she has herpes and said she's "taking care of everything." What can I do to get things out in the open?

Although herpes rarely has serious consequences, the lesions are infectious and tend to reappear. It is important to talk openly with your partner about this sexually transmitted disease. Here are some tips to make things easier:

- *Educate yourself.*
  Be aware that herpes is rarely dangerous. Learn when the disease is most contagious (during the eruption and blister stage), and realize that herpes can be spread even during the non-eruption, non-blister periods—traditionally defined as safe periods.
- *Choose the right time to talk.*
  Discuss herpes with your partner only after you have gotten to know each other.
- *Listen to your partner.*
  Be prepared to answer any questions that he or she may have.
- *Together, put things in perspective.*
  Keep a positive outlook.
  Remember that you are not alone.
  Be aware that using a condom and abstaining from coitus during the most infectious period can prevent transmission of the disease.
  Although there is no known cure, research continues on an antiviral drug.
  Join a local support group together.

InfoLinks

www.herpeszone.com/MainMenu.htm

Syphilis

Syphilis is a serious disease that, left untreated, can cause death. The chance of contracting syphilis during a single sexual encounter with an infected partner is now about 30%. Syphilis takes a well-established course after it is contracted.

Infection

The syphilis bacterium, *Treponema pallidum,* is a spirochete. It is transmitted from an infected person to a new host through intimate contact. Moist, warm tissue, such as that lining the reproductive, urinary, and digestive tracts, offers an ideal environment for the agent.

Incubation

Syphilis incubates without symptoms for 10 to 90 days, followed by the characteristic primary stage of the disease.

Primary Stage

The primary stage of syphilis lasts 1 to 5 weeks. A small, raised, painless sore called a *chancre* forms at this time. This highly infectious lesion is not easily identified in 90% of women and 50% of men; thus these people generally do not seek treatment. The chancre heals in 4 to 8 weeks.

Secondary Stage

The extremely contagious secondary stage of the disease occurs 6 to 12 weeks after initial infection. The infectious agents are now systemic, so symptoms may include a generalized body rash, a sore throat, or a patchy loss of hair. A blood test (VDRL) will be positive, and treatment can be effectively administered. If untreated, the second stage subsides within 2 to 6 weeks. A pregnant woman can easily transmit syphilis to her fetus during this stage. Congenital syphilis often results in stillbirth or an infant born with a variety of life-threatening complications. Early treatment of infected pregnant women can prevent congenital syphilis.

Latent Stage

After the secondary stage subsides, an extended period of noninfectiousness occurs. The infectious agents remain dormant within the body cells, and the infected person displays few clinical signs during this state.

Late Stage

Syphilis can recur for a third time 15 to 25 years after initial contact. In late-stage syphilis, tissue damage is profound and irreversible. The person suffers damage to the cardiovascular system, central nervous system, eyes, and skin, and death from the effects of the disease is likely.

Treatment

Depending on the stage, syphilis is treated with varying doses of Benzathine penicillin G.

---

reportable disease, is far lower than that of gonorrhea. In 1950 a record 217,558 cases of syphilis were reported in this country. The number of cases then fell steadily to fewer than 80,000 cases in 1980. From 1980 through 1990 the incidence climbed, reaching nearly 140,000 cases in 1990. Another decline then began, and in 1993 the number of cases dropped to 101,259. In 2000 the CDC reported that syphilis had fallen to the lowest level (5,972) in 42 years.

In spite of this downward trend, an increasing number of today's cases have been associated with HIV infections, largely among gay men in several larger cities. Syphilis cases among women continue to drop. See the Star box above for more information on this disease. Observers have noted an alarming increase in infant syphilis in children born to mothers who use drugs and support their habit through sexual activity.

Pubic Lice

Three types of lice infect humans: The head louse, the body louse, and the pubic louse all feed on the blood of the host. Except for the relatively uncommon body louse, these tiny insects do not carry diseases. They are, however, very annoying.

Pubic lice, also called crabs, attach themselves to the base of the pubic hairs, where they live and lay their eggs (nits). These eggs move into a larval stage after one week; after two more weeks, they develop into mature adult crab lice.

People usually notice they have a pubic lice infestation when they suffer intense itching in the genital region. Prescription and OTC creams, lotions, and shampoos are usually effective in killing both the lice and their eggs, although some reports suggest that lice are becoming resistant to OTC treatments.

Lice are not transmitted exclusively through sexual contact, but also by contact with bedsheets and clothes that may be contaminated. If you develop a pubic lice infestation, you must thoroughly treat yourself, your clothes, your sheets, and your furniture.

Vaginal Infections

Two common pathogens produce uncomfortable vaginal infections in women. The first is the yeast or fungus pathogen *Candida (Monilia) albicans,* which produces the yeast infection often called *thrush.* These organisms, commonly found in the vagina, seem to multiply rapidly when some unusual stressor (pregnancy, use of birth control pills or antibiotics, diabetes) affects a woman's body. This infection, now called vulvovaginal candidiasis (VVC),[44] is signaled by a white or cream-colored vaginal discharge that resembles cottage cheese. Vaginal itching and vulvar swelling are also commonly reported. Current treatment is based on the use of one of several prescription and OTC azole drugs.

Recently introduced nonprescription azole-based products offer effective home treatment. One should first consult with a physician before using these new products for the first time. (Men rarely report this monilial infection, although some may report mildly painful urination or a barely noticeable discharge at the urethral opening or beneath the foreskin of the penis.)

The protozoan Trichomonas vaginalis also produces a vaginal infection. This parasite can be transmitted through sexual intercourse or by contact with contaminated (often damp) objects, such as towels, clothing, or toilet seats, that may contain some vaginal discharge. In women, this infection, called *trichomoniasis,* or "trich," produces a foamy, yellow-green, foul-smelling discharge that may be accompanied by itching, swelling, and painful urination. Although topically applied treatments with limited effectiveness for trichomoniasis are available, only one highly effective oral medication is currently on the market.[44] Men infrequently contract trichomoniasis but may harbor the organisms without realizing it. They also should be treated to minimize reinfection of partners.[44]

The vagina is warm, dark, and moist, an ideal breeding environment for a variety of organisms. Unfortunately, some highly promoted commercial products seem to increase the incidence of vaginal infections. Among these are tight panty hose (without cotton panels), which tend to increase the vaginal temperature, and commercial vaginal douches, which can alter the acidic level of the vagina. Both of these products might promote infections.

Women are advised to wipe from front to back after every bowel movement to reduce the opportunity for direct transmission of pathogenic agents from the rectum to the vagina. Avoiding public bathrooms when possible is also a good practice. Of course, if you notice any unusual discharge from the vagina, you should report this to your physician.

Cystitis and Urethritis

Cystitis, an infection of the urinary bladder, and urethritis, an infection of the urethra, occasionally can be caused by a sexually transmitted organism. Such infections can also be caused by the organisms that cause vaginitis and organisms found in the intestinal tract. A culture is required to identify the specific pathogen associated with a particular case of cystitis or urethritis. The symptoms are pain when urinating, the need to urinate frequently, a dull aching pain above the pubic bone, and the passing of blood-streaked urine.

Physicians can easily treat cystitis and urethritis with antibiotics when the specific organism has been identified. A newly introduced drug, Monurol, which requires only a single dose, has proved effective. Few complications result from infections that are treated promptly. If cystitis or urethritis is left untreated, the infectious agent could move upward in the urinary system and infect the ureters and kidneys. These upper-urinary-tract infections are more serious and require more extensive evaluation and aggressive treatment. Therefore one should obtain medical care immediately upon noticing symptoms.

A recent study involving urinary tract infections in mice, whose urinary tract infections are virtually identical to those in humans, demonstrated that the bacteria involved often avoid complete antibiotic elimination. This occurs when the bacteria clump into pods that are then covered by a "bio-film" produced by the organisms.[47] The film retards further antibody effectiveness, allowing the infection to be re-established when antibiotics have been cleared from the body.

Preventing cystitis and urethritis depends to some degree on the source of the infectious agent. One can generally reduce the incidence of infection by urinating completely (to fully empty the urinary bladder) and by drinking ample fluids to flush the urinary tract. Drinking cranberry juice has been found to reduce urinary tract infections.

TALKING POINTS Honesty regarding past sexual experiences is a critical issue in a decision to introduce sexual intimacy into a new relationship. What questions would you feel comfortable being asked by another person, and what questions would you be prepared to ask that person?

Taking Charge of Your Health

- Since microorganisms develop resistance to antibiotics, continue taking all such medications until gone, even when the symptoms of the infection have subsided.
- Check your current immunization status to make sure you are protected against preventable infectious diseases.
- If you are a parent, take your children to receive their recommended immunizations as necessary.

- Because of the possibility of contracting HIV/AIDS and sexually transmitted diseases, incorporate disease prevention into all your sexual activities.
- Use the Personal Assessment on page 361 to determine your risk of contracting a sexually transmitted disease.
- If you have ever engaged in high-risk sexual behavior, get tested for HIV.

Summary

- We have made progress in reducing the incidence of some forms of infectious disease, but other infectious conditions are becoming more common.
- A variety of pathogenic agents are responsible for infectious conditions.
- A chain of infection with six potential links characterizes every infectious condition.
- Most infectious conditions progress through five distinct stages.
- One can acquire immunity for some diseases through both natural and artificial means. Children should be immunized according to a schedule.
- The immune system's response to infection relies on cellular and humoral elements.
- The common cold and influenza produce many similar symptoms but differ in their infectious agents, incubation period, prevention, and treatment.
- Tuberculosis and pneumonia are potentially fatal infections of the respiratory system.
- Mononucleosis and chronic fatigue syndrome are infections that produce chronic tiredness.
- Bacterial meningitis, a potentially fatal infection of the linings that cover the brain, is of increasing concern on college campuses.
- Lyme disease is a bacterial infection contracted through outdoor activities.
- Hantavirus pulmonary syndrome is caused by a virus carried by deer mice; human-to-human transmission has also been reported.

- Newly arrived in this country, the West Nile virus is a vector-borne infection that is now widely distributed in the United States.
- Toxic shock syndrome is a bacterial infection generally arising from the improper use of tampons.
- Hepatitis B (serum hepatitis) is a bloodborne infectious condition that produces serious liver damage. Other varieties are hepatitis A, C, D, and E.
- SARS is a potentially fatal respiratory infection that reached North America from Asia.
- HIV/AIDS is a widespread, incurable viral disease transmitted through sexual activity, through intravenous drug use, in infected blood products, or across the placenta during pregnancy.
- The definitive diagnosis of AIDS can be based on the presence of specific conditions or a reduced number of helper T cells.
- HIV and AIDS are currently best treated with a drug cocktail, using protease inhibitors and reverse-transcriptase inhibitors in addition to three new categories of antiviral medications; an effective vaccine for prevention has not been developed. Concerns are rising regarding the unchecked spread of HIV/AIDS in areas of Africa and Asia.
- There are a variety of sexually transmitted conditions, many of which do not produce symptoms in most infected women and many infected men.
- Safer sex practices can reduce the risk of contracting STDs.

Review Questions

1. What are the agents responsible for the most familiar infectious conditions?
2. Describe the six links in the chain of infection.
3. What are the five stages that characterize the progression of infectious conditions?

4. What are the two principal cellular-chemical components of the immune system, and how do they cooperate to protect the body from infectious agents, foreign protein, and abnormal cells?

5. How are the common cold and influenza similar? How do they differ in their causative agents, incubation period, prevention, and treatment?

6. What symptoms make mononucleosis and chronic fatigue syndrome similar? What aspects of each are different?

7. Why is bacterial meningitis of greater concern on the college campus than elsewhere?

8. Why is outdoor activity a risk factor for contracting Lyme disease?

9. During what type of activities would persons most likely expose themselves to a hantavirus infection? What is the reservoir for the hantavirus?

10. What role do birds play in the transmission of the West Nile virus? What insect is the vector?

11. What group of persons seems most susceptible to the development of toxic shock syndrome? In what way is the infection most directly linked to the menstrual cycle?

12. How is hepatitis B transmitted, and which occupational group is at greatest risk of contracting this infection? How do forms A, C, D, and E compare with hepatitis B?

13. What is SARS? Where was the site of origin and how did it most likely reach North America?

14. How is HIV transmitted? How are HIV/AIDS currently treated, and how effective is the treatment? In what areas of the world does the HIV/AIDS epidemic seem virtually unchecked? In terms of STD prevention, how can sexual practices be made safer?

15. What specific infectious diseases could be classified as STDs?

16. Why are women more often asymptomatic for STDs than men?

17. To what extent and in what manner can STD transmission be prevented?

References

1. Hamann B. *Disease identification, prevention, and control,* 2nd ed. McGraw-Hill, 2001.

2. Salidin KS. *Anatomy and physiology: unity of form and function,* 2nd ed. McGraw-Hill, 2001.

3. Parkham P. *The immune system.* Garland Publishing, 2000.

4. Vander A, Sherman J, and Luciano D. *Human physiology: the mechanisms of body function.* McGraw-Hill, 2004.

5. Korbling M, Estrov Z, Champlin R. Adult stem cells and tissue repair. *Bone Marrow Transplant* 32 Suppl 1:S23–24, 2003.

6. Burt RK, Traynor AE. SLE—hematopoietic stem cell transplantation for systemic lupus erythematosus. *Arthritis Res Ther* 5(5):207–209, 2003.

7. Ooi J, et al. Unrelated cord blood transplantation for adult patients with de novo acute myeloid leukemia. *Blood* August 21, 2003 (Epub).

8. Latkovic MS. The morality of human embryonic stem cell research and President Bush's decision: how should Catholics think about such things? *Linacre Q* 69(4):289–315, 2002.

9. Gershon D. Complex political, ethical and legal issues surround research on human embryonic stem cells. *Nature* 422(6934):928–929, 2003.

10. Straetemans M, et al. Review of randomized controlled trials on pneumococcal vaccination for prevention of otitis media. *Pediatr Infect Dis J* 22(6):515–524, 2003.

11. DeStefano F, et al. Childhood vaccinations, vaccination timing, and risk of type 1 diabetes mellitus. *Pediatrics* 108(6):E112, 2001.

12. DeStefano F, et al. Childhood vaccinations and risk of asthma. *Pediatr Infect Dis J* 21(6):498–504, 2002.

13. DeStefano F, Thompson WW. MMR vaccination and autism: is there a link? *Expert Opin Drug Saf* 1(2);115–120, 2002.

14. Immunization safety review: vaccinations and sudden unexpected death in infancy. *News.* The National Academies, 2003 http://www.nap.edu

15. McQuillan GM, et al. Serologic immunity to diphtheria and tetanus in the United States. *Ann Intern Med* 136(9):660–666, 2002.

16. Prevention and control of influenza, recommendations of the Advisory Committee on Immunization Practices (ACIP). *MMWR* 52, RR-08, 2003.

17. Division of Tuberculosis Elimination—2001 Surveillance Report. National Center for HIV, SID, and TB Prevention. CDC, 2003. http://www.cdc.gov/nchstp.tb/surv/surv2001/content/T1.htm

18. Geng E, et al. Changes in the transmission of tuberculosis in New York City from 1900 to 1999. *N Engl J Med* 346(19):1453–1458, 2002.

19. Ewer K, et al. Comparison of T-cell based assay with tuberculin skin test for diagnosis of mycobacterium tuberculosis infection in a school tuberculosis outbreak. *Lancet* 361(9364):1168–1173, 2003.

20. Oosterheert JJ, et al. Severe community-acquired pneumonia: what's in a name? *Curr Opin Infect Dis* 16(2):153–159, 2003.

21. Sisk JE, et al. Cost-effectiveness of vaccination against invasive pneumococcal disease among people 50 through 64 years of age: role of comorbid

conditions and race. *Ann Intern Med* 1389(12):960–968, 2003.

22. Godshall SE, Kirchner JT. Infectious mononucleosis: Complexities of a common syndrome. *Postgrad Med* 107(7):183–184, 2000.

23. National Institute of Allergy and Infectious Disease (NIAID). *Chronic fatigue syndrome-etiological theories.* NIAID, 2000. **http://www.niaid.nih.gov/publications/cfs/etie.htm**

24. *Fibromyalgia basics: symptoms, treatments and research,* 1999, **www.fmnetnews.com/pages/basic.html**

25. *Diagnostic criteria for fibromyalgia and CFS,* 1999, **www.fmnetnews.com/pages/criteria.html**

26. Bruce MG, et al. Risk factors for meningococcal disease in college students. *JAMA* 286(6):688–693, 2001.

27. *Meningococcaly disease.* Division of Bacterial and Mycotic Diseases. Centers for Communicable Disease and Prevention, 2003

28. Nowakowski J, et al. Long-term follow-up with culture-confirmed Lyme disease. *Am J Med* 115(2):91–96, 2003.

29. Allan BF, Keesing F, Ostfeld RS. Effect of forest fragmentation on Lyme disease risk. *Conservation Biology* 17(1):267–272, 2003.

30. Armstrong GL, Bell BP. Hepatitis A virus infections in the United States: model-based estimates and implications for childhood immunizations. *Pediatrics* 109(5):839–845, 2002.

31. Dudclos P. Safety of immuni(s)ation and adverse events following vaccination against hepatitis B. *Expert Opin Drug Saf* 2(3):225–231, 2003.

32. Thomas DL, et al. The natural history of hepatitis C virus infection: host, viral, and environmental factors. *JAMA* 284(4):450–456, 2000.

33. *WHO: SARS outbreak "over the peak" around the world, including China.* Intelihealth: *Health News* (The Associated Press), June 5, 2003.

34. Summary table of SARS cases by country, 1 November 2002–7 August 2003. World Health Organization. August 15, 2003. **http://www.who.int/entity/crs/sars/country/en/country2003_08_15.pdf**

35. *HIV/AIDS Surveillance Report, Centers for Disease,* Centers for Disease Control and Prevention. 13(2):1–47(inclusive), 2001.

36. Ogundele MO, Coulter JB. HIV transmission through breastfeeding: Problems and prevention. *AnnTrop Paediatr* 23(2):91–106, 2003.

37. Edwards S, Crane C. Oral sex and the transmission of viral STIs. *JAMA* 74(1):6–10, 1998.

38. Cox FD. *The aids booklet,* 6th ed. McGraw-Hill, 2000.

39. Hirsch MS, et al. Antiretroviral drug resistance testing in adult HIV-1 infection: recommendations of an International AIDS society—USA Panel. *JAMA* 283(18):2417–2426, 2000.

40. Gulick RM (Presentor). *Current status of new antiretroviral drugs in development.* Topics in HIV Medicine. International AIDS Society-USA. Washington, DC, May 2002.

41. Hui D. HIV protease inhibitors and atherosclerosis. *J Clin Invest* 111(3):317–318, 2003.

42. HIV gp120 vaccine—VaxGen: AIDSVAX, AIDSVAX B/B, AIDSVAX B/E, HIV gp120 vaccine—Genentech, HIV gp120 vaccine AIDSVAX—VaxGen, HIV vaccine AIDSVAX-VaxGen. *Drug R.D.* 4(4):249–243, 2003.

43. Global estimates of the HIV/AIDS epidemic, as of end 2002. December 2002. **http://www.avert.org/worldstats.htm**

44. Centers for Disease Control and Prevention. Sexually transmitted diseases treatment guidelines 2002. *MMWR* 51:(No. RR-6) [inclusive page numbers], 2002.

45. STD Surveillance 2001. National Center for HIV, STD, and TB Prevention. Centers for Disease Control and Prevention, 2001. **http://www.cdc.gov/std/stats/TOC2001.htm**

46. Alcohol policy and sexually transmitted disease rates—United States 1981–1995. *MMWR* 49(16):346–349, 2000.

47. Anderson GG, et al. Intracellular bacterial biofilm-like pods in urinary tract infections. *Science* 301(5629): 105–107, 2003.

As We Go to Press

Today Nigeria, a country in which polio was eradicated, has recently experienced cases of polio; with additional infections currently reported in neighboring countries that were, until recently, polio free.

The western Africa reemergence of polio can be traced to a northern area of Nigeria in which local Islamic clergy began circulating the idea that the polio immunization program sponsored by the national government was using contaminated vaccines for the purpose of creating infertility in women. Growing resistance to the program ensued, and by August 2003, the program was terminated in the region's capital, Abuja. Intervention by the national government, the World Health Organization, and world Islamic leaders, has, to this date, proven ineffective in rebuilding trust in the polio immunization program.

Within a few months of the discontinuation of the Nigerian program, new cases of polio infection were reported from neighboring countries of the Ivory Coast, Ghana, Burkina Faso, Chad, Cameroon, and the Central African Republic. In response, a variety of world organizations, including Rotary International, UNICEF, and the CDC announced plans to assist these countries in becoming polio-free again.

Prior to the spread of the infection to the countries named above, only India, Pakistan, Afghanistan, Egypt, Niger, and Nigeria were reporting new cases of polio.

the changing picture of infectious disease

Just a generation ago, many scientists believed we were wiping out infectious disease. Armed with improved sanitation, better hygiene practices, antibiotics, and pesticides, humankind had malaria, cholera, and tuberculosis (TB) on the run and smallpox and polio well on the way to extinction. In fact, infectious diseases were in decline until 1980, but as we enter the next century, the tide is turning. Ebola, HIV, Marburg virus, Lassa fever, Legionnaires' disease, hantavirus, and hepatitis C are but a few of the more than thirty new pathogens researchers have identified in the last few decades.

Previously unknown microbes have been evolving for thousands of years in animals and insects. They become threatening to humans only when conditions are right for transmission of the diseases from animals, including insects, to us, through a process called zoonosis.

Recent Global Epidemics

The Ebola virus struck in the African countries of Zaire and Sudan in 1976, and again in Sudan in 1979. In 1995 Ebola revisited Zaire, but in Gabon in 1996 it was recognized and stopped before it could take hold. In October 2000, Ebola reappeared in Uganda after not being reported in Africa for several years. The source of Ebola in nature is unclear. Monkeys do become infected but die quickly, as do humans. To be an effective reservoir or source of disease, an animal must be able to tolerate the disease organism and therefore remain active and alive for a longer time in which the virus can be spread. For example, monkeys may be the source of human immunodeficiency virus (HIV) because they harbor a similar virus, simian immunodeficiency virus

(SIV), but don't become sick. Of course, HIV/AIDS is a dangerous virus, but Ebola is more infective and runs a shorter disease course. As one author put it, "Ebola does in ten days what it takes AIDS ten years to accomplish."[1] This is terrible for the nine out of ten people infected with Ebola who die in a matter of days, but ironically by making its victims so sick so quickly, Ebola limits its own spread. Being deathly ill limits the social interactions of carriers.

Many other diseases also pose threats.[2] After a heat wave in 1988, mosquitos carrying dengue (pronounced "ding-ee") spread through Mexico. In 1991 an epidemic of cholera in South America killed 5,000 of the 500,000 people infected. A record year for infectious disease occurred in 1993, possibly set into effect by weather patterns associated with El Niño, which warmed the waters in the tropical Pacific. A year later, epidemic bubonic plague swept through India. In the summer of 1996, a dengue outbreak began in Latin America. By the time it ended, 140,000 people from Argentina to Texas had been infected, and 4,000 of those infected had died.[1]

Occurrence of New Infectious Diseases in the United States and Elsewhere

As the 1996 dengue outbreak illustrates, infectious disease is not just a problem for developing countries. In 1989 an airborne strain of Ebola, which fortunately was not dangerous to humans, was brought to Virginia in Philippine crab-eating monkeys that were to be distributed to research labs across the United States.

Hantavirus became an American problem in 1993. Following an extremely rainy year that was good for vegetation,

the rodent population exploded in the Four Corners area of New Mexico, Arizona, Colorado, and Utah. The rodent population spread hantavirus to sixteen states. This virus killed half of the ninety-four people it infected.[3] More recently, the first case of hantavirus transmission between humans occurred in Argentina. Apparently eighteen people, including five physicians, contracted the disease after having contact with sick patients.

The 1994 earthquake in Southern California provided more evidence to support the theory that new infectious diseases can spread to humans during environmental disturbances. The earthquake exposed a soil fungus that infected 200 people and killed 3.

Today zoonosis-related infections seem even more common as the American public becomes increasingly familiar with conditions such as Lyme disease, West Nile virus infections, SARS (sudden acute respiratory syndrome), and Monkey Pox. Even more recently, potential zoonotic infectious agents have been identified, such as bacterial pathogens in fish raised through aquaculture (rainbow trout in Italy),[4] avian (bird) influenza in China,[5] and flying squirrel-associated typhus in this country.[6] Of course, the relationship of these latter infections to the greater American public remains to be seen.

Leading the Fight for Public Health

The United States leads the international health community with its premier monitoring and response services provided by the Centers for Disease Control and Prevention (CDC).[7] Of course, international cooperation is vital, but we have seen why disease vigilance is in our own interest as well. To move from the reactive system now in place to a predictive one, some specific goals must be met.

A global network of epidemiological field stations should be established to detect and characterize outbreaks early, both here and abroad. Insect carriers of disease need to be managed in a variety of ways, including but not solely relying on pesticides. Further, insecticides and pesticides must be developed that are both effective and environmentally safe. Safe food and water must be made available to everyone, and new antibiotics and vaccines need to be developed. These goals are hard to achieve, particularly in the face of episodes of armed conflict within and between countries, growing religious intolerance that becomes transformed into national disputes, and a global economy that continues to separate the affluent developed countries from those far less developed and affluent.

Having entered a new millennium, Americans may encounter the threat of emerging diseases associated with biological weapons and regional armed conflict. This threat looms even larger when one realizes that some countries view these disease organisms as agents of war and are capable of using them as such. With about a dozen countries in possession or pursuit of biological weapons arsenals, the understanding of deadly pathogens becomes a matter of national security as well as global health. Interestingly in this regard, the principal reason that the United States military personnel gave in 2000 for not reenlisting in the armed forces was their fear of receiving the required Anthrax vaccine developed for use by American forces in order to protect personnel from Anthrax-based biological warfare.

For Discussion . . .

In your view, what is the most important step we can take to fight infectious disease? Do you think the United States does more than its share in monitoring these diseases? What kinds of precautions might prevent zoonosis infections from taking hold in this country? Do you know anyone who works in the public health field? If so, what does he or she do?

1. Monastersky R. Health in the hot zone. *Science News* 1996; 149(14):218–219.
2. Gubler DJ. Resurgent vector-borne diseases as a global health problem. *Emerg Infect Dis* 1998; 4(3):442–450.
3. Anon. Climate creates a hot zone. *Environment* 1996; 37(10):27.
4. Ghittino C, et al. Emerging pathologies in aquaculture: effects on production and food safety. *Vet Res Common.* 2003 Sep; 27 Suppl 1:471–479.
5. Sims LD, et al. Avian influenza in Hong Kong 1997–2002. *Avian Dis.* 2003; 47(3 Suppl):832–838.
6. Reynolds MG, et al. Flying squirrel-associated typhus, United States. *Emerg Infect Dis.* 2003 Oct; 9(10):1341–1343.
7. Preventing emerging infectious diseases: a strategy for the 21st century: overview of the updated plan. *MMWR* (suppl) 1998; 47(15):1–14.

InfoLinks

www.who.Int

www.cdc.gov/ncidod

personal assessment

what is your risk of contracting a sexually transmitted disease?

A variety of factors interact to determine your risk of contracting a sexually transmitted disease (STD). This inventory is intended to provide you with an estimate of your level of risk.

Circle the number of each row that best characterizes you. Enter that number on the line at the end of the row (points). After assigning yourself a number in each row, total the number appearing in the points column. Your total points will allow you to interpret your risk for contracting an STD.

Age

1	3	4	5	3	2	Points
0–9	10–14	15–19	20–29	30–34	35+	_____

Sexual Practices

0	1	2	4	6	8	
Never engage in sex	One sex partner	More than one sex partner but never more than one at a time	Two to five sex partners	Five to ten sex partners	Ten or more sex partners	_____

Sexual Attitudes

0	1	8	1	7	8	
Will not engage in nonmarital sex	Premarital sex is okay if it is with future spouse	Any kind of premarital sex is okay	Extramarital sex is not for me	Extramarital sex is okay	Believe in complete sexual freedom	_____

Attitudes toward Contraception

1	1	6	5	4	8	
Would use condom to prevent pregnancy	Would use condom to prevent STDs	Would never use a condom	Would use the birth control pill	Would use other contraceptive measure	Would not use anything	_____

Attitudes toward STD

3	3	4	6	6	6	
Am not sexually active so I do not worry	Would be able to talk about STD with my partner	Would check out an infection to be sure	Would be afraid to check out an infection	Can't even talk about an infection	STDs are no problem— easily cured	_____

YOUR TOTAL POINTS _____

Interpretation

5–8	Your risk is well below average
9–13	Your risk is below average
14–17	Your risk is at or near average
18–21	Your risk is moderately high
22+	Your risk is high

To Carry This Further . . .

Having taken this Personal Assessment, were you surprised at your level of risk? What is the primary reason for this level? How concerned are you and your classmates and friends about contracting an STD?

chapter thirteen

understanding sexuality

Chapter Objectives

After reading this chapter, you will be able to:

▌explain the genetic basis and gonadal basis of sexuality.

▌describe the psychosocial basis of sexuality, including gender identity, gender preference, gender adoption, and initial adult gender identification.

▌define androgyny and discuss its role in our society.

▌explain the components of the male and female reproductive systems.

▌trace the menstrual cycle and identify the hormones that control the cycle.

▌identify the four stages of the human sexual response pattern.

▌discuss the refractory period and how it affects male sexual performance.

▌discuss the impact of aging on both male and female sexual performance.

▌define the three categories of sexual orientation.

▌identify and discuss a few of the various lifestyles and relationships presented in this chapter.

Online Learning Center Resources

www.mhhe.com/hahn7e

Log on to our Online Learning Center (OLC) for access to these additional resources:

- Chapter key terms and definitions
- Learning objectives
- Student interactive question-and-answer sites
- Self-scoring chapter quiz
- Online assessments
- Key term flash cards

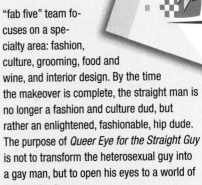

Talking It Over

"I Need Answers about Sex . . ."

OK, admit it. You don't know everything about sex. Why should you? If you're like most college students, your parents probably had a difficult time telling you about the "birds and the bees." Sure, they tried to tell you about what makes a baby, but they probably shied away from talking about topics like sexual expression, oral sex, sexual performance, homosexuality, and masturbation. It's no wonder that you still have questions about sex. Fortunately, you can get many answers online.

CommunicationLinks

www.intelihealth.com
www.goaskalice.columbia.edu
www.webmd.com

Eye on the Media

Mainstream TV Shows with Gay Themes

"The times they are a-changing" is an apt reflection of some new cable TV shows. For the summer/fall 2003 schedule, gay men are coming out in abundance. Although the sit-com *Will and Grace* has been around for a number of years (and successfully opened mainstream eyes to some aspects of gay life), in 2003 the Bravo network launched two new reality shows that featured very different approaches.

In *Queer Eye for the Straight Guy,* five gay men are on a mission to transform a "style-deficient and culture-deprived straight man from drab to fab," according to the Bravo website.[1] These men extol the virtues of a life of style, taste, and class. Each member of the "fab five" team focuses on a specialty area: fashion, culture, grooming, food and wine, and interior design. By the time the makeover is complete, the straight man is no longer a fashion and culture dud, but rather an enlightened, fashionable, hip dude. The purpose of *Queer Eye for the Straight Guy* is not to transform the heterosexual guy into a gay man, but to open his eyes to a world of style and culture.

The *Queer Eye for the Straight Guy* series was created by David Collins, a gay man, and developed by David Metzler, a straight man. Apparently this blend has given the show a fresh, creative, humorous appeal. In its fourth airing on Bravo, the July 29, 2003 show earned the cable network its highest-ever rating. By mid-August, the team had done a makeover for Jay Leno, the *Tonight Show* band, and the show's set, and *Queer Eye for the Straight Guy* seemed poised to make a real run at mainstream television.

The Bravo network also produced television's first gay dating series, *Boy Meets Boy* in 2003.[2] In this reality series, the leading man is presented with fifteen potential mates who will try to win his affection. Group dates and individual one-to-one dates give the leading man and his suitors the chance to get to know each other. At the end of each episode, some of the suitors are gradually eliminated by the leading man in a premise similar to that of heterosexual dating shows like *The Bachelor.*

The biggest surprise in *Boy Meets Boy* is that some of the men are straight men posing as gay men. While this juxtaposition is taking place, viewers get to decide for themselves who is the most deserving suitor. The show, like *Queer Eye* has the potential to challenge the viewers' preconceived notions of what it's like to be gay.

[1]Bravo TV: About the Show: "Queer Eye for the Straight Guy," **www.bravotv.com/Queer_Eye_for_the_Straight_Guy/,** accessed August 27, 2003.

[2]Bravo TV: About the Show: "Boy Meets Boy," **www.bravotv.com/Boy_Meets_Boy/,** accessed August 27, 2003.

Currently, we have reached an understanding of both the biological and psychosocial factors that contribute to the complex expression of our **sexuality.** As a society, we are now inclined to view human behavior in terms of a complex script written on the basis of both biology and conditioning. Reflecting this understanding is how we use the words "male" or "female" to refer to the biological roots of our sexuality and the words "man" or "woman" to refer to the psychosocial roots of our sexuality. This chapter explores human sexuality as it relates to the dynamic interplay of the biological and psychosocial bases that form your **masculinity** or **femininity.**

Biological Bases of Human Sexuality

Within a few seconds after the birth of a baby, someone—a doctor, nurse, or parent—emphatically labels the child: "It's a boy," or "It's a girl." For the parents and society as a whole, the child's **biological sexuality** is being displayed and identified. Another female or male enters the world.

Genetic Basis

At the moment of conception, a Y-bearing or an X-bearing sperm cell joins with the X-bearing ovum to establish the true basis of biological sexuality.[1] A fertilized ovum with sex chromosomes XX is biologically female, and a fertilized ovum bearing the XY sex chromosomes is biologically male. Genetics forms the most basic level of an individual's biological sexuality.

Gonadal Basis

The gonadal basis for biological sexuality refers to the growing embryo's development of **gonads.**[2] Male em-

bryos develop testes about the seventh week after conception, and female embryos develop ovaries about the twelfth week after conception.

Structural Development

The development of male or female reproductive structures is initially determined by the presence or absence of hormones produced by the developing testes—androgens and the müllerian inhibiting substance (MIS). With these hormones present, the male embryo starts to develop male reproductive structures (penis, scrotum, vas deferens, seminal vesicles, prostate gland, and Cowper's glands).

Because the female embryo is not exposed to these male hormones, it develops the characteristic female reproductive structures: the uterus, fallopian tubes, vagina, labia, and clitoris.

Biological Sexuality and the Childhood Years

The growth and development of the child in terms of reproductive organs and physiological processes have traditionally been thought to be "latent" during the childhood years. However, a gradual degree of growth

> **Key Terms**
>
> **sexuality** the quality of being sexual; can be viewed from many biological and psychosocial perspectives.
>
> **masculinity** behavioral expressions traditionally observed in males.
>
> **femininity** behavioral expressions traditionally observed in females.
>
> **biological sexuality** male and female aspects of sexuality.
>
> **gonads** male or female sex glands; testes produce sperm and ovaries produce eggs.

occurs in both girls and boys. The reproductive organs, however, will undergo more greatly accelerated growth at the onset of **puberty** and will achieve their adult size and capabilities shortly.

Puberty

The entry into puberty is a gradual maturing process for young girls and boys. For young girls, the onset of menstruation, called **menarche,** usually occurs at about age 12 or 13 but may come somewhat earlier or later.[3] Early menstrual cycles tend to be **anovulatory.** Menarche is usually preceded by a growth spurt that includes the budding of breasts and the growth of pubic and underarm hair.[4]

Young males follow a similar pattern of maturation, including a growth spurt followed by a gradual sexual maturity. However, this process takes place about 2 years later than in young females. Genital enlargement, underarm and pubic hair growth, and a lowering of the voice commonly occur. The male's first ejaculation is generally experienced by the age of 14, most commonly through **nocturnal emission** or masturbation. For many young boys, fully mature sperm do not develop until about age 15.

Reproductive capability only gradually declines over the course of the adult years. In the woman, however, the onset of **menopause** signals a more definite turning off of the reproductive system than is the case for the male adult. By the early to mid-fifties, virtually all women have entered a postmenopausal period, but for men, relatively high-level **spermatogenesis** may continue for a decade or two.[4]

The story of sexual maturation and reproductive maturity cannot, however, be solely focused on the changes that take place in the body. The psychosocial processes that accompany the biological changes are also important.

Psychosocial Bases of Human Sexuality

If growth and development of our sexuality were to be visualized as a stepladder (Figure 13-1), one vertical rail of the ladder would represent our biological sexuality. The rungs would represent the sequential unfolding of the genetic, gonadal, and structural components.

Because humans, more than any other life form, can rise above a life centered on reproduction, a second dimension (or rail) to our sexuality exists—our **psychosocial sexuality.** The reason we possess the ability to be more than reproductive beings is a question for the theologian or philosopher. We are considerably more complex than the functions determined by biology. The process that transforms a male into a man and a female into a woman begins at birth and continues to influence us through the course of our lives.

Figure 13-1 Our sexuality develops through biological and psychosocial stages.

Gender Identity

Although expectant parents may prefer to have a child of one **gender** over the other, they know that this matter is determined when the child is conceived. External genitals "cast the die," and femininity or masculinity is traditionally

Key Terms

puberty achievement of reproductive ability.

menarche (muh **nar** key) time of a female's first menstrual cycle.

anovulatory (an **oh** vyu luh tory) not ovulating.

nocturnal emission ejaculation that occurs during sleep; "wet dream."

menopause decline and eventual cessation of hormone production by the female reproductive system.

spermatogenesis (sper mat oh **jen** uh sis) process of sperm production.

psychosocial sexuality masculine and feminine aspects of sexuality.

gender general term reflecting a biological basis of sexuality; the male gender or the female gender.

reinforced by the parents and society in general. By age 18 months, typical children have both the language and the insight to correctly identify their gender. They have established a **gender identity.**[5] The first rung rising from the psychosocial rail of the ladder has been climbed.

Gender Preference

During the preschool years, children receive the second component of the *scripting* required for the full development of psychosocial sexuality—the preference for the gender to which they have been assigned. The process through which **gender preference** is transmitted to the child is a less subtle form of the practices observed during the gender identity period (the first 18 months). Many parents begin to control the child's exposure to experiences traditionally reserved for children of the opposite gender. This is particularly true for boys; parents will often stop play activities they perceive as being too feminine.

Gender Adoption

The process of reaching an initial adult gender identification requires a considerable period of time. The specific knowledge, attitudes, and behavior characteristic of adults must be observed, analyzed, and practiced. The process of acquiring and personalizing these "insights" about how men and women think, feel, and act is reflected by the term **gender adoption,** the first and third rungs below the initial adult gender identification rail of the ladder in Figure 13-1.

In addition to developing a personalized version of an adult sexual identity, it is important that the child—and particularly the adolescent—construct a *gender schema* for a member of the opposite gender. Clearly, the world of adulthood, involving intimacy, parenting, and employment, will require that men know women and women know men. Gender adoption provides an opportunity to begin to assemble this equally valuable "picture" of what the other gender is like.

Initial Adult Gender Identification

By the time young people have climbed all of the rungs of the sexuality ladder, they have arrived at the chronological point in the life cycle when they need to construct an initial adult **gender identification.** You might notice that this label seems remarkably similar to the terminology used to describe one of the developmental tasks being used in this textbook. In fact, the task of forming an initial adult identity is closely related to developing an initial adult image of oneself as a man or a woman. Although most of us currently support the concept of

"person" in many gender-neutral contexts (for some very valid reasons), we still must identify ourselves as either a man or a woman.

Transsexualism

Students are often intrigued by a gender identity variance that is first noticed during one or two of the psychosocial stages just discussed. Transsexualism is a variance of the most profound nature because it represents a complete rejection by an individual of his or her biological sexuality. The male transsexual believes that he is female and thus desires to be the woman that he knows he is. The female transsexual believes that she is male and wants to become the man that she knows she should be. Psychiatrists, sex therapists, and transexuals do not view transsexualism as a homosexual orientation.

For transsexuals, the periods of gender preference and gender adoption are perplexing as they attempt, with limited success, to resolve the conflict between what their mind tells them is true and what their body displays. Adolescent and young adult transsexuals often cross-dress, undertake homosexual relationships (which they view as being heterosexual relationships), experiment with hormone replacement therapy, and sometimes actively pursue a **sex reassignment operation.** Thousands of these operations have been performed at some of the leading medical centers in the United States.

Androgyny: Sharing the Pluses

Over the last 25 years our society has increasingly accepted an image of a person who possesses both masculine and feminine qualities. This accepted image has taken years to develop because our society traditionally

---

Key Terms

gender identity recognition of one's gender.

gender preference emotional and intellectual acceptance of one's own gender.

gender adoption lengthy process of learning the behavior that is traditional for one's gender.

gender identification achievement of a personally satisfying interpretation of one's masculinity or femininity.

sex reassignment operation surgical procedure designed to remove the external genitalia and replace them with genitalia appropriate to the opposite gender.

Just as women have broken into traditionally male careers, many men have taken on jobs and tasks that were once considered women's exclusive domain.

has reinforced rigid masculine roles for men and rigid feminine roles for women.

In the past, from the time a child was born, we assigned and reinforced only those roles and traits that were thought to be directly related to his or her biological gender. Boys were not allowed to cry, play with dolls, or help in the kitchen. Girls were not encouraged to become involved in sports; they were told to learn to sew, cook, and baby-sit. Men were encouraged to be strong, expressive, dominant, aggressive, and career oriented, and women were encouraged to be weak, shy, submissive, passive, and home oriented.

These traditional biases have resulted in some interesting phenomena related to career opportunities. Women were denied jobs requiring above-average physical strength, admittance into professional schools requiring high intellectual capacities, such as law, medicine, and business, and entry into most levels of military participation. Likewise, men were not encouraged to enter traditionally feminine careers, such as nursing, clerical work, and elementary school teaching.

For a variety of reasons, the traditional picture has changed. **Androgyny,** or the blending of both feminine and masculine qualities, is more clearly evident in our society now than ever before. Today it is quite common to see men involved in raising children (including changing diapers) and doing routine housework. It is also quite common to see women entering the workplace in jobs traditionally managed by men and participating in sports traditionally played by men. Men are not scoffed at when they are seen crying after a touching movie. Women are not laughed at when they choose to assert themselves. The disposal of numerous sexual stereotypes has probably benefited our society immensely by relieving people of the pressure to be 100% "womanly" or 100% "macho."

Research data suggest that androgynous people are more flexible and independent, have greater self-esteem, have more positive attitudes toward sexuality, and show more social skills and motivation to achieve.[5] This should encourage you to be unafraid to break the gender role stereotype.

 TALKING POINTS How could you demonstrate to your grandmother that the blending of gender roles is a positive development?

Reproductive Systems

The most familiar aspects of biological sexuality are the structures that compose the reproductive systems. Each structure contributes to the reproductive process in unique ways. Thus, with these structures, males have the ability to impregnate. Females have the ability to become pregnant, give birth, and nourish infants through breastfeeding. Many of these structures are also associated with nonreproductive sexual behavior.

Male Reproductive System

The male reproductive system consists of external structures of genitals (the penis and scrotum) and internal

---

Key Terms

androgyny (an **droj** en ee) the blending of both masculine and feminine qualities.

Figure 13-2 The male reproductive system.
A, Side view, **B,** Front view.

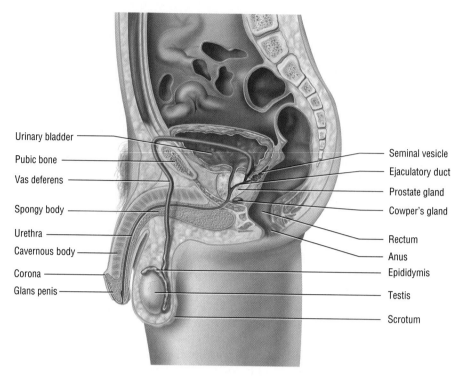

Urinary bladder

Pubic bone

Vas deferens

Spongy body

Urethra

Cavernous body

Corona

Glans penis

Seminal vesicle

Ejaculatory duct

Prostate gland

Cowper's gland

Rectum

Anus

Epididymis

Testis

Scrotum

A

Shaft of penis

Glans penis

Scrotum

Anus

B

structures (the testes, various passageways or ducts, seminal vesicles, the prostate gland, and the Cowper's glands) (Figure 13-2, *A*). The *testes* (also called *gonads* or *testicles*) are two egg-shaped bodies that lie within a saclike structure called the *scrotum*.[6] During most of fetal development, the testes lie within the abdominal cavity. They descend into the scrotum during the last 2 months of fetal life.

The testes are housed in the scrotum because a temperature lower than the body core temperature is required for adequate sperm development. The walls of the scro-

tum are composed of contractile tissue and can draw the testes closer to the body during cold temperatures (and sexual arousal) and relax during warm temperatures. Scrotal movements allow a constant, productive temperature to be maintained in the testes (Figure 13-2, *B*).

Each testis contains an intricate network of structures called *seminiferous tubules*. Within these 300 or so seminiferous tubules, the process of sperm production (spermatogenesis) takes place. Sperm cell development starts at about age 11 in boys and is influenced by the release of the hormone **ICSH (interstitial cell-stimulating hormone)** from the pituitary gland. ICSH does primarily what its name suggests: it stimulates specific cells (called *interstitial cells*) within the testes to begin producing the male sex hormone *testosterone.* Testosterone in turn is primarily responsible for the gradual development of the male secondary sex characteristics at the onset of puberty. By the time a boy is approximately 15 years old, sufficient levels of testosterone exist so that the testes become capable of full spermatogenesis.

Before the age of about 15, most of the sperm cells produced in the testes are incapable of fertilization. The production of fully mature sperm *(spermatozoa)* is triggered by another hormone secreted by the brain's pituitary gland—**FSH (follicle-stimulating hormone).** FSH influences the seminiferous tubules to begin producing spermatozoa that are capable of fertilization.

Spermatogenesis takes place around the clock, with hundreds of millions of sperm cells produced daily. The sperm cells do not stay in the seminiferous tubules but rather are transferred through a system of ducts that lead into the *epididymis.* The epididymis is a tubular coil that attaches to the back side of each testicle. These collecting structures house the maturing sperm cells for 2 to 3 weeks. During this period the sperm finally become capable of motion, but they remain inactive until they mix with the secretions from the accessory glands (the seminal vesicles, prostate gland, and Cowper's glands).

Each epididymis leads into an 18-inch passageway known as the *vas deferens.* Sperm, moved along by the action of hairlike projections called *cilia,* can also remain in the vas deferens for an extended time without losing their ability to fertilize an egg.

The two vasa deferens extend into the abdominal cavity, where each meets with a *seminal vesicle*—the first of the three accessory structures or glands. Each seminal vesicle contributes a clear, alkaline fluid that nourishes the sperm cells with fructose and permits the sperm cells to be suspended in a movable medium. The fusion of a vas deferens with the seminal vesicle results in the formation of a passageway called the *ejaculatory duct.* Each ejaculatory duct is only about 1 inch long and empties into the final passageway for the sperm—the urethra.

This juncture takes place in an area surrounded by the second accessory gland—the *prostate gland.* The prostate gland secretes a milky fluid containing a variety of substances, including proteins, cholesterol, citric acid, calcium, buffering salts, and various enzymes. The prostate secretions further nourish the sperm cells and also raise the pH level, making the mixture quite alkaline. This alkalinity permits the sperm to have greater longevity as they are transported during ejaculation through the urethra, out of the penis, and into the highly acidic vagina.

The third accessory glands, the Cowper's glands, serve primarily to lubricate the urethra with a clear, viscous mucus. These paired glands empty their small amounts of preejaculatory fluid during the plateau stage of the sexual response cycle. Alkaline in nature, this fluid also neutralizes the acidic level of the urethra. Viable sperm cells can be suspended in this fluid and can enter the female reproductive tract before full ejaculation by the male.[7] This may account for many of the failures of the "withdrawal" method of contraception.

The sperm cells, when combined with secretions from the seminal vesicles and the prostate gland, form a sticky substance called **semen.**[8] Interestingly, the microscopic sperm actually makes up less than 5% of the seminal fluid discharged at ejaculation. Contrary to popular belief, the paired seminal vesicles contribute about 60% of the semen volume, and the prostate gland adds about 30%.[1] Thus the fear of some men that a **vasectomy** will destroy their ability to ejaculate is completely unfounded (see Chapter 14).

Key Terms

ICSH (interstitial cell-stimulating hormone) (in ter stish ul) a gonadotropic hormone of the male required for the production of testosterone.

FSH (follicle-stimulating hormone) a gonadotropic hormone required for initial development of ova (in the female) and sperm (in the male).

semen secretion containing sperm and nutrients discharged from the urethra at ejaculation.

vasectomy surgical procedure in which the vasa deferens are cut to prevent the passage of sperm from the testicles; the most common form of male sterilization.

During *emission* (the gathering of semen in the upper part of the urethra), a sphincter muscle at the base of the bladder contracts and inhibits semen from being pushed into the bladder and urine from being deposited into the urethra.[9] Thus semen and urine rarely intermingle, even though they leave the body through the same passageway.

Ejaculation takes place when the semen is forced out of the penis through the urethral opening. The involuntary, rhythmic muscle contractions that control ejaculation result in a series of pleasurable sensations known as *orgasm.*

The urethra lies on the underside of the penis and extends through one of three cylindrical chambers of erectile tissue (two cavernous bodies and one spongy body). Each of these three chambers provides the vascular space required for sufficient erection of the penis. When a male becomes sexually aroused, these areas become congested with blood (*vasocongestion*). After ejaculation or when a male is no longer sexually stimulated, these chambers release the blood into the general circulation and the penis returns to a **flaccid** state.

The *shaft* of the penis is covered by a thin layer of skin that is an extension of the skin that covers the scrotum. This loose layer of skin is sensitive to sexual stimulation and extends over the head of the penis, except in males who have been circumcised. The *glans* (or head) of the penis is the most sexually sensitive (to tactile stimulation) part of the male body. Nerve receptor sites are especially prominent along the *corona* (the ridge of the glans) and the *frenulum* (the thin tissue at the base of the glans).

Female Reproductive System

The external structures (genitals) of the female reproductive system consist of the mons pubis, labia majora, labia minora, clitoris, and vestibule (Figure 13-3). Collectively these structures form the *vulva* or vulval area. The *mons pubis* is the fatty covering over the pubic bone. The mons pubis (or mons veneris, "mound of Venus") is covered by pubic hair and is quite sensitive to sexual stimulation. The *labia majora* are large longitudinal folds of skin that cover the entrance to the vagina, whereas the *labia minora* are the smaller longitudinal skin folds that lie within the labia majora. These hairless skin folds of the labia minora join at the top to form the *prepuce.* The prepuce covers the glans of the *clitoris,* which is the most sexually sensitive part of the female body.

A rather direct analogy can be made between the penis and the clitoris. In terms of the tactile sensitivity, both structures are the most sensitive parts of the male and female genitals. Both contain a glans and a shaft (although the clitoral shaft is beneath the skin surface). Both organs are composed of erectile tissue that can become engorged with blood. Both are covered by skin folds (the clitoral pre-

puce of the female and the foreskin of the male), and both structures can collect **smegma** beneath these tissue folds.[5]

The *vestibule* is the region enclosed by the labia minora. Evident here are the urethral opening and the entrance to the vagina (or vaginal orifice). Also located at the vaginal opening are the *Bartholin's glands,* which secrete a minute amount of lubricating fluid during sexual excitement.

The *hymen* is a thin layer of tissue that stretches across the opening of the vagina. Once thought to be the only indication of virginity, the intact hymen rarely covers the vaginal opening entirely. Openings in the hymen are necessary for the discharge of menstrual fluid and vaginal secretions. Many hymens are stretched or torn to full opening by adolescent physical activity or by the insertion of tampons. In women whose hymens are not fully ruptured, the first act of sexual intercourse will generally accomplish this. Pain may accompany first intercourse in females with relatively intact hymens.

The internal reproductive structures of the female include the vagina, uterus, fallopian tubes, and ovaries. The *vagina* is the structure that accepts the penis during sexual intercourse. Normally the walls of the vagina are collapsed, except during sexual stimulation, when the vaginal walls widen and elongate to accommodate the erect penis. Only the outer third of the vagina is especially sensitive to sexual stimulation. In this location, vaginal tissues swell considerably to form the **orgasmic platform.**[10] This platform constricts the vaginal opening and in effect "grips" the penis (or other inserted object)—regardless of its size.[5] So the belief that a woman receives considerably more sexual pleasure from men with large penises is not supported from an anatomical standpoint.

The *uterus* (or *womb*) is approximately the size and shape of a small pear. This highly muscular organ is capable of undergoing a wide range of physical changes, as evidenced by its enlargement during pregnancy, its contraction during menstruation and labor, and its movement during the orgasmic phase of the female sexual response

---

Key Terms

flaccid (fla sid) nonerect; the state of erectile tissue when vasocongestion is not occurring.

smegma cellular discharge that can accumulate beneath the clitoral hood and the foreskin of an uncircumcised penis.

orgasmic platform expanded outer third of the vagina that grips the penis during the plateau phase of the sexual response pattern.

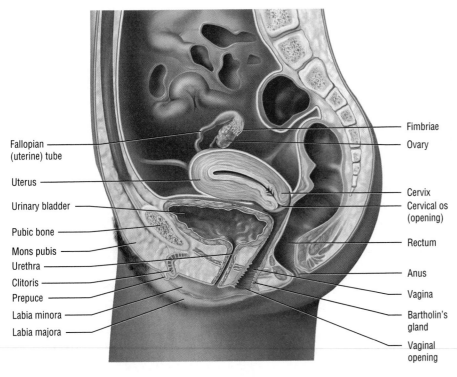

Figure 13-3 The female reproductive system. **A,** Side view, **B,** Front view.

Fallopian (uterine) tube

Uterus

Urinary bladder

Pubic bone

Mons pubis

Urethra

Clitoris

Prepuce

Labia minora

Labia majora

Fimbriae

Ovary

Cervix

Cervical os (opening)

Rectum

Anus

Vagina

Bartholin's gland

Vaginal opening

A

Mons pubis

Prepuce

Clitoris

Urethra

Labia majora

Labia minora

Vaginal opening

Perineum

Anus

B

cycle. The primary function of the uterus is to provide a suitable environment for the possible implantation of a fertilized ovum, or egg. This implantation, should it occur, will take place in the innermost lining of the uterus—the *endometrium.* In the mature female, the endometrium undergoes cyclic changes as it prepares a new lining on a near-monthly basis.

The lower third of the uterus is called the *cervix.* The cervix extends slightly into the vagina. Sperm can enter

the uterus through the cervical opening, or *cervical os.* Mucous glands in the cervix secrete a fluid that is thin and watery near the time of ovulation. Mucus of this consistency apparently facilitates sperm passage into the uterus and deeper structures. However, cervical mucus is much thicker during certain points in the menstrual cycle (when pregnancy is improbable) and during pregnancy (to protect against bacterial agents and other substances that are especially dangerous to the developing fetus).

The upper two thirds of the uterus is called the *corpus,* or *body.* This is where implantation of the fertilized ovum generally takes place. The upper portion of the uterus opens into two *fallopian tubes,* or *oviducts,* each about 4 inches long. The fallopian tubes are each directed toward an *ovary.* They serve as a passageway for the ovum in its week-long voyage toward the uterus. Usually, conception takes place in the upper third of the fallopian tubes.

The ovaries are analogous to the testes in the male. Their function is to produce the ovum, or egg. Usually, one ovary produces and releases just one egg each month. Approximately the size and shape of an unshelled almond, an ovary produces viable ova in the process known as *oogenesis.* The ovaries also produce the female sex hormones through the efforts of specific structures within the ovaries. These hormones play multiple roles in the development of female secondary sex characteristics, but their primary function is to prepare the endometrium of the uterus for possible implantation of a fertilized ovum. In the average healthy female, this preparation takes place about 13 times a year for a period of about 35 years. At menopause, the ovaries shrink considerably and stop nearly all hormonal production.

Menstrual Cycle

Each month or so, the inner wall of the uterus prepares for a possible pregnancy. When a pregnancy does not occur (as is the case throughout most months of a woman's fertile years), this lining must be released and a new one prepared. The breakdown of this endometrial wall and the resultant discharge of blood and endometrial tissue is known as *menstruation* (or *menses*) (Figure 13-4). The cyclic timing of menstruation is governed by hormones released from two sources: the pituitary gland and the ovaries.

Girls generally have their first menstrual cycle, the onset of which is called *menarche,* sometime around age 12 or 13. Body weight, nutrition, heredity, and overall health are factors related to menarche. After a girl first menstruates, she may be anovulatory for a year or longer before a viable ovum is released during her cycle. This cyclic activity will continue until about age 45 to 55.

This text refers to a menstrual cycle that lasts 28 days. However, few women display perfect 28-day cycles. Most women fluctuate by a few days to a week around this 28-day pattern, and some women vary greatly from this cycle.

Your knowledge about the menstrual cycle is critical for your understanding of pregnancy, contraception, menopause, and issues related to the overall health and comfort of women (see the Star box on this page for a discussion of endometriosis). Although at first this cycle may sound like a complicated process,

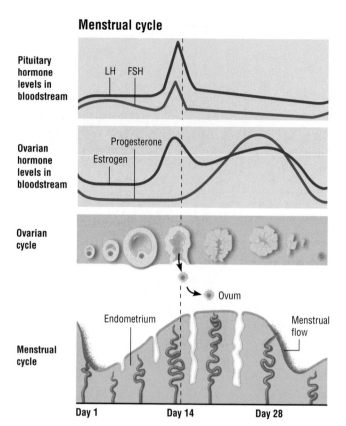

Menstrual cycle

Pituitary hormone levels in bloodstream — LH FSH

Ovarian hormone levels in bloodstream — Progesterone Estrogen

Ovarian cycle

 Ovum

Endometrium Menstrual flow

Menstrual cycle

Day 1 Day 14 Day 28

Figure 13-4 The menstrual cycle involves the development and release of an ovum, supported by hormones from the pituitary, and the buildup of the endometrium, supported by hormones from the ovary, for the purpose of establishing a pregnancy.

Endometriosis

Endometriosis is a condition in which endometrial tissue that normally lines the uterus is found growing within the pelvic cavity. Because the tissue remains sensitive to circulating hormones, it is the source of pain and discomfort during the latter half of the menstrual cycle. Endometriosis is most commonly found in younger women and is sometimes related to infertility in women with severe cases.

In addition to painful cramping before and during menstruation, the symptoms of endometriosis include low back pain, pain during intercourse, painful bowel movements, heavy menstrual flow, and difficulty becoming pregnant.*

Treatment of endometriosis largely depends on its extent. Drugs to suppress ovulation, including birth control pills, may be helpful in mild cases. For more severe cases, surgical removal of the tissue or a hysterectomy may be necessary. For some women, endometriosis is suppressed during pregnancy and does not return after pregnancy.

*WebMD content article. *Your guide to endometriosis,* **www.MY.WEBMD. COM/CONTENT/ARTICLE/46/2953_501htm.** accessed July 10, 2003.

each segment of the cycle can be studied separately for better understanding.

The menstrual cycle can be thought of as occurring in three segments or phases: the menstrual phase (lasting about 1 week), the preovulation phase (also lasting about 1 week), and the postovulation phase (lasting about 2 weeks). Day 1 of this cycle starts with the first day of bleeding, or menstrual flow.

The *menstrual phase* signals the woman that a pregnancy has not taken place and that her uterine lining is being sloughed off. During a 5- to 7-day period, a woman will discharge about ¼ to ½ cup of blood and tissue. (Only about 1 ounce of the menstrual flow is actual blood.) The menstrual flow is heaviest during the first days of this phase. Since the muscular uterus must contract to accomplish this tissue removal, some women have uncomfortable cramping during menstruation. Most women, however, report more pain and discomfort during the few days before the first day of menstrual flow. (See the following discussion of premenstrual syndrome [PMS].)

Today's methods of absorbing menstrual flow include the use of internal tampons and external pads. Caution must be exercised by the users of tampons to prevent the possibility of toxic shock syndrome (TSS) (see Chapter 12). Since menstrual flow is a positive sign of good health, women are encouraged to be normally active during menstruation.

The *preovulation phase* of the menstrual cycle starts about the time menstruation stops. Lasting about 1 week, this phase is first influenced by the release of FSH from the pituitary gland. FSH circulates in the bloodstream and directs the ovaries to start the process of maturing approximately 20 primary ovarian *follicles.* Thousands of primary egg follicles are present in each ovary at birth. These follicles resemble shells that house immature ova. As these follicles ripen under FSH influence, they release the hormone estrogen. Estrogen's primary function is to direct the endometrium to start the development of a thick, highly vascular wall. As the estrogen levels increase, the pituitary gland's secretion of FSH is reduced. Now the pituitary gland prepares for the surge of the **luteinizing hormone (LH)** required to accomplish ovulation.[11]

In the days immediately preceding ovulation, one of the primary follicles (called the *graafian follicle*) matures fully. The other primary follicles degenerate and are absorbed by the body. The graafian follicle moves toward the surface of the ovary. When LH is released in massive quantities on about day 14, the graafian follicle bursts to release the fully mature ovum. The release of the ovum is **ovulation.** Regardless of the overall length of a woman's cycle, ovulation occurs 14 days before her first day of menstrual flow.

The ovum is quickly captured by the fingerlike projections (*fimbriae*) of the fallopian tubes. In the upper third of the fallopian tubes, the ovum is capable of being fertilized in a 24- to 36-hour period. If the ovum is not fertilized by a sperm cell, it will begin to degenerate and eventually will be absorbed by the body.

After ovulation, the *postovulation phase* of the menstrual cycle starts when the remnants of the graafian follicle restructure themselves into a **corpus luteum.** The corpus luteum remains inside the ovary, secreting estrogen and a fourth hormone called *progesterone.* Progesterone, which literally means "for pregnancy," continues to direct the endometrial buildup. If pregnancy occurs, the corpus luteum monitors progesterone and estrogen levels throughout the pregnancy. If pregnancy does not occur, high levels of progesterone signal the pituitary gland to stop the release of LH and the corpus luteum starts to degenerate on about day 24. When estrogen and progesterone levels diminish significantly by day 28, the endometrium is discharged from the uterus and out the vagina. The postovulation phase ends, and the menstrual phase begins. The cycle is then complete.

PMS PMS is characterized by psychological symptoms, such as depression, lethargy, irritability, and aggressiveness, or somatic symptoms, such as headache, backache, asthma, and acne, that recur in the same phase of each menstrual cycle, followed by a symptom-free phase in each cycle. Some of the more frequently reported symptoms of PMS include tension, tender breasts, fainting, fatigue, abdominal cramps, and weight gain.

The cause of PMS appears to be hormonal. Perhaps a woman's body is insensitive to a normal level of progesterone, or her ovaries fail to produce a normal amount of progesterone. These reasons seem plausible because PMS types of symptoms do not occur during pregnancy, during which natural progesterone levels are very high, and because women with PMS seem to feel much better after receiving high doses of natural progesterone in suppository form. When using oral contraceptives that supply synthetic progesterone at normal levels, many women

---

Key Terms

luteinizing hormone (LH) (**loo** ten eye zing) a gonadotropic hormone of the female required for fullest development and release of ova; ovulating hormone.

ovulation the release of a mature egg from the ovary.

corpus luteum (**kore** pus **loo** tee um) cellular remnant of the graafian follicle after the release of an ovum.

report relief from some symptoms of PMS. However, the effectiveness of the most frequently used form of treatment, progesterone suppositories, is now being questioned.

Until the effectiveness of progesterone has been fully researched, it is unlikely that the medical community will deal with PMS through any approach other than a relatively conservative treatment of symptoms through the use of *analgesic drugs* (including *prostaglandin inhibitors*), diuretic drugs, dietary modifications (including restriction of caffeine and salt), vitamin B_6 therapy, exercise, and stress-reduction exercises.

Fibrocystic Breast Condition In some women, particularly those who have never been pregnant, stimulation of the breast tissues by estrogen and progesterone during the menstrual cycle results in an unusually high degree of secretory activity by the cells lining the ducts. The fluid released by the secretory lining finds its way into the fibrous connective tissue areas in the lower half of the breast, where in pocketlike cysts the fluid presses against neighboring tissues. In many women, excessive secretory activity produces a fibrocystic breast condition characterized by swollen, firm or hardened, tender breast tissue before menstruation.

Women who experience a more extensive fibrocystic condition can be treated with drugs that have a "calming" effect on progesterone production. In addition, occasional draining of the fluid-filled cysts can bring relief.

Menopause

For the vast majority of women in their late forties through their mid-fifties, a gradual decline in reproductive system function, called *menopause,* occurs. Menopause is a normal physiological process, not a disease process. It can, however, become a health concern for some middle-aged women who have unpleasant side effects resulting from this natural stoppage of ovum production and menstruation.

As ovarian function and hormone production diminish, a period of adjustment must be made by the hypothalamus, ovaries, uterus, and other estrogen-sensitive tissues. The extent of menopause as a health problem is determined by the degree to which **hot flashes,** night sweats, insomnia, vaginal wall dryness, depression and melancholy, breast changes, and the uncertainty of fertility are seen as problems.

In comparison with past generations, today's midlife women are much less likely to find menopause to be a negative experience. The end of fertility, combined with children leaving the home, makes the middle years a period of personal rediscovery for many women.

For women who are troubled by the changes brought about by menopause, physicians may prescribe **hormone replacement therapy (HRT).** This can relieve many symptoms and offer benefits to help reduce the in-

cidence of osteoporosis (see Chapter 4). However, some forms of HRT have recently been found to increase the risk of breast cancer and cardiovascular problems.[12,13]

Human Sexual Response Pattern

Although history has many written and visual accounts of the human's ability to be sexually aroused, it was not until the pioneering work of Masters and Johnson[14] that the events associated with arousal were clinically documented. Five questions posed by these researchers gave direction to a series of studies involving the scientific evaluation of human sexual response:

Do the Sexual Responses of Males and Females Have a Predictable Pattern?

The answer to the first question posed by the researchers was an emphatic yes. A predictable sexual response pattern was identified;[14] it consists of an initial **excitement stage,** a **plateau stage,** an **orgasmic stage,** and a **resolution stage.** Each stage involves predictable changes in the structural characteristics and physiological function of reproductive and nonreproductive organs in both the male and the female. These changes are shown in Figure 13-5.

Is the Sexual Response Pattern Stimuli-Specific?

The research of Masters and Johnson clearly established a no answer to the second question concerning stimuli

---

Key Terms

hot flashes temporary feelings of warmth experienced by women during and after menopause, caused by blood vessel dilation.

hormone replacement therapy (HRT) medically administered estrogen and progestin to replace hormones lost as the result of menopause.

excitement stage initial arousal stage of the sexual response pattern.

plateau stage second stage of the sexual response pattern; a leveling off of arousal immediately before orgasm.

orgasmic stage third stage of the sexual response pattern; the stage during which neuromuscular tension is released.

resolution stage fourth stage of the sexual response pattern; the return of the body to a preexcitement state.

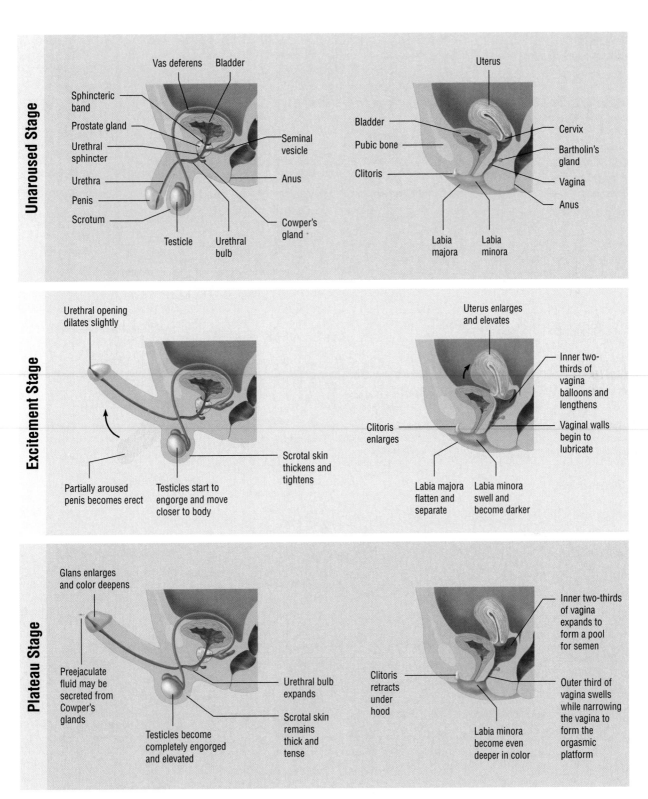

Figure 13-5 The sexual response pattern in men and women.

SENSATION OF ORGASM

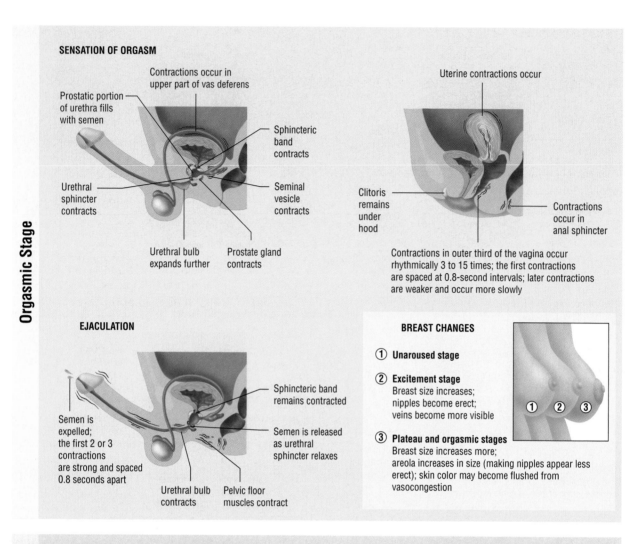

Contractions occur in upper part of vas deferens

Prostatic portion of urethra fills with semen

Sphincteric band contracts

Urethral sphincter contracts

Seminal vesicle contracts

Urethral bulb expands further

Prostate gland contracts

Uterine contractions occur

Clitoris remains under hood

Contractions occur in anal sphincter

Contractions in outer third of the vagina occur rhythmically 3 to 15 times; the first contractions are spaced at 0.8-second intervals; later contractions are weaker and occur more slowly

EJACULATION

Semen is expelled; the first 2 or 3 contractions are strong and spaced 0.8 seconds apart

Sphincteric band remains contracted

Semen is released as urethral sphincter relaxes

Urethral bulb contracts

Pelvic floor muscles contract

BREAST CHANGES

① **Unaroused stage**

② **Excitement stage**
Breast size increases; nipples become erect; veins become more visible

③ **Plateau and orgasmic stages**
Breast size increases more; areola increases in size (making nipples appear less erect); skin color may become flushed from vasocongestion

① ② ③

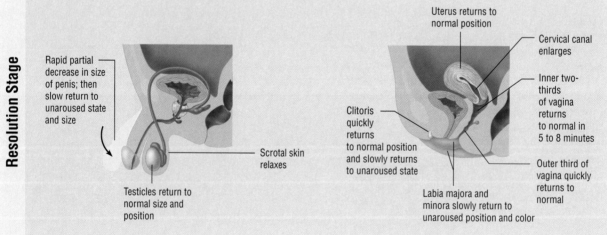

Rapid partial decrease in size of penis; then slow return to unaroused state and size

Scrotal skin relaxes

Testicles return to normal size and position

Uterus returns to normal position

Cervical canal enlarges

Inner two-thirds of vagina returns to normal in 5 to 8 minutes

Clitoris quickly returns to normal position and slowly returns to unaroused state

Outer third of vagina quickly returns to normal

Labia majora and minora slowly return to unaroused position and color

Figure 13-5 *Continued*

specificity. Their findings demonstrated that numerous senses can supply the stimuli necessary for initiating the sexual response pattern. Although touching activities might initiate arousal in most people and maximize it for the vast majority of people, in both males and females, sight, smell, sound, and *vicariously formed stimuli* can also stimulate the same sexual arousal patterns.

What Differences Occur in the Sexual Response Pattern?

Differences between Males and Females

Several differences are observable when the sexual response patterns of males and females are compared:

- With the exception of some later adolescent males, the vast majority of males are not multiorgasmic. The **refractory phase** of the resolution stage prevents most males from experiencing more than one orgasm in a short period, even when sufficient stimulation is available.

- Females possess a **multiorgasmic capacity.** Masters and Johnson found that as many as 10% to 30% of all female adults routinely experience multiple orgasms.

- Although they possess multiorgasmic potential, about 10% of all female adults are *anorgasmic*—that is, they never experience an orgasm.[14] For many anorgasmic females, orgasms can be experienced when masturbation, rather than **coitus,** provides the stimulation.

- When measured during coitus, males reach orgasm far more quickly than do females. However, when masturbation is the source of stimulation, females reach orgasm as quickly as do males.[14]

More important than any of the differences pointed out is the finding that the sexual response patterns of males and females are far more alike than they are different. Not only do males and females experience the four basic stages of the response pattern, but they also have similar responses in specific areas, including the **erection** and *tumescence* of sexual structures; the appearance of a **sex flush;** the increase in cardiac output, blood pressure, and respiratory rate; and the occurrence of *rhythmic pelvic thrusting.*[14]

Differences among Subjects within a Same-Gender Group

When a group of subjects of the same gender was studied in an attempt to answer questions about similarities and differences in the sexual response pattern, Masters and Johnson noted considerable variation. Even when

Sexual Performance Difficulties and Therapies

Despite the predictability of the human sexual response pattern, many people find that at some point in their lives, they are no longer capable of responding sexually. The inability of a person to perform adequately is identified as a sexual difficulty or dysfunction. Sexual difficulties can have a negative influence on a person's sense of sexual satisfaction and on a partner's satisfaction. Fortunately, most sexual difficulties can be resolved through strategies that use individual, couple, or group counseling. Many sexual performance difficulties stem from psychogenic (originating in the mind) factors.

variables such as age, race, education, and general health were held constant, the extent and duration of virtually every stage of the response pattern varied.

Differences within the Same Individual

For a given person the nature of the sexual response pattern does not remain constant, even when observed over a relatively short period. A variety of internal and external factors can alter this pattern. The aging process, changes in general health status, levels of stress, altered environmental settings, use of alcohol and other drugs, and behavioral changes in a sexual partner can cause one's own sexual response pattern to change from one sexual experience to another. Sexual performance difficulties and therapies are briefly discussed in the Star box on this page.

What Are the Basic Physiological Mechanisms Underlying the Sexual Response Pattern?

The basic mechanisms in the fourth question posed by Masters and Johnson are now well recognized. One factor,

Key Terms

refractory phase that portion of the male's resolution stage during which sexual arousal cannot occur.

multiorgasmic capacity potential to have several orgasms within a single period of sexual arousal.

coitus (CO ih tus) penile-vaginal intercourse.

erection the engorgement of erectile tissue with blood; characteristic of the penis, clitoris, nipples, labia minora, and scrotum.

sex flush the reddish skin response that results from increasing sexual arousal.

vasocongestion, or the retention of blood or fluid within a particular tissue, is critically important in the development of physiological changes that promote the sexual response pattern. The presence of erectile tissue underlies the changes that can be noted in the penis, breasts, and scrotum of the male and the clitoris, breasts, and labia minora of the female.

A second mechanism now recognized as necessary for the development of the sexual response pattern is that of *myotonia,* or the buildup of *neuromuscular tonus* within a variety of body structures.[9] At the end of the plateau stage of the response pattern, a sudden release of the accumulated neuromuscular tension gives rise to the rhythmic muscular contractions and pleasurable muscular spasms that constitute orgasm, as well as ejaculation in the male.[3]

What Role Is Played by Specific Organs and Organ Systems Within the Sexual Response Pattern?

The fifth question posed by Masters and Johnson, which concerns the role played by specific organs and organ systems during each stage of the response pattern, can be readily answered by referring to the material presented in Figure 13-5. As you study this figure, remember that direct stimulation of the penis and either direct or indirect stimulation of the clitoris are the principal avenues toward orgasm. Also, intercourse represents only one activity that can lead to orgasmic pleasure.[15]

Patterns of Sexual Behavior

Although sex researchers may see sexual behavior in terms of the human sexual response pattern just described, most people are more interested in the observable dimensions of sexual behavior. Complete the Personal Assessment on page 391 to determine whether your own attitudes toward sexuality are traditional or nontraditional.

Celibacy

Celibacy can be defined as the self-imposed avoidance of sexual intimacy. It is synonymous with sexual abstinence. There are many reasons people could choose not to have a sexually intimate relationship. For some, celibacy is part of a religious doctrine. Others might be afraid of sexually transmitted diseases. For most, however, celibacy is preferred simply because it seems appropriate for them. Celibate people can certainly have deep, intimate relationships with other people—just not sexual relationships. Celibacy may be short-term or last a

lifetime, and no identified physical or psychological complications appear to result from a celibate lifestyle.

TALKING POINTS You have decided to remain celibate until you're ready to make a lifetime commitment to someone. How would you explain this to the person you are now dating?

Masturbation

Throughout recorded history, **masturbation** has been a primary method of achieving sexual pleasure. Through masturbation, people can explore their sexual response patterns. Traditionally, some societies and religious groups have condemned this behavior based on the belief that intercourse is the only "right" sexual behavior. With sufficient lubrication, masturbation cannot do physical harm. Today masturbation is considered by most sex therapists and researchers to be a normal source of self-pleasure.

Fantasy and Erotic Dreams

The brain is the most sensual organ in the body. In fact, many sexuality experts classify **sexual fantasies** and **erotic dreams** as forms of sexual behavior. Particularly for people whose verbal ability is highly developed, the ability to create imaginary scenes enriches other forms of sexual behavior.

When fantasies occur in conjunction with another form of sexual behavior, the second behavior may be greatly enhanced by the supportive fantasy. Both women and men fantasize during foreplay and intercourse. Masturbation and fantasizing are inseparable activities.

Erotic dreams occur during sleep in both men and women. The association between these dreams and ejaculation resulting in a nocturnal emission (wet dream) is readily recognized in males. In females, erotic dreams can lead not only to vaginal lubrication but to orgasm as well.

Shared Touching

Virtually the entire body can be an erogenous (sexually sensitive) zone when shared touching is involved. A soft,

> ### Key Terms
>
> **masturbation** self-stimulation of the genitals.
>
> **sexual fantasies** fantasies with sexual themes; sexual daydreams or imaginary events.
>
> **erotic dreams** dreams whose content elicits a sexual response.

light touch, a slight application of pressure, the brushing back of a partner's hair, and gentle massage are all forms of communication that heighten sexual arousal.

Genital Contact

Two important uses can be identified for the practice of stimulating a partner's genitals. The first is that of being the tactile component of **foreplay.** Genital contact, in the form of holding, rubbing, stroking, or caressing, heightens arousal to a level that allows for progression to intercourse.

The second role of genital contact is that of *mutual masturbation to orgasm.* Stimulation of the genitals so that both partners have orgasm is a form of sexual behavior practiced by many people, as well as couples during the late stage of a pregnancy. For couples not desiring pregnancy, the risk of conception is virtually eliminated when this becomes the form of sexual intimacy practiced.

As is the case of other aspects of intimacy, genital stimulation is best enhanced when partners can talk about their needs, expectations, and reservations. Practice and communication can shape this form of contact into a pleasure-giving approach to sexual intimacy.

Oral-Genital Stimulation

Oral-genital stimulation brings together two of the body's most erogenous areas: the genitalia and the mouth. Because oral-genital stimulation can involve an exchange of body fluids, the risk of disease transmission is real. Small tears of mouth or genital tissue may allow transmission of disease-causing pathogens. Only couples who are absolutely certain that they are free from all sexually transmitted diseases (including HIV infection) can practice unprotected oral sex. Couples in doubt should refrain from oral-genital sex or carefully use a condom (on the male) or a latex square to cover the female's vulval area. Increasingly, latex squares (dental dams) can be obtained from drug stores or pharmacies.

Three basic forms of oral-genital stimulation are practiced.[5] **Fellatio,** in which the penis is sucked, licked, or kissed by the partner, is the most common of the three. **Cunnilingus,** in which the vulva of the female is kissed, licked, or penetrated by the partner's tongue, is only slightly less frequently practiced.

Mutual oral-genital stimulation, the third form of oral-genital stimulation, combines both fellatio and cunnilingus. When practiced by a heterosexual couple, the female partner performs fellatio on her partner while her male partner performs cunnilingus on her. Gay couples can practice mutual fellatio or cunnilingus.

Intercourse

Sexual intercourse (coitus) refers to the act of inserting the penis into the vagina. Intercourse is the sexual behavior that is most directly associated with **procreation.** For some, intercourse is the only natural and appropriate form of sexual intimacy.

The incidence and frequency of sexual intercourse is a much-studied topic. Information concerning the percentages of people who have engaged in intercourse is readily available in textbooks used in sexuality courses. Data concerning sexual intercourse among college students may be changing somewhat because of concerns about HIV infection and other STDs, but a reasonable estimate of the percentage of college students reporting sexual intercourse is between 60% and 75%.

These percentages reflect two important concepts about the sexual activity of college students. The first is that a large majority of college students is having intercourse. The second concept is that a sizeable percentage (25% to 40%) of students is choosing to refrain from intercourse. Indeed, the belief that "everyone is doing it" may be a bit shortsighted. From a public health standpoint, we believe it is important to provide accurate health information to protect those who choose to have intercourse and to actively support a person's right to choose not to have intercourse.

Couples need to share their expectations concerning sexual techniques and frequency of intercourse.[6] Even the "performance" factors, such as depth of penetration, nature of body movements, tempo of activity, and timing of orgasm are of increasing importance to many couples. Issues concerning sexually transmitted diseases (including HIV infection) are also critically important for couples who are contemplating intercourse. These factors also need to be explored through open communication.

There are a variety of books (including textbooks) that provide written and visually explicit information on intercourse positions. Four basic positions for intercourse—male above, female above, side by side, and rear entry—each offer relative advantages and disadvantages.

Key Terms

foreplay activities, often involving touching and caressing, that prepare individuals for sexual intercourse.

fellatio (feh **lay** she oh) oral stimulation of the penis.

cunnilingus (cun uh **ling** gus) oral stimulation of the vulva or clitoris.

procreation reproduction.

Anal Sexual Activity

Some couples practice **anal intercourse,** in which the penis is inserted into the rectum of a partner. Anal intercourse can be performed by both heterosexual couples and gay men. According to a year 2000 report in the journal *Archives of Sexual Behavior,* about 20 to 25 percent of college students have experienced anal intercourse.[16] The anal sphincter muscles contract tightly and tend to resist entry. Thus, couples who engage in anal intercourse must do so slowly, gently, and with adequate amounts of water-based lubricants. Because of the danger of tearing tissues in the rectal area, HIV transmission risk is increased if the inserting male is infected.[3] Unless it is absolutely certain that both partners are uninfected, the inserting male should always wear a condom. Even with a condom, disease transmission is possible, since during anal intercourse, condoms are more likely to tear than during penis-vaginal intercourse. Couples practicing anal sex must not follow anal insertion with insertion into the mouth or vagina because of the likelihood of transmitting infectious agents.

For many people, anal intercourse is not only unpleasant, but simply unnatural for humans. For others, the anal area is just another part of the human body that is especially sensitive to stimulation, and they enjoy the pleasurable sensations that come from intercourse or the insertion of a well-lubricated finger or sex toy. Some people enjoy kissing ("rimming") or touching in the anal area, but this should occur only when the anal area has been fully cleansed or covered with a sheet of protective plastic wrap. As with all sexual behavior, couples need to communicate clearly their feelings about any activity. If one partner is uncomfortable about an activity and wants to stop, his or her feelings must be supported by the other person. A desire for a particular sexual activity must not turn into sexual coercion or a sexual assault.

Until recently, thirteen states had laws on the books that banned **sodomy** (another term for anal sex as well as certain other sexual practices). However, a U.S. Supreme Court ruling *(Lawrence and Garner v Texas)* in June 2003 invalidated a Texas law that banned private consensual sex (in this case, sodomy) between adults of the same sex. Legal experts expect this Texas ruling to eventually invalidate the laws of the twelve other states that banned sodomy in one form or another.[17]

Sexuality and Aging

Students are often curious about how aging affects sexuality. This is understandable because we live in a society that idolizes youth and demands performance. Many younger people become anxious about growing older because of what they think will happen to their ability to express their sexuality. Interestingly, young adults are willing to accept other physical changes of aging (such as the slowing down of basal metabolism, reduced lung capacity, and even wrinkles) but not those changes related to sexuality.

Most of the research in this area suggests that older people are quite capable of performing sexually. As with other aspects of aging, certain anatomical and physiological changes will be evident, but these changes do not necessarily reduce the ability to enjoy sexual activity.[5] Most experts in sexuality report that many older people remain interested in sexual activity. Furthermore, those who are exposed to regular sexual activity throughout a lifetime report being most satisfied with their sex lives as older adults.

As people age, the likelihood of alterations in the male and female sexual response cycles increases. In the postmenopausal women, vaginal lubrication commonly begins more slowly, and the amount of lubrication usually diminishes. However, clitoral sensitivity and nipple erection remain the same as in earlier years. The female capacity for multiple orgasms remains the same, although the number of contractions that occur at orgasm typically is reduced.

In the older man, physical changes are also evident. This is thought to be caused by the decrease in the production of testosterone between the ages of 20 and 60 years. After age 60 or so, testosterone levels remain relatively steady. Thus many men, despite a decrease in sperm production, remain fertile into their eighties.[5] Older men typically take longer to achieve an erection (however, they are able to maintain their erection longer before ejaculation), have fewer muscular contractions at orgasm, and ejaculate less forcefully than they once did. The volume of seminal fluid ejaculated is typically less than in earlier years, and its consistency is somewhat thinner. The resolution phase is usually longer in older men. In spite of these gradual changes, some elderly men engage in sexual intercourse with the same frequency as do much younger men.

Sexual Orientation

Sexual orientation refers to the direction in which people focus their sexual interests. People can be attracted to opposite-gender partners (heterosexuality), same-gender partners (homosexuality), or partners of both genders (bisexuality).

Key Terms
anal intercourse a sexual act in which the erect penis is inserted into the rectum of a partner.
sodomy generally refers to anal or oral sex; a legal term whose definition varies according to state law.

The distinctions among the three categories of sexual orientation are much less clear than their definitions below will suggest. Most people probably fall somewhere along a continuum between exclusive heterosexuality and exclusive homosexuality. As far back as 1948, Kinsey presented just such a continuum.[18]

Heterosexuality

Heterosexuality (or heterosexual orientation) refers to an attraction to opposite-gender partners. (*Heteros* is a Greek word that means "the other.") A heterosexual person is sometimes called *straight*. Throughout the world, this is the most common sexual orientation. For reasons related to species survival, heterosexuality has its most basic roots in the biological dimension of human sexuality. Beyond its biological roots, heterosexuality has significant cultural and religious support in virtually every country in the world. Worldwide, laws related to marriage, living arrangements, health benefits, child rearing, financial matters, sexual behavior, and inheritance generally support relationships that are heterosexual in nature. However, this may be gradually changing. See the Focus On article on page 389 for an update on gay marriage.

Homosexuality

Homosexuality (or homosexual orientation) refers to an attraction to same-gender partners. (*Homos* is a Greek word that means "the same.") The term *gay* refers either to males or females, while the word *lesbian* is used only in reference to females.

What percentage of the population is gay? This is difficult to determine accurately, since many people refuse to reveal their orientations and prefer to remain "in the closet." However, it is probably safe to say that the number of gay people in our society is probably much greater than most people realize. Kinsey estimated that about 2% of American females and 4% of American males were exclusively homosexual.[18,19] More recent estimates place the overall figure to be about 10% of the population. Clearly, the expression of same-gender attraction is widespread.

Bisexuality

People who have the ability to be attracted to either gender are referred to as *bisexual*. Bisexuals generally are in one of three groups: those who are (1) genuinely attracted emotionally and physically to both genders, (2) those who are gay, but feel the need to behave heterosexually, and (3) those who are aroused physically by the same gender but attracted emotionally to the opposite gender. Some participate in a bisexual lifestyle for an extended period of time, while others move on more quickly to a more exclusive orientation.

The size of the bisexual population is unknown. See the Learning from Our Diversity box (page 382) that describes some of the challenges for bisexual men and women.

Origins of Sexual Orientation

Students often wonder "what makes a person gay?" This question has no simple answer. (College sexuality textbooks devote entire chapters to this topic.) Some research has pointed to differences in the sizes of certain brain structures as a possible biological or anatomical basis for homosexuality.[20] Other research proposes possible genetic, environmental, hormonal, or other foundations.

However, for sexual orientation in general, no single theory has emerged that fully explains this complex developmental process. The consensus of scientific opinion is that people do not choose their sexual orientation. Thus, being straight or being gay is something that "just happens." Indeed, most gays and lesbians report that no specific event triggered them into becoming gay. Many gays also indicate that their orientations seemed different from those of other children as far back as their prepuberty years.

Given the many challenges of being gay in a mostly straight world, it would seem logical that gays and lesbians do not make conscious efforts to choose to become gay. (Who would want to be a magnet for taunts, discrimination, and physical violence?) In a similar manner, it is highly likely that heterosexual persons do not actually choose to become straight. Sexual orientation is something that just unfolds in a person's life. See the Discovering Your Spirituality box (page 382) for insight into some of the issues that gays and lesbians face.

Love

Love may be one of the most elusive yet widely recognized concepts that describe some level of emotional attachment to another. Various forms of love include friendship, erotic, devotional, parental, and altruistic love. Two types of love are most closely associated with dating and mate selection: *passionate love* and *companionate love*.

Passionate love, also described as romantic love or **infatuation,** is a state of extreme absorption in another person. It is characterized by intense feelings of tenderness, elation, anxiety, sexual desire, and ecstasy. Often appearing early in a relationship, passionate love typically

---

Key Terms

infatuation a relatively temporary, intensely romantic attraction to another person.

Learning from Our Diversity

The Challenges for Bisexuals

People whose sexual orientation is toward both men and women are termed bisexuals. This can be a confusing label, however. For example, if a man has had one sexual experience with a man, but all of his other sexual experiences are with women, does this mean he is bisexual? And what about the woman who has sequential relationships with men, followed by an occasional relationship with a woman? Is she bisexual? What about people who are sexually attracted to one gender, but are emotionally more attracted to the other gender? The labels can get confusing and can make one wonder about the value of any label describing sexual orientation. This is just one of the many challenges facing bisexual people.

Some experts suggest that bisexuals (those who have had at least one sexual experience with a man and one with a woman) probably outnumber exclusive homosexuals (those who have had sexual experience *only* with persons of their own gender).[1] One might think that this larger group would be better understood by society, but that seems not to be the case. Bisexuals may have a larger field of potential partners, but this benefit may be offset by the difficulty fitting into society.

Heterosexual people, gay males, and lesbians may not view bisexuality as acceptable, believing that the bisexual person is just incapable of making the decision to go one way or the other.[2] They may accuse the bisexual person of wanting the best of both worlds, as if "having it all" (in terms of sexual possibilities and experiences) is an inappropriate,

bad thing. Then there is the issue of telling a new dating partner that you are attracted to both men and women. Some new partners may find this reality a distinct "turnoff." The hostility that bisexual persons arouse can provide a real challenge.

For these reasons, numerous college and university counseling centers are expanding their outreach programs to include programs for bisexual students. If you are interested, you might check into the offerings of your campus counseling center to see if they provide educational information, support groups, or specialized counseling for bisexual students. Many campuses also have student groups that focus on gay, lesbian, bisexual, and transgendered students.

Interestingly, it appears that more and more bisexual students are "coming out" despite the challenges they may face. Perhaps this has been encouraged by the public pronouncements of bisexuality by well-known movie stars, such as Drew Barrymore.[3] In the near future, we may find more public acceptance for people who are bisexual. Would you consider increased public acceptance of bisexuality to be a good or bad thing?

1. Hyde JS and DeLamater JD. *Understanding human sexuality,* ed. 8. 2003, McGraw-Hill.
2. Kelly GF. *Sexuality today: the human perspective,* 7th ed. 2004, McGraw-Hill.
3. Celebrity news. *Drew Barrymore: "I am bisexual,"* 17 July 2003, **http://us.imdb.com/wn?20030717#6,** accessed 23 July 2003.

Discovering Your Spirituality

Coming Out—Then What?

If you are openly gay, when you finally told your family and friends about your sexual orientation, a lot of things changed. But one thing probably stayed the same—you still feel like an outsider. Most of the couples holding hands on campus are young men and women. TV sitcoms are centered on heterosexual couples. They may include a gay character, but usually in a minor role. Popular magazines—through their ads, their features, their entire focus—are telling you how to be attractive to the opposite sex.

Being openly gay has probably made you wonder about some of the mixed messages you receive. The person who says it's OK that you're gay also seems to feel sorry for you—because you can't have a "normal" life and enjoy some of the things she does. Your mother makes remarks that suggest she still has hopes that someday you'll marry her best friend's son.

Feeling good about being gay in a straight world doesn't come easily. You've got to work at it. Start by finding support among your gay friends. Knowing that you're not alone is important—especially right after coming out. Realizing that other good, whole people are gay helps to reinforce your self-esteem. Joining a campus gay organization is good for ongoing support, but don't limit yourself to that group. To

grow as an individual, you also need to interact with and be part of heterosexual society.

Focus on what you value about yourself. Are you creative? Someone who gets things accomplished? A dependable friend? Think about the contributions you make—to your family, school, friends, church, and community. Remind yourself that you're a worthy person.

What do your friends appreciate about you? Do they value your advice? Like your sense of humor? Admire your courage? Think you're a strong leader?

Reinforcing the fact that you're a whole, worthy person is up to you. Listen to the "tapes" that are constantly playing in your head—both positive and negative. Edit out the negative thoughts, and turn up the volume on the positive ones. Take charge of what you think about yourself, rather than accepting what others think you are or should be.

TALKING POINTS How would you react if a close family member told you that he or she was gay? How could you be supportive or at least communicate your feelings without anger or criticism?

does not last very long. Passionate love is driven by the excitement of being closely involved with a person whose character is not fully known.

If a relationship progresses, passionate love is gradually replaced by companionate love. This type of love is less emotionally intense than passionate love. It is characterized by friendly affection and a deep attachment that is based on extensive familiarity with the partner. This love is enduring and capable of sustaining long-term, mutual growth. Central to companionate love are feelings of empathy for, support of, and tolerance of the partner. Complete the Personal Assessment on page 393 to determine whether you and your partner are truly compatible.

Recognizing Unhealthy Relationships

Clearly, not all dating relationships will continue. Many couples recognize when a partnership is nearing an end, and they reach a mutual decision to break off the relationship. This is a traditional, natural way for people to learn about their interactions with others. They simply decide to split up and move on.

However, sometimes people do not recognize or heed the warning signs of an unstable relationship, so they stay involved long after the risks outweigh the benefits. These warning signs include abusive behavior, including both emotional and physical abuse (see Chapter 16). Another red flag is excessive jealousy about a partner's interactions with others. Sometimes excessive jealousy evolves into controlling behavior, and one partner attempts to manage the daily activities of the other partner. By definition, controlling behavior limits your creativity and freedom.

Other warning signs are dishonesty, irresponsibility, lack of patience, and any kind of drug abuse. We certainly do not want to see these qualities in those we have initially judged to be "nice people," even though these unappealing characteristics may be obvious to others. If you suspect that any of these problems may be undermining your relationship, talk about your concerns with one or two trusted friends, and seek the advice of a professional counselor at your college or university. Try to realize that ending your relationship might be the best thing you could do for yourself.

 TALKING POINTS Your sister is in an unhealthy relationship but doesn't seem to see the warning signs. How could you alert her to the potential dangers?

Intimacy

When most people hear the word **intimacy,** they immediately think about physical intimacy. They think about shared touching, kissing, and even intercourse. However, sexuality experts and family therapists prefer to view intimacy more broadly, as any close, mutual, verbal or nonverbal behavior within a relationship. In this sense, intimate behavior can range from sharing deep feelings and experiences with a partner to sharing profound physical pleasures with a partner.

Intimacy is present in both love and friendship. You have likely shared intimate feelings with your closest friends, as well as with those you love. Intimacy helps us feel connected to others and allows us to feel the full measure of our own self-worth.

 TALKING POINTS Your teenage son equates intimacy with sex. How would you explain the emotional intimacy involved in marriage?

Lifestyles and Relationships

A variety of informal and formal lifestyles and relationships exist in our society. Here are a few of the most common ones.

> **Key Terms**
>
> **intimacy** any close, mutual, verbal or nonverbal behavior within a relationship.

Singlehood

One lifestyle option for adults is *singlehood.* For many people, being single is a lifestyle that affords the potential for pursuing intimacy, if desired, and provides an uncluttered path for independence and self-directedness. Other people, however, are single because of divorce, separation, death, or the absence of an opportunity to establish a partnership. The U.S. Bureau of the Census indicates that 42% of women and 38% of men over the age of 18 are currently single.[21]

Many different living arrangements are seen among singles. Some single people live alone and choose not to share a household. Other arrangements for singles include cohabitation, periodic cohabitation, singlehood during the week and cohabitation on the weekends or during vacations, or the *platonic* sharing of a household with others. For young adults, large percentages of single men and women live with their parents.

Like habitation arrangements, the sexual intimacy patterns of singles are individually tailored. Some singles practice celibacy, others pursue intimate relationships in a **monogamous** pattern, and others may have multiple partners. As in all interpersonal relationships, including marriage, the levels of commitment are as variable as the people involved.

Cohabitation

Cohabitation, or the sharing of living quarters by unmarried people, represents another alternative to marriage. According to the U.S. Bureau of the Census, the number of unmarried, opposite-gender couples living together tripled between 1980 and 2000, from 1.6 million couples to over 4.8 million couples. The number of reported same-gender couples totaled nearly 600,000 in the year 2000.[21]

Although cohabitation may seem to imply a vision of sexual intimacy between roommates, several forms of shared living arrangements can be viewed as cohabitation. For some couples, cohabitation is only a part-time arrangement for weekends, during summer vacation, or on a variable schedule. In addition, **platonic** cohabitation can exist when a couple shares living quarters but does so without establishing an intimate relationship. Close friends and people of retirement age might be included in a group called *cohabitants.*

How well do cohabitation arrangements fare against marriage partnerships in terms of long-term stability? A recent 2002 report prepared by the CDC's National Center for Health Statistics[22] indicated that unmarried cohabitations are generally less stable than marriages. The probability of a first marriage ending in separation or divorce within 5 years was found to be 20%, but the probability of a premarital cohabitation breaking up

within 5 years was 49%. After 10 years, the probability of a first marriage ending was 33%, compared to 62% for cohabitations.

Gay and Lesbian Partnerships

To believe that adult partnerships are reserved only for heterosexual couples is to avoid reality. In the United States and in many parts of the world, gays and lesbians are forming partnerships that, in many ways, mimic those of heterosexuals. It no longer is unusual to see same-sex men and women openly living together in one household. Gay and lesbian couples buy houses together and share property rights. As businesses restructure their employee benefits packages, gays and lesbians are covering their partners on health care plans and making them beneficiaries on their insurance policies and retirement plans.

A search of the literature will indicate that gay and lesbian partnerships have many of the same characteristics and problems of heterosexual couples.[3] Like straight couples, they struggle with interpersonal issues related to their relationship and their lifestyle. They work to decide how best to juggle their financial resources, their leisure time, and their friends and extended families. If they live together in an apartment or house, they must decide how to divide the household tasks.

If children are present in the household, they must be cared for and nurtured. These children could have come from an adoption, a previous heterosexual relationship, or, in the case of a lesbian couple, from artificial insemination. Research indicates that children raised in lesbian or gay families overwhelmingly grow up with a heterosexual orientation, and are like other children from heterosexual families in terms of their adjustment, mental health, social skills, and peer acceptance.[3]

One area in which gays and lesbians differ from heterosexual couples is in their ability to obtain a legal marriage. This inequity has been the focus of a national

---

Key Terms

monogamous (mo **nog** a mus) paired relationship with one partner.

cohabitation sharing of a residence by two unrelated, unmarried people; living together.

platonic (pluh **ton** ick) close association between two people that does not include a sexual relationship.

debate over same-sex marriage. For an extended discussion about same-sex marriage, turn to the Focus On article on page 389.

Single Parenthood

Unmarried young women becoming pregnant and then becoming single parents is a continuing reality in the United States. A new and significantly different form of single parenthood is, however, also a reality in this country: the planned entry into a single parenthood by older, better educated people, the vast majority of whom are women.

In contrast to the teenaged girl who becomes a single parent through an unwed pregnancy, the more mature woman who desires single parenting has usually planned carefully for the experience. She has explored several important concerns, including questions about how she will become pregnant (with or without the knowledge of a male partner or through artificial insemination), the need for a father figure for the child, the effect of single parenting on her social life, and its effect on her career development. Once these questions have been resolved, no legal barriers stand in the way of her becoming a single parent.

A very large number of women and a growing number of men are becoming single parents through a divorce settlement or separation agreement. Additionally, increasing numbers of single persons are adopting children. In 2000, single women headed up 7.6 million households with children under age 18. In contrast, single men headed up 1.8 million households in 2000 with children under age 18.[21]

A few single parents have been awarded children through adoption. The likelihood of a single person's receiving a child this way is small, but more people have been successful recently in single-parent adoptions.

Marriage

Just as there is no single best way for two people to move through dating and mate selection, marriage is also a variable undertaking. In marriage, two people join their lives in a way that affirms each as an individual and both as a legal pair. Some are able to resolve conflicts constructively (see the Changing for the Better box). However, for a large percentage of couples, the demands of marriage are too rigorous, confining, and demanding. They will find resolution for their dissatisfaction through divorce or extramarital affairs. For most, though, marriage will be an experience that alternates periods of happiness, productivity, and admiration with periods of frustration, unhappiness, and disillusionment with the partner. Each of you who marries will find the experience unique in every regard. The Changing for the Better box on page 386 presents some advice for improving marriage.

Marriage is a form of emotional and legal bonding.

Changing for the Better

Resolving Conflict Through Better Communication

Whenever I have a disagreement with my girlfriend, both of us say hurtful things and end up feeling bad. How can we resolve our conflicts in a positive way?

Here are some successful ways to manage conflict:

- Show mutual respect. Try to remain calm.
- Identify and resolve the real issue.
- Be a good listener.
- Seek areas of agreement.
- Do not interrupt.
- Mutually participate in decision making.
- Be cooperative and specific.
- Focus on the present and future—not the past.
- Don't try to assign blame.
- Say what you are thinking and feeling.
- When talking, use sentences that begin with "I."
- Avoid using sentences that start with "you" or "why."
- Set a time limit for discussing problems.
- Accept responsibility.
- Schedule time together.

Currently, certain trends regarding marriage are evident. The most obvious of these is the age at first marriage. Today men are waiting longer than ever to marry. The average age at first marriage for men is 27 years.[23] In addition, these new husbands are better educated than in the past and are more likely to be established in their careers. Women are also waiting longer to get married and tend to be more educated and career oriented than they were in the past. Recent statistics indicate that the median age at first marriage for women is 25 years.[23]

Marriage still appeals to most adults. Currently, 76% of adults age 18 and older are either married, widowed, or divorced.[23] Thus only about one-quarter of today's adults have not married. Within the last decade, the percentage of adults who have decided not to marry has nearly doubled.

Divorce

Marriages, like many other kinds of interpersonal relationships, can end. Today, marriages—relationships begun with the intent of permanence "until death do us part"—end through divorce nearly as frequently as they continue.

Why should approximately half of marital relationships be so likely to end? Unfortunately, marriage experts cannot provide one clear answer. Rather, they suggest that divorce is a reflection of unfulfilled expectations for marriage on the part of one or both partners, including the following:

- The belief that marriage will ease your need to deal with your own faults and that your failures can be shared by your partner

- The belief that marriage will change faults that you know exist in your partner
- The belief that the high level of romance of your dating and courtship period will be continued through marriage
- The belief that marriage can provide you with an arena for the development of your personal power, and that once married, you will not need to compromise with your partner
- The belief that your marital partner will be successful in meeting all of your needs

If these expectations seem to be ones you anticipate through marriage, then you may find that disappointments will abound. To varying degrees, marriage is a partnership that requires much cooperation and compromise. Marriage can be complicated. Because of the high expectations that many people hold for marriage, the termination of marriage can be an emotionally difficult process to undertake.

Concern is frequently voiced over the well-being of children whose parents divorce. Different factors, however, influence the extent to which divorce affects children. Included among these factors are the gender and age of the children, custody arrangements, financial support, and the remarriage of one or both parents. For many children, adjustments must be made to accept their new status as a member of a blended family.

 TALKING POINTS A couple you know well is going through a divorce. How could you show support for each person without taking sides?

Taking Charge of Your Health

- Take the Personal Assessment on page 391 to understand your sexual attitudes better.
- Use the Personal Assessment on page 393 to find out how compatible you and your partner are.
- If being around someone whose sexual orientation is different from yours makes you feel uncomfortable, focus on getting to know that person better as an individual.
- If you are in an unhealthy relationship, take the first step toward getting out of it through professional counseling or group support.

- If you are in a sexual relationship, communicate your sexual needs to your partner clearly. Encourage him or her to do the same so that you will both have a satisfying sex life.
- Consider whether your lifetime plan will involve marriage, singlehood, or cohabitation. Evaluate your current situation in relation to that plan.

Summary

- Biological and psychosocial factors contribute to the complex expression of our sexuality.
- The structural basis of sexuality begins in the growing embryo and fetus. Structural sexuality changes as one moves through adolescence and later life.
- The psychosocial processes of gender identity, gender preference, and gender adoption form the basis for an initial adult gender identification.
- The complex functioning of the male and female reproductive structures is controlled by hormones.
- The menstrual cycle's primary functions are to produce mature ova and to develop a supportive environment for the fetus in the uterus.

- The sexual response pattern consists of four stages: excitement, plateau, orgasmic, and resolution.
- Three sexual orientations are heterosexuality, homosexuality, and bisexuality.
- Many older people remain interested and active in sexual activities. Physiological changes may alter the way in which some older people perform sexually.
- Abusive behavior, extreme jealousy, controlling behaviors, dishonesty, and drug abuse are warning signs of an unhealthy relationship.
- A variety of lifestyles and relationships exist in our society.
- A large majority of adults will marry at some time.
- Many marriages will end in divorce.

Review Questions

1. Describe the following foundations of our biological sexuality: the genetic basis, the gonadal basis, and structural development.
2. Define and explain the following terms: gender identity, gender preference, gender adoption, initial adult gender identification, and transsexualism.
3. Identify the major components of the male and female reproductive systems. Trace the passageways for sperm and ova.
4. Explain the menstrual cycle. Identify and describe the four main hormones that control the menstrual cycle.

5. What similarities and differences exist between the sexual response patterns of males and females?
6. What is the refractory period?
7. How do myotonia and vasocongestion differ?
8. What are some of the dangers related to anal sex?
9. Approximately what percentage of today's college students report having had sexual intercourse?
10. Explain the differences between heterosexuality, homosexuality, and bisexuality. How common are each of these sexual orientations in our society?

References

1. Thibodeau GA, Patton KT. *Anatomy and physiology,* 5th ed. Mosby, 2003.
2. Sherwood L. *Human physiology: from cells to systems,* 5th ed. Brooks/Cole, 2004.
3. Hyde JS, DeLamater, JD. *Understanding human sexuality,* 8th ed. McGraw-Hill, 2003.
4. Allgeier ER, Allgeier AR. *Sexual interactions,* 5th ed. Houghton Mifflin, 2000.
5. Crooks R, Baur K. *Our sexuality,* 8th ed. Wadsworth, 2001.
6. LeVay S, Valente, SM. *Human sexuality.* Sinauer Associates, Inc., 2003.

7. Kelly GF. *Sexuality today: the human perspective,* 7th ed. McGraw-Hill, 2004.

8. Masters WH, Johnson VE, Kolodny RC. *Human sexuality,* 5th ed. Addison Wesley, 1997.

9. Strong B, DeVault C, Sayad BW, Yarber WL. *Human sexuality: diversity in contemporary America,* 4th ed. McGraw-Hill, 2001.

10. Greenberg JS, Bruess CE, Haffner DW. *Exploring the dimensions of human sexuality: 2002 update.* Jones and Bartlett, 2002.

11. Hatcher RA, et al. *Contraceptive technology,* 17th ed. Ardent Media, 1998.

12. Writing Group for the Women's Health Initiative Investigators. Risks and benefits of estrogen plus progestin in healthy postmenopausal women: principal results from the Women's Health Initiative Randomized Controlled Trial. *Journal of the American Medical Association,* Vol 288: No 3 (July 17, 2002), 321–333.

13. Hormone therapy is no heart helper. *Harvard Heart Letter,* Vol 13: No 2 (October 2002), 2–4.

14. Masters W, Johnson V. *Human sexual response.* Lippincott, Williams and Wilkins, 1966.

15. Bruess CE, Haffner DW, Greenberg JS. *Exploring the dimensions of human sexuality, 2002 update.* Jones and Bartlett, 2002.

16. Baldwin JI, Baldwin JD. Heterosexual anal intercourse: an understudied, high-risk sexual behavior. *Archives of Sexual Behavior* 29(4), 357–373, 2000.

17. *Supreme Court strikes down Texas sodomy law,* **www.cnn.com/2003/LAW/06/26/scotus.sodomy/index/html,** (June 27, 2003), accessed July 22, 2003.

18. Kinsey AC, Pomeroy WB, Martin CE. *Sexual behavior in the human male,* reprint edition. Indiana University Press, 1998.

19. Kinsey AC, et al. *Sexual behavior in the human female,* reprint edition. Indiana University Press, 1998.

20. Allen LS, Gorski RA. Sexual orientation and the size of the anterior commissure in the human brain. *Pract Nat Acad Sci USA* 89(15): 7199–7202, 1992.

21. U.S. Bureau of the Census. *Statistical abstract of the United States: 2002,* ed. 122. U.S. Government Printing Office, 2002.

22. Bramlett MD, Mosher WD. *Cohabitation, marriage, divorce, and remarriage in the United States.* U.S. Centers for Disease Control and Prevention, National Center for Health Statistics, Vital Health Statistics, 23(22), 2002.

23. Fields J, Casper LM. America's families and living arrangements: March 2000. *Current Population Reports* (U.S. Census Bureau) P20–537, p. 9, 2001.

As We Go to Press

Questions concerning "when life begins" have been debated for many years. This chapter has provided much technical information concerning the biological underpinnings of human life. *As we go to press,* President Bush signed the April 2004 federal law called the Unborn Victims of Violence Act or UVVA. This law provides penalties for anyone convicted of harming a fetus while committing certain federal crimes, such as participating in a terrorist attack or a drug-related shooting.

The significance of this bill cannot be underestimated. In effect, the UVVA recognizes that a fertilized egg, embryo, or fetus has separate legal status from the pregnant women. Opponents of this bill claim that its ultimate intention is to undermine the 1973 Supreme Court *Roe v. Wade* decision and elevate the legal status of a fetus to give it separate legal rights as a person. This recognition could eventually pave the way for a reversal of *Roe v. Wade.*

Proponents of the bill believe that an assault on a pregnant woman harms two victims and should result in two offenses against the perpetrator. It will be interesting to see how frequently federal prosecutors will attempt to enforce this law and whether its application will ever form the basis of an attempt to overthrow *Roe v. Wade.* What's your prediction about the impact of this new federal law?

same-sex marriages

What is the definition of a marriage? Must the marriage partners be only a man and a woman? Would allowing same-sex marriages weaken our society? Or would it make for a stronger society that is capable of recognizing commitments that legally bond men with men and women with women? These questions are being debated now on a scale that could not have been predicted even 5 years ago.

Same-sex marriages would grant gay couples an array of legal and economic benefits, including joint parental custody, insurance and health benefits, joint tax returns, alimony and child support, inheritance of property, hospital visitation rights, family leave, and a spouse's Social Security and retirement benefits.

Same-sex unions have been debated for many years. Some U.S. clergy were presiding over gay "marriages" in the 1980s, and hundreds of companies, businesses, associations, and universities now offer benefits to same-sex partners of employees. Gay publications debated the subject in the 1950s. In his book *Same-Sex Unions in Premodern Europe,* the late John Boswell, a Yale University historian, suggested that ancient marriage ceremonies provide evidence that Greeks and medieval Christians celebrated same-sex relationships.[1]

The year 2000 became a defining year in the debate over same-sex marriages. In April 2000, the Vermont legislature passed the nation's first "civil union" law, which granted legal status to gay and lesbian couples. The law was signed into effect on July 1, 2000. By October 2000, the Health Department in Vermont had registered over 800 civil unions, with three-quarters of the couples coming from out-of-state.[2] This trend has continued since the law has been in effect. By the summer of 2003, 85% of Vermont's civil unions were granted to out-of-state couples.[3]

Legalization of same-sex marriage would grant gay couples a wide range of legal and economic rights.

The law permits same-sex couples to obtain civil union licenses from the town clerk, similar to the way opposite-sex couples obtain marriage licenses. A judge, justice of the peace, or clergy member certifies the civil unions. Divorces between civil union partners are called "dissolutions" and are handled in family court, similar to opposite-sex divorces.[4]

Vermont's law confers on same-sex couples all the benefits that the state presently allows heterosexual married couples. However, Vermont's law does not affect federal programs, such as Social Security. Additionally, civil unions that take place in Vermont are not generally recognized by other states. In fact thirty seven states and the federal government have passed laws that deny the recognition of gay and lesbian marriages. These laws are called Defense of Marriage Acts (DOMAs) and define marriage as the union of one man with one woman.[5]

By the summer of 2003, legal issues concerning same-sex marriage were making weekly headlines, not just in America, but in countries the world over. After the Canadian provinces of British Columbia and Ontario passed laws permitting same-sex marriage in June, the Canadian federal government put forth national legislation that was expected to make same-sex marriages available in all of Canada sometime in 2004.[6] If this were to happen, Canada would be following the path set by Germany (in 2001),[7] Holland (in 2001), and Belgium (in January 2003).[8]

In the United States, a State Supreme Court ruling in Massachusetts was expected in late summer 2003 in a case (*Goodridge v Department of Public Health*) in which seven gay and lesbian couples sued to have Massachusetts expand the definition of marriage to include same-sex couples. Another same-sex marriage suit was pending in New Jersey. While efforts to promote same-sex marriages in Hawaii and Alaska were unsuccessful, the California legislature was in the process of broadening the definition of domestic partnerships to include committed gay and lesbian couples. Such legislation, if passed, would grant to same-sex couples about one-third of the "rights, privileges, and obligations that the state automatically grants to married couples."[8]

Opponents of same-sex marriage were concerned that a June 2003 U.S. Supreme Court ruling (*Lawrence and Garner v Texas*) which struck down a Texas sodomy law banning private consensual sex between same-sex adults would open the door, eventually, for gay and lesbian marriages. The ruling effectively overturned similar sodomy laws that were still on the books in twelve other states.[9] At the time of this writing, efforts were underway among some members of the U.S. Congress to draft a constitutional amendment banning gay marriage. While President Bush was somewhat reluctant to support such an amendment, he did "support the notion that marriage is between a man and a woman."[10]

The July 2003 release of a Vatican document calling for Catholic politicians worldwide to oppose same-sex unions and marriages further added to the explosive nature of this debate. Political observers believe that this issue will be highly prominent in the 2004 political elections in the United States, perhaps on a par with issues involving the economy, foreign policy, and military capability. Indeed, politicians can expect to be asked where they stand on the issue of same-sex marriages.

Activists on both sides of this issue believe that this may be the greatest gay rights debate in history. Where do you stand on this issue? Should gay partners be granted the same legal right to marriage as heterosexual couples, or do you believe that legal marriage should be limited to its traditional definition of a union between a man and a woman?

References:

1. Boswell J. *Same-sex unions in pre-modern Europe,* reprint ed. Vintage Books, 1994.
2. *Civil unions are legal in Vermont.* **www.gaycivilunions.com,** accessed 2 December 2000.
3. Grossman J. *Will other states recognize Vermont's civil unions?* **www.cnn. com/2003/law/05/20/findlaw. analysis.grossman.civilunions.txt/,** 20 May 2003, accessed 22 July 2003.
4. *The Vermont Guide to Civil Unions.* **www.sec.state.vt.us/pubs/ civilunions.html,** accessed 2 December 2000.
5. *FRC ready to respond to historic 'gay marriage' decision in Massachusetts,* media advisory, Family Research Council, **www.frc.org.org/?I= PR03G03,** 10 July 2003, accessed 22 July 2003.
6. Schneider B. *Canada acts on same-sex marriages,* **www.cnn.com/2003/ allpolitics/06/20/ip.pol.opinion. canada.marriages/index.html,** 20 June 2003, accessed 22 July 2003.
7. *German gay marriage law backed.* **www.cnn.com/2002/world/europe/ 07/17/germany.marriage/index.html,** 17 July 2002, accessed 22 July 2003.
8. *Overview: same-sex marriages,* **www.religioustolerance.com/hom_ marr.htm,** accessed 22 July 2003.
9. *Supreme Court strikes down Texas sodomy law,* **www.cnn.com/2003/law/ 06/26/scotus.sodomy/index.html,** 27 June 2003, accessed 22 July 2003.
10. *Bush uncertain about gay marriage ban,* **www.cnn.com/2003/allpolitics/ 07/02/bush.gay/index.html,** 2 July 2003, accessed 22 July 2003.

personal assessment

sexual attitudes: a matter of feelings

Respond to each of the following statements by selecting a numbered response (1–5) that most accurately reflects your feelings. Circle the number of your selection. At the end of the questionnaire, total these numbers for use in interpreting your responses.

1 Agree strongly
2 Agree moderately
3 Uncertain
4 Disagree moderately
5 Disagree strongly

Men and women have greater differences than they have similarities.	1	2	3	4	5
Homosexuality and bisexuality are immoral and unnatural.	1	2	3	4	5
Our society is too sexually oriented.	1	2	3	4	5
Pornography encourages sexual promiscuity.	1	2	3	4	5
Children know far too much about sex.	1	2	3	4	5
Education about sexuality is solely the responsibility of the family.	1	2	3	4	5
Dating begins far too early in our society.	1	2	3	4	5
Sexual intimacy before marriage leads to emotional stress and damage to one's reputation.	1	2	3	4	5
Sexual availability is far too frequently the reason that people marry.	1	2	3	4	5
Reproduction is the most important reason for sexual intimacy during marriage.	1	2	3	4	5
Modern families are too small.	1	2	3	4	5

Family planning clinics should not receive public funds.	1	2	3	4	5
Contraception is the woman's responsibility.	1	2	3	4	5
Abortion is the murder of an innocent child.	1	2	3	4	5
Marriage has been weakened by the changing role of women in society.	1	2	3	4	5
Divorce is an unacceptable means of resolving marital difficulties.	1	2	3	4	5
Extramarital sexual intimacy will destroy a marriage.	1	2	3	4	5
Sexual abuse of a child does not generally occur unless the child encourages the adult.	1	2	3	4	5
Provocative behavior by the woman is a factor in almost every case of rape.	1	2	3	4	5
Reproduction is not a right but a privilege.	1	2	3	4	5

YOUR TOTAL POINTS _____

Interpretation

20–34 points	A very traditional attitude toward sexuality
35–54 points	A moderately traditional attitude toward sexuality
55–65 points	A rather ambivalent attitude toward sexuality
66–85 points	A moderately nontraditional attitude toward sexuality
86–100 points	A very nontraditional attitude toward sexuality

To Carry This Further . . .

Were you surprised at your results? Compare your results with those of a roommate or close friend. How do you think your parents would score on this assessment?

personal assessment

how Compatible are you?

This quiz will help test how compatible you and your partner's personalities are. You should each rate the truth of these twenty statements based on the following scale. Circle the number that reflects your feelings. Total your scores and check the interpretation following the quiz.

1 Never true
2 Sometimes true
3 Frequently true
4 Always true

We can communicate our innermost thoughts effectively.	1	2	3	4
We trust each other.	1	2	3	4
We agree on whose needs come first.	1	2	3	4
We have realistic expectations of each other and of ourselves.	1	2	3	4
Individual growth is important within our relationship.	1	2	3	4
We will go on as a couple even if our partner doesn't change.	1	2	3	4
Our personal problems are discussed with each other first.	1	2	3	4
We both do our best to compromise.	1	2	3	4
We usually fight fairly.	1	2	3	4
We try not to be rigid or unyielding.	1	2	3	4
We keep any needs to be "perfect" in proper perspective.	1	2	3	4
We can balance desires to be sociable and the need to be alone.	1	2	3	4
We both make friends and keep them.	1	2	3	4
Neither of us stays down or up for long periods.	1	2	3	4
We can tolerate the other's mood without being affected by it.	1	2	3	4
We can deal with disappointment and disillusionment.	1	2	3	4
Both of us can tolerate failure.	1	2	3	4
We can both express anger appropriately.	1	2	3	4
We are both assertive when necessary.	1	2	3	4
We agree on how our personal surroundings are kept.	1	2	3	4

YOUR TOTAL POINTS _____

Interpretation

20–35 points	You and your partner seem quite incompatible. Professional help may open your lines of communication.
36–55 points	You probably need more awareness and compromise.
56–70 points	You are highly compatible. However, be aware of the areas where you can improve.
71–80 points	Your relationship is very fulfilling.

To Carry This Further . . .

Ask your partner to take this test too. You may have a one-sided view of a "perfect" relationship. Even if you scored high on this assessment, be aware of areas where you can still improve.

chapter fourteen

managing your fertility

Talking It Over

Choosing a Childless Lifestyle

There are many reasons a couple may choose not to have children. Here are some of the advantages and disadvantages:

Pros:

- more time for travel or work
- spontaneity remains possible
- uninterrupted privacy and intimacy
- easier to leave a bad relationship
- no contribution to overpopulation
- no worries of raising a child in a dangerous world
- less financial burden

Cons:

- possible regret over decision in the future
- feelings of selfishness and guilt

- no child/parent intimacy
- aloneness in old age
- no heirs
- no grandchildren for you or your parents
- loss of friends your own age who are parents

Can you think of other reasons for choosing to remain childless?

CommunicationLinks

www.now2000.com/cbc
www.childfree.com.au/
www.nokidding.net/

Eye on the Media

Information Online—Birth Control and Sexuality

The Internet offers a number of resources for locating information about contraception, birth control, and related topics. Planned Parenthood Federation of America provides one of the most comprehensive sites at **www.plannedparenthood.org.** Here you can find a wide selection of pamphlets, books, newsletters, and videotapes, as well as links to other websites.

If you're looking for birth control information, click on Planned Parenthood's "Frequently Asked Questions," "Health Info,"

"Fact Sheets," "Sexual Health Glossary," and "Links." Some of the frequently asked questions are:

- Am I pregnant?
- What can I do if I am pregnant?
- Do I have a sexually transmitted disease?
- What are the laws in my state about teens' access to abortion services and birth control?
- How can I get access to birth control?

Of course, answers follow each of these questions. Planned Parenthood believes that when people are empowered with knowledge, they are better able to make sound decisions about their health and sexuality.

The "Fact Sheets" option at Planned Parenthood's website provides various reports on specific topics, such as abortion, birth control, family planning, sexually transmitted diseases, and teen pregnancy and abortion. The "Sexual Health Glossary" is a listing of hundreds of terms related to sexuality. The "Links" option lists twenty-five topical categories, each one displaying links to related websites.

Three additional online sites offer reliable information about sexuality and reproductive choices. The first is the Alan Guttmacher Institute website at **www.agi-usa.org.** This institute is dedicated to protecting the reproductive choices of women and men throughout the world. It fulfills its mission by disseminating information and the results of scientific research on the subject. The Guttmacher Institute's menu of options includes abortion, law and public policy, pregnancy and birth, prevention and contraception, sexual behavior, and sexually transmitted diseases and youth.

The American Social Health Association's website is **www.ashastd.org.** This organization is dedicated to stopping the spread of sexually transmitted diseases. ASHA operates a network of national hotlines that answers over 2 million calls each year. The website's menu offers selections on sexually transmitted diseases, frequently asked questions, a sexual health glossary, and support groups.

The Sex Information and Education Council of the United States is a nonprofit organization dedicated to developing, collecting, and disseminating information about sexuality. SIECUS has its website at **www.siecus.org.** This organization promotes comprehensive sexuality education and advocates the right of individuals to make responsible sexual choices. SIECUS publishes and distributes thousands of pamphlets, booklets, and bibliographies each year to professionals and the general public.

If you wish to search for information about certain sexuality topics from a pro-life perspective, you might wish to examine the website for The Ultimate Pro-life Resource List at **www.prolifeinfo.org.** This site is supported by the non-profit Women and Children First organization. The Ultimate Pro-life Resource List provides links to information related to abortion alternatives, Roe vs. Wade, euthanasia and assisted suicide, pregnancy help, pro-life news and pro-life organizations.

How you decide to control your **fertility** will have an important effect on your future. Your understanding of information and issues related to fertility control will help you make responsible decisions in this complex area.

For traditional-age students, these decisions may be fast approaching (see Discovering Your Spirituality on page 397 for a discussion of decision making about sex and the spiritual dimension of sexuality). Frequently, nontraditional students are parents who have had experiences that make them useful resources for other students in the class.

Birth Control vs. Contraception

Any discussion about the control of your fertility should start with an explanation of the subtle differences between the terms **birth control** and **contraception.** Although many people use the words interchangeably, they reflect different perspectives about fertility control. *Birth control* is an umbrella term that refers to all of the procedures you might use to prevent the birth of a child. Birth control includes all available contraceptive measures, as well as all sterilization, and abortion procedures.

Contraception is a much more specific term for any procedure used to prevent the fertilization of an ovum. Contraceptive measures vary widely in the mechanisms they use to accomplish this task. They also vary considerably in their method of use and their rate of success in preventing conception. A few examples of contraceptive methods are the use of condoms, oral contraceptives, spermicides, and diaphragms.

Beyond the numerous methods mentioned, certain forms of sexual behavior not involving intercourse could be considered forms of contraception. For example, mutual masturbation by couples virtually eliminates the possibility of pregnancy. This practice, as well as additional forms of sexual expression other than intercourse (such as

> **Key Terms**
>
> **fertility** the ability to reproduce.
>
> **birth control** all of the methods and procedures that can prevent the birth of a child.
>
> **contraception** any method or procedure that prevents fertilization.

There's More to Sex than You Thought . . .

Are you ready for sex? If you're not sure, take time to think it over. If you start having sex before you're ready, you might feel guilty. You might feel bad because you realize this step isn't right for you now. Or your religious upbringing may make you feel as though you're doing something wrong. You also may not be ready for the emotional aspects of a sexual relationship. Most important, you will probably have difficulty handling the complexities of an unplanned pregnancy or a sexually transmitted disease.

If you do feel ready for sex, you still have a choice. Sex may be OK for you now. It may be personally fulfilling, something that enhances your self-esteem. Alternatively, you can choose to abstain from sex until later—another way of enhancing your self-esteem. You'll feel empowered by making the decision for yourself, rather than doing what is expected. Being strong enough to say "no" can also make you feel good about yourself. For some, making this decision may reflect a renewed commitment to spiritual or religious concerns.

If you're married, sex is a good way of connecting as a couple. It's something that the two of you alone share. It's a time to give special attention to each other—taking a break from the kids, your jobs, and your other responsibilities. It's a way of saying: "This relationship is important—it's something I value."

Going through a pregnancy together is another opportunity for closeness. From the moment you know that you're going to be parents, you're connected in a new way. Your focus becomes the expected child. You'll watch the fetus grow on ultrasound, go to parenting and Lamaze classes together, visit the doctor together, mark the various milestones, and share new emotions. When your child is born, you'll be connected as never before.

Whether you're thinking about starting to have sex, making the decision to wait, or examining the sexual life you have now, you can't ignore the possibilities and the consequences. Is the time right for you? Are you doing this for yourself or for someone else? What do you think you will gain from waiting? Do you expect your future partner to also have made the decision to wait? What do you expect to get from a sexual relationship—pleasure, intimacy, love? What do you expect to give? Do you want an emotional commitment? Do you view sex and love as inseparable? Do you understand how sex can enhance your spirituality? Taking time to consider these questions can make you feel good about yourself—no matter what you decide.

---

kissing, touching, and massage), has been given the generic term **outercourse.** Not only does outercourse protect against unplanned pregnancy, it may also significantly reduce the transmission of sexually transmitted diseases (STDs), including HIV infection.

Theoretical Effectiveness vs. Use Effectiveness

People considering the use of a contraceptive method need to understand the difference between the two effectiveness rates given for each form of contraception. *Theoretical effectiveness* is a measure of a contraceptive method's ability to prevent a pregnancy when the method is used precisely as directed during every act of intercourse. *Use effectiveness,* however, refers to the effectiveness of a method in preventing conception when used by the general public. Use effectiveness rates take into account factors that lower effectiveness below that based on "perfect" use. Failure to follow proper instructions, illness of the user, forgetfulness, physician (or pharmacist) error, and a subconscious desire to experience risk or even pregnancy are a few of the factors that can lower the effectiveness of even the most theoretically effective contraceptive technique.

Effectiveness rates are often expressed in terms of the percentage of women users of childbearing age who do not become pregnant while using the method for 1 year. For some methods the theoretical- and use-effectiveness rates are vastly different; the theoretical rate is always higher than the use rate. Table 14.1 presents data concerning effectiveness rates, advantages, and disadvantages of many birth control methods.

Selecting Your Contraceptive Method

In this section, we discuss some of the many factors that should be important to you as you consider selecting a contraceptive method. Remember that no method possesses equally high marks in all of the following areas. It is important that you and your partner select a contraceptive method that is both acceptable and effective, as determined by your unique needs and

Key Terms
outercourse sexual activity that does not involve intercourse.

Table 14.1 Effectiveness Rates of Birth Control for 100 Women during 1 Year of Use

Method	Estimated Effectiveness		Advantages	Disadvantages
	Theoretical	**Use**		
No method (chance)	15%	15%	Inexpensive	Totally ineffective
Withdrawal	96%	81%	No supplies or advance preparation needed; no side effects; men share responsibility for family planning	Interferes with coitus; very difficult to use effectively; women must trust men to withdraw as orgasm approaches
Periodic abstinence Calendar Basal body temperature Cervical mucus method Symptothermal	91%–99%	75%	No supplies needed; no side effects; men share responsibility for family planning; women learn about their bodies	Difficult to use, especially if menstrual cycles are irregular, as is common in young women; abstinence may be necessary for long periods; lengthy instruction and ongoing counseling may be needed
Cervical cap (no prior births)	91%	80%	No health risks; helps protect against some STDs and cervical cancer	Limited availability in some areas
Spermicide (gel, foam, suppository, film)	94%	74%	No health risks; helps protect against some STDs; can be used with condoms to increase effectiveness considerably	Must be inserted 5 to 30 minutes before coitus; effective for only 30 to 60 minutes; some concern about nonoxynol-9
Diaphragm with spermicide	94%	80%	No health risks; helps protect against some STDs and cervical cancer	Must be inserted with jelly or foam before every act of coitus and left in place for at least 6 hours after coitus; must be fitted by health care personnel; some women may find it awkward or embarrassing to use; some concern about nonoxynol-9
Male condom Male condom with spermicide	97% 99%	86% 95%	Easy to use; inexpensive and easy to obtain; no health risks; very effective protection against some STDs; men share responsibility for family planning	Must be put on just before coitus; some men and women complain of decreased sensation; some concern about nonoxynol-9
Female condom	95%	79%	Relatively easy to use; no prescription required; polyurethane is stronger than latex; provides some STD protection; silicone-based lubrication provided; useful when male will not use a condom	Contraceptive effectiveness and STD protection not as high as with male condom; couples may be unfamiliar with a device that extends outside the vagina; more expensive than male condoms
IUD ParaGard Progestasert Mirena	 99%+ 98% 99%	 99%+ 98% ?	Easy to use; highly effective in preventing pregnancy; does not interfere with coitus; repeated action not needed; depending on the device, can be effective for 1, 5 or 10 years	May increase risk of pelvic inflammatory disease (PID) and infertility in women with more than one sexual partner; not usually recommended for women who have never had a child; must be inserted by health care personnel; may cause heavy bleeding and pain in some women
Contraceptive ring (estrogen-progestin)	99%+	n/a	Easy to use after learning how to insert; remains in place for 3 weeks	Like other hormonal methods, does not protect against STDs; requires a physician's prescription; possibility of CV problems in a small percentage of users
Contraceptive patch	99%+	n/a	Easy to apply; must be changed weekly for 3 weeks	(Same as above)
Combined pill	99%+	95%	Easy to use; highly effective in preventing pregnancy; does not interfere with coitus; regulates menstrual cycle; reduces heavy bleeding and menstrual pain; helps protect against ovarian and endometrial cancer	Must be taken every day; requires medical examination and prescription; minor side effects such as nausea or menstrual spotting; possibility of CV problems, in a small percentage of users
Minipill (progestin only)	99%+	95%		
Depo-Provera (3 month)	99%+	99%+	Easy to use; highly effective for an extended period; continued use prevents menstruation	Requires supervision by a physician; administered by injection; some women experience irregular menstrual spotting and weight gain in early months of use
Tubal ligation	99%+	99%+	Permanent; removes fear of pregnancy	Surgery-related risks; generally considered irreversible
Vasectomy	99%+	99%+	Permanent; removes fear of pregnancy	Generally considered irreversible

Adapted from Hatcher RA et al: *Contraceptive Technology*, 17th rev. ed, 1998. Ardent Media, Inc.

expectations. Completing the Personal Assessment on page 427 will help you make this decision.

For a contraceptive method to be acceptable to those who wish to exercise a large measure of control over their fertility, the following should be given careful consideration:

- *It should be safe.* The contraceptive approach you select should not pose a significant health risk for you or your partner.
- *It should be effective.* Your approach must have a high success rate in preventing pregnancy.
- *It should be reliable.* The form you select must be able to be used over and over again with consistent success.
- *It should be reversible.* Couples who eventually want to have a family should select a method that can be reversed.
- *It should be affordable.* The cost of a particular method must fit comfortably into a couple's budget.
- *It should be easy to use.* Complicated instructions or procedures can make a method difficult to use effectively.
- *It should not interfere with sexual expression.* An ideal contraceptive fits in comfortably with a couple's intimate sexual behavior.

 TALKING POINTS The method of birth control your partner prefers doesn't allow for spontaneous sex. How would you explain that this decreases your enjoyment?

Current Birth Control Methods

Withdrawal

Withdrawal, or **coitus interruptus,** is the contraceptive practice in which the erect penis is removed from the vagina just before ejaculation of semen. Theoretically this procedure prevents sperm from entering the deeper structures of the female reproductive system. The use effectiveness of this method, however, reflects how unsuccessful this method is in practice (see Table 14.1).

There is strong evidence to suggest that the clear preejaculate fluid that helps neutralize and lubricate the male urethra can contain *viable* (capable of fertilization) sperm.[1] This sperm can be deposited near the cervical opening before withdrawal of the penis. This phenomenon may in part explain the relatively low effectiveness of this method. Furthermore, withdrawal does not protect users from the transmission of STDs.

Periodic Abstinence

There are four approaches included in the birth control strategy called **periodic abstinence:** (1) the calendar method, (2) the basal body temperature (BBT) method, (3) the Billings cervical mucus method, and (4) the symptothermal method.[2] All four methods attempt to determine the time a woman ovulates. Figure 14-1 shows a day-to-day fertility calendar used to estimate fertile periods. Most research indicates that an ovum is viable for only about 24 to 36 hours after its release from the ovary. (Once inside the female reproductive tract, some sperm can survive up to a week.)

When a woman can accurately determine when she ovulates, she must refrain from intercourse long enough for the ovum to begin to disintegrate. Of course, some couples are trying to become pregnant, and their goal will be to find the most fertile days that unprotected intercourse could produce a pregnancy.

Fertility awareness, rhythm, natural birth control, and *natural family planning* are terms interchangeable with periodic abstinence. Remember that periodic abstinence methods *do not* provide protection against the spread of STDs and HIV infection.

Periodic abstinence is the only acceptable method endorsed by the Roman Catholic Church. For some people who have deep concerns for the spiritual dimensions of their health, the selection of a contraceptive

Key Terms

withdrawal (coitus interruptus) a contraceptive practice in which the erect penis is removed from the vagina before ejaculation.

periodic abstinence birth control methods that rely on a couple's avoidance of intercourse during the ovulatory phase of a woman's menstrual cycle; also called *fertility awareness, rhythm,* or *natural family planning.*

Figure 14-1 Periodic abstinence (fertility awareness or natural family planning) can combine use of the calendar, basal body temperature measurements, and Billings mucus techniques to identify the fertile period. Remember that most women's cycles are not consistently perfect 28-day cycles, as shown in most illustrations.

Days of menstrual cycle

1
2
3
4
5
6
7
8
9
10
11
12
13
14
15
16
17
18
19
20
21
22
23
24
25
26
27
28

Menstruation—relatively safe for sexual intercourse

Sperm deposited during these days may remain viable at ovulation

Unprotected intercourse should not occur

Ovulation

Unprotected intercourse should not occur

Ovum may remain viable through this point

Relatively safe for unprotected intercourse

method other than periodic abstinence may indicate a serious compromise of beliefs.

The **calendar method** requires close examination of a woman's menstrual cycle for at least eight cycles. Records are kept of the length (in days) of each cycle. A *cycle* is defined as the number of days from the first day of menstrual flow in one cycle to the first day of menstrual flow in the next cycle.

To determine the days she should abstain from intercourse, a woman should subtract 18 from her shortest cycle; this is the first day she should abstain from intercourse in an upcoming cycle. Then she should subtract 11 from her longest cycle; this is the last day she must abstain from intercourse in an upcoming cycle.[3]

The *basal body temperature method* requires a woman (for about 3 or 4 successive months) to take her body temperature every morning before she rises from bed. A finely calibrated thermometer, available in many drugstores, is used for this purpose. The theory behind this method is that a distinct correlation exists between body temperature and the process of ovulation. Just before ovulation, the body temperature supposedly dips and then rises about 0.5° to 1.0° F for the rest of the cycle. The

woman is instructed to refrain from intercourse during the interval when the temperature change takes place.

Drawbacks of this procedure include the need for consistent, accurate readings and the realization that all women's bodies are different. Some women may not fit the temperature pattern projection because of biochemical differences in their bodies. Also, body temperatures can fluctuate because of a wide variety of illnesses and physical stressors. Temperature kits are available in drugstores and cost about $10.

The *Billings cervical mucus method* is another periodic abstinence technique. Generally used with other periodic abstinence techniques, this method requires a woman to evaluate the daily mucous discharge from her

---

Key Terms

calendar method a form of periodic abstinence in which the variable lengths of a woman's menstrual cycle are used to calculate her fertile period.

Vaginal Contraceptive Film

A unique spermicide delivery system developed in England is vaginal contraceptive film (VCF). Vaginal contraceptive film is a sheet containing nonoxynol-9 that is inserted over the cervical opening. Shortly after insertion of the VCF, it dissolves into a gel-like material that clings to the cervical opening. The VCF can be inserted up to an hour before intercourse. Over the course of several hours, the material will be washed from the vagina in the normal vaginal secretions.

This spermicide is a nonprescription form of contraception that is as effective as other spermicidal foams and gels. Users should be aware that the nonoxynol-9 spermicide may not be as effective against STDs as was formerly thought. A box of 12 sheets costs about $12.

Vaginal contraceptive film.

cervix. Users of this method become familiar with the changes in both appearance (from clear to cloudy) and consistency (from watery to thick) of their cervical mucus throughout their cycles. Women are taught that the unsafe days are when the mucus becomes clear and is the consistency of raw egg whites. Such a technique of ovulation determination must be learned from a physician or family planning professional.

The *symptothermal method* of periodic abstinence combines the use of the BBT method and the cervical mucus method.[3] Couples using the symptothermal method are already using a calendar to chart the woman's body changes. Thus some family planning professionals consider the symptothermal method a combination of all of the periodic abstinence approaches.

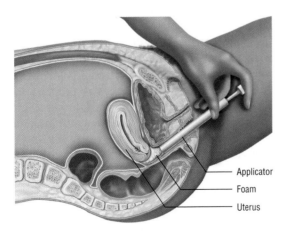

Applicator
Foam
Uterus

Figure 14-2 Spermicidal foams, gels, and suppositories are placed deep into the vagina in the region of the cervix no longer than 30 minutes before intercourse.

Vaginal Spermicides

Spermicides are agents that are capable of killing sperm. When used alone, they offer a moderately effective form of contraception for the woman who is sexually active on an infrequent basis. Modern spermicides are generally safe (but see precaution below), reversible forms of contraception that can be obtained without a physician's prescription in most drugstores and supermarkets. Spermicides are relatively inexpensive. Applicator kits cost about $8 and refills cost around $4 to $8 (Figure 14-2).

Spermicides, which are available in foam, cream, jelly, film, or suppository form, are made of water-soluble bases with a spermicidal agent in the base. Spermicides are commonly used with other contraceptives, such as diaphragms, cervical caps, and condoms.

Spermicides are not specific to sperm cells; they also attack other cells. Until recently, nonoxynol-9, the most commonly used spermicidal agent, was thought to protect women from developing **pelvic inflammatory disease (PID).** Health professionals believed that nonoxynol-9 provided this protection by attacking and killing pathogens which caused various STDs.

Key Terms
spermicides chemicals capable of killing sperm.
pelvic inflammatory disease (PID) a generalized infection of the pelvic cavity that results from the spread of an infection through a woman's reproductive structures.

However, the latest research indicates that nonoxynol-9 is not very effective in killing other pathogens. Nonoxynol-9 may actually *increase* the likelihood of disease transmission, including HIV transmission, because it can cause skin irritations and abrasions in a small percentage of users.[4] These irritated areas and abrasions can provide the avenue for passage into the bloodstream.

For this reason, couples should not depend on vaginal spermicides to stop the spread of infections from person to person. Condoms, when used consistently and correctly, provide much better disease protection and contraceptive effect than spermicides used alone. The latest research also indicates that condoms coated with nonoxynol-9 do not have enough of the spermicide to serve as a back-up contraceptive if the condom breaks.[5] Thus, some health centers and family planning agencies have stopped distributing condoms with nonoxynol-9 in the lubricant. If you and/or your partner have concerns about your use of spermicides, you should seek advice from your physician or health center.

Condoms

Colored or natural, smooth or textured, straight or shaped, plain or reservoir-tipped, dry or lubricated—the latex condom is approaching an art form. This is perhaps an exaggeration. Still, the familiar **condom** remains a safe, effective, reversible contraceptive device. All condoms manufactured in the United States must be approved by the FDA.[6]

For couples who are highly motivated in their desire to prevent a pregnancy, the effectiveness of a condom can approach that of an oral contraceptive—especially if condom use is combined with a spermicide. For couples who are less motivated, the condom can be considerably less effective.

The condom offers substantial protection against STDs. For both the man and the woman, chlamydial infections, gonorrhea, HIV infection, and other STDs are less likely to be acquired when the condom is used correctly

Female condom.

(see the Changing for the Better box on page 403). Some lubricated condoms also contain a spermicide. However, recent research indicates that the use of the spermicide nonoxynol-9 may irritate tissues in some users and actually increase the likelihood of disease transmission.[5] Also, the small amount of spermicide present in the condom's lubricant is not enough to consistently prevent conception if the condom should break. Current recommendations are to use dry condoms or lubricated condoms without spermicide. Also, any additional lubricants used should be water-based lubricants.

The FDA has approved both male and female types of polyurethane condoms. At the time of this writing, at least three brands of polyurethane male condoms and one female condom (Reality) are available as one-time-use condoms.[3] These condoms are good alternatives for people who have an allergic sensitivity to latex estimated to be up to 7% of the population.[7] Also, they are thinner and stronger than latex condoms and can be used with oil-based lubricants. Currently, these condoms are believed to provide protection against STDs that is close to that of latex condoms. The contraceptive effectiveness of polyurethane condoms remains somewhat less than that of the male latex condom.[8,9]

The Reality female condom is a soft, loose-fitting polyurethane sheath containing two polyurethane rings (see photo). Reality is inserted like a diaphragm to line the inner walls of the vagina. The larger ring remains outside the vagina, and the external portion of the condom provides some protection to the labia and the base of the penis. Reality is coated on the inside with a silicone-based lubricant. Additional lubricant is provided for the outside

Male condoms.

Key Terms

condom a latex shield designed to cover the erect penis and retain semen on ejaculation; "rubber."

Putting on a condom seems so easy. Is there anything else I need to know about condom use?

These simple directions for using condoms correctly, in combination with your motivation and commitment to regular use, should provide you with reasonable protection:

- Keep a supply of condoms at hand. Condoms should be stored in a cool, dry place so that they are readily available at the time of intercourse. Condoms that are stored in wallets or automobile glove compartments may not be in satisfactory condition when they are used. Temperature extremes are to be avoided. Check the condom package for the expiration date.
- Do not test a condom by inflating or stretching it. Handle it gently and keep it away from sharp fingernails.
- For maximum effectiveness, put the condom on before genital contact. Either the man or the woman can put the condom in place. Early application is particularly important in the prevention of STDs. Early application also lessens the possibility of the release of preejaculate fluid into the vagina.
- Unroll the condom on the erect penis. For those using a condom without a reservoir tip, a ½-inch space should be left to catch the ejaculate. To leave this space, pinch the tip of the condom as you roll it on the erect penis. Do not leave any air in the tip of the condom.
- Lubricate the condom if this has not already been done by the manufacturer. When doing this, be certain to use a water-soluble lubricant and not a petroleum-based product such as petroleum jelly. Petroleum can deteriorate the latex material. Other oil-based lubricants, such as mineral oil, baby oil, vegetable oil, shortening, and certain hand lotions, can quickly damage a latex condom. Use water-based lubricants only!
- After ejaculation, be certain that the condom does not become dislodged from the penis. Hold the rim of the condom firmly

Pinch the end of the condom to leave ½ inch of space at the tip.

against the base of the penis during withdrawal. Do not allow the penis to become flaccid (soft) while still in the vagina.
- Inspect the condom for tears before throwing it away. If the condom is damaged in some way, immediately insert a spermicidal agent into the vagina or consider using emergency contraception (see page 409).

of the sheath. This lubricant does not contain a spermicide. Female and male condoms should not be used together since they might adhere to each other and cause slippage or displacement. Female condoms cost about $2.50.

Diaphragm

The **diaphragm** is a soft rubber cup with a springlike metal rim that, when properly fitted and correctly inserted by the user, rests in the top of the vagina. The diaphragm covers the cervical opening (Figure 14-3). During intercourse the diaphragm stays in place quite well and cannot usually be felt by either partner.

The diaphragm is always used with a spermicidal cream or jelly. The diaphragm should be covered with an adequate amount of spermicide inside the cup and around the rim. When used properly with a spermicide, the diaphragm is a relatively effective contraceptive, and when combined with the man's use of a condom, its effectiveness is even greater.

Key Terms

diaphragm a soft rubber cup designed to cover the cervix.

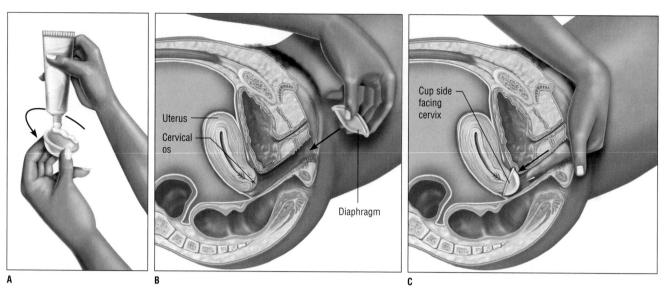

Figure 14-3 A, Spermicidal cream or jelly is placed into the diaphragm. **B,** The diaphragm is folded length-wise and inserted into the vagina. **C,** The diaphragm is then placed against the cervix so that the cup portion with the spermicide is facing the cervix. The outline of the cervix should be felt through the central part of the diaphragm.

Diaphragms must always be fitted and prescribed by a physician.[10] The cost of obtaining a diaphragm and keeping a supply of spermicide may be higher than that of other methods. Also, a high level of motivation to follow the instructions *exactly* is important.

Diaphragms and other vaginal barrier methods, such as the cervical cap, do not provide reliable protection against STDs and HIV infection. Recent concerns about the spermicide nonoxynol-9 should prompt users to ask their physicians to recommend a cream or jelly to use with a diaphragm. If you are concerned about possible infection, either avoid sexual activity or use a latex condom and spermicide in combination.

Cervical Cap

The **cervical cap** is a small, thimble-shaped device that fits over the entire cervix. The cap is held in place by suction rather than by pushing against anatomical structures (Figure 14-4). As with the diaphragm, a spermicide is used with the cervical cap. The use effectiveness of the cervical cap appears to be approximately equal to that of the diaphragm. As with the diaphragm, the effectiveness of the cervical cap is much higher in women who have never had children. Cervical caps are distributed in the United States through physician prescription.

The cervical cap comes in just four sizes and, thus, may be difficult to fit for some women.[8] A physician must prescribe the cervical cap and show the woman how to use it. With new concerns about the use of the spermicide

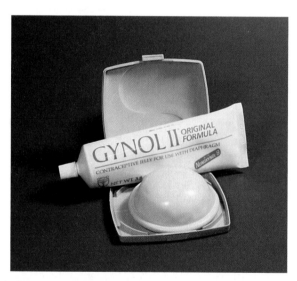

Diaphragm and contraceptive jelly.

nonoxynol-9, women are advised to ask their physicians which contraceptive or cream or jelly they should use with their cervical cap. The cost of a contraceptive cap is similar to that for a diaphragm.

Key Terms

cervical cap a small, thimble-shaped contraceptive device designed to fit over the cervix.

Figure 14-4 After the spermicidal cream or jelly is placed in the cervical cap, the cap is inserted into the vagina and placed against the cervix.

Contraceptive Sponge

The sponge is a small, pillow-shaped polyurethane device containing nonoxynol-9 spermicide. The sponge is dampened with tap water and inserted deep in the vagina to cover the cervical opening. This device provides contraceptive protection for up to 24 hours, regardless of the number of times intercourse occurs. After the last act of intercourse, the device must be left in place for at least 6 hours. Once removed, the sponge must be discarded. The sponge must not be left in place for longer than 24 to 30 hours because of the risk of toxic shock syndrome. Used alone, the sponge does not provide reliable protection against STDs and HIV infection.(Consult your physician if you are concerned about the use of nonoxynol-9.)

Prior to its removal from the market in 1995, when the manufacturer refused to upgrade its physical plant to

Cervical cap.

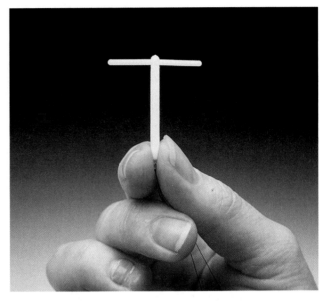

Progestasert IUD.

meet new government safety regulations, the Today Sponge was the most popular female over-the-counter contraceptive. However, a different company, Allendale Pharmaceuticals, purchased the rights to the product and, at the time of this writing, is in the final stages of receiving FDA approval to return the Today Sponge to the U.S. market by early 2004.[11] The sponge is currently available in Canada. For the latest information on this product, see the Allendale website at **www.todayssponge.com.**

Intrauterine Device (IUD)

The **intrauterine device (IUD)** is the most popular reversible contraceptive method in the world, although the number of users in the United States is relatively small. The IUD is a safe, highly effective method of birth control. Experts still do not understand exactly how the IUD prevents pregnancy, but research suggests that IUDs may prevent conception or may prevent a fertilized ovum from implanting in the uterus. IUDs that contain synthetic hormones may cause the cervical mucus to thicken, thus reducing sperm movement into the uterus. Hormonal IUDs could also cause the uterine lining to become thinner and not permit a fertilized ovum to implant.[12]

> **Key Terms**
>
> **intrauterine device (IUD)** a small, plastic, medicated or unmedicated contraceptive device that prevents pregnancy when inserted in the uterus.

Two types of IUDs are available in the United States: T-shaped IUDs containing progestin (Progestasert and Mirena) and a T-shaped IUD wrapped with copper wire (ParaGard). The two hormone-producing IUDs substantially reduce menstrual blood loss, but the copper IUD may increase blood flow at menstruation. About 20% of women who use the Mirena IUD will stop having their periods.[13]

The Progestasert provides highly effective contraceptive protection for 1 year, the Mirena for 5 years, and the ParaGard for up to 10 years. Only a skilled physician can prescribe and insert an IUD. As with many other forms of contraception, IUDs do not offer protection against STDs, including the AIDS virus.[14]

As Table 14.1 indicates, IUDs are very effective birth control devices, surpassed in effectiveness only by abstinence, sterilization, and hormonal contraceptives. Two uncommon but potentially serious side effects of IUD use are uterine perforation (in which the IUD imbeds itself into the uterine wall) and PID (which is a life-threatening infection of the abdominal cavity). The choice of over 100 million women worldwide, IUDs are used by fewer than 1% of women at risk of pregnancy in the United States. The cost for an IUD ranges from $175 to $400, which includes an exam, insertion, and a follow-up visit.[12]

Oral Contraceptives

Introduced in the late 1950s, the **oral contraceptive pill** provides one of the highest effectiveness rates of any single reversible contraceptive method used today. "The pill" is the method of choice for 17 million women in the United States. A successful male version has not yet been developed. (See the Learning from Our Diversity box on page 407.)

Use of the pill requires a physical examination by a physician and a prescription. Since oral contraceptives are available in a wide range of formulas, follow-up examinations are important to ensure that a woman is receiving an effective dosage with as few side effects as possible. Determining the right prescription for a particular woman may require a few consultations.

All oral contraceptives contain synthetic (laboratory-made) hormones. The typical *combined pill* uses both synthetic estrogen and synthetic progesterone in each of twenty-one pills. With *triphasic pills,* the level of estrogen remains constant, but the level of progestin varies every 7 days. In 2003 the FDA approved the newest oral contraceptive (Seasonale) that contains active hormones for 84 days (12 weeks) followed by 1 week of pills containing inactive ingredients.[16] Women using this contraceptive pill would expect to have only four menstrual periods each year. This pill could become a highly popular choice for women. Estrogen levels remain constant during the cycle.

Oral contraceptives.

As with many forms of contraception, *oral contraceptives do not provide protection from the transmission of STDs or HIV infection.* Furthermore, the use of antibiotics lowers the pill's contraceptive effectiveness.

Oral contraceptives function in several ways. The estrogen in the pill tends to reduce ova development. The progesterone in the pill helps reduce the likelihood of ovulation (by lowering the release of luteinizing hormone). The progesterone in the pill also causes the uterine wall to develop inadequately and helps thicken cervical mucus, thus making it difficult for sperm to enter the uterus.

The physical changes produced by the oral contraceptive provide some beneficial side effects in women. Since the synthetic hormones are taken for 21 days and then are followed by **placebo pills** or no pills for 7 days, the menstrual cycle becomes regulated. Even women who have irregular cycles immediately become "regular." Since the uterine lining is not developed to the extent seen in a nonuser, the uterus is not forced to contract with the same amount of vigor. Thus menstrual cramping is reduced, and the resultant menstrual flow is diminished. Research indicates that oral contraceptive use may provide protection against anemia, PID, noncancerous breast tumors, recurrent ovarian cysts, ectopic pregnancy, endometrial cancer, ovarian cancer, and osteoporosis (thinning of the bones).[3]

The negative side effects of the oral contraceptive pill can be divided into two general categories: (1) unpleasant and (2) potentially dangerous. The unpleasant side effects

---

Key Terms

oral contraceptive pill a pill taken orally, composed of synthetic female hormones that prevent ovulation or implantation; "the pill."

placebo pills pills that contain no active ingredients.

Learning from Our Diversity

The Male Contraceptive Pill

Having males be responsible for the medical control of fertility would be a big shift in the sexuality responsibility roles for men and women. Forty-five years after the breakthrough of the female contraceptive pill, researchers are gaining confidence that a version of a male contraceptive pill will be commercially available in the not-too-distant future, perhaps between 5 and 10 years.*

For decades, difficulties have surrounded the development of a male contraceptive pill. Although many people believe that the primary reason for the slow development was the fact that the researchers were male, the most plausible explanations deal with male physiology. The typical male ejaculate contains between 300 and 500 million sperm cells. A contraceptive method that is over 99% effective would still leave thousands and thousands of sperm cells available. In contrast, female contraceptives must block the viability of only one egg each cycle, arguably an easier task.

The drug being tested that blocks sperm development is actually a female hormone. While it is effective at blocking sperm production, it also reduces the amount of testosterone that the male produces. Without adequate levels of testosterone, the male sex drive diminishes considerably. For this reason, researchers are testing the effects of

replacement androgen, often in the form of an injection or an implant. It is also possible that a slow release patch, similar to the nicotine replacement patch, could be used in the future.

Critics claim that a safe, effective, and inexpensive form of male contraception already exists in the form of a vasectomy. They argue, why not use an approach that already has shown its effectiveness for years? Besides, are women going to trust a man who claims he is using an oral contraceptive pill? Would the pill also have to make a man's eyeballs turn blue as proof that he was using an effective method? When would a woman know that a man is being truthful? Unfortunately, the track record for honesty among couples in sexual relationships isn't particularly good.

Within the next decade, the obstacles that prevent a safe and effective male contraceptive pill from being manufactured may be overcome. But questions will still remain, especially for women, since after all is said and done, they will always be the ones who must bear the brunt (as well as the joy) of pregnancy, labor, and childbirth.

*Health news: Will men use a contraceptive pill? Will women trust them? InteliHealth Online, 29 August 2000, www.intelihealth.com/enews?296075.

---

generally subside within 2 or 3 months for most women. A number of women report some or many of the following symptoms:

- Tenderness in breast tissue
- Nausea
- Mild headaches
- Slight, irregular spotting
- Weight gain
- Fluctuations in sex drive
- Mild depression
- More frequent vaginal infections

TALKING POINTS You've tried two different types of oral contraceptives and had unpleasant side effects with both. Your doctor says you should consider another birth control method, but you disagree. How could you talk to him about this in a matter-of-fact way?

The potentially dangerous side effects of the oral contraceptive pill are most often seen in the cardiovascular system. Blood clots, strokes, hypertension, and heart attack seem to be associated with the estrogen component of the combined pill. However, when compared with the risk to

nonusers, the risk of dying from cardiovascular complications is only slightly increased among healthy young oral contraceptive users.

Additionally, the present consensus is that oral contraceptive users place themselves at slightly increased risk of developing breast cancer and cervical cancer. However, it must be emphasized that this risk is quite small. Most health professionals agree that the risks related to pregnancy and childbirth are much greater than those associated with oral contraceptive use. Certainly, a woman who is contemplating the use of the pill must discuss all of the risks and benefits with her physician.

There are some **contraindications** for the use of oral contraceptives. If you have a history of blood clots, migraine headaches, liver disease, a heart condition, high blood pressure, obesity, diabetes, epilepsy, or anemia, or if you have not established regular menstrual cycles, the pill probably should not be your contraceptive

---

Key Terms

contraindications factors that make the use of a drug inappropriate or dangerous for a particular person.

choice. A complete and accurate health history is important before a woman starts to take the pill.

Two additional contraindications are well understood by the medical community. Cigarette smoking and advancing age are highly associated with an increased risk of potentially serious side effects. Increasing numbers of physicians are not prescribing oral contraceptives for their patients who smoke. The risk of cardiovascular-related deaths is enhanced in women over age 35. The risk is even higher in female smokers over age 35.

For the vast majority of women, however, the pill, when properly prescribed, is safe and effective. Careful scrutiny of a woman's health history and careful follow-up examinations when a problem is suspected are essential elements that can provide a margin of safety. The ease of administration, the relatively low cost, and the effectiveness of the pill make it a sound choice for many women. Monthly pill packs cost between $15 and $35. An exam may cost $35 to $125.[17]

Minipills

Some women prefer not to use the combined oral contraceptive pill. To avoid some of the potentially serious side effects of the combined pill, some physicians are prescribing **minipills.** These oral contraceptives contain no estrogen—only low-dose progesterone.[18] The minipill seems to work by thickening cervical mucus, preventing ovulation, and perhaps preventing implantation of the fertilized ovum. The effectiveness of the minipill is slightly lower than that of the combined pill. *Breakthrough bleeding* and **ectopic pregnancy** are more common in minipill users than in combined-pill users.

Injectable Contraceptives

Depo-Provera is a highly effective (99%+) injectable, progesterone contraceptive that provides protection for three months. This hormone shot works by thickening the cervical mucus to keep sperm from joining the egg, preventing the release of the egg, and preventing a fertilized egg from implanting in the uterus.

The most common side effects of Depo-Provera are irregular bleeding and spotting followed by *amenorrhea* (the absence of periods).[3] When the woman's body adjusts to the presence of this drug, breakthrough bleeding diminishes, and the most common side effect is amenorrhea. Many women see this as a desirable effect. Women who stop using Depo-Provera may experience infertility for a period of up to 1 year. The cost of Depo-Provera ranges from $30 to $75 per injection.

In the year 2000, the Pharmacia Corporation received FDA approval to produce a monthly injectable contraceptive called Lunelle. Lunelle combined the hormones estrogen and progestin in its once-a-month shot.

However, Pharmacia stopped production and distribution of Lunelle in October 2002.

Subdermal Implants

This now-discontinued form of contraception used six soft plastic rods filled with synthetic progesterone. Using a local anesthetic, a physician implanted these rods just beneath the skin of a woman's upper or lower arm. The rods released low levels of the hormone for 5 years. In 2002 Wyeth Pharmaceuticals stopped the production and release of subdermal implants.

The Contraceptive Ring

One of the newest contraceptives on the market is the vaginal **contraceptive ring** (NuvaRing). Available by prescription in 2001, NuvaRing is a thin polymer ring (2⅛ inches in diameter and 1/8 inch thick) that contains synthetic estrogen and progestin. Users insert this device deep into the vagina where it remains for 3 weeks. At the end of the third week, the device is removed for a week and the woman has her period. The NuvaRing provides effective contraception (98–99% effective when used properly) for the entire 4-week time frame.[19]

The ring functions in a manner similar to the oral contraceptive pill: it reduces the chances of ovulation and thickens cervical mucus. Women who use the ring cannot at the same time use cervical caps or diaphragms as a backup method. The contraceptive ring does not protect against sexually transmitted diseases, including the virus that causes HIV/AIDS. The costs of the contraceptive ring are about $30–$35 per month for the device and $35–$125 for the exam.[17]

The Contraceptive Patch

In 2002 the Ortho Evra **contraceptive patch** became available to women. This patch contains continuous levels

---

Key Terms

minipills low-dose progesterone oral contraceptives.

ectopic pregnancy a pregnancy in which the fertilized ovum implants at a site other than the uterus, typically in the fallopian tubes.

contraceptive ring thin, polymer contraceptive device containing estrogen and progestin; placed deep within the vagina for a three-week period.

contraceptive patch contraceptive skin patch containing estrogen and progestin; replaced each week for a three-week period.

The NuvaRing contraceptive ring is a flexible ring about 2⅛ inches in diameter. When inserted into the vagina, it delivers a low dose of hormones similar to those found in oral contraceptives.

of estrogen and progestin delivered from a 1¾-inch square patch that is applied weekly to one of four areas on the woman's body: the buttocks, abdomen, upper chest (front and back, excluding the breasts), or upper outer arm.[20] The patch remains attached even while a woman bathes, swims, or exercises. After 3 weeks of patches, the woman uses no patch for the fourth week, during which time the woman has her period. The patch functions in a manner similar to the oral contraceptive pill. Like all hormonal measures of contraception, the patch does not protect against sexually transmitted diseases, including the virus that causes HIV/AIDS.

Emergency Contraception

Emergency contraception is designed to prevent pregnancy after unprotected vaginal intercourse such as when a condom breaks, when a couple uses no method of contraception, or when someone forces another to have intercourse. This method is also called post-coital or "morning after" contraception. Emergency contraception is available in two forms: emergency hormonal contraception and the insertion of an IUD. Both forms of contraception can be prescribed (or carried out) only by a physician.

As of September 2003, five states (Alaska, California, Hawaii, New Mexico, and Washington) had enacted laws that permit a pharmacist to provide emergency contraception to customers in the absence of a prescription by a physician. However, the pharmacist is required to act within a collaborative agreement with a physician. This agreement clearly identifies the circumstances under which the pharmacist can dispense the emergency contraception.[21]

Emergency hormonal contraception involves the use of two doses of certain oral contraceptives.[3] The most commonly used oral contraceptives are the combined pills (Preven), which contain both synthetic estrogen and progesterone. The first dose of pills is taken within 72 hours of unprotected intercourse. A second dose is taken 12 hours later. If progesterone-only pills (Plan B) are used for emergency contraception, the first dose must be taken within 48 to 72 hours after unprotected intercourse.

The insertion of an IUD is a less commonly used, but highly effective, form of emergency contraception. To function as a contraceptive, however, the IUD must be inserted within 5 days after unprotected intercourse.

Sterilization

All of the contraceptive mechanisms or methods already discussed have one quality in common: they are reversible. Although microsurgical techniques are providing medical breakthroughs, **sterilization** should generally be considered an irreversible procedure. When you decide to use sterilization, you are

---

Key Terms

sterilization generally permanent birth control techniques that surgically disrupt the normal passage of ova or sperm.

Figure 14-5 The most frequently used forms of male and female sterilization. **A,** Vasectomy. **B,** Tubal ligation.

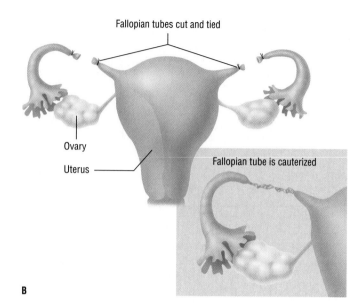

Fallopian tubes cut and tied

Ovary

Uterus

Fallopian tube is cauterized

B

Vas deferens cut and tied on each side

A

giving up control of your own fertility because you will no longer be able to produce offspring.

Therefore, couples considering sterilization procedures usually must undergo extensive discussions with a physician or family planning counselor to identify their true feelings about this finality. Sterilization does not protect one against sexually transmitted diseases, including HIV infection.

The male sterilization procedure is called a *vasectomy*. Accomplished with a local anesthetic in a physician's office, this 20- to 30-minute procedure consists of the surgical removal of a section of each vas deferens. After a small incision is made through the scrotum, the vas deferens is located and a small section is removed. The remaining ends are either tied or *cauterized* (Figure 14-5, *A*).

Immediately after a vasectomy, sperm may still be present in the vas deferens. A backup contraceptive is recommended until a physician microscopically examines a semen specimen. This examination usually occurs about 6 weeks after the surgery. After a vasectomy, men can still produce male sex hormones, get erections, have orgasms, and ejaculate. (Recall that sperm account for only a small portion of the semen.) Some men even report increased interest in sexual activity, since their chances of impregnating a woman are virtually eliminated.

What happens to the process of spermatogenesis within each testicle? Sperm cells are still being produced, but they are destroyed by specialized white blood cells called *phagocytic leukocytes.* The cost of a vasectomy ranges from $240 to $520.[17]

The most common method of female sterilization is *tubal ligation.* During this procedure, the fallopian tubes are cut and the ends are tied back. Some physicians cauterize the tube ends to ensure complete sealing (Figure 14-5, *B*). The fallopian tubes are usually reached through the abdominal wall. In a *minilaparotomy,* a small incision is made through the abdominal wall just below the navel. The resultant scar is quite small and is the basis for the term *band-aid surgery.*

Female sterilization requires about 20 to 30 minutes, with the patient under local or general anesthesia. The use of a *laparoscope* has made female sterilization much simpler than in the past. The laparoscope is a small tube equipped with mirrors and lights. Inserted through a single incision, the laparoscope locates the fallopian tubes before they are cut, tied, or cauterized. When a laparoscope is used through an abdominal incision, the procedure is called a *laparoscopy.*

Women who are sterilized still produce female hormones, ovulate, and menstruate. However, the ovum cannot move down the fallopian tube. Within a day of its release, the ovum will start to disintegrate and be absorbed by the body. Freed of the possibility of becoming pregnant, many sterilized women report an increase in sex drive and activity. Tubal ligation costs range from $1,000 to $2,500.[17]

Two other procedures produce sterilization in women. *Ovariectomy* (the surgical removal of the ovaries) and *hysterectomy* (the surgical removal of the uterus) accomplish sterilization. However, these procedures are used to remove diseased (cancerous, cystic, or hemorrhaging) organs and are not considered primary sterilization techniques.

 TALKING POINTS You and your husband have children, and you'd like to stop taking the pill for health reasons. Your husband says you're pressuring him to have a vasectomy. How can you keep the dialogue going in a cooperative way?

Abortion

Regardless of the circumstances under which pregnancy occurs, women may now choose to terminate their pregnancies. No longer must women who do not want to be pregnant seek potentially dangerous, illegal abortions. On the basis of current technology and legality, women need never experience childbirth. The decision is theirs to make.

Abortion should never be considered a first-line, preferred form of fertility control. Rather, abortion is a final, last-chance undertaking. It should be used only when responsible control of one's fertility could not be achieved. The decision to abort a fetus is a highly controversial, personal one—one that needs serious consideration by each woman.

On the basis of the landmark 1973 U.S. Supreme Court case *Roe v. Wade*, the United States joined many of the world's most populated countries in legalizing abortions.

Each year, approximately 1.3 million women in the United States make the decision to terminate a pregnancy.[15] Thousands of additional women probably consider abortion but elect to continue their pregnancies.

Clearly, abortion is a political issue. It will be interesting to see how future abortion-related decisions will unfold. Special interest groups on both sides of the issue, the Supreme Court, state legislatures, federal agencies (such as the FDA and the Department of Health and Human Services), the Congress, and the president all have a say in the abortion debate in this country. Regardless of the eventual outcomes of this debate, here are the present abortion procedures available in the United States.

 TALKING POINTS You're unexpectedly pregnant, but abortion doesn't seem like a good choice for you. Your boyfriend, your family, and your friends all have strong but conflicting opinions about the situation. How can you show that you value their advice but still make it clear that the final decision needs to be yours alone?

First-Trimester Abortion Procedures

Menstrual extraction. Also referred to as *menstrual regulation*, *menstrual induction*, and *preemptive abortion*, menstrual extraction is a process carried out between the fourth and sixth week after the last menstrual period (or in the days immediately after the first missed menstrual period). This procedure is generally performed in a physician's office with a local anesthetic or *paracervical anesthetic* used. A small plastic *cannula* is inserted through the undilated cervical canal into the cavity of the uterus. Once the cannula is in position, a small amount of suction is applied by a hand-held syringe. By rotating and moving the cannula across the uterine wall, the physician can withdraw the endometrial tissue.

Key Terms

abortion induced premature termination of a pregnancy.

Vacuum Aspiration Induced abortions undertaken during the sixth through ninth weeks of pregnancy are generally done through *vacuum aspiration* of the uterine contents. Vacuum aspiration is the most commonly performed abortion procedure. This procedure is similar in nature to menstrual extraction. Unlike menstrual extraction, however, vacuum aspiration may require **dilation** of the cervical canal and the use of a local anesthetic. In this more advanced stage of pregnancy, a larger cannula must be inserted into the uterine cavity. This process can be accomplished by using metal dilators of increasingly larger sizes to open the canal. After aspiration by an electric vacuum pump, the uterine wall may also be scraped to confirm complete removal of the uterine contents.

Dilation and Curettage (D & C) When a pregnancy is to be terminated during the ninth through fourteenth weeks, vacuum aspiration gives way to a somewhat similar procedure labeled **dilation and curettage,** or more familiarly, **D & C.** D & C usually requires a general anesthetic, not a local anesthetic.[3]

Like vacuum aspiration, the D & C involves the gradual enlargement of the cervical canal through the insertion of increasingly larger metal dilators. When the cervix has been dilated to a size sufficient to allow for the passage of a *curette,* the removal of the endometrial tissue can begin. The curette is a metal instrument resembling a spoon, with a cup-shaped cutting surface on its end. As the curette is drawn across the uterine wall, the soft endometrial tissue and fetal parts are scraped from the wall of the uterus. (The D & C is also used in the medical management of certain health conditions of the uterine wall, such as irregular bleeding or the buildup of endometrial tissue.)

As in the case of menstrual extraction, both vacuum aspiration and D & C are very safe procedures for the woman. The need to dilate the cervix more fully in a D & C increases the risk of cervical trauma and the possibility of perforation, but these risks are reported to be low. Bleeding, cramping, spotting, and infections present minimal controllable risks when procedures are done by experienced clinicians under clinical conditions.

Medical Abortion Mifepristone and methotrexate are drugs that a woman can use under medical supervision to induce a **medical abortion** during the first trimester. Formerly known as RU-486, mifepristone blocks the action of progesterone and causes the uterine lining and any fertilized egg to shed.[23] Under FDA guidelines, women must use mifepristone within 49 days of their last menstrual period. Women take three pills at the first doctor visit and then return 48 hours later to take a second drug, misoprostol, which causes menstruation to occur, usually within about 5 hours. A third visit to a physician is necessary to ensure that the woman is recovering well from the medical abortion. Blood tests or an ultrasound exam will verify that the abortion was successful.

Methotrexate is a drug used since the 1950s for cancer treatment.[24] However, physicians sometimes use this drug in an off-label manner to induce a first term abortion.[3] Typically, a woman receives an injection of methotrexate and, during a second office visit 3 to 7 days later, receives prostoglandin. The fetal contents are expelled, usually within a day, but some methotrexate abortions take up a week to occur. A follow-up office visit is necessary. Medical abortions cost about the same as a first-term surgical abortion ($350–$575).[17]

Second-Trimester Abortion Procedures

When a woman's pregnancy continues beyond the fourteenth week of gestation, termination becomes a more difficult matter. The procedures at this stage are more complicated and take longer to complete. Complications are also more common.

Dilation and Evacuation Vacuum aspiration and D & C can be combined in a procedure called *dilation and evacuation (D & E)* during the earliest weeks of the second trimester (Figure 14-6). The use of D & E increases the likelihood of trauma and postprocedural complications, since larger instruments and greater dilation are required. After about 16 weeks, more intensive procedures will be required to terminate the late second-trimester pregnancy.[3]

Hypertonic Saline Procedure From the sixteenth week of gestation to the end of the second trimester, intrauterine injection of a strong salt solution into the amniotic sac is the procedure most frequently used. The administration of intrauterine **hypertonic saline solution** requires a skilled operator so that the needle used to introduce the salt solution enters the amniotic sac.

Key Terms

dilation gradual expansion of an opening or passageway, such as the cervix.

dilation and curettage (D & C) a surgical procedure in which the cervical canal is dilated to allow the uterine wall to be scraped.

medical abortion an abortion caused by the use of prescribed drugs.

hypertonic saline solution a salt solution with a concentration higher than that found in human fluids.

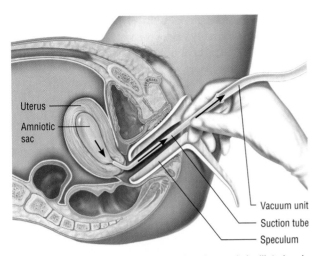

Figure 14-6 During dilation and evacuation, the cervix is dilated and the contents of the uterus are aspirated (removed by suction). This procedure is used to perform abortions up to 16 weeks' gestation.

Once the needle is in place, some amniotic fluid is withdrawn, allowing the saline solution to be injected.

Some physicians support the saline procedure by dilating the cervix with *laminaria* or another dilatory product and administering the hormone oxytocin to stimulate uterine contractions. The onset of uterine contractions will expel the dehydrated uterine contents within 24 to 36 hours.

Prostaglandin Procedure The use of prostaglandin is the third type of abortion procedure used during the second trimester. Prostaglandins are hormonelike chemicals that have a variety of useful effects on human tissue. Produced naturally within the body, these substances influence the contractions of smooth muscle. Since the uterine wall is composed entirely of smooth muscle, it is particularly sensitive to the presence of prostaglandins. When prostaglandin is administered in sufficient quantity (through either a uterine intramuscular injection or a vaginal suppository), uterine contractions become strong enough to expel the fetal contents.

Third-Trimester Abortion Procedures

If termination of a pregnancy is required in the latter weeks of the gestational period, a surgical procedure in which the fetus is removed (*hysterotomy*) or a procedure in which the entire uterus is removed (*hysterectomy*) can be undertaken. These procedures are more complicated and involve longer hospitalization, major abdominal surgery, and an extended period of recovery.

In the late 1990s, the U.S. House of Representatives and the U.S. Senate voted to ban a rarely used third-trimester abortion procedure referred to as dilation and extraction. Lawmakers felt that this procedure, also called *partial-birth abortion*, was too gruesome to be permitted. President Clinton vetoed this ban, and because the Senate failed to override his veto, the ban on partial birth abortion did not become law. Federal efforts to ban this procedure are continuing.

At the state level, however, efforts to enact laws had been more successful. At the time of this writing (in September 2003), thirty-one states had enacted laws related to partial birth abortion. However, in nineteen of these states, court orders had specifically blocked the enforcement of the laws. Partial birth ban laws in nine states (Indiana, Mississippi, Montana, North Dakota, Oklahoma, South Carolina, South Dakota, and Tennessee) had not yet been challenged in the courts. Only four states (Georgia, Kansas, New Mexico, and Utah) had partial birth ban statutes that were considered clearly enforceable.[25]

Post-Abortion Syndrome

Some women who have an abortion may be faced with the consequence of psychological difficulties in the years that follow the abortion. The term **post-abortion syndrome** refers to "the suggested long-term negative psychological effects of abortion."[26] It is possible that these difficulties may arise soon after the abortion or may not surface until years later. The signs and symptoms of post-abortion syndrome are not unlike those of the more well-known post-traumatic stress disorder. (However, it should be noted that the American Psychiatric Association and other organizations do not recognize post-abortion syndrome as an identifiable illness.)

Women having post-abortion syndrome may experience some or all of the following effects: difficulties with personal relationships, substance abuse problems, nightmares, sexual difficulties, communication problems, damage to self-esteem, and, possibly, suicide.[26] These symptoms may range from mild to severe and may be lengthy in duration.

Fortunately, there are abortion follow-up services that can be helpful to women who believe they are suffering from the consequences of abortion. Individual and group counseling, as well as post-abortion support groups, can help women cope with difficult, complicated feelings. Look for these services through your medical care provider, or check your local phone book for helpful resources.

Key Terms

post-abortion syndrome the long-term negative psychological effects of abortion.

A Final Word About Birth Control

In the heat of passion, people often fail to think rationally about the potential outcomes of unprotected sex. Therefore, the time to prepare for the romantic moment is *before* you are in a position where you don't want to think about the possibility of an unintended result. If you choose to be sexually active, find a form of protection that works well for you and use it consistently. If you choose not to be sexually active, realize that this is a viable choice that can be 100% effective.

Pregnancy

Pregnancy is a condition that requires a series of complex yet coordinated changes to occur in the female body. This discussion follows pregnancy from its beginning, at fertilization, to its conclusion, with labor and childbirth.

Physiological Obstacles and Aids to Fertilization

Many sexually active young people believe that they will become pregnant (or impregnate someone) only when they want to, despite their haphazard contraceptive practices. Because of this mistaken belief, many young people are not sold on the use of contraceptives. It is important for young adults to remember that from a species survival standpoint, our bodies were designed to promote pregnancy. It is estimated that about 85% of sexually active women of childbearing age will become pregnant within 1 year if they do not use some form of contraception.[3]

With regard to pregnancy, each act of intercourse can be considered a game of physiological odds. There are obstacles that may reduce a couple's chance of pregnancy, including the following:

Obstacles to Fertilization

1. *The acidic level of the vagina is destructive to sperm.* The low pH of the vagina will kill sperm that fail to enter the uterus quickly.
2. *The cervical mucus is thick during most of the menstrual cycle.* Sperm movement into the uterus is more difficult, except during the few days surrounding ovulation.
3. *The sperm must locate the cervical opening.* The cervical opening is small compared with the rest of the surface area where sperm are deposited.
4. *Half of the sperm travel through the wrong fallopian tube.* Most commonly, only one ovum is released at ovulation. The two ovaries generally "take turns" each month. The sperm have no way of "knowing" which tube they should enter. Thus it is probable that half will travel through the wrong tube.
5. *The distance sperm must travel is relatively long compared with the tiny size of the sperm cells.* Microscopic sperm must travel about 7 or 8 inches once they are inside the female.
6. *The sperm's travel is relatively "upstream."* The anatomical positioning of the female reproductive structures necessitates an "uphill" movement by the sperm.
7. *The contoured folds of the tubal walls trap many sperm.* These folds make it difficult for sperm to locate the egg. Many sperm are trapped in this maze.

There are also a variety of aids that tend to help sperm and egg cells join. Some of these are listed below.

Aids to Fertilization

1. *An astounding number of sperm are deposited during ejaculation.* Each ejaculation contains about a teaspoon of semen.[18] Within this quantity are between 200 and 500 million sperm cells. Even with large numbers of sperm killed in the vagina, millions are able to move to the deeper structures.
2. *Sperm are deposited near the cervical opening.* Penetration into the vagina by the penis allows for the sperm to be placed near the cervical opening.
3. *The male accessory glands help make the semen nonacidic.* The seminal vesicles, prostate gland, and Cowper's glands secrete fluids that provide an alkaline environment for the sperm. This environment helps sperm be better protected in the vagina until they can move into the deeper, more alkaline uterus and fallopian tubes.
4. *Uterine contractions aid sperm movement.* The rhythmic muscular contractions of the uterus tend to cause the sperm to move in the direction of the fallopian tubes.
5. *Sperm cells move rather quickly.* Despite their tiny size, sperm cells can move relatively quickly—just about 1 inch per hour. Powered by sugar solutions from the male accessory glands and the whiplike movements of their tails, sperm can reach the distant third of the fallopian tubes in less than 8 hours as they swim in the direction of the descending ovum.
6. *Once inside the fallopian tubes, sperm can live for days.* Some sperm may be viable for up to a week after reaching the comfortable, nonacidic environment of the fallopian tubes. Most sperm, however, will survive an average of 48 to 72 hours. Thus they can "wait in the wings" for the moment an ovum is released from the ovary (Figure 14-7).
7. *The cervical mucus is thin and watery at the time of ovulation.* This mucus allows for better passage of sperm through the cervical opening when the ovum is most capable of being fertilized.

Labels on figure:
- Fallopian tube
- **Fertilization**
- Sperm cells
- Ovum
- Graafian follicle
- Follicle
- Corpus luteum
- Primary follicles
- Ovary
- Zygote dividing as it travels toward uterus
- Blastocyst is implanted in endometrium (at 8 days)
- Embryo (at 4 weeks)
- Uterine cavity
- Endometrium
- Cervix

Figure 14-7 After its release from the follicle, the ovum begins its week-long journey down the fallopian tube. Fertilization generally occurs in the outermost third of the tube. Now fertilized, the ovum progresses toward the uterus, where it embeds itself in the endometrium. A pregnancy is established.

Human Cloning: An Ethical Dilemma?

Today's most controversial issue related to parenting is reproduction through **human cloning.** With the 1997 breakthrough cloning of the Scottish sheep Dolly, the possibility of human cloning emerged within the scientific community. To clone a human, the procedure would involve the following steps:[27]

- Doctors would surgically retrieve an egg from the female donor.
- The nucleus of this egg would be removed.
- A cell is taken from a cloning subject (a male or female).
- Through an electrical jolt, the cloning subject's cell is fused with the **enucleated egg.** This creates a clonal zygote. Shortly after, this clonal zygote divides over and over and develops into a clonal embryo.
- The clonal embryo is implanted in the womb of a surrogate mother.
- After 9 months, a genetically matched reproduction of the cloning subject is born.

Although this step-by-step process may seem simple, this has never been accomplished with human subjects.[27]

In fact, to produce Dolly, the cloned sheep, it took scientists 277 attempts. The technical expertise to clone humans has not been fully developed, although some scientists believe it could be on the near horizon, if public policy would fully support this area of research.

However, public policy currently does not support human cloning. A few states have passed laws banning human cloning. The U.S. Food and Drug Administration (FDA) has warned researchers that any attempts at human cloning must first get FDA approval, which the FDA claims will not be forthcoming. Both the American Society for Reproductive Medicine and the National Academy of Sciences have voiced their opposition to human cloning.[28] Many public opinion polls have indicated that Americans are overwhelmingly against the use of cloning to produce babies.[29]

> **Key Terms**
>
> **human cloning** the replication of a human being.
>
> **enucleated egg** an ovum with the nucleus removed.

However, the potential use of a particular type of cloning has received much more popular public support in America. This is the use of cloning to reproduce body parts, tissues, and specific organs for use in medical transplant procedures. A baby is never reproduced in this cloning procedure.[28] In organ and tissue cloning, sometimes called **therapeutic cloning,** the clonal embryo is not implanted into a surrogate mother, but allowed to grow (divide) into a number of premature cells called **stem cells.** These stem cells have the potential to grow into any kind of body cell.

Theoretically, scientists could develop techniques that would cause these stem cells to grow into tissues or organs that would match the tissues or organs in the person who donated the genetic material. Because of this genetic match, these cloned organs would not be rejected after the transplant surgery. In essence, this technology permits a person's own body to be a human repair kit. Some predict that, in the not too distant future, scientists will be able to grow replacement organs like hearts, livers, and skin and replacement neurons for persons who suffer from Parkinson's or Alzheimer's disease.

On the other side of the fence are those who wonder if cloning represents "science gone mad". Some believe that any kind of cloning is unethical because it interferes with nature. Altering a woman's eggs, reprogramming cells, and tampering with embryos is something that is *simply wrong.* Regardless of the position you take on this issue, you can expect to see more scientific advances regarding cloning, especially therapeutic cloning.

Signs of Pregnancy

Aside from pregnancy tests done in a professional laboratory, a woman can sometimes recognize early signs and symptoms. The signs of pregnancy have been divided into three categories:

Presumptive Signs of Pregnancy

Missed period after unprotected intercourse the previous month

Nausea on awakening (morning sickness)

Increase in size and tenderness of breasts

Darkening of the areolar tissue surrounding the nipples

Probable Signs of Pregnancy

Increase in the frequency of urination (the growing uterus presses against the bladder)

Increase in the size of the abdomen

Cervix becomes softer by the sixth week (detected by a pelvic examination by clinician)

Positive pregnancy test

Positive Signs of Pregnancy

Determination of a fetal heartbeat

Feeling of the fetus moving (*quickening*)

Observation of fetus by ultrasound or optical viewers

Agents That Can Damage a Fetus

A large number of agents that come into contact with a pregnant woman can affect fetal development. Many of these (rubella and herpes viruses, tobacco smoke, alcohol, and virtually all other drugs) are discussed in other chapters of this text. The best advice for a pregnant woman is to maintain close contact with her obstetrician during pregnancy and to consider carefully the ingestion of any OTC drug (including aspirin, caffeine, and antacids) that could harm the fetus.

It is also important for all women to avoid exposure to radiation during the pregnancy. Such exposure, most commonly through excessive X rays or radiation fallout from nuclear testing, can irreversibly damage fetal genetic structures.

Childbirth: The Labor of Delivery

Childbirth, or *parturition,* is one of the true peak life experiences for both men and women. Most of the time, childbirth is a wonderfully exciting venture into the unknown. For the parents, this intriguing experience can provide a stage for personal growth, maturity, and insight into a dynamic, complex world.

During the last few weeks of the third **trimester,** most fetuses will move deeper into the pelvic cavity in a process called *lightening.* During this movement, the fetus's body will rotate and the head will begin to engage more deeply into the mother's pelvic girdle. Many women will report that the baby has "dropped."

Another indication that parturition may be relatively near is the increased reporting of *Braxton Hicks contractions.*[6] These uterine contractions, which are of mild intensity and often occur at irregular intervals, may be felt throughout a pregnancy. During the last few weeks of pregnancy (*gestation*), these mild contractions

---

Key Terms

therapeutic cloning the use of certain human replication techniques to reproduce body tissues and organs.

stem cells premature cells that have the potential to turn into any kind of body cell.

trimester a 3-month period; human pregnancies encompass three trimesters.

Figure 14-8 Labor, or childbirth, is a three-stage process. During effacement and dilation, the first stage (**A**), the cervical canal is gradually opened by contractions of the uterine wall. The second stage (**B**), delivery of the fetus, encompasses the actual delivery of the fetus from the uterus and through the birth canal. The delivery of the placenta, the third stage (**C**), empties the uterus, thus completing the process of childbirth.

First Stage

A

Placenta

Umbilical cord

Uterus

Cervical opening

Birth canal

Uterine contractions thin the cervix and enlarge the cervical opening.

Second Stage

B

Perineum

Uterine contractions are aided by mother's voluntary contractions of abdominal muscles.

Fetus moves through dilated cervical opening and birth canal.

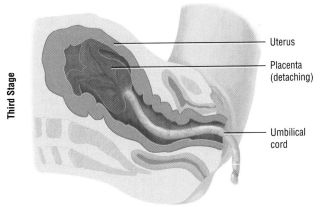

Third Stage

C

Uterus

Placenta (detaching)

Umbilical cord

Placenta detaches from uterine wall and is delivered through the birth canal.

can occur more frequently and may cause a woman to feel as if she is going into labor (**false labor**).

Labor begins when uterine contractions become more intense and occur at regular intervals. The birth of a child can be divided into three stages: (1) *effacement* and dilation of the cervix, (2) delivery of the fetus, and (3) delivery of the placenta (Figure 14-8). For a woman

Key Terms

false labor conditions that resemble the start of true labor; may include irregular uterine contractions, pressure, and discomfort in the lower abdomen.

having her first child, the birth process lasts an average of 12 to 16 hours. The average length of labor for subsequent births is much shorter—from 4 to 10 hours on the average. Labor is very unpredictable: labors that last between 1 and 24 hours occur daily at most hospitals.

Stage One: Effacement and Dilation of the Cervix

In the first stage of labor the uterine contractions attempt to thin (efface) the normally thick cervical walls and to enlarge (dilate) the cervical opening.[30] These contractions are directed by the release of prostaglandins and the hormone oxytocin into the circulating bloodstream.

The first stage of labor is often the longest. The cervical opening must thin and dilate to a diameter of 10 cm before the first stage of labor is considered complete.[22] Often this stage begins with the dislodging of the cervical mucous plug. The subsequent *bloody show* (mucous plug and a small amount of blood) at the vaginal opening may indicate that effacement and dilation have begun. Another indication of labor's onset may be the bursting or tearing of the fetal amniotic sac. "Breaking the bag of waters" refers to this phenomenon, which happens in various measures in expectant women.

The pain of the uterine contractions becomes more intense as the woman moves through this first stage of labor. As the cervical opening effaces and dilates from 0 to 3 cm, many women report feeling happy, exhilarated, and confident. In the *early phase of the first stage* of labor, the contractions are relatively short (lasting from 15 to 60 seconds) and the intervals between contractions range from 20 minutes to 5 minutes as labor progresses. However, these rest intervals will become shorter and the contractions more forceful when the woman's uterus contracts to dilate 4 to 7 cm.

In this *second phase of the first stage* of labor, the contractions usually last about 1 minute each and the rest intervals drop from about 5 minutes to 1 minute over a period of 5 to 9 hours.

The *third phase of the first stage* of labor is called *transition*. During transition, the uterus contracts to dilate the cervical opening to the full 10 cm required for safe passage of the fetus out of the uterus and into the birth canal (vagina).[2] This period of labor is often the most painful part of the entire birth process. Fortunately, it is also the shortest phase of most labors. Lasting between 15 and 30 minutes, transition contractions often last 60 to 90 seconds each. The rest intervals between contractions are short and vary from 30 to 60 seconds.

An examination of the cervix by a nurse or physician will reveal whether full dilation of 10 cm has occurred.

Until the full 10 cm dilation, women are cautioned not to "push" the fetus during the contractions. Special breathing and concentration techniques help many women cope with the first stage of labor.

Stage Two: Delivery of the Fetus

Once the mother's cervix is fully dilated, she enters the second stage of labor, the delivery of the fetus through the birth canal. Now the mother is encouraged to help push the fetus out (with her abdominal muscles) during each contraction. In this second stage the uterine contractions are less forceful than during the transition phase of the first stage and may last 60 seconds each, with a 1- to 3-minute rest interval.

This second stage may last up to 2 hours in first births.[18] For subsequent births, this stage will usually be much shorter. When the baby's head is first seen at the vaginal opening, *crowning* is said to have taken place. Generally the back of the baby's head appears first. (Infants whose feet or buttocks are presented first are said to be delivered in a *breech position*.) Once the head is delivered, the baby's body rotates upward to let the shoulders come through. The rest of the body follows quite quickly. The second stage of labor ends when the fetus is fully expelled from the birth canal.

Stage Three: Delivery of the Placenta

Usually within 30 minutes after the fetus is delivered, the uterus will again initiate a series of contractions to expel the placenta (or *afterbirth*). The placenta is examined by the attending physician to ensure that it was completely expelled. Torn remnants of the placenta could lead to dangerous *hemorrhaging* by the mother. Often the physician will perform a manual examination of the uterus after the placenta has been delivered.

Once the placenta has been delivered, the uterus will continue with mild contractions to help control bleeding and start the gradual reduction of the uterus to its normal, nonpregnant size. This final aspect of the birth process is called **postpartum.** External abdominal massage of the lower abdomen seems to help the uterus contract, as does an infant's nursing at the mother's breast.

Key Terms

postpartum the period after the birth of a baby, during which the uterus returns to its prepregnancy size.

Cesarean Deliveries

A **cesarean delivery** (cesarean birth, C-section) is a procedure in which the fetus is surgically removed from the mother's uterus through the abdominal wall. This type of delivery, which is completed in up to an hour, can be performed with the mother having a regional or a general anesthetic. A cesarean delivery is necessary when either the health of the baby or the mother is at risk.

Although a cesarean delivery is considered major surgery, most mothers cope well with the delivery and postsurgical and postpartum discomfort. The hospital stay is usually a few days longer than for a vaginal delivery. In 2002, the percentage of cesarean deliveries reached an all-time high of 26.1% of all births in the U.S.[31]

 TALKING POINTS Are there people in your life that you can comfortably ask, "What was it like to go through labor and delivery?" Will you feel open enough to express any personal concerns you might have about your own fears of this process?

Infertility

Most traditional-age college students are interested in preventing pregnancy. However, increasing numbers of other people are trying to do just the opposite: they are trying to become pregnant. It is estimated that about one in six couples has a problem with *infertility*. These couples wish to become pregnant but are unable to do so.

Why do couples experience infertility? The reasons are about evenly balanced between men and women. About 10% of infertility has no detectable cause.[1] The most common male complication is insufficient sperm production and delivery. A number of approaches can be used to increase sperm counts. Among the simple approaches are the application of periodic cold packs on the scrotum and the replacement of tight underwear with boxer shorts. When a structural problem reduces sperm production, surgery can be helpful. Frequent intercourse (more than once every 36 hours) tends to lower sperm counts.[32] Most experts (fertility endocrinologists) suggest that couples have intercourse at least a couple of times in the week preceding ovulation.

Men can also collect (through masturbation) and save samples of their sperm to use in a procedure called *artificial insemination by partner*. Near the time of ovulation, the collected samples of sperm are then deposited near the woman's cervical opening. In the related procedure called *artificial insemination by donor*, the sperm of a donor are used. Donor semen is screened for the presence of pathogens, including the AIDS virus.

Causes of infertility in women center mostly on obstructions in the reproductive tract and the inability to ovulate. The obstructions sometimes result from tissue damage (scarring) caused by infections. Chlamydial and gonorrheal infections often produce fertility problems. In certain women the use of IUDs has produced infections and PID; both of these increase the chances of infertility. Other possible causes of structural abnormalities include scar tissue from previous surgery, fibroid tumors, polyps, and endometriosis. A variety of microsurgical techniques may correct some of these complications.

One of the most recent innovative procedures involves the use of **transcervical balloon tuboplasty.** In this procedure, a series of balloon-tipped catheters are inserted through the uterus into the blocked fallopian tubes. Once inflated, these balloon catheters help open the scarred passageways.

When a woman has ovulation difficulties, pinpointing the specific cause can be very difficult. Increasing age produces hormone fluctuations associated with lack of ovulation. Being significantly overweight or underweight also has a serious effect on fertility. However, in women of normal weight who are not approaching menopause, it appears that ovulation difficulties are caused by lack of synchronization between the hormones governing the menstrual cycle. Fertility drugs can help alter the menstrual cycle to produce ovulation. Clomiphene citrate (Clomid), in oral pill form, or injections of a mixture of LH and FSH taken from the urine of menopausal women (Pergonal) are the most common fertility drugs available. Both are capable of producing multiple ova at ovulation. (See Focus On article on page 424.)

Assisted Reproductive Technologies (ART)

For couples who are unable to conceive after drug therapy, surgery, and artificial insemination, the use of one of four assisted reproductive technologies (ART) can be helpful. One option is *in vitro fertilization and embryo transfer (IVF-ET)*. This method is sometimes referred to as the "test tube" procedure. Costing around $10,000 per attempt, IVF-ET consists of surgically retrieving fertilizable ova from the woman and combining them in a glass dish with sperm. After several days,

---

> **Key Terms**
>
> **cesarean delivery** surgical removal of a fetus through the abdominal wall.
>
> **transcervical balloon tuboplasty** the use of inflatable balloon catheters to open blocked fallopian tubes; a procedure used for some women with fertility problems.

the fertilized ova are transferred into the uterus. IVF-ET accounts for 98% of all ART procedures.[33]

A second test tube procedure is called *gamete intrafallopian transfer (GIFT)*. Similar to IVF-ET, this procedure involves depositing a mixture of retrieved eggs and sperm directly into the fallopian tubes.

Fertilized ova (zygotes) can also be transferred from a laboratory dish into the fallopian tubes in a third procedure called *zygote intrafallopian transfer (ZIFT)*. One advantage of this procedure is that the clinicians are certain that ova have been fertilized before the transfer to the fallopian tubes. GIFT and ZIFT combined account for fewer than 2% of ART procedures.[33]

The fourth (and newest) procedure is *intracytoplasmic sperm injection* (ICSI). This is a laboratory procedure in which a single sperm cell is injected into a woman's retrieved egg. The fertilized egg is then transplanted into the woman's uterus. The cost and technical expertise involved in ICSI make it a seldom-used procedure for infertile couples.

Surrogate Parenting

Surrogate parenting is another option that has been explored, although the legal and ethical issues surrounding this method of conception have not been fully resolved. Surrogate parenting exists in a number of forms. Typically, an infertile couple will make a contract with a woman (the surrogate parent), who will then be artificially inseminated with semen from the expectant father.

In some instances the surrogate will receive an embryo from the donor parents. In some cases, women have served as surrogates for their close relatives. The surrogate will carry the fetus to term and return the newborn to the parents. Because of the concerns about true "ownership" of the baby, surrogate parenting may not be a particularly viable or legal option for many couples.

TALKING POINTS You have tried for a couple of years to get pregnant, and now you are ready to consider some of the newest options to increase the chances of conception. Your partner seems unwilling to spend much money for these high-tech procedures. You are ready to spend some of your retirement savings in this effort. How can you and your partner best come to an agreement on this issue?

A Final Word About Infertility

The process of coping with infertility problems can be an emotionally stressful experience for a couple. Hours of waiting in physicians' offices, having numerous examinations, scheduling intercourse, producing sperm samples, and undergoing surgical or drug treatments place multiple burdens on a couple. Knowing that other couples are able to conceive so effortlessly adds to the mental strain. Fortunately, support groups exist to assist couples with infertility problems. Some of these groups are listed in the Star box above.

What can you do to reduce the chances of developing infertility problems? Certainly avoiding infections of the reproductive organs is one crucial factor. Barrier methods of contraception (condoms, diaphragm) with a spermicide reportedly cut the risk of developing infertility in half. The use of an IUD should be carefully considered, and the risk from multiple partners should encourage responsible sexual activity. Men and women should be aware of the dangers from working around hazardous chemicals or consuming psychoactive drugs. Maintaining overall good health and having regular medical (and, for women, gynecological) checkups are also good ideas. Finally, since infertility is linked with advancing age, couples may not want to indefinitely delay having children.

Taking Charge of Your Health

- Use the Personal Assessment on page 427 to help you determine which birth control method is best for you.
- Talk to your doctor about the health aspects of different types of birth control before making your decision.
- If the method of birth control you are currently using is unsatisfactory to you or your partner, explore other options.

- Reduce your risk of infertility by choosing a birth control method carefully, protecting yourself from infections of the reproductive organs, and maintaining good overall health.
- If you plan to have children, set a time frame that takes into account decreased fertility with advancing age.

Summary

- *Birth control* refers to all of the procedures that can prevent the birth of a child.
- *Contraception* refers to any procedure that prevents fertilization.
- Each birth control method has both a theoretical-effectiveness rate and a use-effectiveness rate. For some contraceptive approaches, these rates are similar (such as hormonal methods), and for others the rates are very different (such as condoms, diaphragms, and periodic abstinence).
- Many factors should be considered when deciding which contraceptive is best for you.
- Sterilization (vasectomy and tubal ligation) is generally considered an irreversible procedure.

- Currently, abortion remains a woman's choice under the guidelines of the 1973 *Roe v. Wade* decision.
- Abortion procedures vary according to the stage of the pregnancy.
- Several physiological factors can be either aids or obstacles to fertilization.
- Human cloning raises many ethical issues.
- Pregnant women should avoid agents that can harm the fetus.
- Childbirth takes place in three distinct stages.
- For couples with fertility problems, numerous strategies can be used to help conception take place.

Review Questions

1. Explain the difference between the terms *birth control* and *contraception*. Give examples of each.
2. Explain the difference between theoretical and use-effectiveness rates. Which one is always higher?
3. Identify some of the factors that should be given careful consideration when selecting a contraceptive method. Explain each factor.
4. For each of the methods of birth control, explain how it works and its advantages and disadvantages.
5. How do minipills differ from the combined oral contraceptive?
6. How does the contraceptive patch differ from the contraceptive ring?

7. What is emergency contraception?
8. How are tubal ligation and vasectomy accomplished?
9. Identify and describe the different abortion procedures that are used during each trimester of pregnancy. What is a medical abortion?
10. What are some obstacles and aids to fertilization presented in this chapter? Can you think of others?
11. Identify and describe the events that occur during each of the three stages of childbirth. Approximately how long is each stage?
12. What can be done to reduce chances of infertility? Explain IVF-ET, GIFT, ZIFT, and ICSI procedures.

References

1. McAnulty RD, Burnette MM. *Exploring human sexuality: making healthy decisions.* Allyn and Bacon, 2001.
2. Strong B, DeVault C, Sayad BW, Yarber WL. *Human sexuality: diversity in contemporary America,* 4th ed. McGraw-Hill, 2001.
3. Hatcher RA, et al. *Contraceptive technology,* 17th ed. Ardent Media, 1998.
4. WebMD Medical News. *Warning for spermicide nonoxynol-9* (January 17, 2003), **www.my.webmd.com/content/article/59/66773.htm,** accessed September 15, 2003.
5. Davis JL. *Spermicide promotes HIV,* WebMD Medical News (September 26, 2002), **www.webmd.com/content/article/50/40570.htm,** accessed September 15, 2003.
6. Allgeier ER, Allgeier AR. *Sexual interactions,* 5th ed. Houghton Mifflin, 2000.
7. DeNoon D. *Best condoms still latex.* WebMD Health (March 21, 2003), **www.my.webmd.com/content/article/62/71710,htm,** accessed September 11, 2003.
8. Planned Parenthood Federation of America. *Your contraceptive choices,* **www.plannedparenthood.org,** accessed September 10, 2003.
9. Steiner MJ, et al. Contraceptive effectiveness of a polyurethane condom and a latex condom: a randomized controlled trial. *Obstetrics and Gynecology,* March 2003, 101(3):539–547.
10. Greenberg JS, Bruess CE, Haffner DW. *Exploring the dimensions of human sexuality.* Jones and Bartlett, 2000.
11. Allendale Pharmaceuticals, telephone interview, September 11, 2003.
12. Planned Parenthood Federation of America. *Your contraceptive choices: IUD,* **www.plannedparenthood.org/bc/cchoices3.html#IUD,** accessed September 12, 2003.
13. Berlex Laboratories Website. *Changes in menstruation,* **www.mirena-us.com,** accessed September 15, 2003.
14. Crooks R, Baur K. *Our sexuality,* 8th ed. Wadsworth, 2001.
15. U.S. Bureau of the Census. *Statistical abstract of the United States: 2002,* 122nd ed. U.S. Government Printing Office.
16. U.S. Food and Drug Administration. *FDA approves Seasonale oral contraceptive,* FDA Talk Paper, (September 5, 2003), **www.fda.gov/bbs/topics/ANSWERS/2003/ANS01251.html,** accessed September 8, 2003.
17. Planned Parenthood Federation of America. *Birth control,* **www.plannedparenthood.org/bc/,** accessed September 10, 2003.
18. Hyde JS, DeLamater JD. *Understanding human sexuality,* 8th ed. McGraw-Hill, 2003.
19. Columbia University Health Education Program. *The NuvaRing—another birth control option,* **www.goaskalice.columbia.edu,** (November 11, 2002), accessed September 10, 2003.
20. Ortho-McNeil Pharmaceutical. *The first birth control patch receives FDA approval* (press release November 20, 2001), **www.ortho-mcneil.com/news/archive/pr/news_evra.htm,** accessed November 27, 2001.
21. The Alan Guttmacher Institute. *State policies in brief: Access to emergency contraception,* (September 1, 2003), **www.agi-usa.org/pubs/spib_EC.pdf,** accessed September 7, 2003.
22. Kelly GF. *Sexuality today: the human perspective,* 7th ed. McGraw-Hill, 2004.
23. *FDA approves 'abortion pill.'* (September 28, 2000), **www.cnn.com/health/women/09/28/abortion.pill,** accessed October 15, 2000.
24. Creinin MD, et al. Mifepristone and misoprostol and methotrexate/misoprostol in clinical practice for abortion. *American Journal of Obsterics and Gynecology,* March 2003, 188(3):664–669.
25. The Alan Guttmacher Institute. *State policies in brief: Bans on 'partial-birth' abortion* (September 1, 2003), **www.agi-usa.org/pubs/spib_BPBA.pdf,** accessed September 7, 2003.
26. Blonna R, Levitan J. *Healthy sexuality.* Morton Publishing Co., 2000.
27. Bonsor K. *How human cloning will work,* **www.science.howstuffworks.com/human-cloning.htm,** accessed 24 September 2003.
28. DeNoon D. *Cloning FAQs and fiction,* **www.my.webmd.com/content/article/57/66221.htm,** (6 January 2003), accessed 24 September 2003.
29. Warner J. *Most Americans against human cloning,* **www.my.webmd.com/content/article/59/66746.htm,** (16 January 2003), accessed 24 September 2003.
30. LeVay S, Valente SM. *Human sexuality.* Sinauer Associates, Inc, 2003.
31. National Center for Health Statistics. U.S. birth rate reaches record low: births to teens continue 12-year decline; cesarean deliveries reach an all-time high, *NCHS Press Release* (25 June 2003), **www.cdc.gov/nchs/releases/03news/lowbirth.htm,** accessed 1 October 2003.
32. WebMd. *Health guide A-Z: infertility—home treatment,* **www.my.webmd.com/content/healthwise/130/32439,** accessed 2 October 2003.
33. WebMd. *A couple's guide: trying to conceive,* **www.my.webmd.com/content/article/73/87996,** accessed 3 October 2003.

The political circumstances surrounding the so-called "partial birth abortion" procedures have changed very much since the manuscript for this edition (see page 413) was finished. The U.S. Congress passed the "Partial-Birth Abortion Ban Act" and in November 2003 President George W. Bush signed the bill into law. Shortly thereafter, a number of organizations (including the American Civil Liberties Union, the National Abortion Federation, and Planned Parenthood Federation of America) went to court and won temporary restraining orders to effectively block the immediate implementation of the new law.

As we go to press in April 2004, three trials (in California, New York, and Nebraska) are under way that challenge the wording and constitutionality of the new law. Critics of the law claim that the wording is vague and fails to protect women's health and reproductive choices. Proponents of the law contend that the procedure is not medically necessary to protect a woman's health and that it causes undue, inhumane pain to the fetus.

By the time you read this, verdicts in these suits will likely have been rendered. Do you know the current status of this law?

supertwins: the boom in multiple births

During World War II their parents gave them patriotic names, such as Franklin, Delano, and Roosevelt, or Franklin D. (for Roosevelt) and Winnie C. (a girl named for Winston Churchill).[1] You may know them as Rachel, Richard, Rebecca, and Ryan or Courtney, Britanny, and Tiffany. They're supertwins—multiple-birth siblings such as triplets, quadruplets, quintuplets, and even sextuplets and more. From 1989 to 1993, an average of 1,057 sets of triplets, 241 sets of quads, and 32 sets of quints were born each year in the United States.[1] More recently, the McCaugheys of Iowa gave birth to septuplets on November 19, 1997. All of their septuplets are home and doing well. Nkem Chukwu and her husband Lyke Louis Udobi of Texas were not as lucky with their octuplets. One of the eight died shortly after delivery in 1998.

Such multiple births are controversial for several reasons, including the increased risk they bring to the mother and the fetuses.

The Good, the Bad, and the Unusual

A special type of bonding occurs among multiple-birth siblings that ranges from reading one another's moods to saving another's life, as in the case of twin girls Brielle and Kyrie.[1,2] Kyrie, at 2 pounds 3 ounces, was doing well, but Brielle, the smaller twin, at 2 pounds, had had trouble breathing, an irregular heart rate, and a low blood oxygen level since birth. Then Brielle's condition suddenly became critical. The hospital staff tried every medical procedure they thought might help, to no avail. As a last resort, they put the girls in the same incubator, as some European hospitals do. Amazingly, Brielle's condition immediately improved and within

minutes her blood oxygen level was the best it had been since birth. Studies have confirmed that double bedding of multiple-birth babies reduces the length of their hospital stay.[2]

On the darker side, sometimes multiple births, or the prospect of them, are exploited by parents. The Dionne quintuplets, now 60 years old, were the middle 5 of 13 children. When their father sold the rights to exhibit his daughters, the Ontario government made them wards of the state. But the government ended up exploiting them in a bizarre glass playground Quintland-type display, which attracted 10,000 visitors a month. When they were returned to their parents, they were made to feel guilty for their unusual birth and the ensuing familial discord.[3] The surviving quints have written a book about their experiences and have helped teach the world that multiples are not something to be exploited.

Recently, in England, a woman abused fertility drugs by taking them even though she was already fertile and ignoring her physician's instructions while on the drugs. She became pregnant with eight fetuses. She refused to undergo multifetal pregnancy reduction, which would have given the remaining fetuses a better chance of survival, because she had sold her story to a tabloid and would get more money for each baby born. All eight fetuses died at 19 weeks' gestation.[4]

Fertility Drugs and Techniques

Since the birth of the first "test tube baby" (conceived by in vitro fertilization) in 1978, the number of assisted pregnancies and multiple births has escalated. The use of fertility drugs and techniques that stimulate

ovulation sometimes causes the release of multiple eggs per cycle.[1,5]

The infertility rate among married couples is 8.5%. While this rate has remained relatively constant in recent years, the number of couples seeking help for infertility has tripled.[6] Less than half of the couples who receive fertility treatment ever give birth, but one-fourth of those who *do* achieve a pregnancy give birth to more than one child.[1,6] This happens for a number of reasons. First, some fertility drugs are so strong that they cause multiple eggs to be released during one cycle. Second, some treatments are developed too quickly and are administered under too little supervision.[7] And third, fertility services are so competitive and lucrative ($67,000 to $114,000 per delivery.[3]) that many clinics go to great lengths to increase the likelihood of pregnancy, such as implanting up to eight embryos in a woman's uterus. In the United Kingdom, a doctor can lose his or her license for implanting more than three embryos, but no such laws have been passed in the United States.[8] Usually, few or no embryos develop; if too many develop, however, multifetal pregnancy reduction is often suggested.[7] This abortion procedure is usually performed by injecting potassium chloride into the most accessible embryos to increase the odds of survival for the others.[9]

The whole process of fertility treatment has been described as an emotional roller coaster.[1] The parents often want children desperately but can't conceive naturally. The drugs and hormones women are given to promote pregnancy can cause great emotional distress. If a couple does achieve a pregnancy, exhilaration can turn to fear when they find out how many embryos are developing. Will they be able to care for that many children? What if some or all of the babies are sick, or die? Should some be aborted to give the others a better chance? Many fertility clinics do an unsatisfactory job of counseling couples about the likelihood of success and the risks associated with the procedures, so couples often must answer these tough questions without all the information they need.[7]

Medical Complications

After conception, the fertility specialist's job is finished. Everything that goes on during the course of pregnancy and delivery is in the hands of another physician, usually an obstetrician with a specialty in high-risk pregnancy. These physicians must discuss with the parents any risks and concerns that were not addressed earlier.[7]

Each additional fetus shaves roughly 3.5 weeks off the normal 40-week gestation period.[9] Prematurity brings with it a host of problems. The babies are about a third of the weight or less of single babies and much more likely to be ill. The death rate before or soon after birth is 19 times higher for triplets than single babies.[1] From birth to 28 days, the death rate for multiples is still 7 times higher than for singles.[7] Surviving babies suffer higher rates of cerebral palsy and other neurological problems.[10]

Of course, multiple babies have longer hospital stays and are more likely to require intensive care during their stay than single babies. Although the issue of "drive-through" deliveries, in which mother and baby are released within 24 hours, has become a controversial topic lately, the average stay for a single baby is 4.6 days, compared with 8.2 days for twins and 34 days for triplets.[1,6] During their stays, 15% of single infants need intensive care, while 50% of twins and 75% of triplets, quads, and quints require this level of care.[6] Research has shown that most of the heavy use of medical resources in multiple births is due to lower gestational age and lower birth weight.[11]

Multiple births also increase the mother's need for care. The risks of cesarean delivery, anemia, hypertension, postpartum hemorrhage, and kidney failure are all greater in mothers of supertwins.[1,6] And this specialized care is extremely expensive: The estimated cost of a single birth is $9,850, compared with $37,950 for twins and $109,764 for triplets.[6] Hospital costs for quints can easily exceed half a million dollars.[1] If an insurance company covers this cost, we all pay in the form of increased premiums and deductibles. If they do not pay, it can spell financial ruin for the family. And these medical and financial complications all occur even before the newborns come home.

Public and Private Life

Parents of supertwins say the stress kicks in after about six months. Until then, they're busy just trying to meet their constant needs, which during the first three months involves feeding each of three to six babies seven to eight times per day.[1] Because of the stress of the babies' medical problems, financial strain, and pure exhaustion, child abuse is 2.5 to 9 times more likely in families with twins, compared with singles, and parents of supertwins are more likely to divorce.[1,7]

However, some people take it all in stride. One father of quintuplets regards the parenting of his five 3 ½ and one 7-month-old babies as character building. He's manufactured his own stairstep stroller, and he and his wife handle the 20 minutes of buckling, toy stowing, negotiating with the kids, and answering the questions of strangers whenever they go somewhere, with smiles of their faces.[1]

Some strangers beam at the sight of this unusual family, while others grimace and turn away. When people lightly tell their mother, "I'm glad it's you and not me," she answers in all seriousness, "Me too." The father sums up their situation this way: "Sure, it's a lifestyle change, but you take one day at a time, people help, and things work out."[1]

Family, friends, strangers, and even local and national companies do help

out. Discounts on diapers and baby food, two years' worth of free formula, a night's stay at a local motel, discounts on vans, and money to start college funds are examples of public generosity to the families of quads and quints. But along with public generosity comes public nosiness. One family answered a knock on the door from a senior citizens' tour bus group that wanted the parents to wake up the kids for a picture. More commonly, strangers think they can touch the children or ask personal questions of the parents, such as "Are they natural?" and "So, have you had your tubes tied?" and so on.[1]

Two nonprofit support groups help families cope with the unique stressors that multiple-birth families face. The Triplet Connection, based in California, and Mothers of Supertwins (MOST), based in New York, were both founded in the 1980s by triplet moms to provide reliable, accessible information to the families of supertwins.[1] With the sincere help of most people and organizations like these, parents can increase the odds that the more will truly be the merrier.

For Discussion . . .

Do you know any sets of twins or supertwins? How are their lives and those of their parents different from other families? What would you do if you or your partner were pregnant with supertwins? Do you think society has an obligation to help support supertwin families?

References

1. Jackson DD. People say, you poor thing and I'm thinking I have four healthy kids. *Smithsonian* 27(6):30–39, 1996.
2. Sheehan N. A sister's helping hand. *Reader's Digest* 148(889): 155–156, 1996.
3. Came B. A family tragedy. *Maclean's* 107:40–43, 1994.
4. Luscombe B. Eight at once is too many. *Time* 148(18):103, 1996.
5. Anonymous. Where are they now? *Time* 148(7):18, 1996.

6. Anonymous. The high cost of having some babies gets higher by the numbers. *Science News* 146(6):95, 1994.

7. Anonymous. And baby makes three or more: the ethics of fertility treatment are mainly a private matter. *The Economist* 340(7979):16, 1996.

8. Seligmann J. Fewer bundles of pain. Fertility doctors introduce reforms to reduce premature and multiple births. *Newsweek* 127(10):63, 1996.

9. Cowley G, Springen K. More is not merrier: when fertility drugs work too well. *Newsweek* 128(9): 49, 1996.

10. Doyle P. The outcome of multiple pregnancy. *Hum Reprod* (11 Suppl) 4:110–117, 1996.

11. Ettner SL, Christiansen CL, Callahan TL, Hall JE. How low birth weight and gestational age contribute to increased inpatient costs for multiple births. *Inquiry* 34(4):325–339, 1997–1998.

personal assessment

which birth control method is best for you?

To assess which birth control method would be best for you, answer the following questions, and check the interpretation below.

	Do I:	Yes	No
1.	Need a contraceptive right away?	____	____
2.	Want a contraceptive that can be used completely independent of sexual relations?	____	____
3.	Need a contraceptive only once in a great while?	____	____
4.	Want something with no harmful side effects?	____	____
5.	Want to avoid going to the doctor?	____	____
6.	Want something that will help protect against sexually transmitted diseases?	____	____
7.	Have to be concerned about affordability?	____	____
8.	Need to be virtually certain that pregnancy will not result?	____	____
9.	Want to avoid pregnancy now but want to have a child sometime in the future?	____	____
10.	Have any medical condition or lifestyle that may rule out some form of contraception?	____	____

Interpretation

If you have checked *Yes* to number:

1. Condoms and spermicides may be easily purchased without prescription in any pharmacy.
2. Sterilization, oral contraceptives, hormone injections, rings, or patches, cervical caps, and periodic abstinence techniques do not require that anything be done just before sexual relations.
3. Diaphragms, condoms, or spermicides can be used by people who have coitus only once in a while. Periodic abstinence techniques may also be appropriate but require a high degree of skill and motivation.
4. IUD use should be carefully discussed with your physician. Sometimes the use of oral contraceptives or hormone products results in some minor discomfort and may have harmful side effects.
5. Condoms and spermicides do not require a prescription from a physician.
6. Condoms help protect against some sexually transmitted diseases. Nonoxynol-9 may increase STD transmission in some users. No method (except abstinence) can guarantee complete protection.
7. Be a wise consumer: check prices, ask pharmacists and physicians. The cost of sterilization is high, but there is no additional expense for a lifetime.
8. Sterilization provides near certainty. Oral contraceptives, hormone injections, rings or patches or a diaphragm-condom-spermicide combination also give a high measure of reliable protection. Periodic abstinence, withdrawal, and douche methods should be avoided. Outercourse may be a good alternative.
9. Although it is sometimes possible to reverse sterilization, it requires surgery and is more complex than simply stopping use of any of the other methods.
10. Smokers and people with a history of blood clots should probably not use oral contraceptives or other hormone approaches. Some people have allergic reactions to a specific spermicide or latex material. Some women cannot be fitted well with a diaphragm or cervical cap. The woman and her health care provider will then need to select another suitable means of contraception.

To Carry This Further . . .

There may be more than one method of birth control suitable for you. Always consider whether a method you select can also help you avoid an STD. Study the methods suggested above, and consult Table 14.1 to determine what techniques may be most appropriate.

chapter fifteen

becoming an informed health care consumer

Talking It Over

Health Care: Where Do You Stand?

Health care is more than a political "hot potato." It's a high-priority issue that affects everyone, even if you're young and healthy. You probably realize that the U.S. health care system isn't perfect. What can you, as a college student, do?

- Keep yourself informed by reading and talking about health care issues.
- Write e-mails about your health care concerns to your legislators.

- Consider where candidates stand on health care issues when you vote.
- Join an advocacy group that is working to improve health care.

CommunicationLinks

www.health.gov/healthypeople
www.capweb.net

Eye on the Media

The Internet—Your New Health Superstore

In 2000, an estimated 33 million Americans explored the Internet in search of information, products, and services related to their health. A majority, an estimated 53%, will search for information about specific conditions, such as cancer or hypertension. Smaller but still impressive percentages of people will look for information about dieting and nutrition, fitness, women's health, and pharmaceuticals. In fact, the health books, supplements, medications, and devices found through these visits generated sales of about $1.7 billion in 2003.

The biggest challenge for you as a health consumer is determining the credibility of the information you find on the Internet. How can you know that this information (and accompanying products or services) is trustworthy

Health care providers often evaluate you by criteria from their area of expertise. The nutritionist knows you by the food you eat. The physical fitness professional knows you by your body type and activity level. In the eyes of the expert in health consumerism, you are the product of the health information you believe, the health-influencing services you use, and the products you consume. When you make your decisions about health information, services, and products after careful study and consideration, your health will probably be improved. However, when your decisions lack insight, your health, as well as your pocketbook, may suffer.

Health Information

The Informed Consumer

What aspects of health do people seem most interested in having information about? To which products and services do they most want access? In a 2001 poll conducted for the Kaiser Family Foundation to determine the health interests of American youth (15 to 24 years of age), the following areas were found: diseases (50%), sexual health (44%), weight loss/gain (25%), drugs and alcohol (23%), depression/mental illness (23%), violence (23%), smoking (19%), eating disorders (15%), acne/skin care (15%), local clinics (15%), and sexual assault (10%).[1] In light of the breadth of these interest areas and the complexity associated with each, it is very likely that most people turn to a variety of sources for the information and access that they seek. In the section that follows you will be introduced to several sources of health-related information. Complete the Personal Assessment on page 457 to rate your own skills as a consumer of health-related information, products, and services.

Sources of Information

Your sources of information on health topics are as diverse as the number of people you know, the number of publications you read, and the number of experts you see or hear. No single agency or profession regulates the quantity or quality of the health-related information you receive. Readers will quickly recognize that all are familiar sources and that some provide more accurate and honest information than others.

Family and Friends

The accuracy of information you get from a friend or family member may be questionable. Too often the information your family and friends offer is based on "common knowledge" that is wrong. In addition, family members or friends may provide information they believe is in your best interest rather than facts that may have a more negative effect on you.

Advertisements and Commercials

Many people spend much of every day watching television, listening to the radio, and reading newspapers or magazines. Because many advertisements are health oriented, these are significant sources of information. The primary purpose of advertising, however, is to sell products or services. One newer example of this intertwining of health information with marketing is the "infomercial," in which a compensated studio audience watches a skillfully produced program that trumpets the benefits of a particular product or service. In spite of the convincing nature of these infomercials, however, the validity of their information is often questionable.

In contrast to advertisements and commercials, the mass media routinely offer public service messages that give valuable health-related information.

Labels and Directions

Federal law requires that many consumer product labels, including all medications and many kinds of food (see Chapter 5), contain specific information. For example, when a pharmacist dispenses a prescription medication, he or she must give a detailed information sheet describing the medication.

Many health care providers and agencies give consumers informative information about their health problems or printed directions for preparing for screening procedures. Generally, information from these sources is accurate and current and is given with the health of the consumer foremost in mind.

Folklore

Because it is passed down from generation to generation, folklore about health is the primary source of health-related information for some people.

The accuracy of health-related information obtained from family members, neighbors, and coworkers is difficult to evaluate. As a general rule, however, one should exercise caution relying on its scientific soundness. A blanket dismissal is not warranted, however, because folk wisdom is occasionally supported by scientific evidence. In addition, the emotional support provided by the suppliers of this information could be the best medicine some people could receive. In fact, for some ethnic groups, indigenous health care is central to overall health care. Even though many Americans would consider this form of care "folk medicine," it is highly valued and trusted by those who find it familiar.

Testimonials

People strongly want to share information that has benefited them. Others may base their decisions on such testimonials. However, the exaggerated testimonials that accompany the sales pitches of the medical quack or the "satisfied" customers appearing in advertisements and on commercials and infomercials should never be interpreted as valid endorsements.

Mass Media

Health programming on cable television stations, stories in lifestyle sections of newspapers, health care correspondents appearing on national network news shows, and the growing number of health-oriented magazines are sources of health information in the mass media.

Specific reliance on the mass media sources can be seen in a survey conducted for the National Council on Aging, when it was reported that for persons between the ages of 46 and 64, television was the most widely turned to source of health-related information (36%), while magazines (34%), newspapers (17%), the Internet (8%), and radio (2%) followed behind.[2]

Health-related information in the mass media is generally accurate, but it is sometimes presented so quickly or superficially that its usefulness is limited.

Practitioners

The health care consumer also receives much information from individual health practitioners and their professional associations. In fact, today's health care practitioner so clearly emphasizes patient education that finding one who does not offer some information to a patient would be difficult. Education improves patient **compliance** with health care directives, which is important to the practitioner and the consumer.

Online Computer Services

The development of computer technology in the last decade has opened new sources of health information. Today, more than 100 million Americans (out of 270 million) have access to online services. However, the extent to which the Internet is used to access health-related information seems uncertain. A recent study found that only about 20% of American adults sought health-related information on the Internet during 2002,[3] while two earlier studies suggested much higher percentages (75%–80% and 40%). Regardless of the extent of its use, the Internet offers expansive collections of information, including text and video, to people interested in health.

To make certain that this increasingly important source of health information provides the most reliable information possible, twenty of the most frequently visited health-related sites joined forces in creating a code

---

Key Terms

compliance willingness to follow the directions provided by another person.

Discussing Web-Based Health Information with Your Physician

How should health-related information gleaned from the Internet be used, particularly when communicating with health care providers? Howard LeWine, MD, offers the following suggestions*:

- Inform your health care provider that you are accessing the Internet for information related to your particular area of concern. Know the name of the site you're using; your provider might already be familiar with the site, or wish to access it in preparation for your discussion.
- Do not bombard your provider with questions whenever you come across information that might be related to your health concern. Keep notes and discuss all of your findings at one time.
- Be prepared to *discuss* your information with your provider; don't use Web information to second-guess his or her position. Bear in mind that health concerns are too complex to generalize from the kind of one-size-fits-all information provided by even the most reliable websites, and must be evaluated on a case-by-case basis by a physician who has actually examined you.
- Always recognize that health-related information involves knowledge from many disciplines and uses highly technical language; media-based sources may grossly oversimplify in an effort to be accessible to lay persons.

*LeWine H: Quick tips for using online health information with your physician. *Harvard Special Commentary.* October 9, 2002, **www.intelihealth.com.**

Communication Between Patients and Their Health Care Providers

In the complex world of modern health care, it is of critical importance that patients communicate important information to their health care providers, and, in turn, that they understand as fully as possible the information that they receive from the providers. Below are ten valuable suggestions from the joint commission on Accreditation of Healthcare Organizations and the U.S. Government's Agency for Healthcare Research and Quality.

- Take part in every decision about your health care.
- If you are not prepared to ask questions on your own behalf, ask a family member or friend to fill this role for you.
- Tell your physician and pharmacist about every drug you are taking, including prescription drugs, OTC drugs, vitamins, supplements, and herbal products—bring them with you.
- Make certain that you get the results of every test and understand what they mean.
- If you do not hear about test results, never assume that everything is all right. Call your doctor's office and ask.
- Whenever possible, choose a hospital where many patients receive the same procedure that you are to receive. Ask your physician or the hospital for the actual numbers.
- Ask hospital personnel if they have washed their hands before they begin touching you.
- If you are having surgery, make sure that you, your physician, and your surgeon all agree on what will be done during the operation.
- Insist that your surgeon write his or her initials or words such as "yes" or "this side" on the part of the body to be operated on. Put "no" on the opposite body part.
- When you are discharged, ask your doctor to explain your treatment plan, including changes in medications, restrictions on activity, and additional therapies you will need.

In many situations involving medical care, carefully communicated comments and questions between providers and patients can be the basis of the successful resolution of a health problem, versus unnecessary delay, pain, discomfort, or even death.

Source: Ellis L. *How you can help guard against errors.* June 28, 2002. **http://www.intelihealth.com**

of ethics to ensure that information (and products sold via the sites) was valid and reliable. This voluntary code of ethics was implemented in November 2000.

Health Reference Publications

A substantial portion of all households own or subscribe to a health reference publication, such as the *Encyclopedia of Complementary Health Practices,*[4] the *Physicians' Desk Reference* (PDR),[5] or a newsletter such as *The Harvard Medical School Health Letter* or *The Johns Hopkins Medical Letter: Health After 50.* Some consumers also use personal computer programs and videocassettes featuring health-related information.

Reference Libraries

Public and university libraries continue to be popular sources of health-related information. One can consult with reference librarians and check out audiovisual collections and printed materials.

TALKING POINTS A family member considers herself good at diagnosing health problems. Since she hasn't been wrong in years, she no longer relies on physicians. What questions could you ask her to point out the dangers associated with her approach?

Consumer Protection Agencies and Organizations

Federal Agencies

Office of Consumer Affairs, Food and Drug Administration

U.S. Department of Health and Human Services
5600 Fishers Lane
Rockville, MD 20857
(301) 827-5006

www.fda.gov/oca/aboutoca.htm

Federal Trade Commission
Consumer Inquiries
Public Reference Branch
6th Street and Pennsylvania Avenue
Washington, DC 20580
(202) 326-2222

www.ftc.gov

Fraud Division
Chief Postal Inspector
U.S. Postal Inspection Service
475 L'Enfant Plaza
Washington, DC 20260-2166
(202) 268-4299

www.usps.gov

Consumer Information Center
Pueblo, CO 81009
(719) 948-3334

www.pueblo.gsa.gov

U.S. Consumer Product Safety Commission Hotline
(800) 638-CPSC

Consumer Organizations

Consumers Union of the U.S., Inc.
101 Truman Avenue
Yonkers, NY 10703
(914) 378-2000

www.consumerreports.org

Professional Organizations

American Medical Association
515 N. State Street
Chicago, IL 60610
(312) 464-5000

www.ama-assn.org

American Hospital Association
1 N. Franklin Street
Chicago, IL 60606
(312) 422-3000

www.aha.org

American Pharmaceutical Association
2215 Constitution Avenue, NW
Washington, DC 20037
(202) 628-4410

www.aphanet.org

Consumer Advocacy Groups

A variety of nonprofit consumer advocacy groups patrol the health care marketplace (see the Star box above). These groups produce and distribute information designed to help the consumer recognize questionable services and products. Large, well-organized groups, such as The National Consumers' League and Consumers Union, and smaller groups at the state and local levels champion the right of the consumer to receive valid and reliable information about health care products and services.

Voluntary Health Agencies

Volunteerism and the traditional approach to health care and health promotion are virtually inseparable. Few countries besides the United States can boast so many national voluntary organizations, with state and local affiliates, dedicated to improving health through research, service, and public education. The American Cancer Society, the American Red Cross, and the American Heart Association are voluntary (not-for-profit) health agencies. Consumers can, in fact, expect to find a voluntary

health agency for virtually every health problem. College students should also note that volunteerism on their part, perhaps with a health agency like the Red Cross or the AHA, is both a personally satisfying experience and an activity viewed favorably by potential employers.

Government Agencies

Government agencies are also effective sources of information to the public. Through meetings and the release of information to the media, agencies such as the Food and Drug Administration, Federal Trade Commission, United States Postal Service, and Environmental Protection Agency publicize health issues. Government agencies also control the quality of information sent out to the buying public, particularly through labeling, advertising, and the distribution of information through the mail. The various divisions of the National Institutes of Health regularly release research findings and recommendations to clinical practices, which in turn reach the consumer through clinical practitioners.

State governments also distribute health-related information to the public. State agencies are primary sources of information, particularly in the areas of public health and environmental protection. For an example of health care activism at work, see the Learning from Our Diversity box above.

Qualified Health Educators

Health educators work in a variety of settings and offer their services to diverse groups. Community health educators work with virtually all of the agencies mentioned in this section; patient educators function in primary care settings; and school health educators are found at all educational levels. Health educators are increasingly being employed in a wide range of wellness-based programs in community, hospital, corporate, and school settings.

Health Care Providers

The sources of health information just discussed can greatly help us make decisions as informed consumers. The choices we make about physicians, health services, and medical payment plans will reflect our commitment to remaining healthy and our trust in specific people who are trained in keeping us healthy. Refer to the Changing for the Better box on page 435 for tips on choosing a physician.

Why We Consult Health Care Providers

Most of us seek care and advice from medical and health practitioners when we have a specific problem. A bad cold, a broken arm, or a newly discovered lump can motivate us to consult a health care professional. Yet *diagnosis* and *treatment* are only two reasons that we might require the services of health care providers.

We also might encounter health practitioners when we undergo *screening*. Screening most often involves a cursory (or noninvasive) collection of information that can quickly be compared to established standards, themselves often based on gender, age, race, or the presence of

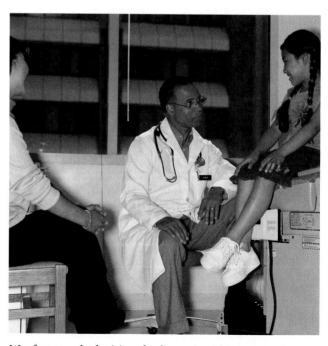

We often consult physicians for diagnosis and treatment of common ailments.

We're moving to a new town at the beginning of the summer. What will my parents and I need to know about choosing a new doctor?

- Talk with people about their health care providers. Most likely they will identify some providers that they would recommend, or not recommend.
- Talk with people in the health care field. They will generally find ways to "suggest" practitioners without violating professional practice standards.
- Call local hospitals for recommendations. They will usually provide several names of physicians who they know are taking new patients.
- Contact the websites listed in the InfoLinks at the end of this box for additional information on health care providers.

During your initial visit:

- Obtain a description of the physician's medical background, such as education, residencies, and specialty areas.
- How does the physician keep up with new developments in the medical profession?
- What are the normal office hours? What should be done if help is needed after normal office hours?
- What is included in a comprehensive physical examination?
- How does the physician feel about second and third opinions?
- With which hospitals is the physician affiliated?
- With which specialists is the physician associated?
- What is the physician's fee schedule?

After your initial visit, ask yourself:

- Was I comfortable with the physician's age, gender, race, and national origin?
- Was I comfortable with the physician's demeanor? Did I find communication with the physician to be understandable and reassuring? Were all my questions answered?
- Did the physician seem interested in having me as a patient?
- Are the physician's training and practice specialty in an area most closely associated with my present needs and concerns?
- Does the physician have staff privileges at a hospital I prefer?
- Does the physician's fee-for-service policy in any way exclude or limit my ability to receive necessary services?
- Did the physician take a complete medical history as a part of my initial visit? Did the physician address prevention, health promotion, or wellness during my visit?
- Did I sense that the physician was unusually reluctant or eager to try new medical procedures or medications?
- When the physician is unavailable, are any colleagues on call 24 hours a day? Did I feel that telephone calls from me would be welcomed and returned in a reasonable time?

If you have answered yes to most of these questions, you have found a physician with whom you should feel comfortable.

InfoLinks

www.healthgrades.com
www.nahdo.org

---

pre-existing conditions. Your earliest experience with screening may have been in elementary school, where physicians, nurses, audiologists, and dentists sometimes examine all children for normal growth and development patterns. As an adult, your screening is more likely to be done on an individual basis by a physician's staff as a routine portion of every office visit when they collect baseline information such as height, weight, and blood pressure measurements. You may also encounter community-based screening when you stop at your local shopping mall's health fair and have your blood pressure taken or cholesterol checked. Although screening should be considered much less precise than actual diagnosis, screening serves to identify people who should seek further medical examination.

Consultation is a fourth reason that knowledgeable consumers seek health care providers. A consultation is the use of two or more professionals to deliberate a person's specific health problem or condition. Consultations are especially helpful when **primary care health providers,** such as family practice physicians, gynecologists, pediatricians, internists, and general practice dentists, require the opinion of specialists. Using additional practitioners as consultants can also help reassure patients who may have doubts about their own condition or about the abilities of their physician.

Prevention is a fifth reason we might seek a health care provider. With the current emphasis on trying to stop problems before they begin, using health care

---

Key Terms

primary care health providers health care providers who generally see patients on a routine basis, particularly for preventive health care.

---

providers for prevention is becoming more common. People want information about how to prevent needless risks and promote their health, and they seek such advice from physicians, nurses, dentists, exercise physiologists, patient educators, and other health promotion specialists.

When prevention becomes a routine component of your personal health care, you will annually receive, in addition to the baseline measurements of height, weight, and blood pressure, more in-depth assessments such as a blood chemistry assessment, lipid profile, and cardiogram. Women will also likely receive a ViraPap test, breast examination, mammography, and pelvic examination, while men will likely receive a Prostate Specific Antibody (PSA) test, digital prostate examination, and testicular examination.

Physicians and Their Training

In every city and many smaller communities, the local telephone directory lists physicians in a variety of medical specialties. These health care providers hold the academic degree of Doctor of Medicine (MD) or Doctor of Osteopathy (DO).

At one time, **allopathy** and **osteopathy** were clearly different health care professions in terms of their healing philosophies and modes of practice. Today, however, MDs and DOs receive similar educations and engage in very similar forms of practice. Both can function as primary care physicians or as board-certified specialists. Their differences are in the osteopathic physician's greater tendency to use manipulation in treating health problems. In addition, DOs often perceive themselves as being more holistically oriented than MDs.

Medical and osteopathic physicians undergo a long training process. After they are accepted into professional schools, students generally spend 4 or more years in intensive training that includes advanced study in the preclinical medical sciences and clinical practice. When they complete this phase of training, the students are awarded the MD or DO degree and then take the state medical license examination. Most newly licensed physicians complete a residency at a hospital. Residency programs vary in length from 3 to 4 years. When they conclude their residency programs, including board-related examinations, physicians are granted board-certified status. Interestingly, since the late 1990s, applications for medical schools have been in a state of decline, and that, in turn, influences residency programs.[6] In addition to state and specialty board certification, comprehensive national certification of physicians is a frequently discussed possibility. At this time, no nationally required and all-encompassing certification of physician competency is required.

Complementary, Alternative, and Integrative Care Practitioners

In addition to medical and osteopathic physicians, several other forms of health care offer alternatives within the large health care market. Included within this group of complementary or alternative forms of practice are chiropractic, acupuncture, homeopathy, naturopathy, herbalism, reflexology, and ayurveda.[7] Although the traditional medical community has long scoffed at these fields of practice as ineffective and unscientific, many people use these forms of health care and believe strongly that they are as effective as (or more effective than) allopathic and osteopathic medicine. As a result of this belief, today many physicians are better informed about complementary care methods and more comfortable discussing them with patients. Following are brief descriptions of some of the more popular of these complementary care fields and the practitioners that function within them.

Chiropractic

Historically (and, to varying degrees, today) the underlying premise of chiropractic is that misalignment or subluxation of the spinal (vertebral) column is the primary cause of illness, and, thus, its realignment is the appropriate treatment for illness. Accordingly, chiropractic medical practice is primarily limited to vertebral adjustments, where manual manipulation of the spine its used to correct misalignments. Recent studies have shown that **chiropractic** treatment of some types of low-back pain can be more effective than conventional care. With about 50,000 practitioners in the United States, chiropractic is the third-largest health profession, used by 15 to 20 million people. Some chiropractors use only spinal manipulation, while others use additional medical technologies, including dietary supplementation and various noninvasive technologies similar to those used by physical therapists and athletic trainers, including massage.

In spite of the fact that chiropractors undergo nearly the same number of years of training as do primary care physicians and take courses closely aligned with those

> ### Key Terms
>
> **allopathy** (ah **lop** ah thee) a system of medical practice in which specific remedies (often pharmaceutical agents) are used to produce effects different from those produced by a disease or injury.
>
> **osteopathy** (os tee **op** ah thee) a system of medical practice in which allopathic principles are combined with specific attention to postural mechanics of the body.
>
> **chiropractic** manipulation of the vertebral column to relieve misalignments and cure illness.

taken by physicians, current laws restrict the scope of chiropractic practice to those techniques initially consistent with the original theoretical basis of their discipline, "one cause—one cure of all illnesses and diseases." Unless carefully controlled research, as specified by the National Center for Complementary and Alternative Medicine,[8] finds spinal subluxation/manipulation to be a salient cause/cure of illness (which seems unlikely), chiropractic medicine is likely to remain a user-friendly, highly popular but highly limited approach to health care.

Acupuncture

Acupuncture is, for Americans, the most familiar component of the 3,000-year-old Chinese medical system. This system is based on balancing the active and passive

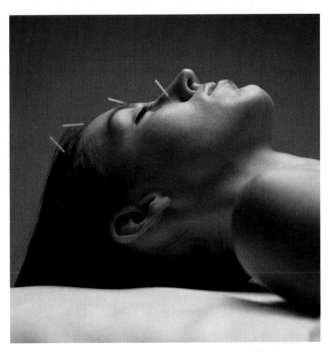

Acupuncture has received increasing acceptance within the Western medical community.

forces with the patient's body to strengthen the qi ("chee"), or life force. The system also employs herbs, food, massage, and exercise.

Acupuncturists place hair-thin needles at certain points in the body to stimulate the patient's qi. These points are said to correspond to different organs and bodily functions and, when stimulated, help the body's own defenses fight illness. More specifically, the scientific communities suggest that acupuncture speeds up the electrical conductivity within the central and peripheral nervous systems, enhances the production of biological opiates, and alters the production of specific neurotransmitters within various areas of the nervous system.[9]

Of all the Chinese therapies, acupuncture is the most widely accepted in the West. Researchers have produced persuasive evidence of acupuncture's effectiveness as an anesthetic and as an antidote to chronic pain, migraines, dysmenorrhea, and osteoarthritis.[10]

Reflexology

Reflexology uses principles similar to those of acupuncture but focuses on treating certain disorders through massage of the soles of the feet. To date, however, there is relatively little data regarding its effectiveness, when evaluated under carefully controlled conditions. The National Center for Complementary and Alternative Medicine has yet to fund carefully controlled research into the effectiveness of reflexology.

Homeopathy

Widely accepted in Europe, **homeopathy** is the leading alternative therapy in France. Homeopathy uses infinitesimal doses of herbs, minerals, or even poisons to stimulate the body's curative powers. The theory on which homeopathy is based, the *law of similars,* contends that if large doses of a substance can cause a problem, tiny doses can trigger healing. A few small studies showed homeopathy to be at least somewhat effective in treating hay fever, diarrhea, and flu symptoms, but members of the scientific community call the studies flawed or preliminary and suggest that the placebo effect was occurring. Much more

> ### Key Terms
>
> **acupuncture** insertion of fine needles into the body to alter electroenergy fields and cure disease.
>
> **reflexology** massage applied to specific areas of the feet to treat illness and disease in other areas of the body.
>
> **homeopathy** (hoe mee **op** ah thee) the use of minute doses of herbs, minerals, or other substances to stimulate healing.

informative, however, are reports from three meta-analysis studies, funded by the National Center for Complementary and Alternative Medicine, involving the reassessment of 240 individual studies, in which it was concluded that major methodology weaknesses existed in most studies of homeopathy studies conducted to date. It was further concluded that on the basis of these studies there was no strong evidence in favor of homeopathy over conventional treatment methods. The Center recommended that larger, more carefully controlled studies be conducted.[11]

An interesting new dimension to the marketing of homeopathy as an effective alternative to conventional medical care relates to the contention of some homeopathy physicians that the "molecular essence" of their homeopathic medicines can be sent via the Internet, thus allowing treatment to occur through cyberspace.[12]

Naturopathy

The core of naturopathic medicine is what Hippocrates called *medicatrix naturae,* or the healing power of nature. Proponents of **naturopathy** believe that when the mind and the body are in balance and receiving proper care, with a healthy diet, adequate rest, and minimal stress, the body's own vital forces are sufficient to fight off disease. Getting rid of an ailment is only the first step toward correcting the underlying imbalance that allowed the ailment to take hold, naturists believe. Correcting the imbalance might be as simple as rectifying a shortage of a particular nutrient, or as complex as reducing overlong work hours, strengthening a weakened immune system, and identifying an inability to digest certain foods.

Herbalism

Herbalism may be the world's oldest and most widely used healing form. Herbalists make herbal brews for treating a variety of ills, such as depression, anxiety, and hypertension. In some cases, scientific research supports the herbalists' beliefs. For example, studies have found St. John's wort to be more effective than a placebo and one of the older tricyclic antidepressants in alleviating mild depression, and that garlic reduces cholesterol and blood pressure, while black cohosh (a member of the buttercup family) and soy can relieve hot flashes and other menopause symptoms.

However, the potential side effects of many dietary supplements have raised questions about the dangers associated with particular herbs, especially of products containing ephedra, a stimulant used to enhance athletic performance or stimulate weight loss.[13] The Food and Drug Administration began to consider taking increased control over the testing and safety of all dietary supplements following the ephedra-related death of Baltimore Orioles pitcher Steve Belcher in February 2003; more than 150 deaths have been linked to the supplement.[14] In December 2003, after extensive studies, the FDA officially banned the sale and use of

ephedra, to be implemented in April 2004.[15] However, it is important to recognize that most supplements are not studied in this manner, and that virtually no regulation of the supplements industry currently exists.

Ayurveda

Even older than Chinese medicine, India's **ayurveda** takes a preventive approach and focuses on the whole person. This system employs diet, tailored to the patient's constitutional type, or dosha; herbs; yoga and breathing exercises; meditation; massages; and purges, enemas, and aromatherapy. Practitioners of ayurveda report success in treating rheumatoid arthritis, headaches, and chronic sinusitis.

. . .

If you would like to consult a practitioner in one of the alternative disciplines but you don't know where to start, see the Changing for the Better box on page 439 for some tips on choosing a provider in alternative medicine.

At the urging of many people in both the medical and complementary health care fields, the National Institutes of Health requested federal funding to establish a scientific center for the study of alternative medical care. Today the National Center for Complementary and Alternative Medicine assembles information about alternative approaches to medical care and provides a framework for well-controlled research into the effectiveness of each approach. The first substantial recommendation regarding an alternative form of care, acupuncture, was released in 1998.

It will be interesting to note whether all the branches of complementary medical care will want their theories of treatment and prevention tested under the rigorous criteria used by the National Center for Complementary and Alternative Medicine and to see how they respond if the results are not favorable.

Restricted-Practice Health Care Providers

We receive much of our health care from medical physicians. However, most of us also use the services of various health care specialists who also have advanced graduate-level training. Among these professionals are dentists, psychologists, podiatrists, and optometrists.

Key Terms

naturopathy (na chur **op** ah thee) a system of treatment that avoids drugs and surgery and emphasizes the use of natural agents to correct underlying imbalances.

herbalism an ancient form of healing in which herbal preparations are used to treat illness and disease.

ayurveda (ai yur **vey** da) traditional Indian medicine based on herbal remedies.

I'm interested in exploring complementary approaches to medicine, but I feel uncertain about how to proceed. What steps should I take?

Perhaps you are one of the millions of people who feel that their doctors don't encourage them to ask questions, don't seek their opinion about their medical condition, or don't take a thorough medical history. Perhaps you want advice on improving your health rather than just a quick diagnosis and prescription.

For whatever reasons, millions of Americans are turning to complementary medical practitioners, such as doctors of naturopathy, Chinese medicine, or ayurveda. Unfortunately, the patient looking for these alternatives faces other problems: practitioners' training may be weak, they might not be licensed or covered by insurance, they are hard to find, and they usually are not permitted to prescribe drugs unless they also happen to be medical doctors. This means that you must do some legwork to find a good provider who can meet your needs.

Consider the following tips for finding the practitioner who is right for you.

- *Don't forget the family physician.* Family-practice medicine is enjoying a surge in the United States, and many of these doctors tend to think holistically.
- *Find a physician who believes in complementary therapies.* Your doctor's attitude toward the treatment can be just as important as your own.
- *Give the treatment time.* Complementary therapies encourage the body to do its own healing. This often takes time. Seek a physician who is confident in your self-healing ability, so you won't become discouraged if it takes some time.
- *Request natural healing.* Natural healing tends to change the internal conditions so that pathogens are less likely to gain a

foothold; conventional medicine seeks to destroy the pathogen. Natural healing searches for the causes of symptoms, while conventional medicine treats symptoms.

- *Know your disease.* Find books that describe your conditions and offer complementary as well as conventional treatments. This way you can discuss your treatment with your physician and create an effective treatment plan.
- *Treat yourself.* Don't overuse your health care provider, whether conventional or complementary. For many conditions, you can be your own best doctor; of course, persistent or severe symptoms should send you to the physician.
- *Learn whether the treatment is covered by insurance.* Coverage of complementary treatment differs sharply by state. Some insurance groups are beginning to pay for more complementary medicine, and HMOs are hiring some complementary specialists.
- *Talk to professional associations.* Most of the more established complementary fields have associations that can give you a list of providers. Use it as a start.
- *Interview the practitioner.* Before making an appointment, talk with the doctor over the telephone. Then, in the practitioner's office, take notes, even use a tape recorder, to make certain you understand. Watch for a practitioner who is a good listener, a good communicator, and open-minded.

InfoLinks

http://nccam.nih.gov

Dentists (Doctor of Dental Surgery, DDS) deal with a wide range of diseases and impairments of the teeth and oral cavity. Dentists undergo undergraduate predental programs that emphasize the sciences, followed by 4 additional years of study in dental school and, with increasing frequency, an internship program. State licensure examinations are required. As with physicians, dentists can also specialize by completing a postdoctoral master's degree in fields such as oral surgery, **orthodontics,** and **prosthodontics.** Dentists are also permitted to prescribe therapy programs (such as the treatment of temporomandibular joint [TMJ] dysfunction) and drugs that pertain to their practices (primarily analgesics and antibiotics).

As discussed in Chapter 2, *psychologists* provide services to help patients understand behavior patterns or perceptions. More than forty states have certification or licensing laws that prohibit unqualified people from using

the term *psychologist.* The consumer should examine a psychologist's credentials. Legitimate psychologists have received advanced graduate training (often leading to a PhD or EdD degree) in clinical, counseling, industrial, or educational psychology. Furthermore, these practitioners will have passed state certification examinations and, in many states, will have met further requirements that allow

Key Terms

orthodontics a dental specialty that focuses on the proper alignment of the teeth.

prosthodontics a dental specialty that focuses on the construction and fitting of artificial appliances to replace missing teeth.

them to offer health services to the public. Psychologists may have special interests and credentials from professional societies in individual, group, family, or marriage counseling. Some are certified as sex therapists.

Unlike psychiatrists, who are medical physicians, psychologists cannot prescribe or dispense drugs. They may refer to or consult with medical physicians about clients who might benefit from drug therapy.

Podiatrists are highly trained clinicians who practice podiatric medicine, or care of the feet (and ankles). Although not MDs or DOs, doctors of podiatric medicine (DPM) treat a wide variety of conditions related to the feet, including corns, bunions, warts, bone spurs, hammertoes, fractures, diabetes-related conditions, athletic injuries, and structural abnormalities. Podiatrists perform surgery, prescribe medications, and apply orthotics (supports or braces), splints, and corrective shoes for structural abnormalities of the feet.

Doctors of podiatric medicine follow an educational path similar to that taken by MDs and DOs, consisting of a 4-year undergraduate preprofessional curriculum, 4 additional years of study in a podiatric medical school, and an optional residency of 1 or 2 years. Board-certified areas of specialization include surgery, orthopedics, and podiatric sports medicine. Hospital affiliation generally requires board certification in a specialized area.

Optometrists are eye specialists who primarily treat vision problems associated with **refractory errors.** They examine the eyes and prescribe glasses or contact lenses to correct visual disorders. Additionally, optometrists prescribe prescription medications, such as antibiotic drops for application in the eye. Optometrists sometimes attempt to correct certain ocular muscle imbalances with specific exercise regimens. Optometrists must complete undergraduate training and additional years of coursework at one of sixteen accredited colleges of optometry in the United States or two Canadian colleges before taking a state licensing examination.

Nurse Professionals

Nurses constitute a large group of health professionals who practice in a variety of settings. Their responsibilities usually depend on their academic preparation. Registered nurses (RNs) are academically prepared at two levels: (1) the technical nurse, and (2) the professional nurse. The technical nurse is educated in a 2-year associate degree program. The professional nurse receives 4 years of education and earns a bachelor's degree. Both technical and professional nurses must successfully complete state licensing examinations before they can practice as RNs.

In light of the important role that nurse professionals play in today's health care system, it is worrisome that a significant shortage of nurses exists. On the basis of enrollment data for nursing programs in this country, and the number of nurses who have apparently left the workforce for various reasons, the current shortage of registered nurses is estimated to be 110,000. Projecting through 2008, it is estimated that the shortage will have increased to 450,000.[16] Compounding the shortage of nurses is an equally acute shortage of nursing faculty to staff the nursing education programs that currently exist. As can be imagined, the demand for nurses has increased salaries, generated competition between health care institutions to recruit nurses, and increased the nurse-to-patient ratio to dangerously high levels in many areas of the country. In this final regard, it is estimated that as many as 20,000 unnecessary deaths that occur annually in American hospitals and nursing facilities can be attributed to the shortage—about one-fifth of all deaths attributed to medical errors.[17]

Many professional nurses continue their education and earn master's and doctoral degrees in nursing or other health-related fields. Some professional nurses specialize in a clinical area (such as pediatrics, gerontology, public health, or school health) and become certified as *advanced practice nurses* (APNs). Currently four APN fields, including nurse midwives, nurse anesthetists, nurse practitioners, and nurse case managers, can be found in larger communities. Working in close association with physicians, APNs perform an array of diagnositic, treatment, and administrative activities once limited to physicians. The ability of these highly trained nurses to function at this level gives communities additional primary care providers and frees physicians to deal with more complex cases.

Licensed practical nurses (LPNs) are trained in hospital-based programs that last 12 to 18 months. Because of their brief training, LPNs' scope of practice is limited. Most LPN training programs are gradually being phased out.

Allied Health Care Professionals

Our primary health care providers are supported by a large group of allied health care professionals, who are often responsible for highly technical services and procedures. These professionals include respiratory and inhalation therapists, radiographic technologists, nuclear medicine technologists, pathology technicians, general medical technologists, operating room technicians, emergency medical technicians, physical therapists, occupational therapists, cardiac rehabilitation therapists, dental

---

Key Terms

refractory errors abnormal patterns of light wave transmission through the structures of the eye.

technicians, physician assistants, and dental hygienists. Depending on the particular field, the training for these specialty support areas can take from 1 to 5 years of post-secondary school study. Programs include hospital-based training leading to a diploma through associate, bachelor's, and master's degrees. Most allied health care professionals must also pass state or national licensing examinations.

Self-Care/Home Care

The emergence of the **self-care movement** suggests that many people are becoming more responsible for maintaining their health. They are developing the expertise to prevent or manage many types of illness, injuries, and conditions. They are learning to assess their health status and treat, monitor, and rehabilitate themselves in a manner that was once thought possible only through a physician or some other health care specialist.

The benefits of this movement are that self-care can (1) reduce health care costs, (2) provide effective care for particular conditions, (3) free physicians and other health care specialists to spend time with other patients, and (4) increase interest in health-related activities.

Self-care is an appropriate alternative to professional care in three areas. First, self-care may be appropriate for certain acute conditions that have familiar symptoms and are limited in their duration and seriousness. Common colds and flu, many home injuries, sore throats, and non-allergic insect bites are often easily managed with self-care. That said, there are some symptoms that might seem somewhat familiar that should not be responded to through self-care, but rather by seeing a physician promptly. These include feeling of pressure or squeezing in the chest, a sudden severe headache, markedly blurred vision, difficulty talking or walking, dizziness and confusion, blood in urine or stool, unrelieved depression, and a cough with a yellow-green discharge.[18] Self-care might be useful at some point, but not until the symptoms have been evaluated by a physician.

A second area in which self-care might be appropriate is therapy. For example, many people administer injections for diabetes mellitus, allergies, and migraine headaches and continue physical therapy programs in their homes. Asthma and hypertension are also conditions that can be managed or monitored with self-care.

A third area in which self-care has appropriate application is health promotion. Weight loss programs, physical conditioning activities, smoking cessation, and stress-reduction programs are particularly well suited to self-care (see the Discovering Your Spirituality box on page 442).

As the U.S. population ages, it is becoming increasingly common for family members to provide home care to older relatives. As the number of frail older people increases, home care can significantly reduce the need for institutional care. Home care also can be delivered by home health care specialists. In fact, this form of care is proving so cost-effective that some insurance programs, including *Medicare* and *Medicaid,* cover portions of the cost of home health care for older adults. (See the Star box on Medicare and Medicaid on page 446.)

With the rapid development of the home health care industry during the 1980s and 1990s, concerns mounted about the lack of regulation over aspects of the industry, particularly the background and training of personnel, and the existence of fraud in the billing of services to Medicare and Medicaid. In 1999 the Healthcare Integrity and Protection Data Bank was established to better supervise the billing by home health care providers for services covered under Medicare and Medicaid.[19]

A decision to provide family-based home care, particularly for older adults, is often made for admirable and understandable reasons, including love for the relative who needs care and the high cost of professional home care and institutional care. For the millions of families who have made this decision, providing home health care can be highly rewarding. It also can be very demanding, however, because of the needs and limitations of the person who requires care and the compromises the caregivers must make. Particularly when a spouse or family decides to provide care without the assistance of professional caregivers, they can jeopardize their own health long before the recovery or death of the person for whom they are caring. Even when their physical stamina seems unaffected, factors such as fatigue, emotional strain, postponement of personal and family goals, loss of social contact, and even physical abuse of caregivers by those receiving care can be substantial.

Health Care Facilities

Most of us have a general idea of what a hospital is. However, all hospitals are not alike. They usually fall into one of three categories—private, public, or voluntary. *Private hospitals* (or proprietary hospitals) function as profit-making hospitals. They are not supported by tax monies and usually accept only clients who can pay all their expenses. Although there are some exceptions,

---

> **Key Terms**
>
> **self-care movement** the trend toward individuals' taking increased responsibility for prevention or management of certain health conditions.

The average life expectancy for women in the United States today is 80 years. For men, it's 76 years. That's a dramatic change from just a century ago. Thanks to tremendous advances in medical science and technology, many people are enjoying healthy, happy, and spiritually fulfilling lives well into their final years.

But this longevity comes with a price tag. It means that making healthful choices every day—including eating a balanced diet, getting exercise and adequate rest, and making opportunities for emotional and spiritual expression—takes on new importance. If you're going to live 10 "extra" years, what do you want to do with that time? Probably many of the things you're doing now, plus some different ones. Are you going to be able to meet the challenge—healthwise?

Taking charge of your health right now, when you're young and healthy, can be one of the most empowering things you do. By consciously choosing a healthy lifestyle—limiting your intake of alcohol, avoiding drugs and cigarette smoking, and limiting your sexual partners—you are building the foundation for good health in your later years.

If you should ever have a serious health problem, you'll be better equipped to handle it if you're used to taking care of yourself. You'll feel comfortable being involved in your treatment decisions and doing whatever you can to control the quality of your life. You'll see your health crisis as a challenge you need to deal with, instead of viewing yourself as a helpless victim.

Taking charge of your own health—by being an informed health care consumer, by choosing a healthy lifestyle, and by fostering a positive attitude—brings a sense of peace. It's knowing that you're doing everything you can to take care of yourself. It's enhancing the quality of your life today and preparing for an active and rewarding tomorrow.

these hospitals are generally smaller than tax-supported voluntary hospitals. Commonly owned by a group of business investors, a large hospital corporation, or a group of physicians, these hospitals sometimes limit their services to a few specific types of illnesses.

Public hospitals are supported primarily by tax dollars. They can be operated by government agencies at the state level (such as state mental hospitals) or at the federal level (such as the Veterans Administration Hospitals and various military service hospitals such as Walter Reed Army Hospital). Large county or city hospitals are frequently public hospitals. These hospitals routinely serve indigent segments of the population. They also function as *teaching hospitals.*

The most commonly recognized type of hospital is the *voluntary hospital.* Voluntary hospitals are maintained as nonprofit public institutions. Often supported by religious orders, fraternal groups, or charitable organizations, these hospitals usually offer a wider range of comprehensive services than do private hospitals or clinics. Voluntary hospitals are supported by patient fees (covered by health insurance), Medicare reimbursement, and Medicaid and public assistance reimbursement.

In the last decade, hospitals, particularly private and voluntary hospitals, have expanded their scope of services. Today hospitals often operate *wellness centers,* stress centers, cardiac rehabilitation centers, chemical dependence programs, health education centers, and satellite centers for well-baby care and care for the homeless. During the 1990s two trends were observed in terms of hospital organization and ownership. These included the acquisition of small hospitals (such as county hospitals and smaller community hospitals) by larger regional hospitals and the reorganization of voluntary hospitals as for-profit hospitals. Both trends reflected the rapid movement of medical care in the direction of *managed care,* the term referring to the more profit-focused, cost-efficient, and third-party-controlled care reflective of the application of corporate strategies to the delivery of health care services.

Other health care facilities include clinics (both private and tax-supported), nursing homes (most of which are private enterprises), and rehabilitation centers. Rehabilitation centers are often supported by charitable organizations devoted to the care of chronically ill or handicapped people, orthopedically injured people, or burn victims.

In recent years, many private, 24-hour drop-in medical emergency and surgical centers have appeared. These clinics have their own professional staffs of physicians, nurses, and allied health professionals.

Patients' Institutional Rights

Regardless of the type of institution in which you are a patient, you have a variety of rights. These are intended to protect you from unnecessary harm and financial loss. The hospital too can expect your cooperation as a patient.

As a patient, you can expect all of the following from the institution:

- To be treated with respect and dignity
- To be afforded privacy and confidentiality consistent with federal and state laws, institutional policies, and the requirements of your insurance carrier

- To be provided services on request, as long as they are reasonable and consistent with appropriate care
- To be fully informed of the identity of the physicians and staff providing care
- To be kept fully updated about your condition, including its management and your prognosis for recovery
- To be informed of any experimental or other research/educational projects that may be utilized in your treatment and to refuse such treatment
- To have the opportunity to specify advance directives (a living will, a life-prolonging statement, or the appointment of a health care representative) in order to facilitate health care decisions
- To receive an explanation of your bill for services regardless of the source of payment
- To present a complaint and receive a response about any aspect of your care or treatment and to have your complaint taken seriously
- To be involved in ethical considerations that arise during the course of your care

The institution can expect you, as a patient:

- To keep all appointments
- To provide all background information pertinent to your condition
- To treat hospital personnel with respect
- To ask questions and seek clarification about matters that affect you
- To follow the treatment prescribed by your physician
- To be considerate and respectful of other patients and to ensure that your visitors are considerate and respectful as well
- To satisfy your financial obligation to health care providers through the provision of insurance information and by arranging credit where applicable

As a patient, you may at any time:

- Refuse treatment
- Seek a second opinion
- Discharge yourself from the institution

Health Care Costs and Reimbursement

There are many avenues for receiving health care. However, being able to pay for quality health care is one of the greatest concerns of the American public. According to the latest available statistics (2002), 41.2 million Americans are without health insurance. Furthermore, Americans are less optimistic today about their ability to maintain adequate health insurance coverage, find reasonably priced health care, and afford long-term homebound or nursing home care than ever before. Unfortunately, the word *crisis* is appropriate to use when talking about our ability to afford high-quality health care today.

Cost is a basic concern about health care. It is estimated that in 2000 Americans spent $1.295 trillion on health care, and by 2007 this expenditure will increase to $2.13 trillion. Stated another way, in 2000 Americans incurred an average of $4,547 per person in health care-related costs. This amount is expected to increase to $7,100 per person by the year 2007. No developed country spends a greater percentage (14.2% in 2000) of its gross domestic product on health care than does America.[20] In 2000, the U.S. Government spent more than $1,424 billion on health care for its citizens; that figure is expected to top $1,907 billion in 2005.[20, 21]

As a result of factors such as the high cost of modern medical technology, an emphasis on long life at any cost, the growing number of older people with chronic conditions that require expensive long-term care, and the AIDS epidemic, controlling the cost of medical care is one of the most complex problems facing the nation. Nevertheless, more than forty different plans have been advanced since 1990 to respond to this problem. These range from only modest changes in the current system, to tax-credit strategies and mandatory employment-based insurance, to a federally controlled national health plan. Today government officials seem to be particularly interested in lowering the cost of prescription drugs for older Americans. In December 2003, President Bush signed the Medicare Prescription Drug Improvement and Modernization Act. Hailed as an answer to rising drug costs for seniors, the act was widely criticized as still being too costly for many seniors.[22]

Health Insurance

Health insurance is a financial agreement between an insurance company and an individual or group for the payment of health care costs. After paying a premium to an insurance company, the policyholder is covered for specific benefits. Each policy is different in its coverage of illnesses and injuries. Merely having an insurance policy does not mean that all health care expenses will be covered. Most health insurance policies require various forms of payments by the policyholder, which includes deductible amounts, fixed indemnity benefits, coinsurance, and exclusions. In 2000 Americans spent $372.8 billion on private health insurance, and they are expected to spend $643.4 billion by 2007.[23]

A *deductible* amount is an established amount that the insuree must pay before the insurer reimburses for services. For example, a person or family may have to pay the first $200 of the year's medical expenses before insurance begins providing any coverage.

A policy with *fixed indemnity* benefits will pay only a specified amount for a particular procedure or service. If the policy pays only $1,000 for an appendectomy and the actual cost of the appendectomy was $1,500, then the policy owner will owe the health care provider $500. A policy with full-service benefits, which pays the entire cost of a particular procedure or service, may be worth the extra cost.

Policies that have *coinsurance* features require that the policy owner and the insurance company share the costs of certain covered services, usually on a percentage basis. One standard coinsurance plan requires that the policyholder pay 20% of the costs above a deductible amount, and the company pays the remaining 80%.

An *exclusion* is a service or expense that is not covered by the policy. Elective or cosmetic surgery procedures, unusual treatment protocols, prescription drugs, and certain kinds of consultations are common exclusions. Illness and injuries that already exist at the time of purchase (preexisting conditions) are often excluded. In addition, injuries incurred during high-risk activities (ice hockey, hang gliding, mountain climbing, intramural sports) might not be covered by a policy.

Health insurance can be obtained through individual policies or group plans. Group health insurance plans usually offer the widest range of coverage at the lowest price and are often purchased cooperatively by companies and their employees. In 2003 companies with health insurance benefits spent on average $6,656.00 for each employee's family health insurance plan—a 28% increase over 2000 costs.[24] Fortunately, no employee is refused entry into a group insurance program. However, when employees leave the company, their previous group coverage can follow them for a prescribed period of time only, usually 18 to 24 months. Today, as many large American companies continue to lay off employees, the eventual loss of health insurance becomes a serious personal and family crisis.

Individual policies can be purchased by one person (or a family) from an insurance company. These policies are often much more expensive than group plans and may provide much less coverage. Still, people who do not have access to a group plan should attempt to secure individual policies, because the financial burdens resulting from a severe accident or illness that is not covered by some form of health insurance can be devastating. Many colleges and universities offer annually renewable health insurance policies that students can purchase. The Changing for the Better box above gives the consumer some questions to consider before purchasing a health insurance policy.

Health Maintenance Organizations

Health maintenance organizations (HMOs) are health care delivery plans under which health care providers agree to meet the covered medical needs of subscribers for a prepaid amount of money. For a fixed monthly fee, enrollees are given comprehensive health care with an emphasis on preventive health care. Enrollees receive their care from physicians, specialists, allied health professionals, and educators who are hired (group model) or contractually retained (network model) by the HMO.

Managed care, and HMOs in particular, was a reaction to the sharply climbing costs of health care in the 1980s. Businesses, which paid a large portion of health care costs through employee-benefit plans, complained that no one in the health care loop had an incentive to control costs. Employers complained that consumers paid only a deductible and a small copayment, giving them little cause to question prices; doctors faced little financial oversight; and insurance companies merely rubber-stamped the bills.

When HMOs presented an alternative, employers began offering their workers incentives to select HMOs over traditional fee-for-service coverage and thus attempted to rein in the runaway costs of health care. HMOs now cover nearly 70 million Americans. Increases in membership continued until 2000, when many HMOs that participated in Medicare supplement plans discontinued participation and, thus, discontinued service to their previously enrolled older adult members. The escalating cost of prescription medications was the principal factor in this decision. In all HMOs the annual cost of membership continues to rise, particularly for persons enrolled in the for-profit HMOs. This increase reflects the rising cost of services that must be provided to members.

HMOs are usually the least expensive but most restrictive type of managed care. The premiums are 8% to 10% lower than traditional plans, they charge no deductibles or coinsurance payments, and copayments are $5 to $10 per visit. However, you are limited to using the doctors and hospitals in the HMO's network, and you must get approval for treatments and referrals.

In theory, HMOs were to be the ideal blend of medical care and health promotion. Today, however, many observers are concerned that too many HMOs are being too tightly controlled by a profit motive in which physicians are being paid large bonuses to *not* refer patients to specialists or are prevented by "gag rules" from discussing certain treatment options with patients because of their costs to the HMOs.

Concerns, in addition to the "gag rules" mentioned above, have also arisen over the years. Among these have been concerns related to the right of members to sue their HMOs for medical negligence, the provision of better ob-gyn coverage, and the development of a more efficient mechanism to appeal denial of services. The latter is among the most distressing aspects of HMO membership to most members.

In spite of the problems just mentioned, HMOs remain, in theory, more cost-efficient than the traditional fee-for-service healthcare model. Cost containment is achieved, in part, because most of the medical services within a group model HMO are centralized, there is little duplication of facilities, equipment, or support staff. Central filing of records gives all the HMO physicians access to a single file for each client. This saves time, administrative costs, and the overlapping of care. HMOs also routinely use health-promotion activities.[25]

Other new approaches to reducing health costs are independent practice associations (IPAs) and preferred provider organizations (PPOs). An IPA is a modified form of an HMO that uses a group of doctors who offer prepaid services out of their own offices and not in a central HMO facility. IPAs are viewed as "HMOs without walls." A PPO is a group of private practitioners who sell their services at reduced rates to insurance companies. When a policyholder chooses a physician who is in that company's PPO network, the insurance company pays the entire physician's fee. When a policyholder selects a non-PPO physician, the insurance company pays only a portion of that physician's fee. Today, more than 80% of Americans with health benefits are enrolled in a managed care plan (HMO, IPA, or PPO).[26] In some areas of the country, such as California, Oregon, and Washington, over 90% of persons with benefits are in managed care plans. For a discussion on Medicare and Medicaid, see the Star box on page 446.

Extended Care Insurance

With the aging of the population and the greater likelihood that nursing home care will be required (at nearly $57,000.00 per year in 2002), insurers have developed

Medicare and Medicaid

Persons over the age of 65 (as well as persons of any age who have specific illnesses or disabilities) are provided with health care through Medicare. Medicare includes hospital insurance, nursing and hospice care, and some home health care, as well as optional coverage (for a monthly fee) for other costs such as medical devices, therapy, and most recently, prescription drugs. Anyone who has paid Medicare taxes while working becomes eligible for Medicare upon turning 65.

Unlike Medicare, *Medicaid* is designed to assist in meeting the health care needs of qualified persons of any age. While Medicare is funded and administered by the federal government, Medicaid is administered by the individual states, using funds provided by both the state and federal government. This means that, while the federal government sets mandatory eligibility and service standards, states are able to set optional eligibility standards tailored to the needs of their citizens. For this reason, standards and services for Medicare recipients can very greatly from state to state. For more information on Medicaid programs in your state, visit the federal government's Medicaid page at **http://cms.hhs.gov/medicaid/,** and click on the link for your state.

Source: U.S. Department of Health and Human Services
http://cms.hhs.gov

extended care policies.[27] When purchased at an early age (by mid-50s), these policies are much more affordable than if purchased when a spouse or family member will soon require institutional care. However, not all older adults will need extensive nursing home care, so an extended care policy could be an unnecessary expenditure.

Access to Health Care

With 41.2 million Americans lacking any health insurance and with nearly a quarter of those with insurance being underinsured, Americans are finding it increasingly difficult to access their country's highly sophisticated health care system. The unemployed poor, working poor, and minorities have the most difficulty accessing health care. African Americans, Hispanic Americans, and Native Americans have the worst health status of all Americans, yet they receive the fewest health care services. Even for older Americans with Medicare, gaping holes exist in the types of care covered (for example, glasses and hearing aids are not covered) and the prices of prescription medications far exceed the coverage provided. Thus, as America enters the twenty-first century, its people are expressing growing concern about the extent to which their

health care needs will be met. As political opposition remains strongly against a national health care system, the United States joins South Africa to make them the only two major industrialized nations lacking a comprehensive and unified approach to meeting the health care needs of their populations.

Health-Related Products

As you might imagine, prescription and over-the-counter (OTC) drugs constitute an important part of any discussion of health-related products.

Prescription Drugs

Caution: Federal law prohibits dispensing without prescription. This FDA warning appears on the labels of approximately three-fourths of all medications. Prescription drugs must be ordered for patients by a licensed practitioner. Because these compounds are legally controlled and may require special skills in their administration, the public's access to these drugs is limited.

Although the *Physicians' Desk Reference* lists more than 2,500 compounds that can be prescribed by a physician, only 200 drugs make up the bulk of the nearly 3,010 million new prescriptions and refills dispensed by 43,600 pharmacies in 2001.[27] Total retail prescription sales of $145 billion for 2000 represents a 15% increase over the previous year's sales. This upward trend reflects in large part the greater variety of prescription medications being prescribed each year by physicians. It is projected that by the year 2012 approximately $446 billion will be spent on prescription medications.[21] The rapid expansion of online pharmacies now occurring is unlikely to influence the number of prescriptions filled, though their presence will likely affect the sales of "brick and mortar" drugstore chains.

Some consumers have fled the U.S. market altogether and chosen to purchase prescription medications in Canada, where prices are substantially lower. For example, a 90-day supply of the prescription drug Zocor, used to lower blood cholesterol, will cost more than $350 at a typical American pharmacy; in Canada, a patient can purchase the same amount of the same medication for $140.[28]

Research and Development of New Drugs

As consumers of prescription drugs, you may be curious about the process by which drugs gain FDA approval. The rigor of this process may be the reason that only about one hundred new drugs are approved annually.

The nation's pharmaceutical companies constantly explore the molecular structure of various chemical compounds in an attempt to discover important new compounds with desired types and levels of biological activity. Once these new compounds are identified, companies begin extensive in-house research with computer simulations and animal testing to determine whether clinical trials with humans are warranted. Of the 125,000 or more compounds under study each year, only a few thousand receive such extensive preclinical evaluation. Even fewer of these are then taken to the FDA to begin the evaluation process necessary to gain approval for further research with humans. When the FDA approves a drug for clinical trials, a pharmaceutical company can obtain a patent, which prevents the drug from being manufactured by other companies for the next 17 years.

The $500 million price tag for bringing a new drug into the marketplace reflects this slow, careful process. If the 7 years of work needed to bring a new drug into the marketplace go well, a pharmaceutical company enjoys the remaining 10 years of legally protected retail sales. Today new "fast-track" approval procedures at the FDA are progressively reducing the development period, particularly for desperately needed breakthrough drugs like those used to treat AIDS. Concern was expressed in 2000 that this "rush to approval" forced the FDA to utilize the services of independent evaluators, many of whom had ties to the pharmaceutical industry that would have influenced their assessments of a drug's readiness for marketing.

Generic versus Brand Name Drugs

When a new drug comes into the marketplace, it carries three names: its **chemical name,** its **generic name,** and its **brand name.** While the 17 year patent is in effect, no other drug with the same chemical formulation can be sold. When the patent expires, other companies can manufacture a drug of equivalent chemical composition and market it under the brand name drug's original generic name. Because extensive research and development are unnecessary at this point, producing generic drugs is far less costly than developing the original brand name drug. Nearly all states allow pharmacists to substitute generic drugs for brand name drugs, as long as the prescribing physician approves. In 2002 the list of approved generic drugs was increased by 80 additional inclusions. For those interested in viewing all of the current approved generics, the FDA updates each month its Generic Drug Approvals list.[29]

 TALKING POINTS Your mother insists on using the brand-name drug that she has used for years to control her arthritis pain, even though her doctor has prescribed a generic version that has recently become available. What might you say to help her consider the less expensive option?

Categories of Over-the-Counter (OTC) Products

- Antacids
- Antimicrobials
- Sedatives and sleep aids
- Analgesics
- Cold remedies and antitussives
- Antihistamines and allergy products
- Mouthwashes
- Topical analgesics
- Antirheumatics
- Hematinics
- Vitamins and minerals
- Antiperspirants
- Laxatives
- Dentrifices and dental products
- Sunburn treatments and preventives
- Contraceptive and vaginal products
- Stimulants
- Hemorrhoidals
- Antidiarrheals
- Dandruff and athlete's foot preparations

Today a variety of reference books are available to inform consumers about the availability of generic drugs and the prescription drugs that they can legally be substituted for.

Over-the-Counter Drugs

When people are asked when they last took some form of medication, for many the answer might be, "I took aspirin (or a cold pill, or a laxative) this morning." In making this decision, people engaged in self-diagnosis, determined a course for their own treatment, self-administered their treatment, and freed a physician to serve people whose illnesses are more serious than theirs. None of this would have been possible without readily available, inexpensive, and effective OTC drugs (see the Star box above).

> **Key Terms**
>
> **chemical name** name used to describe the molecular structure of a drug.
>
> **generic name** common or nonproprietary name of a drug.
>
> **brand name** specific patented name assigned to a drug by its manufacturer.

Figure 15-1 The FDA will soon require over-the-counter drugs to carry standardized labels, such as the one to the right.

Drug Facts

Active Ingredient (in each tablet) | **Purpose**
Chlorpheniramine maleate 2 mg | Antihistamine

Uses temporarily relieves these symptoms due to hay fever or other upper respiratory allergies:

■ sneezing   ■ runny nose   ■ itchy, watery eyes   ■ itchy throat

---

Warnings
Ask a doctor before use if you have

■ glaucoma   ■ a breathing problem such as emphysema or chronic bronchitis
■ trouble urinating due to an enlarged prostate gland

Ask a doctor or pharmacist before use if you are taking tranquilizers or sedatives

When using this product
■ you may get drowsy   ■ avoid alcoholic drinks
■ alcohol, sedatives, and tranquilizers may increase drowsiness
■ be careful when driving a motor vehicle or operating machinery
■ excitability may occur, especially in children

If pregnant or breast-feeding, ask a health professional before use.
Keep out of reach of children. In case of overdose, get medical help or contact a Poison Control Center right away.

Directions

adults and children 12 years and over	take 2 tablets every 4 to 6 hours; not more than 12 tablets in 24 hours
children 6 years to under 12 years	take 1 tablet every 4 to 6 hours; not more than 6 tablets in 24 hours
children under 6 years	ask a doctor

Other information
■ store at 20-25° C (68-77° F)   ■ protect from excessive moisture

---

Inactive ingredients D&C yellow no. 10, lactose, magnesium stearate, microcrystalline cellulose, pregelatinized starch

---

While 2,500 prescription drugs are available, there are perhaps as many as 300,000 different OTC products, routinely classified into twenty-six different families (see the Star box on page 447). Like prescription drugs, nonprescription drugs are regulated by the FDA. However, for OTC drugs, the marketplace is a more powerful determinant of success.

The regulation of OTC drugs is based on a provision in a 1972 amendment to the 1938 Food, Drug, and Cosmetic Act. As a result of that action, OTC drugs were placed in three categories (I, II, and III) based on the safety and effectiveness of their active ingredient(s). Today, only category I OTC drugs that are safe, effective, and truthfully labeled are to be sold. The FDA's drug-classification process also allows some OTC drugs to be made stronger and some prescription drugs to become nonprescription drugs by reducing their strength through reformulation.

Like the proposed label shown in Figure 15-1 above, current labels for OTC products reflect FDA requirements. The labels must clearly state the type and quantity of active ingredients, alcohol content, side effects, instructions for appropriate use, warning against inappropriate use, and risks of using the product with other drugs (polydrug use). Unsubstantiated claims must be carefully avoided in advertisements of these products.

Preparing for Difficult Decisions

Many people do not wish to think about what would happen if they were rendered completely incapacitated and unable to speak for themselves. But determining in advance the kind of treatment you wish to receive in the event of a terminal illness or severe injury can lift a terrible burden off of your family and loved ones, who might be hard pressed to make those decisions for you. For this reason, many people are using legal documents called *advance medical directives* to articulate their wishes regarding lifesaving measures, organ donation, and deciding whether treatment is burdensome or beneficial with hopes for recovery.

One of the most common of these medical directives is the living will, a document that confirms a person's desires to die peacefully and with a measure of dignity should a time arrive when there is little hope for recovery from a terminal illness or severe injury. Living will statutes exist in all fifty states and in the District of Columbia. An estimated 25% of U.S. adults have signed living wills.[30]

A second important document that can assist terminally ill or incapacitated patients is the **medical power of attorney for health care** document. This legal document authorizes another person to make specific health care decisions about treatment and care under specified circumstances, most commonly when patients are in long-term vegetative states and cannot communicate their medical wishes. This document helps inform hospitals and physicians which person will help make the critical medical decisions. Usually this person is a loving relative. It is recommended that people complete both a living will and a medical power of attorney for health care documentation.

It can also be beneficial to think about decisions that would need to be made in the event of your death. One such decision is organ donation. On any given day, more than eighty thousand Americans are on waiting lists for organ transplants. For some, the decision to donate body tissue and organs after death is rewarding and comforting. To become an organ donor, you must fill out an organ donor card indicating your wishes to become an organ donor and specifying what organs and tissues you would like to donate in the event of your death. In many states, you can put this information on your driver's license. However, it is also crucial that you discuss your wishes with family members so that they understand them and are able to inform medical professionals of your wishes if you should die suddenly.

A second decision regards funeral arrangements. The disposition of human remains is a complicated reality in today's world. Factors ranging from public health laws to the emotional needs of survivors dictate that we plan ahead, if time permits. Accordingly, a growing percentage (currently estimated to be 30%) of Americans are preplanning and prepaying for their funerals. Federal Trade Commission laws and some state regulations give structure to the process, but it behooves individual consumers to work carefully with a reputable funeral home.

Although the cost of funerals can vary widely depending on the areas of the country and the individual desires of individuals, the average American funeral, less cemetery plot, grave opening/closing, and marker, is approximately $6,000. Among the specific components of this cost are professional services charges ($1,213), embalming ($420), other preparations of body (cosmetics, hair) ($150), visitation and viewing ($275), funeral service at funeral home ($350), transfer of remains to funeral home (usually from a hospital or nursing home) ($154), hearse for local use ($185), other vehicles (flower car/family car) ($85), acknowledgment cards ($18), casket ($2330), and vault ($950). Cremation of the body, rather than burial or entombment, will lower this cost to some degree.

Today many people wish to pay funeral expenses before their death, thus freeing grieving family members from the task of "guessing" what final arrangements were desired. To make certain that this process can be carried out in a standardized manner that is both professional and fair, the Federal Trade Commission has established the following rules to regulate preplanned and prepaid funerals. According to these rules:

- Funeral directors must provide a list of itemized prices in person and, if you ask, over the phone.
- You have the right to choose the goods and services you want (with some exceptions). The funeral home cannot require you to buy a package of preselected goods and services.
- If a state law requires you to buy a particular item, the funeral provider must disclose it on the price list, with reference to the specific law.
- The funeral provider may not refuse, or charge a fee, to handle a casket you bought elsewhere.
- If you want to buy a casket, the funeral home must provide you with descriptions of the selections and prices before showing you the caskets.
- A funeral provider that offers cremation must make alternative containers available.

Once preplanning is completed and a contract signed, the consumer can prepay for the service or purchase an insurance policy that will cover the funeral costs when death occurs. After prepaying, the purchaser should be certain that the money is deposited by the funeral provider into a funeral trust account at an insured

---

Key Terms

medical power of attorney for health care a legal document that designates who will make health care decisions for people unable to do so for themselves.

(FDIC) lending institution. A copy of all relevant information and documents should be given to responsible family members for safekeeping, rather than being left in a safe deposit box. Additionally, funeral-related instructions should not be written into a will, but rather discussed with family members at a time well before death seems likely.

TALKING POINTS Have you discussed the importance of a living will with your parents or grandparents? How might you approach the subject?

Health Care Quackery and Consumer Fraud

A person who earns money by marketing inaccurate health information, unreliable health care, or ineffective health products is called a fraud, quack, or charlatan. **Consumer fraud** flourished with the old-fashioned medicine shows of the late 1880s. Unfortunately, consumer fraud still flourishes. You need look no further than large city newspapers to see questionable advertisements for disease cures and weight loss products. Quacks have found in health and illness the perfect avenues to make maximum gain with minimum effort.

When people are in poor health, they may be afraid of becoming disabled or dying. So powerful are their desires to live and avoid suffering that people are vulnerable to promises of health improvement or a cure. Even

though many people have great faith in their physicians, they also want access to experimental treatments or products touted as being superior to currently available therapies. When tempted by the promise of help, people sometimes abandon traditional medical care. Of course, quacks recognize this vulnerability and present a variety of "reasons" to seek their help (see the Changing for the Better box above). Gullibility, blind faith, impatience, superstition, ignorance, or hostility toward professional expertise eventually carry the day. In spite of the best efforts of agencies at all levels, no branch of government can protect consumers from their own errors of judgment that so easily play into the hands of quacks and charlatans.

Regardless of the motivation that leads people into consumer fraud, the outcome is frequently the same. First, the consumer loses money. The services or products are grossly overpriced, and the consumers have little recourse to help them recover their money. Second, the consumers often feel disappointed, guilty, and angered by their own carelessness as consumers. Far too frequently, consumer fraud may lead to unnecessary suffering.

> **Key Terms**
>
> **consumer fraud** marketing of unreliable and ineffective services, products, or information under the guise of curing disease or improving health; quackery.

Taking Charge of Your Health

- Keep yourself well informed about current health issues and new developments in health care.
- Analyze the credibility of the health information you receive before putting it into practice.
- Select your health care providers by using a balanced set of criteria (see pages 435 and 439).
- Explore alternative forms of health care, and consider using them as a complement to traditional health care.

- In selecting a health care plan, compare various plans on the basis of several key factors, not simply cost (see page 444).
- Assemble a complete personal/family health history as soon as possible. Be sure to include information from older family members.
- Comply with all directions regarding the appropriate use of prescription and OTC medications.

Summary

- Sources of health information include family, friends, commercials, labels, the Internet, and information supplied by health professionals, as well as others.
- Physicians can be either Doctors of Medicine (MDs) or Doctors of Osteopathy (DOs). They receive similar training and engage in similar forms of practice.
- Although alternative health care providers, including chiropractors, naturopaths, herbalists, and acupuncturists, meet the health care needs of many people, systematic study of these forms of health care is only now under way.
- Restricted-practice health care providers play important roles in meeting the health and wellness needs of the public.
- Nursing at all levels is a critical health care profession. Advanced practice nurses represent the highest level of training within nursing.
- Self-care is often a viable approach to preventing illness and reducing the use of health care providers.
- Our growing inability to afford health care services has reached crisis proportions in the United States.

- More than 41 million Americans, not just the poor, have problems getting health care. Minorities have the most limited access to health care services of all Americans.
- Health insurance is critical to our ability to afford modern health care services.
- HMOs provide an alternative way of receiving health care services, although the influence of the profit motive in their operation is a concern.
- Medicare and Medicaid are governmental plans for paying for health care services.
- The development of prescription medication is a long and expensive process for pharmaceutical manufacturers. The cost of prescription medication is the most rapidly increasing aspect of health care affordability.
- OTC products have a role to play in the treatment of illness, but their safe use is based on following label directions.
- Critical health consumerism, including avoiding health quackery, requires careful selection of health-related information, products, and services.

Review Questions

1. Determine how you would test the accuracy of the health-related information you have received in your lifetime.
2. Identify and describe some sources of health-related information presented in this chapter. What factors should you consider when using these sources?
3. Describe the similarities between allopathic and osteopathic physicians. What is an alternative health care practitioner? Give examples of the types of alternative practitioners.
4. What are the theories underlying acupuncture and ayurveda?
5. Describe the services that are provided by the following limited health care providers: dentists, psychologists, podiatrists, and optometrists. Identify several allied health care professionals. What levels of training and expertise exist within nursing?
6. In what ways is the trend toward self-care evident? What are some reasons for the popularity of this movement?
7. How do private, public, and voluntary (proprietary) hospitals differ.
8. What is health insurance? Explain the following terms relating to health insurance: deductible

amount, fixed indemnity benefits, full-service benefits, coinsurance, exclusion, and preexisting condition.

9. What is a health maintenance organization? How do HMO plans reduce the costs of health care? What are IPAs and PPOs?

10. What do the chemical name, brand name, and generic name of a prescription drug represent? OTC drugs are approved for marketing on the basis of what three factors?

11. What role does Medicare and Medicaid play in meeting the health care needs of the American public?

Which portion of Medicare is universal? What elective option does Medicare offer?

12. What are the two criteria that must be met by an OTC drug? In comparison with prescription medication and OTC drugs, what regulatory control does the FDA have over dietary supplements?

13. What is health quackery? What federal agencies have some ability to limit its presence? What can a consumer do to avoid consumer fraud?

References

1. Rideout V. *Generation Rx.com.* International Communications Research, Kaiser Family Foundation. 2001. **http://www.kff.org/2001/200111211a/GenerationRx.pdf**

2. The National Council on the Aging. Media sources of health info. As reported in *USA Today,* 26 October 1999, 9d.

3. Baker L, et al. Use of the Internet and e-mail for health care information: results from a national survey. *JAMA* 289(18): 2400–2406. 2003.

4. Clark C, Gordon RJ, Harris B (editors). *Encyclopedia of complementary health practice.* Springer. 1999.

5. *Physicians' desk reference pocket guide to prescription drugs.* Simon and Schuster, Inc. 2002.

6. Tieman J. Med school downer, Applications decline for third year in a row, experts cite anti-affirmative action initiatives. *Mod Health* 30(38): 18–19, 2000.

7. Sierpina VS. *Integrative health care: complementary and alternative therapies for the whole person.* F. A. Davis, 2000.

8. National Center for Complementary and Alternative Medicine. National Institutes of Health. September 2003. **http://www.nccam.nih.gov**

9. *Acupuncture: Mechanism of action.* National Center for Complementary and Alternative Medicine, September 2003. **http://www.bccan.nih.gov/health/acupuncture/#nccam**

10. NIH panel issues consensus statement on acupuncture (press release) 5 November 1997. **http://www.gov/news/plr/nov97/od.or.htm**

11. Questions and answers about homeopathy. National Center for Complementary and Alternative Medicine. 2003. **http://www.nih.gov/health/homeopathy/index.htm#a1**

12. Jaroll L. Homeopathic e-mail: can the "memory" of molecules be transmitted via the Internet? *Time,* 153(19), 7 May 1999.

13. Shekelle PG, et al. Efficacy and safety of ephedra and ephedrine for weight loss and athletic performance: a meta-analysis. *JAMA* 289(12): 1537–1545. 2003.

14. Associated Press. U.S. Bans Ephedra, Drug linked to Deaths. December 30, 2003.

15. Fontanarosa PB, Rennie D, DeAngelis CD. The need for regulation of dietary supplements—lessons from ephedra. *JAMA* 289(12): 1568–1570, 2003.

16. Norris S, Morgan R. Providers issue brief: nursing shortages: year end report—2002. *Issue Brief Policy Track Serv,* 1–14, December 31, 2002.

17. Aiken LH, et al. Hospital nurse staffing and patient mortality, nurse burnout, and job satisfaction. *JAMA* 288(16): 1987–1993, 2002.

18. Eastman PD. Now, do-it-yourself care. *AARP Bulletin Online.* January 2002. **http://www.aarp.org.bulletin/yourhealth/articles/a2003-08-05-doityourself.html**

19. *Federal Register.* 64(243): 71041. Rules and Regulations. December 20, 1999.

20. Health Care Financing Administration. *National health care expenditures projections tables—1972–2007, Table 1.* November 2000. **http://www.hcfa.gov/NHE-Proj/t01.htm**

21. *National health care expenditure amounts, and average annual percent change by type of expenditure (Table 2).* Centers for Medicare & Medicaid Services. Department of Health and Human Services. **http://www.cms.hhs.gov/statistics/nhe/projections-2002/t2.asp**

22. Rosenbaum, David E. Bush Signs Law to cover Drugs for the Elderly. *The New York Times,* December 9, 2003.

23. Health Care Financing Administration. *Personal health care expenditures, average percent change, percent distribution and per capita amounts, by source of funds for selected calendar years 1970–2007, Table 2a.* November 2000. **http://www.chfa.gov/stats/NHE-proj/to2b.htm**

24. *Employer health benefits. 2003 annual survey.* The Kaiser Family Foundation and Health Research and Educational Trust. 2003.

25. McKenzie JF, Pinger RR, Kotecki JE. *An introduction to community health,* 4th ed. Jones and Bartlett. 2002.

26. *Statistical abstract of the United States: 2002*, 122nd ed. U.S. Census Bureau. U.S. Department of Commerce, 2003. (Tables Nos. 102 and 1001)
27. *Average annual cost of nursing home care.* The Metlife Assisted Living Market Telephone Survey, 2002. **http://www.massmutual.com/mmfg/pdf/ nursing_home_cost.pdf**
28. What's the Difference? *USA Today,* July 25, 2003, 5A.
29. *Generic drug approvals.* FDA/Center for Drug Evaluation and Research. January 2003.

http://www.fda.gov/cder/ogd/approvals/ default.htm
30. Partnership for caring. Facts about advance directives. **http://www.partnershipforcaring.org,** 10 October 2000.
31. *Funerals: a consumer guide.* Federal Trade Commission, 2002.
32. *Drug consult 2004. The Comprehensive reference for generic and brand name drugs.* Mosby's Drug Consult, 2004. Mosby, 2004.

As We Go to Press

The inability to adequately communicate in one's own language is, by definition, illiteracy. For some this inability is so widespread that even the ability to read or write is absent. For others illiteracy exists only in terms of selected aspects of the language, such as the highly technical language of an academic discipline, or within the jargon of a group based on the uniqueness of experiences or interests. For the typical American, medical (health care) illiteracy is a likely reality.

In a recently released report of a study conducted by the Agency for Healthcare Research and Quality, it was disclosed that 90 million Americans have very little understanding of the instructions given to them by health care practitioners, often involving information critical to prevention or recovery from serious health problems. Underlying this medical illiteracy is a multitude of problems, not all of which are the "fault" of the laypersons. In no particular order, these include:

- the highly technical language of medicine, with long complicated words and terms, many having suffixes derived from Latin.
- the age, illness/discomfort, or sensory impairment of persons receiving medically related instructions.
- the failure of practitioners to "quiz" their patients about "what is it that I just finished instructing you to do?"
- the lack of fluency in English of many patients and the inability of practitioners or their staff to speak languages other than English.
- the absence in the homes of most patients of easy-to-read home health reference books that would make complicated instructions or the abbreviated information on prescription and OTC medication labels easier to understand.

- the complicated legal language associated with health consent forms that often obscure understanding by virtually all persons, except those with medical/ legal backgrounds.

In response to the literacy concerns identified by the report just released, the following recommendations were made by the agency responsible for the study:

. . . Government sponsored research on methods for improving health care literacy.

. . . Health care professional schools should teach their students (future practitioners) how to better communicate with laypersons.

. . . Health care related literacy should be required in elementary through college curricula.

. . . Health care third party payers (insurance companies, Medicare, Medicaid) should strongly encourage providers to increase their efforts in communicating effectively.

In the final analysis, the absence of literacy in the health care field is too dangerous and expensive to allow for continued stagnation. Health care is too important and expensive for the general public to remain compromised in understanding the care they need and are paying for.

using health information on the internet

So you want to find some information on health. Maybe you have a paper due in this class. Maybe you need more information on a condition that you or a loved one has. Or maybe you simply want to take advantage of the latest information on fitness and nutrition to make healthful decisions. No matter what information you're looking for, you can probably find it on the Internet. But be wary as you search—a great deal of misinformation is also available, and it may be hard for the average consumer to separate health fact from health fiction.

You can be relatively certain that government sites and links contain reliable information. In fact, the U.S. Department of Health and Human Services has established a site to provide consumer information. It can be accessed under Health/General Health or directly at **www.healthfinder.gov.** This site was launched in April 1997 to improve consumer access to federal health information online. As Healthfinder points out in its introductory paragraph, information alone can't take the place of health care you may need, but it can make you an informed partner in your own health care. This site leads you to selected online publications, databases, websites, support and self-help groups, government agencies, not-for-profit organizations, and universities that provide reliable health information to the public.

Unfortunately, the government does not have the resources to filter out all false and misleading health care information. Many people mistakenly believe that advertising claims must be true or advertisers would not be allowed to continue making them. Not enough time, money, and regulators are available to assess the validity of each and every health claim. However, health care professionals and consumer advocates can give us the tools we need to determine the reliability of health information for ourselves.

What Is Quackery and How Can You Spot It?

One prominent consumer advocate is Stephen Barrett, a retired physician and nationally renowned author. In 1969 he founded the Lehigh Valley Committee against Health Fraud, which recently changed its name to Quackwatch. Investigation of questionable claims, answering of inquiries, distribution of reliable publications, reporting of illegal marketing, and improvement of the overall quality of health information on the Internet are all tasks that this group takes on.

Quackery is more difficult to spot than most people think. Whereas fraud is deliberate deception and more easily recognized and corrected, quackery involves the use of methods that are not scientifically valid. Information purveyed by quacks cannot be scientifically confirmed or denied, and this is where the problem arises. There is no way to separate the good from the bad or the harmful from the benign or helpful.

Anecdotes and Testimonials

Some alternative health care methods have been accepted by the scientific community, having met reliable criteria for safety and effectiveness. Other methods are in the experimental stages. These methods are unproven but are based on plausible, rational principles and are undergoing responsible testing. But many other alternative health remedies are groundless and completely lack scientific rationale. Instead of scientific tests, people who promote these methods rely on anecdotes and testimonials to "prove" the effectiveness of their products. Perhaps you have noticed that claims of effectiveness are not found on the products themselves, but rather in brochures placed in conspicuous locations very near the products. This use of testimonials is unique to the dietary supplement market and reflects the virtual absence of regulatory power held by the FDA and FTC. The FDA does allow a limited number of claims related to structural/functional benefits and a very small number of disease-related health claims.

Intelligent Consumer Behavior

Americans waste $50 million to $150 million per year on bogus mail-order health remedies. Many of these products are now available on the Internet. You can avoid wasting your money in this way by not buying any of these products without medical advice from your physician or other health care professional. And don't be fooled by money-back guarantees; they're usually as phony as the products that they back.

Be wary of characteristic quackery ploys. Purveyors of quackery may say that they care about you, but their care, even if it were sincere, cannot make useless medicine work. These products are commonly touted as having no side effects. If this is true, then the product is too weak to have any effect at all. Quacks will encourage you to jump on the bandwagon of their time-tested remedy, as if popularity and market longevity are surrogates for effectiveness. When they do claim that their products are backed by scientific studies, these studies turn out to be untraceable, misinterpreted, irrelevant, nonexistent, or based on poorly designed research.

The costs of buying into health care quackery are more than financial. The psychological effects of disillusionment and the physical harm caused by the method itself or by abandoning more effective care are much worse.

HONcode Principles

Any reputable health information site on the Internet subscribes to the HONcode Principles. These principles are put forth and monitored by the Geneva-based Health On the Net Foundation and have arisen from input from webmasters and medical professionals in several countries. According to these principles, any medical advice appearing at a site must meet the following requirements:

- It must be given by medically trained and qualified professionals unless a clear statement is made that the information comes from a non-medically qualified individual or organization.
- The information must be intended to support, not replace, the physician-patient relationship.
- Data relating to individual patients and visitors to a medical website are confidential.
- Site information must have clear references to source data and, where possible, specific links to that data.
- Claims related to the benefit or performance of a treatment, product, or

service must be supported by appropriate, balanced evidence.
- The webmaster's e-mail address should be clearly displayed throughout the website.
- Commercial and noncommercial support and funding for the site should be clearly revealed.
- There must be a clear differentiation between advertising at the site and the original material created by the institution operating the site.

Be skeptical about any health information you find on the Internet that does not meet these criteria. Ask your physician whether the information is accurate, or move on to a more reliable site.

Assessing Health Care Information

The Internet is a valuable health care tool. Reliable information is supplied by government health agencies, research universities, hospitals, disease foundations, and other experts. However, not all health sites are reputable. As the saying goes, you can't believe everything you read, even if it's on the Internet. Anyone can create an online resource that looks professional. Ordinary people who believe they've been helped by a product, companies trying to sell products and services, and even cheats and quacks are all out there spouting their information. To protect yourself, you must be an informed consumer of

information. To evaluate the credibility of an online source, ask yourself the following questions:

1. Who maintains the information?
2. Is it linked to other reputable sources of medical information?
3. When was it last updated?
4. Is it selling a product?

While the Internet cannot and should not replace visits with a physician, reliable information obtained on the Internet can make us more active partners in our own health care. It can give us information we can use to stay healthy and prevent disease. It can help us to ask our doctors the right questions and educate us so that we're not afraid to ask them. It can connect us to people who are experiencing the same things as we are. It can help us learn about our health, receive support from others, and make sound health care decisions based on fact—not fiction.

For Discussion . . .

Which health-related sites have you visited on the Internet? Did you find them informative? Reliable? Fun? What could be done to improve the status of health information on the Internet?

InfoLinks

www.hon.ch
www.nnlm.nlm.nih.gov/gmr/publish/eval.htm

personal assessment

are you a skilled health consumer?

Circle the selection that best describes your practice. Then total your points for an interpretation of your health consumer skills.

1   Never
2   Occasionally
3   Most of the time
4   All of the time

1. I read all warranties and then file them for safekeeping.
   1   2   3   4
2. I read labels for information pertaining to the nutritional quality of food.
   1   2   3   4
3. I practice comparative shopping and use unit pricing, when available.
   1   2   3   4
4. I read health-related advertisements in a critical and careful manner.
   1   2   3   4
5. I challenge all claims pertaining to secret cures or revolutionary new health devices.
   1   2   3   4
6. I engage in appropriate medical self-care screening procedures.
   1   2   3   4
7. I maintain a patient-provider relationship with a variety of health care providers.
   1   2   3   4
8. I inquire about the fees charged before using a health care provider's services.
   1   2   3   4
9. I maintain adequate health insurance coverage.
   1   2   3   4
10. I consult reputable medical self-care books before seeing a physician.
    1   2   3   4
11. I ask pertinent questions of health care providers when I am uncertain about the information I have received.
    1   2   3   4
12. I seek second opinions when the diagnosis of a condition or the recommended treatment seems questionable.
    1   2   3   4
13. I follow directions pertaining to the use of prescription drugs, including continuing their use for the entire period prescribed.
    1   2   3   4
14. I buy generic drugs when they are available.
    1   2   3   4
15. I follow directions pertaining to the use of OTC drugs.
    1   2   3   4
16. I maintain a well-supplied medicine cabinet.
    1   2   3   4

YOUR TOTAL POINTS _____

Interpretation

16–24 points   A very poorly skilled health consumer
25–40 points   An inadequately skilled health consumer
41–56 points   An adequately skilled health consumer
57–64 points   A highly skilled health consumer

To Carry This Further . . .

Could you ever have been the victim of consumer fraud? What will you need to do to be a skilled consumer?

chapter sixteen

protecting your safety

Chapter Objectives

After studying this chapter, you should be able to:

▌ define the terms *intentional* and *unintentional injuries* and give three examples of each.

▌ discuss the different types of domestic violence, including intimate partner violence, child maltreatment, and elder maltreatment.

▌ list some ways to reduce one's risk of becoming a victim of violent crime in your home, in your car, or on campus.

▌ explain the particular way guns contribute to violent crime statistics.

▌ name at least five groups who are targets of hate crimes.

▌ if you are male, list five things you can do to avoid perpetrating a date rape; if you are female, list five things you can do to reduce your risk of becoming a date rape victim.

▌ motor vehicle injuries are the leading cause of injury deaths in the United States. List ten things you can do to reduce your risk of becoming seriously injured in a motor vehicle crash.

▌ compare the risk of a fatal injury occurring while riding a motorcycle to the risk of a fatal injury while riding in a car and explain the difference.

▌ list ten things one can do to prevent injuries from occurring in the home.

▌ explain what identity theft is, and list several steps that you can take to protect yourself from it.

Online Learning Center Resources

www.mhhe.com/hahn7e

Log on to our Online Learning Center (OLC) for access to these additional resources:

- Chapter key terms and definitions
- Learning objectives
- Student interactive question-and-answer sites

- Self-scoring chapter quiz
- Online assessments
- Key term flash cards

Talking It Over

Helping a Friend End Abuse

Although the boyfriend of one of your friends has been threatening her, she isn't taking the situation seriously. What should you say?

- Explain that domestic violence includes emotional, psychological, physical, and sexual abuse in which one person tries to control another.
- Encourage your friend to tell you how she feels about the situation. Getting her to admit that she is frightened is the first step toward recognizing that she needs help.

- Explain that your friend's safety is more important than "loyalty" to her boyfriend.
- Provide information on support that's available.

CommunicationLinks

www.feminista.com/vln4

www.ndvh.org

Eye on the Media

Terrorism on Television: The Tragedy of September 11/The World Trade Center Disaster

Where were you on the morning of September 11, 2001? How did you hear the news about the terror attacks on New York and Washington? The entire nation stood stunned as TV cameras captured a passenger jet crashing into one of New York's twin towers, followed a few minutes later by a second plane that hit the second tower. Soon after, it was reported that a third plane had hit the Pentagon, and a fourth had crashed in a field in Pennsylvania.

Most of the day's horrors were captured by television cameras, as well as by a few film crews who happened to be filming in Manhattan that day. Americans watched in horror as networks played and replayed footage of each plane hitting the World Trade Center, and of the fires that ensued; they saw office workers running for their lives and witnessed fireman and other rescue workers going back into buildings that were clearly unsound to guide people out of the burning towers. And finally, they saw the two towers crumble to the ground.

For three full days the major TV networks suspended their regular programming to cover the disaster in depth. No commercials, no sitcoms, no soap operas, and no David Letterman or Jay Leno for days. When Letterman returned to the air, it wasn't to tell jokes but to have Dan Rather talk about the tragic events, and viewers saw the normally staunch newsman's eyes fill with tears. When *Saturday Night Live* featured New York Mayor Rudolph Giuliani, it was as a respected guest, not as a target for a spoof. By Saturday morning the cartoons were back—for the children. In fact, many networks geared toward children—most notably PBS—tailored their programming to offer them more comforting fare, and provided special public service announcements advising parents on how to help their children feel safe despite their own uncertainty.

In the weeks and months that followed, the media helped provide a sense of unity to a vast, grieving nation. But the constant coverage of the tragedy and its aftermath—including footage of the attacks, and of rescue workers searching the rubble of Ground Zero for the bodies of their fallen comrades—took a toll on many people watching.

People lost sleep and felt depressed. Some worried about having to get on an airplane again. Young children had an especially difficult time—wondering why this happened and whether *they* would be victims of a terrorist attack. Some children touched buildings to make sure they were "safe" before going inside.

Today, Americans are acutely aware of the possibility of terror attacks on our soil. The international news media regularly report on anti-American sentiments in Middle Eastern countries. The Department of Homeland Security continually evaluates the national threat level, with a system ranging from Code Green (low) to Code Red (severe). When the national threat level was raised from Yellow (elevated) to Orange (heightened) in December of 2003, it was major news. Many media outlets—especially the 24-hour news channels—report on the nation's state of alert every day. Continual coverage of the War on Terror—first in Afghanistan and then in Iraq—only add to Americans' concern for their safety and for that of American troops abroad.

Do you worry about another attack? How closely do you follow media coverage of national and international terror issues? Are you aware of the nation's state of alert on any given day? Do you watch the news differently from the way you watched it before September 11, 2001?

As recently as 25 years ago, the suspicious disappearance of a school-aged child or the death of a bystander during a drive-by shooting was virtually unheard of. However, violent crimes are committed so frequently in the United States that it is difficult to watch a television news report or read a newspaper without seeing headlines announcing some heinous murder or other senseless act of violence, including terrorist acts.

Although the overall crime rate has dropped in the last decade, domestic violence continues to be directed at women and children, and many people fear being a random victim of a homicide, robbery, or carjacking. Law enforcement officials contend that gang activities and hard-core drug involvement are significant factors related to continued violent behavior in our society.

Although violence may seem to be focused in urban areas, no community is completely safe. Even people who live in small towns and rural areas now must lock their doors and remain vigilant about protecting their safety. Crime on college campuses remains a threat for all students. Complete the Personal Assessment on page 481 to see whether you are adequately protecting your own safety.

Intentional Injuries

Intentional injuries are injuries that are committed on purpose. Except for suicide (which is self-directed), intentional injuries reflect violence committed by one person acting against another person. Examples include homicide, robbery, rape, suicide, assault, child abuse, spouse abuse, and elder abuse. Each year in the United States, intentional violence results in nearly 50,000 deaths and another 2 million nonfatal injuries.[1]

In 2001, more than 24 million crimes were committed against U.S. residents age 12 and older, according to data collected by the National Crime Victimization Survey. Of these, one in four (5.7 million) were violent crimes (rape, sexual assault, robbery, aggravated assault, and simple assault). The good news is that these figures continue the downward trend in criminal victimization that began in 1994. The violent crime rate in 2001 was about half the rate in 1994.[2,3]

Homicide

Homicide, or murder, is the intentional killing of one person by another. The United States leads the industrialized world in homicide rates. The 2000 murder rate was 5.5 per 100,000 inhabitants. Fortunately, this rate reflected an

---

Key Terms

intentional injuries injuries that are purposely committed by a person.

homicide the intentional killing of one person by another person.

annual decline since 1991, when the homicide rate was 9.8 per 100,000. In fact, this rate was the lowest since 1965.[4]

Criminal justice experts are trying to pinpoint why U.S. homicide rates are dropping. No one answer has emerged, but speculation centers on better community policing efforts; the 1994 passage of the broad Federal Crime Bill; recent legislation, such as the Brady Law; and a variety of tough state laws, such as the "three strikes and you're out" provisions, that mandate life sentences without parole for repeat violent offenders. If recent incarceration rates do not change, an estimated 1 in 20 people (5.1%) will serve time in a state or federal prison. The chances of going to prison are higher for men (9%) than for women (1.1%).[5]

One continuing phenomenon is the extent to which illegal drug activity is related to homicide. A variety of research studies from large cities indicate that 25% to 50% of all homicides are drug related.[6] Most of these murders are associated with drug trafficking, including disputed drug transactions. Nationally, this figure is much lower; for 2000 only 4.4% of homicides were drug related.[7] Additionally, high percentages of both homicide assailants and victims have drugs in their systems at the time of the homicide.[6]

Handguns continue to be the weapon of choice for homicides. It was the proliferation of handguns and their use in violent crimes that led to the passage of the so-called Brady Law.

Domestic Violence

Domestic violence refers to criminal acts of violence committed within a home or homelike setting by people that have some type of relationship with the victim. This text will discuss three forms of domestic violence: intimate partner violence, child maltreatment, and elder maltreatment.

Intimate Partner Violence

Intimate Partner Violence (IPV) refers to violence committed by a current or former spouse or boyfriend or girlfriend. IPV can include murder, rape, sexual assault, robbery, aggravated assault, and simple assault. Violent acts that constitute abuse range from a slap on the face to murder.

A 2001 report released by the Bureau of Justice Statistics revealed some slightly encouraging findings regarding IPV.[8] The report indicated that intimate nonlethal violence had declined 48% since 1993, from a rate of 5.8 nonfatal victimizations per 1,000 persons to just 3 per 1,000 persons. The rate of decline was greater for female victims (49%) than for male victims (42%). Two reasons have been proposed for the decline in intimate partner violence: better services for families at risk and an improved economy during the period covered by the report.[9] Actually, rates of IPV began to edge upward in 2001,[8] perhaps as a result of rising unemployment.

Cell Phone Safety While Driving

Cell phones that fit easily into a pocket or purse are being used in every place imaginable, including restaurants, theaters, subways, parks, golf courses, and, of course, in cars. And it's in cars that the use of cellular phones is most controversial. A variety of studies and reports indicate a four- to nine-fold increase in the potential for car crashes associated with the driver's use of a cell phone. In July 2001, the state of New York passed the country's first *statewide ban* on the use of hand-held cellular phones while driving. Violators of this ban are subject to a $100 fine for the first offense. Since then, at least 24 other states have passed laws regulating cell phone use while operating a motor vehicle.

Research suggests the use of a cell phone decreases driver concentration and delays driver reaction time. The use of mounted, hands-free phones may improve safety, although the safety benefit has been controversial. Experts in traffic safety are careful to point out that there are too many other factors associated with driving to make it fair to blame behind-the-wheel phone use for all or most accidents. These complicating factors include adverse weather conditions, the structural integrity of the cars, the age and health of the drivers, radio, CD, or cigarette use, and interactions between drivers and passengers. The influence of other drivers on the road must also be considered.

If you must use your cell phone in a car, consider these commonsense rules: Get off the main road to a safe parking area to make your call, especially if the call is an important one or one that might upset you. If you must talk while driving, opt for a hands-free phone. Dial when your car is stopped. Keep calls very brief. Don't try to dial or talk in heavy traffic. Keep your eyes on the road. (Or, let a passenger make the call!)

Source: Governors Highway Safety Association: Cell phone restrictions— state and local jurisdictions. 2003. **www.statehighwaysafety.org/html/ state_info/cellphone_laws**

Murders by intimates in 2000 reached the lowest levels since 1976. In 2000 1,687 murders were reported among intimate partners, whereas nearly 3,000 such murders took place in 1976. As has been the case for many years, three of every four victims of intimate murder in 2000 were female.[8]

One serious issue related to domestic violence is the vast underreporting of this crime to law enforcement

Key Terms

intimate partner violence violence committed against a person by her or his current or former spouse, boyfriend, or girlfriend.

authorities. The U.S. Department of Justice estimates that about half of the survivors of domestic violence do not report the crime to police. Too many survivors view these violent situations as private or personal matters and not actual crimes. Despite painful injuries, many survivors view the offenses against them as minor.

It's easy to criticize the survivors of domestic violence for not reporting the crimes committed against them, but this may be unfair. Why do women stay in abusive relationships? Many women who are injured may fear being killed if they report the crime. They may also fear for the safety of their children. Women who receive economic support from an abuser may worry about being left with no financial resources.

However, help is available for victims of intimate abuse. Most communities have family support or domestic violence hot lines that abused people can call for help. Many have shelters where abused women and their children can seek safety while their cases are being handled by the police or court officials. If you are being abused or know of someone who is being injured by domestic violence, don't hesitate to use the services of these local hot lines or shelters. Also, check the resources listed in the Health Reference Guide at the back of this text.

 TALKING POINTS A close friend confides that her boyfriend sometimes "gets rough" with her. She's afraid to talk to him about it because she thinks that will make things worse. What immediate steps would you tell her to take?

Child Maltreatment

Like intimate partner violence, **child maltreatment** tends to be a silent crime. It is estimated that nearly 1 million children are survivors of child abuse and neglect each year.[10] Some children are survivors of repeated crimes, and since many survivors do not report these crimes, the actual incidence of child abuse is difficult to determine.

Child maltreatment includes child abuse and child neglect. Children are abused in various ways. Physical abuse reflects physical injury, such as bruises, burns, abrasions, cuts, and fractures of the bones and skull. Sexual abuse includes acts that lead to sexual gratification of the abuser. Examples include fondling, touching, and various acts involved in rape, sodomy, and incest. Psychological abuse is another form of child abuse. Certainly, children are scarred by family members and others who routinely damage their psychological development. However, this form of abuse is especially difficult to identify and measure.

Child neglect is failure to provide a child with adequate clothing, food, shelter, and medical attention. The incidence of child neglect is approximately three times that of physical abuse and about seven times the incidence of child sexual abuse. Furthermore, child maltreatment

deaths are more often associated with neglect than with any other type of abuse.[10] Educational neglect, such as failure to see that a child attends school regularly, is one of the most common types of child neglect. Each form of abuse can have devastating consequences for the child— both short term and long term.

Research studies in child abuse reveal some noteworthy trends. Abused children are much more likely than nonabused children to grow up to be child abusers themselves. Abused children are also more likely to suffer from poor educational performance, increased health problems, and low levels of overall achievement. Recent research points out that abused children are significantly more likely than nonabused children to become involved in adult crime and violent criminal behavior. Finally, neglected children's rates of arrest for violence were almost as high as those for physically abused children.[11]

It is beyond the scope of this book to discuss the complex problem of reducing child maltreatment. However, the violence directed against children can likely be lessened through a combination of early identification measures and violence prevention programs. Teachers, friends, relatives, social workers, counselors, psychologists, police, and the court system must not hesitate to intervene as soon as child abuse is suspected. The later the intervention, the more likely that the abuse will have worsened. Once abuse has occurred, it is likely to happen again.

Violence prevention programs can help parents and caregivers learn how to resolve conflicts, improve communication, cope with anger, improve parenting skills, and challenge the view of violence presented in movies and television. Such programs may help stop violence before it begins to damage the lives of young children. Figure 16-1 provides simple alternatives parents can choose to avoid hitting a child.

Elder Maltreatment

Among the nation's 35 million elderly people, between 1 to 2 million, have been injured, exploited, or otherwise mistreated.[12,13] Particularly vulnerable are women over the age of 75 years. Nearly half of the abusers are the adult children of the victims, and 85% were family members.[14]

Many elderly people are hit, kicked, attacked with knives, denied food and medical care, and have their Social Security checks and automobiles stolen. This problem reflects a combination of factors, particularly the stress of

> ## Key Terms
>
> **child maltreatment** the act or failure to act by a parent or caretaker which results in abuse or neglect of a child or which places the child in imminent risk of serious harm.

12 alternatives to lashing out at your child.

The next time everyday pressures build up to the point where you feel like lashing out — STOP! And try any of these simple alternatives.

You'll feel better . . . and so will your child.

1. Take a deep breath. And another. Then remember <u>you</u> are the adult . . .

2. Close your eyes and imagine you're hearing what your child is about to hear.

3. Press your lips together and count to 10. Or better yet, to 20.

4. Put your child in a time-out chair. (Remember the rule: one time-out minute for each year of age.)

5. Put yourself in a time-out chair. Think about why you are angry: is it your child, or is your child simply a convenient target for your anger?

6. Phone a friend.

7. If someone can watch the children, go outside and take a walk.

8. Take a hot bath or splash cold water on your face.

9. Hug a pillow.

10. Turn on some music. Maybe even sing along.

11. Pick up a pencil and write down as many helpful words as you can think of. Save the list.

12. Write for parenting information: Parenting, Box 2866, Chicago, IL 60690.

Take Time Out. Don't Take It Out On Your Child.

® National Committee for Prevention of Child Abuse

Ad Council

CHILD ABUSE PREVENTION CAMPAIGN
MAGAZINE AD NO. CA-2835-90—7″ x 10″
Volunteer Agency: Lintas: Campbell-Ewald, Campaign Director: Beth M. Pritchard, S.C. Johnson & Son, Inc.

Figure 16-1 Alternatives to abusing your child.

caring for failing older people by middle-aged children who are also faced with the demands of dependent children and careers. In many cases, the middle-aged children were themselves abused, or there may be a chemical dependence problem. The alternative, institutionalization, is so expensive that it is often not an option for either the abused or the abusers.

Although protective services are available in most communities through welfare departments, elder abuse is frequently unseen and unreported. In many cases, the elderly people themselves are afraid to report their children's behavior because of the fear of embarrassment that they were not good parents to their children. Regardless of the cause, however, elder abuse must be reported to the appropriate protective service so that intervention can occur.

Gangs and Youth Violence

In the last 30 years, gangs and gang activities have been increasingly responsible for escalating violence and criminal activity. Before that time, gangs used fists, tire irons, and,

occasionally, cheap handguns ("Saturday night specials"). Now, gang members don't hesitate to use AK-47s (semi-automatic military assault weapons) that have the potential to kill large groups of people in a few seconds.

The gang problem is most persistent in cities of greater than 25,000 population, where 66% of gang members live.[15] Here, socially alienated and economically disadvantaged youth come to believe that society has no significant role for them. So, they seek support from an association of peers that has well-defined lines of authority. Rituals and membership initiation rites are important in gang socialization. Gangs often control particular territories within a city. Frequently, gangs are involved in criminal activities, commonly illicit drug trafficking, and robberies.

Gangs and youth violence also occur in the suburbs. Sixty-one percent of large suburbs (greater than 100,000 population) reported gang activity. Only 13% of small cities and 7% of rural jurisdictions reported gang activity.[15]

Attempting to control gang and youth violence is expensive for communities. For every gang-related homicide, there are about 100 nonfatal gang-related intentional injuries, so gang violence becomes an expensive health-care proposition. Furthermore, gang and youth violence takes an enormous financial and human toll on law enforcement, judicial, and corrections departments. Reducing gang and youth violence is a daunting task for the nation.

Gun Violence

The tragic effect of gun violence has already been touched on throughout this chapter. Guns are being used more than ever in our society. Gun violence is a leading killer of American teenagers and young men, especially African American men, and the use of semiautomatic assault weapons by individuals and gang members continues. The fatality rate for gun injuries is 30%, much higher than the fatality rate for injuries of all causes (less than 1%).[16] Colleges and universities are not immune to gun violence. A recent study reported that 4.3% of college students had a working firearm at college, of these, nearly half stated that they had a gun for protection.[17] Accidental deaths of toddlers and young children from loaded handguns is another dimension of the violence attributable to guns in our society. In addition, guns are often used in **carjackings** (see the Changing for the Better box on page 465).

> **Key Terms**
>
> **carjacking** a crime that involves a thief's attempt to steal a car while the owner is behind the wheel; carjackings are usually random, unpredictable, and frequently involve handguns.

No one is totally free from the risk of senseless violence—children, adults, or college students. No single group, however, is a more tragic target of violence than the disabled. Despite the protective efforts of laws such as the Fair Housing Amendments Act, the Americans with Disabilities Act, and the Rehabilitation Act, the disabled remain an easily victimized segment of the population.

Because of the high level of vulnerability that disabled persons face, national advocacy groups, such as All Walks Of Life, are working to assist the disabled, their caregivers, and the general population in reducing the risk of violence to this group. However, much can also be accomplished on an individual basis. If you are an able-bodied college student, you can probably implement the following suggestions on your campus:

- Encourage your disabled peers to remain vigilant by staying tuned in to their environment. Remind them that simply because they appear disabled does not guarantee that they will be protected from harm.
- Support your disabled friends in the challenges imposed by their limitations, particularly when they are in unfamiliar environments or experiencing unusual situations.
- Suggest that your peers with disabilities carry, or wear a personal alarm device. Such devices, also frequently carried

by able-bodied students, can be purchased in bookstores or sporting goods stores.
- Remind your disabled friends to inform others about their schedule plans, for example, when they will be away from school and when they are likely to return.
- Encourage people with disabilities to seek the assistance of an escort (security personnel) when leaving a campus building or a shopping mall to enter a large parking area.
- Be an advocate for your disabled friends. For example, if residence hall room doors do not have peepholes at wheelchair height, find out if the doors can be modified.

One additional approach remains controversial. That is the teaching of self-defense techniques to people with disabilities. Groups that advocate instruction to the disabled in the martial arts, such as judo, remind us that "doing nothing will produce nothing." Others contend that a limited ability to use a martial art leads to a false sense of confidence that encourages a disregard for other forms of protection. They further argue that if disabled persons try to counter aggression with ineffectively delivered martial arts techniques, they may anger their attacker and actually increase the aggression against themselves.

The growing use of firearms has prompted serious discussions about enactment of gun control laws. For years, gun control activists have been in opposition with the National Rifle Association (NRA) and its congressional supporters. Gun control activists want fewer guns manufactured and greater controls over the sale and possession of handguns. Gun supporters believe that such controls are not necessary and that people (criminals) are responsible for gun deaths, not simply the guns. This debate will certainly continue.

TALKING POINTS At a campus talk on carjacking, one college student announced that he planned to carry a registered gun to protect himself. How would you respond to his position?

Bias and Hate Crimes

One sad aspect of any society is how some segments of the majority treat certain people in the minority. Nowhere is this more obvious than in **bias and hate crimes.** These crimes are directed at individuals or groups of people solely because of a racial, ethnic, religious, or other difference attributed to these minorities. The targeted individuals are often verbally and physically attacked, their houses are spray painted with various slurs, and many are forced to move from one neighborhood or community to another.

According to Federal Bureau of Investigation (FBI) statistics, there are about 8,000 hate crime incidents in the United States each year. Motivations for hate crimes are biases against race (61%), religion (14%), sexual orientation (13%), and ethnicity (11%).[18]

Typically, the offenders in bias or hate crimes are fringe elements of the larger society who believe that the mere presence of someone with a racial, ethnic, or religious difference is inherently bad for the community, state, or country. Examples in the United States include skinheads, the Ku Klux Klan, and other white supremacist groups. (The case of Matthew Shepard [see the Star box on page 466] drew worldwide attention to hate crimes.) Increasingly, state and federal laws have been enacted to make bias and hate crimes serious offenses.

Key Terms

bias and hate crimes criminal acts directed at a person or group solely because of a specific characteristic, such as race, religion, sexual orientation, ethnic background, or other difference.

There have been several carjacking incidents in my area recently. What can I do to avoid this problem without carrying a gun?

In the last 10 years a new form of violence has reached the streets of America. This crime is commonly called *carjacking.* Unlike auto theft, in which a car thief attempts to steal an unattended parked car, carjacking involves a thief's attempt to steal a car with a driver still behind the wheel.

Most carjacking attempts begin when a car is stopped at an intersection, usually at a traffic light. A carjacker will approach the driver and force him or her to give up the car. Resisting an armed carjacker can be extremely dangerous. Law enforcement officials offer the following tips to prevent carjacking:

- Drive only on well-lit and well-traveled streets, if possible.
- Always keep your doors locked when driving your car.
- Observe traffic that may be following you. If you think that something suspicious is happening, try to locate a police officer or a busy, populated area to seek help.
- If someone approaches your car and you cannot safely drive away, roll the window down only slightly and leave the car running and in gear. If the situation turns bad, use your wits and quickly flee the scene, either in the car or on foot. Remember: your life is worth more than your car.
- If another car taps the rear bumper of your car (a common carjacking maneuver to get you to exit your car) and you feel uncomfortable about getting out of your car, tell the other driver that you are driving to the police station to complete the accident report.

Road Rage

Within the last 10 years, a phenomenon called "road rage" has been on the rise on the streets and highways of the United States. This violence occurs when a driver becomes enraged at the driving behavior of others—cutting off someone, driving too slowly, going through yellow lights and red lights, playing loud music, passing a long line of cars on the shoulder, playing "chicken" as two lanes merge into one. Toss in horn-honking, four-letter words, and hand gestures, and you have all the elements of the daily commuter.

Sometimes road rage has deadly results. It's not unusual for road ragers to force other cars into accidents. Since some drivers carry guns, they may injure or kill other drivers. These tragedies usually are not premeditated. They often happen when a driver loses control under the pressure of a triggering incident.

There is no typical profile of a person who expresses road rage. Although road ragers are frequently young-adult, aggressive males, road rage can be displayed by anyone who drives and is stressed by time constraints, family problems, or job difficulties. One quick way to determine if you are prone to road rage is to tape record your voice while you're driving. If you hear yourself screaming and complaining, you could be considered an aggressive driver. You will need to find ways to calm yourself during your commute.

To avoid becoming a perpetrator or a victim of road rage, follow these recommendations:

- Avoid making hand gestures
- Use your horn sparingly
- Allow plenty of time to reach your destination
- Imagine yourself being videotaped while driving
- Avoid blocking the passing lane
- Avoid switching lanes without signaling
- Use only one parking place
- Avoid parking in a space for disabled people, unless you are disabled
- Refrain from tailgating
- Do not allow your door to hit the parked car next to you
- If you drive slowly, pull over and let others pass
- Avoid the unnecessary use of high-beam headlights
- Do not talk on a car phone while driving
- Avoid making eye contact with aggressive drivers
- Keep your music volume under control

Always drive defensively. Assume that a difficult situation may get out of hand, so conduct yourself in a calm, courteous manner. It's better to swallow your pride and preserve your health than to risk unnecessary danger to yourself or other people on the road.

TALKING POINTS You're in a car with a friend when another driver starts tailgating you very closely. Your friend (the driver) slows down to annoy the tailgater. How would you convince your friend that his action is dangerous?

Stalking

In recent years the crime of stalking has received considerable attention. **Stalking** refers to an assailant's planned efforts to pursue an intended victim. Most stalkers are

---

Key Terms

stalking a crime involving an assailant's planned efforts to pursue an intended victim.

Violence Based on Sexual Orientation

Recent news reports indicate that violence based on sexual orientation continues to occur in the United States. Nowhere is this more clear than in the case of Matthew Shepard, an openly gay University of Wyoming freshman who was murdered in October 1998. Shepard was lured from a Laramie, Wyoming, bar by two young adult men posing as homosexuals. These men beat Shepard severely, stole $20 from him, and tied him to a fence post, where he was left to die. The men were later convicted of kidnapping and murder.

In July 1999, Barry Winchell, an Army private at Fort Campbell, Kentucky, was bludgeoned to death with a bat wielded by fellow private Calvin Glover. Glover, who said he was intoxicated when he committed the crime, was later convicted of premeditated murder in a military court and sentenced to life in prison, with the possibility of parole. Another soldier, charged as an accessory to the crime, apparently had spread rumors among members of the Army unit that Winchell was gay. This accomplice also tried to clean up the scene of the crime. He was sentenced to 12 years in prison.

The murder of Private Winchell prompted calls for a reevaluation of the military's 1993 "don't ask, don't tell" policy concerning homo-

sexuals. Under this policy, gays can serve in the military as long as they do not disclose their sexual orientation. Superiors in the military cannot investigate or expel personnel who keep their sexual orientation to themselves. Some believe this "don't ask, don't tell" policy prevents military authorities from investigating complaints of harassment based on sexual orientation. This policy came up in the year 2000 presidential campaign and could be revised in the future.

Both of these deaths served as a reminder that the federal government has not yet passed the Hate Crimes Prevention Act. Supported by President Clinton, but not passed by Congress at the time of this writing, this proposed legislation would add acts of hatred motivated by sexual orientation, gender, and disability to the list of hate crimes already covered by federal law. Among these crimes already covered are ones motivated by prejudice based on race, religion, color, or national origin.

It will be interesting to see whether this proposed federal legislation will be enacted soon. The public outcry following the deaths of Matthew Shepard and Barry Winchell indicates that much support exists for some version of a Hate Crimes Prevention Act.

---

male. Many stalkers are excessively possessive or jealous and pursue people with whom they formerly had a relationship. Other stalkers pursue people with whom they have had only an imaginary relationship.

Stalkers often go to great lengths to locate their intended victims and frequently know their daily whereabouts. Although not all stalkers plan to batter or kill the person they are pursuing, their presence and potential for violence can create an extremely frightening environment for the intended victim and family. Some stalkers serve time in prison for their offense, waiting years to "get back at" their victims.

Virtually all states have enacted or tightened their laws related to stalking and have created stiff penalties for offenders. In many areas the criminal justice system is proactive in letting possible victims of stalking know, for example, when a particular prison inmate is going to be released. In other areas, citizens are banding together to provide support and protection for people who may be victims of stalkers. It should not come as a surprise that stalking occurs on college campuses. About 13% of college women are stalked in a given year.[19]

If you think you are or someone you know is being stalked, contact the police (or a local crisis intervention hot line number) to report your case and follow their guidance. Be on the alert if someone from a past relationship suddenly reappears in your life or if someone seems to be irrationally jealous of you or overly obsessed with you. Report anyone who continues to pester or intimidate you with phone calls, notes or letters, e-mails, or un-

wanted gifts. Report people who persist in efforts to be with you after you have told them you don't want to see them. Until the situation is resolved, be alert for potentially threatening situations and keep in close touch with friends. Discovering Your Spirituality (page 467) features the question of dealing with fear in our lives.

TALKING POINTS You suspect that someone is stalking you, but your friends think you're being dramatic. How would you get objective advice on what to do?

OnSITE/InSIGHT

Learning to Go: Health

Are you proactive about your personal safety? Click on Learning to Go: Health on the Online Learning Center at **www.mhhe.com/hahn7e** to check out the following lessons:

Lesson 46: Protect yourself from rape and sexual assault.

Lesson 48: Avoid becoming a victim of crime.

Lesson 50: Keep yourself safe at home.

Lesson 51: Play it safe when you're having fun.

Lesson 52: Drive safely and defensively.

Lesson 53: Shield yourself from road rage.

Putting Fear in Perspective

Your elderly neighbor stays locked in her house all day, afraid to open the door to anyone. Too many hours of watching local TV news, you think. But it's not just older people who are living in fear. Parents, women, gays, and minorities are all looking over their shoulders.

Some parents who walked to school when they were children wouldn't think of letting their kids do that. What about child molesters and kidnappers? A young woman at a party guards her drink all night—afraid that someone might put a drug in it. She's afraid of being raped. The gay person who goes to his old neighborhood to visit his grandmother feels uneasy. Is it his imagination, or are people looking at him in a threatening way? An African American man walking down the street hears a racial slur. Should he ignore it, or stop and say something?

All of these situations call for caution. If you're a parent, you need to be careful about your child's safety. But your child can walk to school—accompanied by you, another parent, or an older child. If you're a woman, you can keep an eye on your drink at a party without making that the focus of your attention. If you're a gay man who feels uncomfortable in an unfamiliar part of town, stay focused on where you're going. Walk quickly and confidently, without being intimidated. If you're a minority who's being taunted, keep your dignity and remain calm.

Putting fear in perspective takes practice. First, stay reasonable. Recognize that acts of violence represent the extreme elements of society. There's a good reason you probably haven't met many (or any) murderers, robbers, or rapists. They make up a small segment of society. The people you usually encounter, who are basically good, represent the large majority. Second, be aware. Pay attention to what's going on around you. See things in a neutral way. If you do, you'll realize when an argument is about to turn into a fistfight or worse. Third, use common sense. Don't put yourself at risk, but don't stop living. You can't build your life around avoiding a potential act of violence. Fourth, trust your senses. If someone is walking too close to you and you feel uncomfortable, cross the street and go into a store. Last, practice what-if situations. For example, what would you do if you were in your car at a stoplight and someone held a gun up to your window? Considering your possible actions ahead of time, without dwelling on them, is one way of preparing yourself for real-life threats.

Living in fear is something that happens gradually—as fear takes control of a person's life. But that doesn't need to happen to you. You can take control of fear in a healthy, positive way—to build a life of rich experiences balanced by caution and good sense.

Sexual Victimization

Ideally, sexual intimacy is a mutual, enjoyable form of communication between two people. Far too often, however, relationships are approached in an aggressive, hostile manner. These sexual aggressors always have a victim—someone who is physically or psychologically traumatized. *Sexual victimization* occurs in many forms and in a variety of settings. This section takes a brief look at sexual victimization as it occurs in rape and sexual assault, sexual abuse of children, sexual harassment, and the commercialization of sex.

Rape and Sexual Assault

As violence in our society increases, the incidence of rape and sexual assault correspondingly rises. The victims of these crimes fall into no single category. Victims of *rape* and *sexual assault* include young and old, male and female. They can be the mentally retarded, prisoners, hospital patients, and college students. We all are potential victims, and self-protection is critical. Read the Star box on page 468 concerning myths about rape.

Sometimes a personal assault begins as a physical assault that turns into a rape situation. Rape is generally considered a crime of sexual aggression in which the victim is forced to have sexual intercourse. Current thought about rape characterizes this behavior as a violent act that happens to be carried out through sexual contact. (See the Changing for the Better boxes on page 468 and 469 on rape awareness guidelines and help for the rape survivor.)

Acquaintance and Date Rape

In recent years, closer attention has been paid to the sexual victimization that occurs during relationships. *Acquaintance rape* refers to forced sexual intercourse between individuals who know each other. *Date rape* is a form of acquaintance rape that involves forced sexual intercourse by a dating partner. Studies on a number of campuses suggest that about 20% of college women reported having experienced date rape but a recent report issued by the Bureau of Justice Statistics puts the figure at about 3% per year. This figure includes completed and attempted rapes.[19] A higher percentage of women report being kissed and touched against their will. Alcohol is frequently a significant contributing factor in these rape situations. (See Chapter 8 concerning alcohol's role in campus crime.) Some men have reported being psychologically coerced into intercourse by their female dating partners. In many cases the aggressive partner will display certain behaviors that can be categorized (see the Changing for the Better box on page 470).

Psychologists believe that aside from the physical harm of date rape, a greater amount of emotional damage

Myths about Rape

Despite the fact that we are all potential victims, many of us do not fully understand how vulnerable we are. Rape, in particular, has associated with it a number of myths (false assumptions), including the following:

- Women are raped by strangers. In approximately half of all reported rapes, the victim has some prior acquaintance with the rapist. Increasingly, women are being raped by husbands, dating partners, and relatives.
- Rapes almost always occur in dark alleys or deserted places. The opposite is true. Most rapes occur in or very near the victim's residence.
- Rapists are easily identified by their demeanor or psychological profile. Most experts indicate that rapists do not differ significantly from nonrapists.
- The incidence of rape is overreported. Estimates are that only one in five rapes is reported.
- Rape happens only to people in low socioeconomic classes. Rape occurs in all socioeconomic classes. Each person, male or female, young or old, is a potential victim.
- There is a standard way to escape from a potential rape situation. Each rape situation is different. No one method to avoid rape can work in every potential rape situation. Because of this, we encourage personal health classes to invite speakers from a local rape prevention services bureau to discuss approaches to rape prevention.

may occur. Such damage stems from the concept of broken trust. Date rape victims feel particularly violated because the perpetrator was not a stranger: it was someone they initially trusted, at least to some degree. Once that trust is broken, developing new relationships with other people becomes much more difficult for the date rape victim.

Nearly all victims of date rape seem to suffer from *post-traumatic stress syndrome*. They may have anxiety, sleeplessness, eating disorders, and nightmares. Guilt concerning their own behavior, loss of self-esteem, and judgment of other people can be overwhelming, and the individual may require professional counseling. Because of the seriousness of these consequences, all students should be aware of the existence of date rape.

Date Rape Drugs

As you may recall from Chapter 7, Rohypnol, GHB (liquid ecstasy, G), and ketamine (K, Special K, and Cat) have joined alcohol as forms of date rape intoxicants. For their own safety, students must be vigilant about being duped into consuming substances that increase the likelihood of sexual assault and violence.

Sexual Abuse of Children

One of the most tragic forms of sexual victimization is the sexual abuse of children. Children are especially vulnerable to sexual abuse because of their dependent relationships with parents, relatives, and caregivers (such as babysitters, teachers, and neighbors). Often, children are unable to readily understand the difference between appropriate and inappropriate physical contact. Abuse may range from blatant physical manipulation, including fondling, to oral sex, sodomy, and intercourse.

Because of the subordinate role of children in relationships involving adults, sexually abusive practices often go unreported. Sexual abuse can leave emotional scars that make it difficult to establish meaningful relationships later in life. For this reason, it is especially important for people to pay close attention to any information shared by children that could indicate a potentially abusive situation. Most states require that information concerning child abuse be reported to law enforcement officials.

Sexual Harassment

Sexual harassment consists of unwanted attention of a sexual nature that creates embarrassment or stress. Examples of sexual harassment include unwanted physical contact, excessive pressure for dates, sexually explicit humor, sexual innuendos or remarks, offers of job advancement based on sexual favors, and overt sexual assault. Unlike more overt forms of sexual victimization, sexual harassment may be applied in a subtle manner and can, in some cases, go unnoticed by coworkers and fellow students. Still, sexual harassment produces stress that cannot be resolved until the harasser is identified and forced to stop. Both men and women can be victims of sexual harassment.

Sexual harassment can occur in many settings, including employment and academic settings. On the college campus, harassment may be primarily in terms of the offer of sex for grades. If this occurs to you, think carefully about the situation and document the specific times, events, and places where the harassment took place. Consult your college's policy concerning harassment. Next, you could report these events to the appropriate administrative officer (perhaps the affirmative action officer, dean of academic affairs, or dean of students). You may also want to discuss the situation with a staff member of the university counseling center.

If harassment occurs in the work environment, the victim should document the occurrences and report them to the appropriate management or personnel official. Reporting procedures will vary from setting to setting. Sexual harassment is a form of illegal sex discrimination and violates Title VII of the Civil Rights Act of 1964.

In 1986 the U.S. Supreme Court ruled that the creation of a "hostile environment" in a work setting was sufficient evidence to support the claim of sexual harassment. This action served as an impetus for thousands of women to step forward with sexual harassment allegations. Additionally, some men are also filing sexual harassment lawsuits against female supervisors.

Not surprisingly, this rising number of complaints has served as a wake-up call for employers. From university settings to factory production lines to corporate board rooms, employers are scrambling to make certain that employees are fully aware of actions that could lead to a sexual harassment lawsuit. Sexual harassment workshops and educational seminars on harassment are now common and serve to educate both men and women about this complex problem.

Violence and the Commercialization of Sex

It is beyond the scope of this book to explore whether sexual violence can be related to society's exploitation or commercialization of sex. However, sexually related products and messages are intentionally placed before the public to try to sway consumer decisions. Do you believe that there could be a connection between commercial products, such as violent pornography in films and magazines, and

I've heard that there are warning signs for date rape. What signs should I be alert for?

First, consider your partner's behaviors. Many, but not all, date rapists show one or more of the following behaviors: a disrespectful attitude toward you and others, lack of concern for your feelings, violence and hostility, obsessive jealousy, extreme competitiveness, a desire to dominate, and unnecessary physical roughness. Consider these behaviors as warning signs for possible problems in the future. Reevaluate your participation in the relationship.

Below are some specific ways both men and women can avoid a date rape situation:

Men

- *Know your sexual desires and limits.* Communicate them clearly. Be aware of social pressures. It's OK not to score.
- *Being turned down when you ask for sex is not a rejection of you personally.* Women who say no to sex are not rejecting the person; they are expressing their desire not to participate in a single act. Your desires may be beyond control, but your actions are within your control.
- *Accept the woman's decision.* "No" means "No." Don't read other meanings into the answer. Don't continue after you are told "No!"
- *Don't assume that just because a woman dresses in a sexy manner and flirts that she wants to have sexual intercourse.*

- *Don't assume that previous permission for sexual contact applies to the current situation.*
- *Avoid excessive use of alcohol and drugs.* Alcohol and other drugs interfere with clear thinking and effective communication.

Women

- *Know your sexual desires and limits.* Believe in your right to set those limits. If you are not sure, STOP and talk about it.
- *Communicate your limits clearly.* If someone starts to offend you, tell him so firmly and immediately. Polite approaches may be misunderstood or ignored. Say "No" when you mean "No."
- *Be assertive.* Often men interpret passivity as permission. Be direct and firm with someone who is sexually pressuring you.
- *Be aware that your nonverbal actions send a message.* If you dress in a sexy manner and flirt, some men may assume you want to have sex. This does not make your dress or behavior wrong, but it is important to be aware of a possible misunderstanding.
- *Pay attention to what is happening around you.* Watch the nonverbal clues. Do not put yourself into vulnerable situations.
- *Trust your intuitions.* If you feel you are being pressured into unwanted sex, you probably are.
- *Avoid excessive use of alcohol and drugs.* Alcohol and other drugs interfere with clear thinking and effective communication.

Being aware of your surroundings when using an ATM is important for personal safety.

violence against women? Does prostitution lead directly to violence? Do sexually explicit "900" phone numbers or Internet pornography cause an increase in violent acts? Can the sexual messages in beer commercials lead to acquaintance rape? What do you think?

Identity Theft

Identity theft has been on the rise since the early 1990s. Thieves use falsely obtained names, addresses, and social security numbers to open credit card accounts and bank

Key Terms

identity theft a crime involving the fraudulent use of a person's name, social security number, credit line, or other personal financial or identifying information.

Reducing Your Risk for Identity Theft

The Federal Trade Commission outlines several steps to minimize your risk for identity theft:

- Order a copy of your credit report from each of the three major credit bureaus, and review it carefully to make sure it's accurate.
- Place passwords on your credit card, bank and phone accounts. Avoid obvious passwords such as birthdays, mother's maiden name, or social security numbers.
- Keep personal information in your home secure. Be vigilant about guarding your mail and your trash; consider using a document shredder when discarding sensitive papers like credit card bills. Make sure your home computer has firewall protection.
- Ask about information security procedures in your workplace or at your school.

- Carefully read all your bills to make sure that you recognize all purchases and charges.
- Do not give out your personal information. Be especially wary of e-mail and phone solicitations requesting such information.
- Watch your wallet. Be wary of pickpockets, and carry only the identification and credit cards you need. Do not carry your social security card with you unless it is absolutely necessary.
- If you are a victim of identity theft, visit the FTC's website (**http://www.consumer.gov/idtheft/**) for valuable information on how to file a complaint and restore your credit.

Source: Federal Trade Commission. *ID Theft: When Bad Things Happen to Your Good Name.*

accounts, purchase cell phone services, and secure loans to buy automobiles and other big-ticket items. They might even avoid paying taxes by working under false social security numbers, or use your identity for other purposes—if they are arrested, for example. Identity thefts can drain a person's bank account and ruin their credit rating before a person knows they've become a victim. Often the crime is not discovered until a person wants to make a major purchase—like a house or a car—which requires a credit check.

There are several steps that you can take to avoid becoming a victim of identity theft. The most important step involves ordering copies of your credit reports each year to make sure that there are no fraudulent accounts in your name.[20] Other steps are outlined in the Star box above.

Unintentional Injuries

Unintentional injuries are injuries that have occurred without anyone intending that any harm be done. Common examples include injuries resulting from car crashes, falls, fires, drownings, firearm accidents, recreational accidents, and residential accidents. Each year, unintentional injuries account for nearly 100,000 deaths and 29 million visits to hospital emergency departments.[21]

Unintentional injuries are very expensive for our society, both from a financial standpoint and from a personal and family standpoint. Fortunately, to a large extent it is possible to avoid becoming a victim of an unintentional injury. By carefully considering the tips presented in the safety categories that follow, you will be protecting yourself from many preventable injuries.

Since this section of the chapter focuses on a selected number of safety categories, we encourage readers to

consider some additional, related activities. For further information in the area of safety, consult a safety textbook. Finally, we encourage you to take a first aid course from the American Red Cross or the National Safety Council. These first aid courses incorporate a significant amount of safety prevention information along with the teaching of specific first aid skills.

Residential Safety

Many serious accidents and personal assaults occur in dorm rooms, apartments, and houses. As a responsible adult, you should make every reasonable effort to prevent these tragedies from happening. One good idea is to discuss some of the following points with your family or roommates and implement needed changes:

- Fireproof your residence. Are all electrical appliances and heating and cooling systems in safe working order? Are flammable materials safely stored?
- Prepare a fire escape plan. Install smoke or heat detectors.
- Do not give personal information over the phone.
- Use initials for first names on mailboxes and in phone books.
- Install a peephole and deadbolt locks on outside doors.

> ### Key Terms
>
> **unintentional injuries** injuries that have occurred without anyone's intending that harm be done.

- If possible, avoid living in first floor apartments. Change locks when moving to a new apartment or home.
- Put locks on all windows.
- Require repair people or delivery people to show valid identification.
- Do not use an elevator if it is occupied by someone who makes you feel uneasy.
- Be cautious around garages, laundry rooms, and driveways (especially at night). Use lighting for prevention of assault.

Recreational Safety

The thrills we get from risk-taking are an essential part of our recreational endeavors. But a significant number of injuries occur in recreational settings. Bicycle riding accounted for 412,000 emergency department visits in 2001.[21] Some injuries occur because we fail to consider important recreational safety information. Do some of the following recommendations apply to you?

- Seek appropriate instruction for your intended activity. Few skill activities are as easy as they look.
- Always wear your automobile safety belt.
- Make certain that your equipment is in excellent working order. Use specific safety gear designed for cycling, in-line skating, and scooter use.
- Involve yourself gradually in an activity before attempting more complicated, dangerous skills.
- Enroll in an American Red Cross first aid course to enable you to cope with unexpected injuries.
- Remember that alcohol use greatly increases the likelihood that people will get hurt.
- Protect your eyes from serious injury.

Wearing proper safety gear—including a helmet—is an essential safety measure when biking or skating. Obeying traffic laws and using proper hand signals are equally important.

- Learn to swim. Drowning occurs most frequently to people who never intended to be in the water.
- Obey the laws related to your recreational pursuits. Many laws are directly related to the safety of the participants.
- Be aware of weather conditions. Many outdoor activities turn to tragedy with sudden shifts in the weather. Always prepare yourself for the worst possible weather.

Firearm Safety

Each year more than 13,000 Americans are murdered with guns, nearly 2,000 die in gun-related accidents, and another 200 die from discharged firearms where the intent was not determined.[22] Most murders are committed with handguns. (Shotguns and rifles tend to be more cumbersome than handguns and thus are not as frequently used in murders, accidents, or suicides.) Over half of all murders result from quarrels and arguments between acquaintances or relatives. With many homeowners arming themselves with handguns for protection against intruders, it is not surprising that over half of all gun accidents occur in the home. Children are frequently involved in gun accidents, often after they discover a gun they think is unloaded. Handgun owners are reminded to adhere to the following safety reminders:

- Make certain that you follow the gun possession laws in your state. Special permits may be required to carry a handgun.
- Make certain that your gun is in good mechanical order.
- If you are a novice, enroll in a gun safety course.
- Consider every gun to be a loaded gun, even if someone tells you it is unloaded.
- Never point a gun at an unintended target.

Number of Fatal Motor Vehicle Crashes According to Age of Driver
Crashes per 100,000 drivers

Age	Value
16-20	63
21-24	45
25-34	32
35-44	26
45-54	22
55-64	20
65-69	19
70-up	26

Figure 16-2 Driving is a dangerous activity for those under age 25. What could be done to reduce the number of driving fatalities among this age group?

- Keep your finger off the trigger until you are ready to shoot.
- When moving with a handgun, keep the barrel pointed down.
- Load and unload your gun carefully.
- Store your gun and ammunition safely in a locked container. Use a trigger lock on your gun when not in use.
- Take target practice only at approved ranges.
- Never play with guns at parties. Never handle a gun when intoxicated.
- Educate children about gun safety and the potential dangers of gun use. Children must never believe that a gun is a toy.

Motor Vehicle Safety

The greatest number of injury deaths in the United States take place on highways and streets. Young people (ages 16–24 years) are more likely to be involved in a fatal motor vehicle crash than persons of any other age. (Figure 16-2). The most dangerous time to drive is the period 12 A.M. to 3 A.M. Saturdays and Sundays.[23]

Motor vehicle accidents also cause disabling injuries. With nearly 2 million such injuries each year, concern for the prevention of motor vehicle accidents should be important for all college students, regardless of age. With this thought in mind, we offer some important safety tips for motor vehicle operators:

- Make certain that you are familiar with the traffic laws in your state.

- Do not operate an automobile or motorcycle unless it is in good mechanical order. Regularly inspect your brakes, lights, and exhaust system.
- Do not exceed the speed limit. Observe all traffic signs.
- Always wear safety belts, even on short trips. Require your passengers to buckle up. Always keep small children in child restraints.
- Never drink and drive. Avoid horseplay inside a car.
- Be certain that you can hear the traffic outside your car. Keep the car's radio/music system at a reasonable decibel level.
- Give pedestrians the right-of-way.
- Drive defensively at all times. Do not challenge other drivers. Refrain from drag racing.
- Look carefully before changing lanes.
- Be especially careful at intersections and railroad crossings.
- Carry a well-maintained first aid kit that includes flares or other signal devices.
- Alter your driving behavior during bad weather.
- Do not drive when you have not had enough sleep (see the Focus On article on page 479).

Home Accident Prevention for Children and the Elderly

Approximately 1 person in 10 is injured each year at home. Children and the elderly spend significantly more hours each day at home than do young adults and adults.

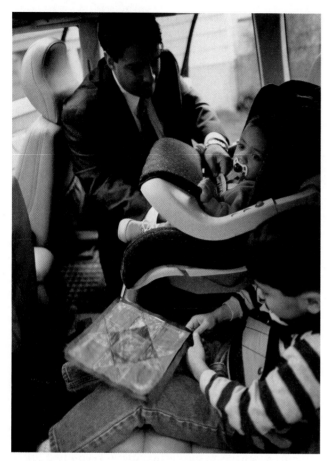

Consistent use of safety restraints during childhood can help make buckling up a lifelong habit.

It is especially important that injury prevention be given primary consideration for these groups (see the Changing for the Better box on page 475). Here are some important tips to remember. Can you think of others?

For Everyone

- Be certain that you have adequate insurance protection.
- Install smoke detectors appropriately.
- Keep stairways clear of toys and debris. Install railings.
- Maintain electrical and heating equipment.
- Make certain that inhabitants know how to get emergency help.

For Children

- Know all the ways to prevent unintentional poisoning.
- Use toys that are appropriate for the age of the child.
- Never leave young children unattended, especially infants.
- Keep any hazardous items (guns, poisons, etc.) locked up.
- Keep small children away from kitchen stoves.

For the Elderly

- Protect from falls.
- Be certain that elderly people have a good understanding of the medications they may be taking. Know the side effects.
- Encourage elderly people to seek assistance when it comes to home repairs.
- Make certain that all door locks, lights, and safety equipment are in good working order.

Campus Safety and Violence Prevention

Although many of the topics in this chapter are unsettling, students and faculty must continue to lead normal lives in the campus environment despite potential threats to our health. The first step in being able to function adequately is knowing about these potential threats. You have read about these threats in this chapter; now you must think about how this information applies to your campus situation.

The campus environment is no longer immune to many of the social ills that plague our society. At one time the university campus was thought to be a safe haven from the real world. Now there is plenty of evidence to indicate that significant intentional and unintentional injuries can happen to anyone at any time on the college campus.

For this reason, you must make it a habit to think constructively about protecting your safety. In addition

I take a common sense approach to safety, but I worry sometimes that I haven't thought about something important. What's the basic checklist for different areas?

Entry

- Install a deadbolt lock on the front door and locks or bars on the windows.
- Add a peephole or small window in the front door.
- Trim bushes so burglars have no place to hide.
- Add lighting to the walkway and next to the front door.
- Get a large dog.

Bedroom and Nursery

- Install a smoke alarm and a carbon monoxide detector.
- Remove high threshold at doorway to avoid tripping.
- Humidifiers can be breeding grounds for bacteria; use them sparingly and follow the manufacturer's cleaning instructions.
- In the nursery, install pull-down shades or curtains instead of blinds with strings that could strangle a child.

Living Room

- Secure loose throw rugs or use ones with nonskid backing.
- Remove trailing wires where people walk.
- Cover unused electrical outlets if there are small children in the home.
- Provide additional lighting for reading, and install adjustable blinds to regulate glare.

Kitchen

- To avoid burns, move objects stored above the stove to another location.
- Install ceiling lighting and additional task lighting where food is prepared.
- Keep heavy objects on bottom shelves or countertops; store lightweight or seldom-used objects on top shelves.
- Promptly clean and store knives.
- Keep hot liquids such as coffee out of children's reach, and provide close supervision when the stove or other appliances are in use.
- To avoid food-borne illness, thoroughly clean surfaces that have come into contact with raw meat.

Bathroom

- A child can drown in standing water; keep the toilet lid down and the tub empty.
- Clean the shower, tub, sink, and toilet regularly to remove mold, mildew, and bacteria that can contribute to illness.
- Store medications in their original containers in a cool, dry place out of the reach of children.
- Add a bath mat or nonskid strips to the bottom of the tub.
- Add grab bars near the tub or shower and toilet, especially if there are elderly adults in the home.
- Keep a first-aid kit stocked with bandages, first-aid ointment, gauze, pain relievers, syrup of Ipecac, and isotonic eyewash; include your physician's and a nearby emergency center's phone numbers.

Stairway

- Add a handrail for support.
- Remove all obstacles or stored items from stairs and landing.
- Repair or replace flooring material that is in poor condition.
- Add a light switch at the top of the stairs.
- If there is an elderly person in the home, add a contrasting color strip to the first and last steps to identify the change of level.

Fire Prevention Tips

- Install smoke detectors on every level of your home.
- Keep fire extinguishers handy in the kitchen, basement, and bedrooms.
- Have the chimney and fireplace cleaned by a professional when there is more than $\frac{1}{4}$ inch of soot accumulation.
- Place space heaters at least 3 feet from beds, curtains, and other flammable objects.
- Don't overload electrical outlets, and position drapes so that they don't touch cords or outlets.
- Recycle or toss combustibles, such as newspapers, rags, old furniture, and chemicals.
- If you smoke, use caution with cigarettes and matches; never light up in bed.
- Plan escape routes and practice using them with your family.

to the personal safety tips presented earlier in this chapter, remember to use the safety assistance resources available on your campus. One of these might be your use of university-approved escort services, especially in the evenings as you move from one campus location to another. Another resource is the campus security department (campus police). Typically, campus police have a 24-hour emergency phone number. If you think you need help, don't hesitate to call this number. Campus security departments frequently offer short seminars on safety topics to student organizations or residence hall groups. Your counseling center on campus might also offer programs on rape prevention and personal protection.

If you are motivated to make your campus environment safer, you might wish to contact an organization that focuses on campus crime. Safe Campuses Now is a nonprofit student group that tracks legislation, provides educational seminars, and monitors community incidents involving students. For information about Safe Campuses Now, including how to start a chapter on your campus, call (706) 354-1115, or see their web page at **www.uga.edu\~safe-campus.** We encourage you to become active in making your campus a safer place to live.

Taking Charge of Your Health

- Use the Personal Assessment on page 481 to determine how well you manage your own safety.
- Assess your behaviors and those of your dating partners for signs of potential date rape by reviewing the "Avoiding Date Rape" box on page 470.
- Check your residence for the safety strategies listed on page 475. Make the necessary changes to correct any deficiencies.
- Review the motor vehicle safety tips on page 473. If you need to make changes to your car or your driving, begin working on them at once.

- Check the recommendations for recreational safety on page 472 and put them into practice. Be assertive about using these measures when you are participating in activities with others.
- Find out about the security services available on your campus, and take advantage of them. Post the 24-hour-help phone number in your room and carry it with you.
- Minimize your risk for identity theft by taking the steps outlined on page 471.

Summary

- Everyone is a potential victim of violent crime.
- Each year in the United States, intentional injuries cause nearly 50,000 deaths and another 2 million non-fatal injuries.
- The homicide rate in the United States has declined significantly since the 1960s.
- Domestic violence includes intimate partner violence, child maltreatment, and elder maltreatment.
- Forms of child maltreatment include child abuse and child neglect. Child neglect is more common than child abuse.
- Youth violence and gang activity are serious social problem, especially in large cities.

- Gun violence continues to be a major contributor to the fatal injury statistics.
- Hate crimes are crimes motivated by bias against other races, religions, ethnicities, or sexual orientation.
- Rape, sexual assault, and sexual harassment are forms of sexual victimization in which victims are often both physically and psychologically traumatized.
- Unintentional injuries are injuries that occur without anyone intending that harm to be done.
- More people die from unintentional injuries than from intentional injuries.
- Motor vehicles are the leading cause of unintentional injury deaths.

Review Questions

1. Identify some of the categories of intentional injuries. How many people are affected each year by intentional injuries?
2. What are some of the most important facts concerning homicide in the United States? How are most homicides committed?
3. Identify the three types of domestic violence discussed in the chapter.
4. What reasons might explain why so many people do not report domestic violence?

5. Aside from the immediate consequences of child maltreatment, what additional problems do many abused and neglected children face in the future?
6. Explain why gangs and gang activities continue to plague our large cities. How do gang activities lower the quality of life in communities?
7. List some examples of groups that are known to have committed bias or hate crimes.
8. Identify some general characteristics of a typical stalker.

9. Explain some of the myths associated with rape. How can date rape be prevented?

10. Identify some examples of behaviors that could be considered sexual harassment. Why are employers especially concerned about educating their employees about sexual harassment?

11. Identify some common examples of unintentional injuries.

12. List some places where unintentional injuries occur. Point out three safety tips from each of the safety areas listed at the end of this chapter.

13. Identify some precautions you can take to reduce your risk of becoming involved in a fatal motor vehicle crash.

14. In what ways can individuals minimize their risk for identity theft?

References

1. Centers for Disease Control and Prevention, National Center for Injury Prevention and Control, WISQARS (Web-based Injury Surveillance Query and Reporting System), March 7, 2003, **www.cdc.gov/ncipc/wisqars/**

2. Bureau of Justice Statistics. *National Crime Victimization Survey: Criminal Victimization 2001, Changes 2000–01 with Trends 1993–2001*. U.S. Department of Justice, NCJ 194610, September 2002.

3. Bureau of Justice Statistics. U.S. Department of Justice, Office of Justice Programs, *National Crime Victimization Survey, Violent Crime Trends, 1973–2001*, **www.ojp.usdoj.gov/bjs/glance/tables/viortrdtab.htm**

4. Bureau of Justice Statistics. *Homicide Trends in the U.S., Long term trends*, U.S. Department of Justice, Office of Justice Programs, November 2002, **www.ojp.usdoj.gov/bjs/homicide/tables/totalstab.htm**

5. Bureau of Justice Statistics. *Criminal offenders statistics: lifetime likelihood of going to state or federal prison*, U.S. Department of Justice, November 2000.

6. Bureau of Justice Statistics. U.S. Department of Justice, Office of Justice Programs, *Homicide Trends in the United States*, November 21, 2002.

7. Bureau of Justice Statistics. U.S. Department of Justice, Office of Justice Programs, *Drug Use and Crime*, January 2000, **www.ojp.usdoj.gov/bjs/dcf/duc.htm#to**

8. Bureau of Justice Statistics. U.S. Department of Justice, Office of Justice, *Crime Data Brief, Intimate Partner Violence, 1993–2001*. NCJ 197838, February 2003.

9. McKenzie JF, Pinger RR, Kotecki JF. *An Introduction to Community Health*, 4th ed. Jones & Bartlett, 2002.

10. United States Department of Health and Human Services, Administration on Children, Youth and Families; *Child Maltreatment 2001*. Washington, D.C.: U.S. Government Printing Office, 2003, **http://www.acf.hhs.gov/programs/cb/publications/cm01/cm01.pdf**

11. National Institute of Justice. *The cycle of violence revisited*. Washington, D.C.: U.S. Department of Justice, Office of Justice Programs, NIJ, Research in Progress Seminar Series, February 1996.

12. U.S. Census Bureau. *The 65 years and over population: 2000, Census 2000 Brief*. U.S. Department of Commerce, Economics and Statistics Administration, 2001, **http://www.census.gov/prod/2001pubs/c2kbr01-10.pdf**

13. National Research Council. *Elder Mistreatment: Abuse, Neglect, and Exploitation in an Aging America*. Washington, D.C.: The National Academies Press, 2003.

14. Office for Victims of Crime, Statistical Overviews. *Elder Abuse and Neglect*. Washington, D.C.: U.S. Department of Justice, Office of Justice Programs, 2001, **www.ojp.usdoj.gov/ovc/ncvrw/2001/stat_over_7.htm**

15. Office of Juvenile Justice and Delinquency Prevention. *OJJDP Fact Sheet: National youth gang survey trends from 1996 to 2000*. Washington, D.C., U.S. Department of Justice, Office of Justice Programs, 2002.

16. Centers for Disease Control and Prevention: *Surveillance for Fatal and Nonfatal Firearm-related Injuries—United States, 1993–1998*. Morbidity and Mortality Surveillance Summaries 50(ss02): 1–32, 2001.

17. Miller M, Hemenway D, Wechsler H. Guns and Gun Threats at College. *J Am Coll Hlth* 51(2): 57–65.

18. Bureau of Justice Statistics. *Special Report: Hate Crimes Reported in NIBRS, 1997–1999*. U.S. Department of Justice, Office and Justice Programs, NCJ 186765, Washington, D.C., 2001.

19. National Institute of Justice. *The Sexual Victimization of College Women*. U.S. Department of Justice, Bureau of Justice Statistics, Washington, D.C., 2001.

20. Federal Trade Commission. ID THEFT: When bad things happen to your good name. **www.consumer.gov/idtheft,** 2002.

21. National Safety Council. *Injury Facts, 2003 Edition*. Itasca, IL, 2003.

22. Minimo AM, Smith BL. *Deaths: Preliminary data for 2000*. National Vital Statistics Reports 49(12): 1–40.

23. National Highway Traffic Safety Administration. *Traffic Safety Facts 2001*. Washington, D.C., U.S. Department of Transportation. DOT HS 809 484, 2002.

A recently released report by the AAA Foundation for Traffic Safety reveals that drivers whose ages are 65 years and older are 1.78 times more likely to die in car crashes than drivers ages 55 to 64. Cognitive skills and vision decline with age the report noted. Drivers over 75 were more than 2.59 times more likely to die in car crashes, while those 85 and over were 3.72 times as likely to die when compared with drivers 55 to 64 years of age. Seniors are also more likely to die involved in left turn crashes as they age.

These statistics are important because the proportion of Americans who are seniors is growing. By 2030 one in five Americans will be 65 or older. Among the many web resources available for seniors is **www.senior drivers.org**

The report noted that teenage drivers remain the age group at highest risk for injury or death in traffic crashes.

Available at **http://www.aaafoundation.org/multimedia/ index.cfm?button-SeniorInjury,** accessed 4/12/04

drowsy driving

Dean was driving home from college late on a moonlit Friday night. His on-campus job kept him working until 9 P.M. after a day of classes. He had stopped to shoot pool with some friends after work and started his hour-long trek home at about 11:30. Just after midnight, Dean turned onto a 15-mile stretch of perfectly straight highway that cut through pastures and fields. The summer night was crystal clear. The radio was playing loudly, there were few oncoming cars, and visibility was good.

"I felt fine," Dean recalled later. "I was a little run down, but I wasn't sleepy at all. I was cruising along listening to tunes, and the next thing I knew I was surrounded by corn. The sound of the stalks hitting the car must have woken me up. It scared the hell out of me. I guess I fell asleep for a few seconds, but I don't know how it could have happened."

The Danger of Driving While Sleepy

Dean experienced a phenomenon that is too often ignored. Falling asleep at the wheel is something that no one thinks will happen to them, yet drowsy driving is estimated to cause up to 200,000 accidents per year on American roads.[1,2] Dean was lucky. His car veered right where a dirt tractor path connected with the road, and he missed a deep ditch by only a few feet. He avoided power poles, trees, and oncoming traffic as well. "Since then, I've put off several late-night trips when I thought I might be too tired. I even took a nap once on an overnight drive when I felt myself drifting," Dean said. "If I hadn't fallen asleep at the wheel before, I probably would have kept driving."

Sleepiness is a significant cause of traffic fatalities. Up to 3% of all yearly vehicular deaths in the United States can be attributed to driving while drowsy, yet Americans remain woefully uneducated to this problem.[1]

Sleepiness undermines a person's ability to make sound decisions and reduces attention span considerably.[2] Any condition that impairs the judgment of drivers should be taken seriously. It has been estimated that 100 million Americans fail to get enough sleep and that up to 50% of all accident-related fatalities (not just driving fatalities) can be attributed to sleep deprivation.[3]

Early Warning Signs

Drivers are often not aware that they are in need of sleep until after they get behind the wheel, or they ignore the signs of sleep deprivation and drive anyway. When drowsiness sets in, drivers are often caught by surprise, and they can fall asleep without realizing it. Being able to recognize the signs of sleep deprivation before we fall victim to it is therefore important. Some of the symptoms of sleep deprivation you should watch out for are:[1,2]

- Struggling against fatigue throughout the day
- Needing caffeine to stay alert, especially on a daily basis
- Falling asleep quickly (within 5 minutes) after stopping to rest
- Having an irritable or argumentative attitude without knowing why
- Needing an alarm clock to wake up in the morning (well-rested people wake up on time naturally)

Tips to Avoid Drowsy Driving

Because of the stealthy manner in which sleep can overtake you, it is important to evaluate your condition before getting behind the wheel and also while you are on the road. It is also important to prevent regular sleep deprivation. We must reduce the risk of falling asleep while driving by using common sense. The following suggestions should help reduce your chances of driving while drowsy:[1]

- Get plenty of sleep. About 8 hours of sleep per night is desirable. If this is not practical, try to catch up on sleep when possible (take naps, sleep more on weekends, etc.).
- Take breaks while driving. Stop at least every 2 hours on long trips. If possible, avoid driving alone so the driving duties can be split. Don't eat heavy meals, and avoid too much caffeine.
- Stay alert. Talk, listen to the radio, sing, or do whatever you can to keep from drifting off. Don't let all of the passengers in the car sleep; having someone to converse with can help keep the driver alert.
- Don't get too comfortable. Getting too relaxed can promote dozing off. Avoid using cruise control. Reduce use of the heater, and keep the windows open when possible.
- Don't drink and drive. This is true anytime, but even a small amount of alcohol in the system can intensify the effects of fatigue on the body.
- If you feel yourself drifting off or you think you may be in danger of falling asleep, stop driving. Dozing off for a few seconds (a phenomenon known as microsleep) is a significant warning sign of fatigue. Don't try to fight through fatigue while driving. Pull off the road at a safe place and take a nap if you need to.

Take time to heed the warning signs of fatigue. Remember that dozing off at the wheel creates a potentially dangerous situation for both yourself and others on or near the road. Being able to recognize when you are at risk of falling asleep and taking steps to avoid driving while drowsy are more than just common sense; they're a necessity for your own and others' personal safety. Getting a few extra winks of sleep and taking the time to ensure you are alert before you get into the driver's seat could save lives.

The National Heart, Lung, and Blood Institute (NHLBI), one of the National Institutes of Health, oversees the National Center on Sleep Disorders Research. This center is an excellent resource for current information, research results, and reports concerning drowsy driving. You can look for links to drowsy driving at the website **www.nhlbi.nih.gov.**

For Discussion . . .

How much sleep do you get each night on average? Do you regularly experience any of the signs of fatigue mentioned in this article? Do you experience fatigue more often during certain times of the day or week? If so, can you think of ways to increase the amount of sleep you get? What would you have to give up to accomplish this goal?

References

1. Matson M. Forgotten menace on our highways, *Reader's Digest*, 144(86), June 1994.
2. Toufexis A. Drowsy America, *Time*, 136(26), Dec 17, 1990.
3. Bennett G. Why you must get more sleep, *McCall's*, 122(3), Dec 1994.

personal assessment

how well do you protect your safety?

This quiz will help you measure how well you manage your personal safety. For each item below, circle the number that reflects the frequency with which you do the safety activity. Then, add up your individual scores and check the interpretation at the end.

3 I regularly do this
2 I sometimes do this
1 I rarely do this

1. I am aware of my surroundings and do not get lost.
   3   2   1
2. I avoid locations in which my personal safety could be compromised.
   3   2   1
3. I intentionally vary my daily routine (such as walking patterns to and from class, parking places, and jogging or biking routes) so that my whereabouts are not always predictable.
   3   2   1
4. I walk across campus at night with other people.
   3   2   1
5. I am careful about disclosing personal information (address, phone number, social security number, my daily schedule, etc.) to people I do not know.
   3   2   1
6. I carefully monitor my alcohol intake at parties.
   3   2   1
7. I watch carefully for dangerous weather conditions and know how to respond if necessary.
   3   2   1
8. I do not keep a loaded gun in my home.
   3   2   1
9. I know how I would handle myself if I were to be assaulted.
   3   2   1
10. I maintain adequate insurance for my health and my property.
    3   2   1
11. I keep emergency information numbers near my phone.
    3   2   1
12. I keep my first aid skills up-to-date.
    3   2   1
13. I use deadbolt locks on the doors of my home.
    3   2   1
14. I use the safety locks on the windows at home.
    3   2   1
15. I check the batteries used in my home smoke detector.
    3   2   1
16. I have installed a carbon monoxide detector in my home.
    3   2   1

17. I use adequate lighting in areas around my home and garage.
    3   2   1
18. I have the electrical, heating, and cooling equipment in my home inspected regularly for safety and efficiency.
    3   2   1
19. I use my car seat belt.
    3   2   1
20. I drive my car safely and defensively.
    3   2   1
21. I keep my car in good mechanical order.
    3   2   1
22. I keep my car doors locked.
    3   2   1
23. I have a plan of action if my car should break down while I am driving it.
    3   2   1
24. I use appropriate safety equipment, such as flotation devices, helmets, and elbow pads, in my recreational activities.
    3   2   1
25. I can swim well enough to save myself in most situations.
    3   2   1
26. I use suggestions for personal safety each day.
    3   2   1

TOTAL POINTS _____

Interpretation
Your total may mean that:

72–78 points	You appear to carefully protect your personal safety.
65–71 points	You adequately protect many aspects of your personal safety.
58–64 points	You should consider improving some of your safety-related behaviors.
Below 58 points	You must consider improving some of your safety-related behaviors.

To Carry This Further . . .
Although no one can be completely safe from personal injury or possible random violence, there are ways to minimize the risks to your safety. Scoring high on this assessment will not guarantee your safety, but your likelihood for injury should remain relatively low. Scoring low on this assessment should encourage you to consider ways to make your life more safe. Refer to the text and this assessment to provide you with useful suggestions to enhance your personal safety. Which safety tips will you use today?

chapter seventeen

the environment and your health

Chapter Objectives

After reading this chapter, you should be able to:

▌ identify several environmental factors that can impact your personal health in either positive or adverse ways.

▌ explain how your personal health is influenced by different environmental factors on several scales, including personal environment, the community and regional environment, and the global environment.

▌ describe specific actions that you can take to minimize health risks associated with your personal environment—your home, your automobile, your workplace.

▌ describe the distinction between a "point source" versus a "nonpoint source" of community/regional air or water pollution.

▌ detail several specific actions that you can take to minimize environmental health risks at the community and regional level.

▌ describe several global environmental health issues, and offer several actions that you might take to foster change.

Online Learning Center Resources

www.mhhe.com/hahn7e

Log on to our Online Learning Center (OLC) for access to theses additional resources:

- Chapter key terms and definitions
- Learning objectives
- Student interactive question-and-answer sites
- Self-scoring chapter quiz
- Online assessments
- Key term flash cards

Talking It Over

Talking—and Acting—Like an Environmentalist

One of your classmates claims to be an avid environmentalist who loves hiking, camping, and other outdoor activities. He is involved with several organizations that lobby the government for environmental reform. So, when you see him drive a large, gas-guzzling SUV up to the recycling center, where he deposits neatly sorted paper, bottles, and cans for recycling, does this image strike you as contradictory? Do you think he recycles to ease a guilty conscience about driving an SUV? Would it matter more if you were standing in the middle of New York City (far from any dirt roads), or in Salt Lake City (surrounded by vast wildlands)? If his love of the great outdoors requires a larger vehicle (to haul camping gear, kayak, etc.), might he have made a more environmentally sound choice?

CommunicationLinks:

www.thedetroitproject.com
http://www.ecocenter.org/auto.shtml

Eye on the Media

Does Eco-Terrorism Really Work to Protect Our Environment?

On August 23, 2003, several automobile dealerships were attacked by arsonists who left graffiti claiming that they destroyed or damaged gas-guzzling SUVs to protect the environment. The unknown perpetrators claimed to be acting in accordance with the Earth Liberation Front, or ELF. According to their Internet website, ELF is an international underground organization that uses "direct action" (called eco-terrorism by others) in the form of economic sabotage to stop the destruction of the natural environment. Since 1997, the ELF in North America has caused over $100 million in damages to entities who profit from the destruction of life and the planet.

Many people are angered by the degradation of our shared natural environment, but is direct action/eco-terrorism ever justified in a democratic society? For some, the degradation or destruction of a local wetland, a forested mountaintop, or a local river or lake is a personal loss, like the death of an old friend. Many people are frustrated by the perception that well-funded corporate interests have bought out our democratic political system so that they can exploit our shared natural lands. Some wonder, "If the system is unfair, why not take direct action to right these wrongs?"

Those who participate in eco-terrorism may feel at the time that they are "part of the solution," but are they really? To shift the course of the global human population toward a more ecologically sustainable path will require many changes, large and small, governmental and personal. Does eco-terrorism really change people's attitudes and behaviors toward protecting our environment? Will eco-terrorism stimulate governments toward more ecologically sound policies, or cause a

societal backlash against all groups who work to protect the environment? Does direct action against environmental "bad guys" discourage their activities, or allow them to claim "victim" status that brings them assistance in proceeding with their destructive practices?

One likely motivation for ELF's acts of economic sabotage is to get environmental problems on the national agenda; to make people more aware and motivated to act in the political process. Certainly, this strategy worked well for the civil rights movement. The TV pictures of peaceful black demonstrators being viciously attacked by white police officers and their dogs caused our entire nation to wake up to the problem of institutional racism. To date, the main results from actions

by ELF are short-lived news stories that show damage to expensive SUVs and burned-out buildings. These news stories never show pictures of environmental damage associated with the manufacture of the SUVs or economic development of natural habitats. All the public sees is waste of resources in the burned hulks of automobiles, the vandalism of extremists. This does not seem to be a particularly effective way to draw public attention to environmental problems. Even worse, some anti-environment commentators use widely televised actions of ELF to discredit the entire environmental movement. Using the media to get environmental issues on the national agenda is a good thing only if it advances positive changes that provide real environmental protection.

Environmental issues are important concerns for many college-age students as they perceive disturbing trends that may affect their future health and well-being. News programs regularly present the latest bad news about over-population, pollution, global warming, damage to the ozone layer, loss of wilderness to economic exploitation, and endangered species. Movies such as *Water World, Blade Runner, Batman, The Matrix,* and *The Terminator* depict fictional futures that are dismal environmental disasters. Some college students join environmental organizations that work to clean up litter, encourage recycling, regulate pollution, control human population growth, and protect endangered species and natural areas. Others feel there is nothing they can do about such monumental environmental issues. They lose hope for a future where the world will be a good place to live and raise a family, and may become depressed and apathetic. The impact of the environment on your health depends on the nature of your environment and your personal responses to that environment.

Your **environment** includes a range of conditions that can influence your health, such as the availability of resources (oxygen, water, food) and environmental characteristics, such as temperature, humidity, toxins, allergens, pathogens, noise, and radiation. Conditions in your environment operate across a wide range of spatial scales, from the air immediately surrounding your body to the global earth, air, and ocean system. Your physical health is influenced primarily by your *personal environment,* comprised of conditions in the home, neighborhood, and workplace, including indoor air, drinking water, toxic building materials and noise. This personal environment is influenced by conditions in the larger *community* and

regional environment, including such conditions as air pollution and water pollution. These local and regional conditions are influenced by conditions of the *global environment,* such as climate and solar radiation.

The goal of this chapter is to help you identify aspects of your environment that can significantly affect your health, and to suggest ways that you can exert personal control over these environmental influences. Different environmental conditions and personal responses will be important at the various spatial scales (home/workplace, community/region, and global). Figure 17-1 displays some environmental problems at various spatial scales, and a range of personal responses that might be appropriate at each level.

The Personal Environment: Home, Neighborhood, Workplace

On average you spend about 90% of your time in your home, workplace, local stores, and entertainment venues.[1] The indoor air you breathe, the water you drink from the tap, and the radiation and noise in your immediate surroundings are environmental factors that have the most direct impact on your health. Some indoor environmental

> **Key Terms**
>
> **environment** the physical conditions (temperature, humidity, light, presence of substances) and other living organisms that exist around your body.

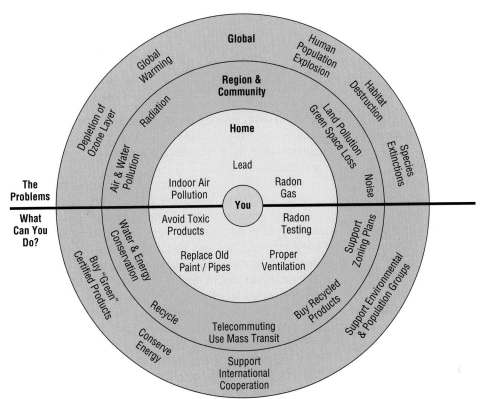

Figure 17-1 Spatial scales of environmental health risks and appropriate personal responses to environmental problems.

problems cause immediate health effects, such as headaches, dizziness, nausea, or allergic reactions. Other environmental problems act in subtle, cumulative ways, causing major health problems such as cancer or neurological damage that may not become apparent until permanent damage is done.

Of all the different environmental influences on your health, you have the greatest control over factors in your personal environment. You are responsible for maintaining your appliances so that they do not produce excessive air pollution. You control the ventilation in your home, allowing you to vent pollutants outside. You choose which products you will purchase, and can avoid products that contain toxic chemicals. You can eliminate tobacco smoke from your home and workspace. You can identify sources of health risk in the workplace and notify those responsible for environmental safety.

Indoor Air Quality

Indoor air quality within buildings can be influenced by a wide range of factors, including ventilation, humidity, gases given off by building construction materials, furniture and flooring materials, and combustion by-products from stoves and furnaces. When there is a problem with one or more of these factors, people in the affected build-

ing can experience a wide range of symptoms, from headaches and itchy eyes to unconsciousness and death. This section covers some of the most important health risks associated with indoor air quality.

Carbon Monoxide

Carbon monoxide is a highly toxic gas that is colorless, odorless, and tasteless, and so is not detectable by the unaided senses. Health effects of carbon monoxide vary from mild discomfort (headaches, dizziness, mental confusion, and nausea) at concentrations below 70 parts per million (ppm) to death at concentrations above 150 ppm. Persons who suffer from heart disease may feel chest pain at low concentrations. Regular exposure to low levels in

---

Key Terms

indoor air quality characteristics of air within homes, workplaces, and public buildings, including the presence and amount of oxygen, water vapor, and a wide range of substances that can have adverse effects on your health.

carbon monoxide a gaseous by-product of the incomplete combustion of natural gas, kerosene, heating oil, wood, coal, gasoline, and tobacco.

Religious Perspectives on Human-Environment Relationships

Lynn White (*Science*, 1967), stated that the root of all the environmental problems today can be found in Judeo-Christian and Islamic scripture. According to scripture of these religious traditions, the purpose of all of creation was to meet the needs and uses of humankind. This established a dualism (human versus not human) that did not exist in earlier religions that perceived divinity in all of creation. White proposed that this dualism encourages exploitation and dominion over nature by humans, resulting in the many environmental problems facing us today.

Earth-based religions of many indigenous cultures of the world (pre-Christian Europe, Native American, African) believed that many or all aspects of the natural world were manifestations of one or more gods. Humans were perceived as being at the mercy of these powerful natural forces, and often performed religious rituals to gain favors or atone for sins against Nature. Many of these cultures appear to have lived in ecological balance with their environment. Whether this balance was the consequence of their religious beliefs, their small populations, their limited technologies, or the combination of these factors is unknown. Modern Earth-based religions (including Paganism, Wicca, Druidism, and Goddess religions) also worship the natural world as a manifestation of the energy of God or Creation. People who follow these religious traditions are often dedicated to protecting the environment.[1]

Traditional Hinduism also lacks the distinction between humankind as separate from the rest of Creation. Hindus believe that humans, gods, and nature are all parts of a single organic whole; God is present in all of Nature. Because divine forces sustain all life on Earth, Hindus believe they should live in harmony with Creation. Any abuse of Nature is considered a sacrilegious act. These traditional beliefs encourage Hindus to live in balance with their environment. However, in their efforts to develop a modern economic system in India, many Hindus have abandoned these traditional beliefs: in recent decades India has suffered from the same environmental degradation as many other developed nations.[2]

In the Islamic tradition, humankind is considered the most favored of God's creation, and all the rest of Creation is deemed subservient to human needs and uses. However, Islamic tradition also holds that all living things in Nature are partners of humankind, deserving of respect and their own existence. Islamic tradition also stipulates that humankind should be good stewards of natural resources and should not pollute clean waters with their wastes. Muslims are encouraged to put the common good ahead of personal benefit, and to be moderate in consumption, including the use of natural resources.[3]

While the Judeo-Christian scripture has passages that could be seen as justifying environmentally destructive behavior, it also has distinctly environment-friendly teachings. In the Judeo-Christian tradition, God created the heavens and Earth, the land and waters, the plants and animals, and humankind. At the end of each day of Creation, the Bible states that God saw each of his creations was "good." Some theologians interpret these statements to mean that the Creator valued all aspects of Creation, not just humankind. Several biblical passages invoke human responsibility to be "good stewards" over the other parts of Creation. However, other passages in the Bible are less environmentally friendly, including statements that humankind should "go forth and multiply" and "subdue the Earth." These passages are often cited by those who seek a religious basis to justify unchecked human population growth and environmental destruction in pursuit of human goals.

The National Religious Partnership for the Environment is an umbrella organization for Christians and Jews who believe that protecting the environment is a mandate well-founded in their scriptural traditions.[4] This association of religious congregations works to increase awareness of the environmental message in the Bible and Torah. A main objective of this association is to enhance the activity of its members in the political process in support of environmental protection. For people who are committed to protecting the environment and dedicated to their Judeo-Christian religion, this organization offers a community of like-minded people working toward similar goals.

[1]Pagan and Earth-based Religions. **http://www.beliefnet.com/index/index_10015.html**
[2]Adhopia A: Hinduism Promotes Environmental Protection. 2001. **http://www.indianest.com/analysis/018.htm**
[3]Alhilaly TH: Islam and Ecology. 1993. **http://www.ummah.com/islam/taqwapalace/fitness/microcosmpage2.html**
[4]National Religious Partnership for the Environment. **http://www.nrpe.org**

---

the home or workplace can cause flu-like symptoms that rapidly disappear after you leave the location where you are exposed.[1] At high concentrations greater than 150 ppm, carbon monoxide poisoning can render you unconscious and then kill you.[2]

You can minimize your exposure to carbon monoxide and risk of poisoning by keeping all appliances that burn gas or other fuels in proper working order and ensuring proper ventilation. You should use the manufacturer-specified fuel in space heaters, and ensure proper ventilation of space heaters, woodstoves, charcoal and gas grills, and fireplaces. You should avoid letting your car idle inside a garage, especially if it is attached to your home.[1] Finally, you should install a carbon monoxide detector that will let you monitor levels of this gas in your home and will sound an alarm if levels exceed safety standards. Every year, 300 people in the United States die from carbon monoxide poisoning,[3] usually due to improperly maintained furnaces or incorrectly used space heaters. A carbon monoxide alarm can prevent this tragedy from happening to you.

Volatile Organic Compounds

Volatile organic compounds (VOCs) are emitted from products such as paint, paint stripper, cleaning solvents, wood preservatives, aerosol sprays, cleaners, disinfectants, insect repellents and pesticides, air fresheners, stored fuels and automotive products, hobby supplies such as wood glue, and recently dry-cleaned clothing. Formaldehyde is a specific VOC that commonly enters the indoor environment due to emissions from pressed wood products (hardwood plywood wall paneling, particleboard, fiberboard) and furniture made with these pressed wood products. Urea-formaldehyde foam used for home insulation can emit this gas into the indoor environment.[4]

The health effects of volatile organic compounds will vary, depending on which specific substance is involved. Immediate effects of many VOCs include irritation to the eyes, nose, and throat, headaches, loss of coordination, and/or nausea. Longer-term exposure to some VOCs can result in damage to the liver, kidney, and central nervous system. Some VOCs are known or suspected carcinogens in animals and/or humans.

There are several ways you can limit your exposure to toxic volatile organic compounds. First, minimize your use of products that contain these substances by choosing cleaning supplies, paints, and glues that do not contain VOCs. If you must use a product that contains VOCs, follow directions and provide for plenty of ventilation. Also, you should buy only as much of the VOC-containing product as you will need for your current project and dispose of the unused portion in an appropriate manner as soon as possible.

Tobacco Smoke

Secondhand tobacco smoke is an indoor air pollutant widely recognized as a major health risk, especially for children. For example, this pollutant can increase the risk for acute asthma attacks that require hospital emergency care. There is some evidence that regular exposure to tobacco smoke increases the risk of developing asthma in the first place.[5] Exposure to tobacco smoke in the home is also associated with increased risk of Sudden Infant Death Syndrome (SIDS), childhood bronchitis, pneumonia and ear infections, cardiovascular disease, and cancer. The health effects of indoor tobacco smoke are covered in more detail in Chapter 9.

Asbestos

Asbestos is a building material that was widely used for insulation, floor tiles, and for its fire retardant and noise-dampening properties. Health effects of asbestos expo-sure include cancers of the lung and abdomen, and irreversible scarring of the lungs that can result in reduced respiratory function. These dire effects most commonly occur only after many years of exposure, usually in the workplace.[6] When the serious health risks associated with exposure to asbestos became known, governmental agencies banned several asbestos products, and manufacturers voluntarily limited other uses of asbestos. Today, asbestos is most commonly found in older buildings, including homes, schools, and factories. The greatest risk of exposure to asbestos occurs when insulation, floor tiles, and other asbestos-containing substances deteriorate, or are damaged during building renovation. These activities release the microscopic asbestos fibers into the air, from which they are inhaled into the lungs. However, intact and undisturbed, asbestos-containing products are relatively safe.[6]

You can minimize your risk of exposure to asbestos fibers by leaving undamaged asbestos-containing materials alone, and by hiring qualified contractors to remove damaged asbestos. Do not try to remove asbestos yourself. Never cut, rip, or use a sander on any material that contains asbestos. Follow manufacturer's recommendations for replacing and disposing of products that contain asbestos.[6]

Biological Pollutants

There are many sources of **biological air pollutants** within your personal environment. Disease-causing viruses and bacteria (common cold, flu, measles) are put into the air when infected people or animals sneeze or cough. Contaminated central air handling systems can be breeding grounds for mold, mildew, and bacteria and can then distribute these contaminants throughout the home. Some people have allergic reactions (itchy eyes, runny nose, sneezing, coughing, stuffy chest, shortness of breath, headache, and/or dizziness) to spores from mold that grows on moist surfaces inside buildings. Some research indicates that exposure to indoor mold can more

---

Key Terms

volatile organic compounds a wide variety of chemicals that contain carbon and readily evaporate into the air.

asbestos a term used to refer to a class of minerals that have a fibrous crystal structure.

biological air pollutants living organisms or substances produced by living organisms that cause disease or allergic reactions, including bacteria, molds, mildew, viruses, dust mites, plant pollen, and animal dander, urine, or feces.

than double your risk of developing adult onset asthma.[5] Pollen from plants around the home or workplace can cause allergic reactions (hay fever) in many people. Household pets, rats, mice, and cockroaches are sources of saliva, urine, feces, and skin dander that can also stimulate strong allergic reactions.[7]

You can minimize your exposure to biological indoor air pollutants by maintaining the relative humidity in your home within the range of 30% to 50%. This will minimize the growth of many microorganisms that can cause health problems. Control indoor air humidity by installing exhaust fans in bathrooms and kitchens (major sources of water vapor), venting places where water vapor accumulates (attics, basements, and crawl spaces), and using air conditioning or a dehumidifier. You should also eliminate standing water, rugs that have been damaged by leaks or floodwater, and any other wet surfaces.[7]

To minimize allergic reactions to biological indoor air pollutants, you should regularly clean and vacuum your home. While this will not completely eliminate dust mites, pollen, and animal dander, cleaning can substantially reduce the amounts of these allergens and the severity of allergy symptoms. Allergic individuals should leave the house while it is being vacuumed because this may temporarily increase airborne levels of mite allergens and other biological contaminants. You should also try to keep your house free of rodents and cockroaches as these pests are sources of potent allergens.[7]

Radon

Radon is an environmental health risk that seeps into buildings from the soil surrounding their foundation. It is invisible, odorless, and tasteless, and can be detected only using radon detectors. Uranium, the source of radon, can be found in most parts of the world, and this element is present in rock and soil in parts of all fifty states of the United States. Once radon is produced by decay of uranium, this gas moves through the ground to the air above. Some radon gas may dissolve into groundwater.

It is estimated that indoor radon is at a level sufficient to increase risk of lung cancer in one of every fifteen homes in the United States.[8] The U.S. Surgeon General has warned that exposure to radon gas is the second leading cause of lung cancer in the United States. The National Academy of Sciences estimates that radon exposure causes about 15,000 lung cancer deaths in the United States every year.[9] This risk from radon is especially high for cigarette smokers. Lung damage is caused by radioactive particles formed as by-products from decay of radon that are inhaled and trapped deep within the lungs. As the particles continue the radioactive decay process, they emit bursts of energy that damage adjacent lung tissue. There are no obvious short-term effects from this damage, but long-term exposure can cause lung cancer.[9] There is some evidence that consuming water that is contaminated by radon gas can increase the risk of stomach cancer. The National Academy of Sciences estimates consumption of radon in drinking water causes 19 stomach cancer deaths per year in the United States.[10]

The key to minimizing the health risk of radon exposure is to have your home tested. You can purchase an inexpensive "do-it-yourself" test kit in some hardware stores and other retail outlets. If you can't find a radon test kit locally, you can purchase one from the National Safety Council's Radon Hotline (800-767-7236). After the kit is exposed to the air in your home for a specified time period, it must be returned to a laboratory for analysis.

If unsafe levels of radon are detected in your home, you should work with a contractor who is certified to install a radon reduction system. This will often involve installing a venting system just below the concrete slab of the house foundation. The venting system will intercept the radon gas before it enters your home and vent it outside, where it can be dissipated by wind. You should also have cracks in the slab, basement walls, or foundation of the home repaired to reduce seepage of radon gas through these spaces. However, just sealing the cracks, without installing the belowground venting system, will not adequately reduce indoor radon levels. If you live in a region where high radon levels are common and you plan to build a new home, you should work with your contractor to install radon-resistant features during construction. The average cost to install a radon venting system in an existing home is $800 to $2,500. The average cost to install radon-resistant features in a new home during construc-

Key Terms

radon a naturally occurring radioactive gas that is emitted during the decay of uranium in soil, rock, and water.

tion is $350 to $500 (a 128% to 400% savings).[8] For a map of radon risk zones in the United States, see **http://www.epa.gov/iaq/radon /zonemap.html.**

Lead

Lead is a toxic metal that was widely used in house paint, as a gasoline additive, and in plumbing solder for metal pipes. As the health consequences of lead toxicity became better known, several of these uses of lead were banned, including lead-based house paint and leaded gasoline. However, lead is a very stable substance that remains in the environment today, long after its use was banned.

Lead exposure most commonly occurs in older homes, built before 1970. Many of these homes contain substantial amounts of lead-based paint, and older metal plumbing may contain lead solder. In late 1991, more than 10 years after lead-based paint was banned, the Secretary of the U.S. Department of Health and Human Services called lead, "the number one environmental threat to the health of children in the United States."[11] Exposure to lead from old paint occurs when the paint breaks down into paint flakes and dust, which are then inhaled or swallowed. This risk is especially high for young children who often put their hands into their mouth. Lead can also leach from solder in old plumbing and be ingested when people drink tap water.[11]

While lead additives in gasoline were banned by 1990, lead from automobile exhaust fumes was already deposited in soils and can still be found in high concentrations near major highways and city streets. Airborne dust from dirt tracked into the house on shoes can transfer this contaminant to the indoor environment.

Lead has serious health effects when ingested or inhaled, especially for children. Lead can affect virtually all organ systems of the body, but is particularly damaging to the nervous system, kidneys, and blood. *Acute lead toxicity* (blood lead level greater than 80 micrograms per deciliter) can lead to convulsions, coma, and death. However, blood lead levels as low as 10 micrograms per deciliter in children can delay physical and mental development, lower IQ, reduce attention span, and increase behavioral problems.[11]

You can minimize your exposure to lead by replacing deteriorated lead house paint and lead soldered plumbing, and by keeping your home clean of roadside dirt that may be contaminated with residual lead from automobile exhaust. If the lead-based paint in your old house is in good condition, leave it alone; it does not pose a hazard *if it is intact*. However, if the old paint is flaking or producing paint dust, you should have it removed by a contractor that is certified for lead abatement. Do not try to remove lead-based paint yourself, as you may inhale large amounts of paint dust or volatilized lead.

Health on the Web

Behavior Change Activities

Learn about Lead Poisoning

Lead poisoning has been a predominant topic in environmental health news in recent years. Lead is a very harmful substance, especially to young children as it is easily absorbed into their bodies. However, lead can be harmful to anyone who comes in contact with large quantities of it. Go to **http://www.wmeac.org/learn/toxics.asp** at the West Michigan Environmental Council and scroll down to the section on Lead. Click on the "self-test" link to learn whether you or your child should be tested for lead poisoning.

Automobiles and Air Pollution

Did you know that if you "top off" your gas tank on a hot day, you are actually creating smog, which you then breathe into your lungs? Did you know that a full bus is six times more energy efficient than each person on the bus driving his or her own car? Learn more fascinating air pollution facts with this air pollution quiz from Car Talk at Cars.com. Go to **http://cartalk.cars.com/About/Pollution-Quiz/**, take the quiz, and then learn how to help fight air pollution!

If you are exposed to lead contamination, eating a balanced diet that is rich in calcium and iron can reduce the effects of lead toxicity.[11] If you live in an older house with metal plumbing, you should have the tap water tested for lead. Lead is not readily excreted by the body, and will tend to accumulate over time. There are chelating drug treatments which help the body to excrete lead and reduce toxicity effects, but they have adverse side effects and are generally used only to treat acute lead toxicity.[12]

Drinking Water

The safety of drinking water in your home is affected by environmental factors both in the home or neighborhood and in the larger community. The water supply for rural homes is often a well that draws from groundwater, and can be much affected by environmental conditions around the home and neighborhood. In urban areas a municipal water supply system draws from rivers or lakes and then treats the water to make it safe to drink. The community/regional environment plays the dominant role in determining the safety of water from municipal suppliers. However, municipal water can be contaminated by the personal environment as it passes through pipes in the home. Environmental health issues relating to drinking water as influenced by conditions in your home and neighborhood will be covered here. Issues related to municipal water supply are presented later in this chapter.

Tap water is a key source of pollutants in the home.

Approximately 23 million people in the United States obtain their drinking water from groundwater (i.e., from private wells), streams, or cisterns that collect rain water.[13] These households are responsible for ensuring the safety of their own drinking water. Private drinking water supplies that rely on surface waters, or wells that tap shallow groundwater layers, are at risk of contamination by pathogens from home septic systems, contaminants from leaking underground fuel storage tanks, improper disposal of various household chemicals (cleaners, automotive fluids, and pesticides), and agricultural chemicals applied to surrounding farm fields.

Nitrate from agricultural fertilizer that leaches into shallow groundwater supplies poses a widespread health risk in rural areas. The U.S. Geological Survey estimates that 10% to 20% of groundwater sources of drinking water may have levels of nitrate contamination that pose risks to human health.[14] Excessive consumption of nitrate in contaminated drinking water can cause serious illness and death. Nitrate interferes with the oxygen-transport function of the blood (methemoglobinemia). This effect is most pronounced in children, resulting in "blue-baby" syndrome.[14,15] Nitrate can also cause reproductive problems and is linked to development of several types of cancer.[16]

Rural wells contaminated by nitrate may also have high levels of other agricultural chemicals. Some researchers have suggested that agricultural pesticides and herbicides can contribute to the development of testicular cancer and reduced sperm production in men, breast cancer in women, and nervous system disorders in children.[16]

Leaching of substances from pipes in the plumbing of older homes is another potential source of contamination to drinking water in the home.[17] Metallic pipes can release toxic metals such as lead and copper into the water. Polyvinyl chloride (PVC) pipes manufactured before 1977 may release toxic vinyl chloride into the water. Vinyl chloride is a known human carcinogen.

Leaching of toxic substances from pipes into the drinking water supply is most problematic in small diameter pipes (less than a 2-inch diameter), with high water temperatures, and when the water is stagnant in the pipes for long periods (more than 24 hours).[17] A relatively easy way to reduce contaminants from household plumbing in your drinking water is to regularly flush fresh water through the plumbing. Let the water run from the tap for a couple of minutes before taking water to drink, especially first thing in the morning and if you have been away from home for long time periods. In some cases it may be advisable to replace the old plumbing, but this can be very expensive.

Private water supplies should be tested annually for nitrate and fecal coliform bacteria. If you suspect there may be a problem with radon or pesticide contamination, you may need to test your water even more frequently.[14] Testing will generally require that you send samples of your water to a laboratory that tests water quality. You can get a listing of local certified laboratories from your local or state public health department. Some local health departments test private water for free. A private laboratory will charge $10 to $20 to perform a nitrate and bacteria test. Testing for pesticides or organic chemicals may cost from several hundred to several thousand dollars. Most laboratories mail back the sample results within a few days, or several weeks if the analyses are more complex. The results will indicate the concentrations of contaminants and indicate whether each contaminant exceeds a drinking water quality standard.

If your drinking water contains contaminants that exceed safety standards, you should retest the water supply immediately and contact your public health department for assistance. High bacteria concentrations can sometimes be easily controlled by disinfecting a well. Water filters may also remove some contaminants. However, other problems may require a new source of water, such as a deeper well. Alternatively, you may need to rely on bottled water until a new water source can be obtained.[13] You can obtain technical assistance with residential drinking water supply problems from the organization Farm*A*Syst/Home*A*Syst (see the websites **http://www.uwex.edu/farmasyst** or **http://www.uwex.edu/homeasyst**).

Noise

Noise can be defined as any undesirable sound. What constitutes "undesirable sound" will vary from one person to the next, but it often involves loud sounds that occur at irregular intervals and are not controllable by the listener.[18] In the personal environment of the home, neighborhood, and workplace, noise may include overly loud music, barking dogs, motorcycles and cars with broken or missing muffler systems, loud machinery, appliances and power tools, airplanes flying overhead, and train whistles.

The health effects of environmental noise depend on the intensity, frequency, and nature of the noise. Excessively loud noise can cause physical damage to sensory tissues in your ears, resulting in partial or total hearing loss that can be temporary or permanent. This physical damage will depend on both the intensity (as measured in decibels) and the duration of exposure to the loud noise. For example, sitting in front of the speaker column at a large rock concert, with noise levels at 120 decibels for over 2 hours, can result in immediate pain and long-term or permanent hearing loss. Ironically, the tissues that are damaged by excessively loud sounds are those responsible for hearing high frequency sounds associated with normal conversation, not the tissues that actually hear the damaging sound. Loud noise sources rob you of one of your most important senses, the ability to hear the unamplified human voice.

Even noise at lower levels can cause adverse health effects. The American Speech-Language-Hearing Association reports that low level noise can elevate blood pressure, reduce sleep, cause fatigue, and disturb digestion. These physical effects of low level noise can impact emotional, intellectual, social, and occupational health. Effects reported by the World Health Organization include increased frustration and anxiety, impaired ability to concentrate, reduced productivity and ability to learn, and increased absenteeism and accidents. These effects of noise can increase your feeling of stress and diminish your ability to tolerate minor irritations; you may exhibit anger and aggression that are out of proportion to the immediate source of your irritation.[18] This antisocial behavior may have negative consequences in your personal relationships and occupational health.

A common source of long-term exposure to loud sound that causes hearing loss in many young people is amplified music. Occasional loud rock music at 110 to 120 decibels may cause only temporary damage. However, daily exposure to such sound levels will cause permanent hearing loss. A number of aging rock stars have admitted to significant hearing loss that they attribute to standing in front of huge amplifiers night after night. Many rock musicians performing today stand behind the main speaker columns or wear ear protection. Jacking up the volume in your headphones, or the powerful amplifier in your car stereo, may be fun today, but is it worth a lifetime of incessant ringing in your ears and diminished hearing later in life? See Changing for the Better on page 492 for tips on reducing the health risks associated with noise pollution.

TALKING POINTS How can you encourage your children to develop sound habits regarding their environment and their personal health? What changes can you make in your own habits to serve as a better example for them?

The Community and Regional Environment

The community and regional environment is comprised of the outdoor air you breathe, local rivers and lakes that provide water and recreation opportunities, surrounding lands (urban, industrial, suburban, rural, agricultural, natural communities), and all the people and other species that live in these areas. A wide range of human activities can degrade this community environment in ways that affect personal health. Air, water, and land pollution include many substances that have significant negative effects on physical health. Loss of natural areas and other recreational and aesthetic "green space" to roads, cities, and industrial development can adversely affect your perceived quality of life, with negative effects on emotional and spiritual health. Degraded environmental conditions in many communities discourage new economic development and may limit occupational health.

While you can exert some influence on the environmental conditions in your community, the influence of any one individual is usually small. Your control over how the community environment affects your personal health is often limited to controlling your exposure to known health risks, such as contaminated water and land, or outdoor air pollution. You can also choose to reduce your own contributions to community/regional air, water, and land pollution through conservation of energy and water and recycling solid waste.

Because one person cannot have a significant impact on community environmental problems, many people join organizations that work to improve the environment and quality of life in their community. By working with others of like mind in the political process and in environmental organizations, you become "part of the solution" to major environmental problems that can affect your health and that of your family. For many people, getting involved in solving local environmental problems can provide significant benefits to emotional and spiritual health.

In this section you will learn about aspects of the community and regional environment that can affect your health, and what you can do to exert some level of personal control over these environmental influences.

Air Pollution

Air pollution includes substances that naturally occur in the air (pollen, microbes, dust, sea salt, volcanic ash) and substances produced by human activities (engine exhaust, ozone, various volatile organic compounds, and acid rain). In this section on community and regional environmental influences on health, we focus on those components of air pollution that are produced within a specific region and that have substantial health effects within that community or region.

The primary sources of human-caused air pollutants are various kinds of internal combustion engines associated with electric power plants, industry, and

Key Terms

air pollution refers to a wide variety of substances found in the atmosphere that can have adverse effects on human health, crop productivity, and natural communities.

Learning from Our Diversity

Native Americans and the Environment

An essay by David Lewis, in *Native America in the Twentieth Century: An Encyclopedia,* published in 1994 by Garland Publishers of New York, describes the historical and modern environmental ethic of Native Americans. Many early environmentalists were inspired by their perceptions of the close relationship between Native Americans and their natural environment. Before contact with Euroamericans, Native American cultures perceived that their spiritual and physical universes were one. They felt connected with the animate and inanimate beings of their environment, and managed its bounty carefully so as not to upset the spirits who kept their world in balance and supplied all necessary resources. They acknowledged the power of the Earth and considered the hunter and hunted as equal partners in the larger scheme of things. They practiced rituals with the animals they killed, the agricultural fields they tended, and the resources they consumed to ensure a continued supply.

Romantic modern misconceptions that Native Americans "left no mark on the land" ignore much cultural and historical evidence that they used fire and water to transform their landscapes.* When necessary, Native Americans adjusted their environments to meet their cultural and material needs. However, Native Americans were careful students of their functional environments. They strived for maximum sustained yield, not maximum production. Their use of natural resources was based on reciprocity and balance.* This approach to stewardship of natural resources is certainly worthy of admiration, and a worthy goal for modern society.

Modern Native American communities are often far removed from their traditional land ethic, a fact that sometimes places them at odds with environmentalists. However, environmental problems on Native American lands must be placed in the perspective of the total destruction of their cultures and environment at the hands of Euroamericans. There are instances when control of natural resources on Indian reservations has been returned to Native Americans, with disastrous environmental consequences. However, these Native American communities have been forced to live on remote, marginal lands, with few apparent natural resources, and lacking virtually all the native plants and animal species upon which their traditional practices depended. These communities suffer in the depths of poverty, and sometimes seek any economic development regardless of the environmental cost. In desperation, some accept toxic waste dumps onto their lands, and others strip the land of its forests to meet the immediate needs of their communities. Often, these environmentally destructive decisions are made by Euroamerican government agents on behalf of their Native American clients.

Another point of disagreement between Native Americans and modern environmentalists involves traditional hunting of species that are now considered threatened or endangered, such as the bald eagle, bowhead whale, and Florida panther. The rights of Native Americans to these traditional hunting practices, intimately connected with their religion and culture, is protected by the American Indian Religious Freedom Act of 1978. Environmentalists who oppose these hunts seem to pick and choose which Native American traditions to admire and which to condemn. They fail to recognize that the religious practice of the hunts is part of a larger tradition that motivated Native Americans to seek balance with their environment.

As Native American communities struggle to meet their most basic needs and maintain their cultural traditions in a hostile modern world, we should be careful about harshly judging their departures from traditional land ethics. There is a diversity of opinion within Native American communities, just as in other communities. Some people seek to be modern, while others yearn for the traditional values of an earlier day. Traditional land ethics are much more recent history for Native Americans than are similar, pre-Christian, Earth-centered religions of Euroamericans. Nonetheless, both communities struggle with the question of how best to manage our environment for present and future generations.

*Lewis DR: Essay on Native American Environmental Issues. In: *Native Americans and the Environment.* 2000. **http://www.cnie.org/nae/docs/intro.html**

---

transportation (trucks, automobiles, and farm/construction equipment). Oil refineries and chemical production factories also contribute to air pollution in some communities. Electric power stations, industrial facilities, and chemical factories are classified as *point sources* that produce large amounts of pollution from a single location. Automobiles, trucks, heavy construction/farm equipment, gas stations, lawn mowers, and charcoal grills are *nonpoint sources* of air pollutants. Individually, nonpoint sources produce relatively small amounts of pollution, but when added together account for a large proportion of community air pollution.

Air pollutants that are directly produced by internal combustion engines include *carbon monoxide, nitrogen dioxide, sulfur dioxide, hydrocarbons and particulate matter.* Carbon monoxide is a toxic gas that impairs respiration, as described under indoor air quality in the previous section. Nitrogen and sulfur oxides interact with water vapor in the air to form small particulates (diameter $<2.5\mu$) that are inhaled into the deepest parts of the lungs. These substances can damage lung tissues, reduce lung capacity, cause coughing and chronic bronchitis, and may worsen such ailments as hypersensitivity to allergens, asthma, emphysema, and heart disease. The U.S. Environmental Protection Agency estimates that over 70 million people in the United States live in counties where levels of small particulate air pollutants exceed human health standards for at least some part of the year.[19] It has been

Smog over a major U.S. city.

estimated that small particulate air pollution causes as many as 50,000 to 100,000 premature deaths in the United States per year.[20] In addition to these direct effects, nitrogen oxides may act as a fertilizer, stimulating pollen production in many plant species (such as ragweed) and worsen pollen-related allergic reactions in humans.[14]

Tropospheric ozone is another important regional air pollutant that is linked to chemicals in exhaust fumes from internal combustion engines. This substance is produced when hydrocarbons, nitrogen oxides, and other small particle matter chemically interact in the presence of sunlight. The result is a brownish haze over affected cities, often called *smog.*

Ozone levels are particularly high in locations with warm, sunny climates (Southern California) and where natural vegetation produces volatile organic compounds that contribute to the photochemical process that produces ozone (eastern U.S.). The U.S. Environmental Protection Agency estimates that over 110 million people in the United States live in counties where ozone levels exceed human health standards for at least some part of the year.[19] Most of these people live in Southern California and near the East Coast between Virginia and southern Maine (see Figure 17-2).

Inhalation of ozone can cause lung damage that reduces lung capacity. This is a particular health risk to individuals who suffer from asthma, emphysema, or heart disease. On days when ozone concentrations are highest, local hospital emergency room visits associated with respiratory distress increase from 10% to 20%.[21] There is also some evidence that childhood exposure to ozone can actually cause children to become asthmatic.[22]

Air toxics are a diverse collection of hazardous air pollutants produced mainly by electric power plants and industrial sources that constitute a widespread

environmental health risk in the United States. When lifetime cancer risks for all carcinogenic air toxics are combined, 20 million people live in areas where the risk exceeds 100 in one million.[23] However, these risk estimates are based on a lifetime of exposure to toxic air pollutant levels in 1996. With continued progress on reducing toxic air pollution, this risk is expected to decrease in the future. Since passage of the Clear Air Act in 1970, much progress has been made in reducing air pollution in the United States. However, further reduction of air pollution poses serious technological, economic, and political challenges. For more information about air toxics, go to the website **http://www.epa.gov/ttn/atw.**

Unfortunately, the degree to which you can control your own exposure to regional air pollution and the associated health risks is limited. In larger urban areas where air pollution levels are high, weather reports often include information about air pollution. If you live in a large city, you should pay attention to air pollution information, often conveyed in color-coded alerts. A "yellow" air pollution alert means people who suffer from respiratory or cardiac diseases, or hypersensitivity to

---

Key Terms

tropospheric ozone ozone is comprised of three oxygen atoms that are bound into a single molecule; tropospheric ozone refers to this substance as it occurs in the lower layer of the atmosphere, close to the ground.

air toxics a class of 188 toxic air pollutants identified by the U.S. Environmental Protection Agency as known or suspected causes of cancer or other serious health effects.

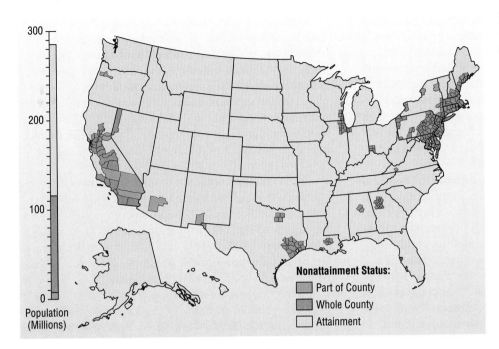

Figure 17-2 Counties classified by EPA as in "nonattainment" of ozone standards in the year 2003.

allergens, should stay indoors. An "orange" alert indicates that everyone should limit their outdoor activities to the minimum possible.

You can also help to lower air pollution levels by limiting contributions from your own automobile, lawn mower exhaust, and charcoal grill. You can car pool, use mass transit, or telecommute (work at home via a computer network) to reduce air pollution associated with automobile exhaust. You can fill your car gas tank, mow your lawn, and use your grill during the cooler evening hours to reduce your contribution to tropospheric ozone. You can conserve electricity to reduce emissions from electric power plants. In areas of the United States where air pollution is especially problematic, local laws may require that you do some of these things on days when conditions result in a "pollution emergency."

Water Pollution

Humankind has had a very schizophrenic relationship with our rivers and lakes. Water is an essential resource for all living things on our planet, including humans and the plants and animals we use for food. We also value our rivers and lakes for their recreational opportunities and aesthetic benefits. Yet we used these water bodies as convenient dumps for sewage and industrial wastes.

The problem of water pollution came to national attention in 1968 when children playing with matches set on fire chemical pollutants that covered the Cuyahoga River in Ohio. The subsequent public outcry resulted in the Clean Water Act of 1972 and the Safe Drinking Water Act of 1974. Since then, substantial progress has been made in reducing water pollution and ensuring safe drinking water supplies.

The job of cleaning rivers and lakes in the U.S. is not complete, and people who come in close contact with contaminated waters or fish from these areas are still at risk for a variety of health problems. Water pollution comes from both point sources (sewer overflows, livestock feedlots, industrial areas, and mines) and from nonpoint sources such as runoff from urban streets and agricultural areas that carries chemicals and animal waste into rivers. Toxic air pollutants can be deposited into water bodies in rainfall. Some of the most troublesome water pollutants in the U.S. today are described below.

Biological water pollutants from untreated sewage and drainage from leaking home septic systems include various species of disease-causing viruses, bacteria, and protozoa. These organisms cause diseases that are at best uncomfortable (diarrhea) and at worst lethal (dysentery, hepatitis, typhoid fever, and cholera). In the late 1800s, diseases associated with contaminated drinking water were the third leading cause of death in the United States.[24]

The largest sources of biological water pollutants in surface waters of the U.S. today are overflows from old combined septic and storm sewers during heavy rainfall events, and animal wastes that are carried by runoff of rainfall from agricultural areas. While much has already been done to eliminate biological pollution, billions of dollars are still required to finish this task.

> **Key Terms**
>
> **biological water pollutants** disease-causing organisms that are found in water.

At present, your personal risk of exposure to biological water pollution in the United States is relatively small. Public health departments monitor local surface waters for the presence of **fecal coliform bacteria** in every county in the U.S. These bacteria are an indicator that water has been contaminated by sewage. All municipal drinking water systems, and many private households, in the U.S. treat their water to kill pathogenic organisms. By the end of the 20th century, deaths due to water pathogens in the drinking water supply were very rare in the U.S.[24]

A wide variety of other **toxic pollutants** can be found in surface and groundwater sources of drinking water. These substances include naturally occurring toxic elements (such as arsenic and mercury) produced by breakdown of minerals. Human activities produce a wide range of toxic chemicals, including metals, solvents, plastics, and PCBs (polychlorinated biphenols). Arsenic and mercury have both natural and human-caused sources. Runoff of *agricultural pesticides* carries toxic substances into rivers where large areas of land are used for crop production.

The dumping of toxic substances into surface waters is now illegal, but some of these toxins are very stable and can be found in large quantities in the sediments of rivers and lakes that were polluted before 1972. Cleaning up these toxic sediments can be very costly. A recent decision to dredge and dispose of PCB-contaminated sediments in the Hudson River near Albany, New York, will cost hundreds of millions of dollars.

Health effects of agricultural chemicals and other toxic substances depend on the specific chemical.[24] Taken as a group, these substances have been linked to adverse effects on the blood, liver, spleen, kidney, adrenal gland, thyroid gland, reproductive system (fertility), and cardiovascular system. Some are known or suspected human *carcinogens* (substances that cause cancer), *mutagens* (substances that cause cell mutations), or *teratogens* (substances that cause birth defects). The risks for these health effects are greatest for workers who come in direct contact with the concentrated chemicals. More insidious are health effects such as cancer and birth defects that develop imperceptibly, after long-term exposure to low concentrations of these chemicals in the environment.

The U.S. Environmental Protection Agency has set **maximum contaminant level (MCL)** standards for the amounts of the biological pollutants, pesticides, and toxic chemicals that are allowed in municipal drinking water supplies.[24] MCLs are set at levels that minimize human health risks, but also take into account the limits of available treatment technology and the costs of meeting the standards. Municipal water suppliers are required to report any violations of MCLs to state and federal environmental agencies.

The best way for you to minimize physical health risks posed by consuming biological or toxic contaminants is to be informed. Municipal water suppliers must report the amounts of biological contaminants, agricultural pesticides, and toxic substances that are detected in their water. You can access your supplier's annual report at **http://www.epa.gov/safewater/dwinfo.htm.** These reports list the mean and range (minimum and maximum) concentrations for all regulated contaminants for all samples analyzed in a year. Look at the maximum value to determine if your water system occasionally fails to meet health standards. If your water supplier fails to meet health standards, consider drinking bottled, boiled, or filtered water until the supplier fixes the problems.

You can also be exposed to toxic substances by eating contaminated fish or wild game. Some toxic substances, such as mercury and PCBs, accumulate to high levels in the bodies of shellfish, fish, and waterfowl that consume contaminated water. This problem can occur even in remote, apparently pristine areas. People who regularly consume wild food animals are at highest risk.

To reduce health risks associated with consuming wild game, you should be aware of health advisories for consuming contaminated fish or game, usually issued by the public health or fish and game state agencies. These advisories are often stated as limits on how much fish or meat should be consumed in a specified time period. Pregnant women should be especially careful of consuming shellfish, fish, or wild game; mercury and PCBs cause birth defects.

You can also be exposed to waterborne pollutants, with associated health risks, as a result of recreational activities. You should be aware of "Don't swim" warnings for your local rivers and lakes, usually issued by the public health department. When backpacking, always filter, boil, or chemically treat drinking water to kill pathogens, even in apparently pristine wilderness areas.

Land Pollution

We do not consume land or soil into our bodies the way we do air and water, but pollution of land can still result in serious adverse health effects. Disposal of toxic wastes often involves burying them in the ground. When done with proper safeguards, this disposal method can be safe. If

---

Key Terms

fecal coliform bacteria a category of bacteria that live within the intestines of warm-blooded animals; the presence of these bacteria is used as an indicator that water has been contaminated by feces.

toxic pollutants substances known to, or suspected of, causing cancer or other serious health problems.

maximum contaminant level the highest concentration of a contaminant that is allowed in drinking water, as established and regulated by the U.S. Environmental Protection Agency.

done improperly, toxic pollutants leach into groundwater or are carried by runoff into surface waters, resulting in significant human health risks.

Most land pollution today is associated with the disposal of **solid waste.** *Municipal solid waste* consists of everyday items such as product packaging, grass clippings, furniture, clothing, bottles, food scraps, newspapers, appliances, paint, and batteries. Other solid waste produced by business and industry includes waste tires, concrete, asphalt, bricks, lumber, and shingles from demolished buildings, and *sewage sludge* (solids remaining after wastewater treatment). In 1999 the U.S. population produced 230 million tons of solid waste, or about 4.6 pounds of waste per person per day (or 1,680 pounds per person per year).[25]

Municipal sanitation departments and private disposal companies are very efficient at removing these wastes from our homes and businesses and putting them someplace where we don't see them. These waste disposal locations include sanitary landfills (wastes are compacted and buried under soil), ocean dumping in garbage barges (with trash sometimes escaping to wash up on beaches), and incinerators (where solid wastes are burned).

While out-of-sight often means out-of-mind, these solid wastes do not "go away," but rather, they accumulate. Many municipal and regional sanitary landfills are reaching their capacity and must be closed. As we run out of places to dump our solid waste, some have proposed that we burn it in large incinerators. However, incinerators release toxic substances into the air and their ash contains concentrated toxic chemicals.

Most of the potential health effects of land pollution have already been described in this chapter under the topics of air and water pollution. Most human exposure to pollutants that are deposited on land occurs when those toxic substances end up in the air or water. You can limit your risk of these health effects by being aware of where solid wastes are disposed, both at the present time and in the past. You should be particularly aware of proximity to a local landfill or waste disposal site if your water source is a private well that draws from groundwater that might be contaminated. In this situation, you should regularly monitor your water for pollutants.

You can reduce your personal contribution to the solid waste problem of your community by following the Three R's: Reduce, Reuse, Recycle. You can consume less and accept less packaging on the products you buy. You can compost yard waste or use a lawn mower with a mulching blade to eliminate grass clippings and leaves. Reusing bottles, zipper-closure storage bags, cloth shopping bags, and cloth diapers reduces solid waste. Newspapers, magazines, aluminum and steel cans, glass bottles, and many plastic containers can be recycled and the materials used to make new products. However, recycling will only work if you also buy products that are made from recycled materials, such as recycled paper and plastic "wood" products.

Loss of Green Space

Loss of **green space** represents another kind of land pollution that can affect your quality of life and health. In many parts of the United States, green space is being converted to housing developments, shopping malls, industrial sites, and highways. Wildlife species disappear from your community and surroundings as their habitats are destroyed.

While development of green space for human uses may provide job opportunities and be beneficial for your occupational health, it can also detract from recreational and aesthetic aspects of your community. If you find that you must travel farther and longer from home or work to find a safe and enjoyable location to jog or bicycle, you may exercise less often. Your sense of "quality of life" is diminished when you no longer see wild animals in your backyard or you feel that your community is becoming ugly.

Some communities have created land-use (zoning) plans that allow for economic development while protecting recreational and aesthetic values in their communities. These zoning plans can be controversial, as they try to balance the rights of private property owners with the welfare of the entire community. You can contribute toward protecting environmental quality in your community by supporting land-use planning and enforceable zone laws that protect green space while allowing for responsible economic development.

Radiation

Radiation is a general term that refers to various forms of energy that are emitted by atoms and molecules when they undergo change, including radio waves, infrared, visible light, ultraviolet, X-rays, and gamma rays. Each kind of radiation has different effects on biological materials and health. **Ionizing radiation** causes damage to biological structures such as DNA that can result in serious adverse health effects. Ionizing radiation is produced

---

Key Terms

solid waste pollutants that are in solid form, including nonhazardous household trash, industrial wastes, mining wastes, and sewage sludge from wastewater treatment plants.

green space areas of land that are dominated by domesticated or natural vegetation, including rural farmland, city lawns and parks, and nature preserves.

ionizing radiation electromagnetic radiation that is capable of breaking chemical bonds, such as X-rays and gamma rays.

The High-Tech Revolution and E-Waste

The much heralded high-tech revolution has a hidden dark side, mountains of accumulating obsolete electronic equipment that contain large amounts of toxic substances. During the period from 1997 to 2007, it is estimated that over 500 million computers must be disposed of. These computers will contain 6.2 billion pounds of plastic, 1.6 billion pounds of lead, 3 million pounds of cadmium, 1.9 million pounds of chromium, and 632,000 pounds of mercury. Lead, cadmium, chromium, and mercury are highly toxic metals, and can cause a wide range of severe health effects if they end up in the air, drinking water, or food supply.[1,2]

Computers contain over 1,000 different substances, many of which are toxic. This makes recycling a complex, labor-intensive process that can cost more than the value of the recycled materials. Only 6% of obsolete computers disposed of after 1998 were recycled. The remainder was deposited in landfills across the country. It is estimated that 70% of heavy metals such as lead and mercury going into U.S. landfills today comes from electronic waste. Several states, including California and Massachusetts, have banned disposal of computer monitors in landfills to protect groundwater.[1] While recycling of computers is seen as the ideal solution to the problem of waste disposal, it is estimated

that 50% to 80% of computers "recycled" before the year 2002 were actually shipped to poor Asian countries. Workers in these countries disassemble computers to recover useful materials for very low wages and with minimal or no protection from the toxic materials to which they are exposed. These countries have weak or poorly enforced environmental regulations, so materials that cannot be recycled are dumped into rivers or burned in open air pits. These practices expose the recycling workers and surrounding local populations to toxic substances.[1]

The practice of shipping toxic computer waste to underdeveloped countries is now banned by an international treaty, but the United States is the only developed nation that has not ratified this treaty. The "free market" justification for the practice of shipping toxic computer waste to underdeveloped countries is that this provides jobs and helps poor people. The question is whether or not it is moral to give poor people the choice between poverty or poisons?[1]

Given that the use of computers and electronics will only increase in the future, many argue that we must develop environmentally responsible computer recycling systems. Recently proposed legislation would require the Environmental Protection Agency to help set

up computer recycling across the United States. The program would be funded by a fee of up to $10 on all retail sales of desktop and laptop PCs and computer monitors. Similar legislation is also appearing in many state legislatures. The electronics industry favors charging consumers the fee when they return their old computers to the manufacturer rather than on new computers. Some computer manufacturers are already initiating computer take-back programs. However, development of a comprehensive national strategy for responsibly addressing the computer waste problem continues as of this writing.

The other, and perhaps most important, approach to the computer waste problem is to develop electronic equipment that is less toxic and more easily recycled. This will require development of, and investment in, new technologies. In our free market system, this will happen only when the electronics manufacturers must share the cost of dealing with computer waste.

[1]Puckett J, et al: Exporting Harm: The High-Tech Trashing of Asia. The Basal Action Network and Silicon Valley Toxics Coalition, 2002.
[2]U.S. Environmental Protection Agency: WasteWise Update: Electronics Reuse and Recycling. 2003. **http://www.epa.gov/wastewise/pubs/ wwupda14.pdf**

---

by nuclear reactions, and sources include medical X-rays, naturally occurring radioactive minerals such as uranium, various radioactive materials used by industry, nuclear reactors and their waste products, and nuclear bomb explosions. **Non-ionizing radiation** most commonly causes adverse health effects simply by heating tissues, resulting in burns. These effects are generally less severe than the effects from ionizing radiation. Sources of non-ionizing radiation include sunlight and electromagnetic fields generated by all electrical and electronic devices. (See Focus On article at the end of the chapter for more on non-ionizing radiation.)

The health effects of exposure to X-rays and gamma radiation depend on many factors, including the duration, type, and dose of radiation, and your individual sensitivity. Heavy exposure to these forms of radiation can occur if you are near a nuclear bomb blast or downwind of a major nuclear reactor accident. In such cases,

exposure can cause *radiation sickness,* including intense fatigue, nausea, weight loss, hair loss, fever, bleeding from the mouth, and compromised immune system, usually resulting in death. Exposure to ionizing radiation can also increase the occurrence of birth defects and cancer.

While your risk of exposure to ionizing radiation is very low, issues related to nuclear power plants and radioactive wastes are often very controversial. Nuclear

Key Terms

non-ionizing radiation electromagnetic radiation that cannot break chemical bonds, but may excite electrons (ultraviolet radiation) or heat biological materials (infrared, radio frequency, and microwave radiation).

reactors generate 20% of the electricity used in the United States. However, many people resist attempts to build new reactors in their community, and do not want radioactive wastes stored in, or transported across, their region. For decades, nuclear reactors in the U.S. have been accumulating highly radioactive wastes on-site in shallow, water-filled temporary holding tanks. During this time, the U.S. government has been working to develop appropriate technologies and find sites to store these wastes permanently. The most likely location is in underground salt caves below Yucca Mountain, Nevada. A major health concern raised about this nuclear waste disposal program is the need to transport large quantities of highly radioactive waste by truck or train across the highways and rails of the U.S. Many people do not want these wastes to be transported through their community, but the current situation is not safe either. This problem will only get worse as older nuclear power plants are retired, and hundreds of tons of radioactive concrete and steel must be disposed of.

 TALKING POINTS How can you approach your political representatives about environmental policy? What are some effective ways of keeping health-related environmental issues on the national agenda?

The Global Environment

The global environment is comprised of the atmosphere, oceans, continental land masses, and all the living organisms that exist on Earth. Interactions among these components of the global environment influence the characteristics of solar radiation at the ground level, climate (temperature, precipitation, seasonal variation), production of food plants and animals, availability of freshwater, energy requirements for heating and cooling of human habitations, the geographic distribution of diseases, the composition of natural communities (deserts, tundra, rain forest), and the survival and extinction of species.

Some of the characteristics of the global environment have obvious and direct effects on human physical health, such as the presence of disease-causing organisms or solar UV radiation that can increase the risk of skin cancer. Other effects of the global environment on personal health are less well documented, such as the adverse effects on emotional or spiritual health associated with the extinction of species or destruction of beautiful natural communities. Many scientists warn that the global environment is being degraded by the combined forces of ever more powerful technology being used by a rapidly increasing global human popula-

tion. In this section we briefly describe major concerns regarding the global environment and how these might affect personal health.

 TALKING POINTS Your sister is a sun worshipper who loves the look of a deep, dark tan. How might you persuade her to protect her skin from the rays of the sun?

Human Population Explosion

Many scientists warn that the human population is increasing at a rate that cannot be sustained by the resources of the Earth. There are currently over 6 billion people in the global human population, and this is projected to increase to over 10 billion in the next 50 years. Every year the world's population grows by about 78 million people, with 97% born into the poorest countries.[26] Consider the vast problems we face with the current population, including depletion of natural resources (freshwater, food, and oil), air and water pollution, conflict and political upheaval, starvation, and destruction of natural communities. Now imagine trying to solve these problems in the 21st century with twice as many people trying to make a living and raise a family on the same Earth.

The effects of the human population explosion on personal health depend on who you are and where you live. Many of the poorer nations of Asia, Africa, and South America will not be able to feed their people; starvation and associated diseases will be major health problems for these populations. Growing populations in dry regions are exceeding their freshwater supply, and hundreds of millions of people must drink from contaminated water sources. Every year, 5 million children die from waterborne diarrhea diseases associated with unsanitary drinking water.[26] By 2025, 2.5 billion people may live in regions where available freshwater is insufficient to meet their needs.

In many extremely poor countries, hungry people will destroy most or all of the remaining natural communities (tropical rain forests, African savanna) in vain efforts to grow food on lands that are not suited for agriculture. Six hundred thousand square miles of forest were cut down worldwide in the 1990s. How much will remain in a world with 10 billion people? Overcultivation of farmlands has already degraded the fertility of a land area equivalent to that of the United States and Canada combined.[26] Hungry people on oceanic islands destroy their coral reefs by using dynamite or cyanide to catch fish. In Africa hungry people hunt wild game for food, putting more species at risk of extinction.

Competition among nations for limited supplies of water and oil is often a root cause of political tensions, terrorism, and war. Political upheaval in the Middle East, recent terrorist attacks on U.S. targets, and the war in Iraq can be partially explained by competition for scarce resources (water, land, and oil). The genocide that killed hundreds of thousands in Rwanda in 1994–95 has been traced to inequitable distribution of land and associated hunger in some parts of that country.[27]

The solutions to the human population growth problem are simple in theory, but often complex in their implementation. Basic population ecology theory states that the rate of population growth can be reduced if: (1) women have fewer children over their lifetime, and (2) if they delay the start of their reproduction. A somewhat counterintuitive pattern is that population growth rate slows when infant survival rate is increased by better health care. Women choose to have fewer children if they are confident that the children they do have will survive.[26]

Simply providing education opportunities to girls can have major and long-lasting effects that act to reduce population growth. Girls who become educated delay having their first child; educated women have half the pregnancies of their uneducated sisters.[26] Educated women are more likely to be able to find employment outside the home. Working women usually have fewer children, and women with an independent income have a greater say about how many children they will have. Access to birth control information and affordable contraception is also needed to allow women to control their family size.

Unfortunately, these proactive initiatives are often held hostage to political and cultural controversies. The sad result is that human populations may ultimately be controlled by increased death rates associated with starvation, disease, and war, rather than reduced birth rates.

Global Climate Change

A wide range of human activities add **greenhouse gases** to the atmosphere that trap heat and cause a net gain of energy and increase in temperature in the Earth system. This increase in global temperature is called the "Greenhouse Effect" or "Global Warming." Human-caused sources of greenhouse gases include both industrial and agricultural activities, including the burning of fuels, conversion of natural communities to human uses, and methane emissions from livestock herds, flooded rice fields, and leaking gas pipelines.[28]

There is growing evidence that increases in atmospheric greenhouse gases are associated with changes in global climate. Chemical analyses of gas bubbles in glacial ice core samples from the polar ice caps indicate that over the past 420,000 years when carbon dioxide and methane concentrations increased, so did atmospheric temperature.[29] Coincident with the current increase in atmospheric concentrations of greenhouse gases, average global surface temperature was higher during the decade of the 1990s than at any other time in recorded history.[28] However, there is still controversy regarding the relative contributions of humans versus natural processes, and whether or not this warming trend is a short-term phenomenon or the beginning of a long-term trend.

Potential effects of climate change on human health include increased heat stress, loss of life in increasingly frequent severe storms and floods, expansion of the range of disease-carrying insects from subtropical regions into temperate regions (such as the United States), increased abundance of waterborne pathogens, decreased air and water quality, and decreased food availability associated with severe weather and water shortages.[28]

Ecological effects of global warming include increased frequency of wildfires and insect pest outbreaks that destroy forests, and widespread death of coral reefs associated with higher water temperature. Many scientists project large-scale decline and extinction of species that cannot adapt to changes in climate and cannot migrate to more suitable areas because of barriers associated with human roads, cities, and farms.[28] These ecological changes could adversely impact emotional and spiritual health as cherished natural wonders are degraded or disappear entirely under the onslaught of climate changes.

The primary means proposed for reducing and reversing global warming associated with human activities is to reduce the burning of fossil fuels such as oil and coal and increase the proportion of our energy needs that are met by other technologies. Many suggest that a combination of energy conservation, increased efficiency of automobiles and electrical appliances, and a gradual shift to alternate power sources for cars (fuel cells and/or hydrogen) and electricity (photovoltaic cells, wind turbines, geothermal energy, nuclear power) can get this job done. These transitions will require major shifts in national and global economies, continuing innovation and technology development, and many small changes in everyday life of humans on planet Earth.

Your ability as an individual to take personal responsibility for addressing the global warming problem is

Key Terms

greenhouse gases a category of gases in the atmosphere that allow solar radiation to pass through the atmosphere to the Earth, but then trap the heat that is radiated from the Earth back toward space; greenhouse gases include water vapor, carbon dioxide, methane, nitrous oxide, and tropospheric ozone.

limited, but all good things must start with individuals willing to do the right thing. You can reduce your personal contribution to global warming by conserving electricity at home, driving the most fuel-efficient automobile that meets your needs, using mass transit where available, recycling/reusing, and purchasing appliances that are rated as highly efficient. Government action will be required to support widespread conservation practices in industry and business. You could join and be active in environmental organizations that work to address global warming. When politicians see their constituents want to protect our common global environment, they may find the political will to do the right thing.

Stratospheric Ozone Depletion

The *stratospheric ozone layer* is a concentration of ozone molecules located about 10 to 25 miles above the Earth's surface. Stratospheric ozone is a naturally occurring gas formed by the interaction of atmospheric oxygen and components of solar radiation. The stratospheric ozone layer protects living organisms on the Earth's surface from harmful solar ultraviolet (UV) radiation. For people, overexposure to UV rays can lead to skin cancer, cataracts (clouding of the lens of the eye), and weakened immune systems. Increased UV can also lead to reduced crop yield and disruptions in the ocean's food chain.

It has been well-documented that chemical reactions between stratospheric ozone and certain human-made air pollutants can significantly reduce the ozone layer, causing increased UV radiation at the Earth's surface. The chemicals that cause ozone depletion include chlorofluorocarbons or CFCs (used as coolants in many air conditioning and refrigeration systems, in insulating foams, and as solvents), halons (used in fire suppression systems), and methyl bromide (used in pesticides).[30]

The vast majority of this depletion of the ozone layer occurs in the atmosphere above the north and south polar regions, with up to a 60% loss over Antarctica. These decreases in the stratospheric ozone layer have been associated with as much as a 50% increase in UV radiation at the ground level in Antarctica.[33] The ozone layer has decreased by 5% to 10% above the United States.[30]

In response to the well-documented links between certain air pollutants and depletion of the ozone layer, an international ban on the production of halons and CFCs went into effect in the mid-1990s. As the amounts of ozone-depleting chemicals in the atmosphere decrease, the ozone layer is expected to recover to natural levels by the year 2050.[30]

To limit your risk of skin cancer and other UV-related health problems, you should limit your exposure to direct sunlight, and when you are outside you should

When you buy sunglasses, look for the UV-Protection rating.

wear sunscreen on exposed skin. You should also wear sunglasses that are rated as eliminating over 95% of UV radiation.

Loss of Natural Habitats and Species Extinctions

On every continent, an exploding human population armed with ever more powerful technology is altering or completely taking over the habitats of other species that share our planet. Sixteen to 23% of the total land surface of Earth has been converted entirely for human uses, including row crop fields, grazing lands, and urban/industrial areas. As much as 40% to 50% of the land surface has been transformed or degraded by human activities.[31]

The Earth has lost almost half (7.5 billion acres) of its original forest cover to human exploitation. Every year, another 40 million acres is cleared for farming or logged for timber. Only 20% of the original forest cover on Earth remains ecologically intact and able to support its full complement of species, mostly in the northern parts of Canada and Siberia. In the lower 48 states of the United States, only 1% of the original pristine forest present at the time of European settlement remains today, located in three scattered parks/wilderness areas.[32]

As much as 30% of the African continent is at risk for **desertification,** mainly due to overgrazing by livestock,

---

Key Terms

desertification a process that converts lands that historically supported grasslands, shrublands, or dry forest to nonproductive desert.

excessive brush and tree cutting for fuel, and inappropriate agricultural practices.[33] This problem is most severe when expanding populations of poor people try to feed themselves using nonsustainable food production methods on dry lands.

The worldwide human population currently uses 50% of the Earth's freshwater runoff, 70% of which is used for agricultural irrigation. In some major river drainages, water diversion is so great that no water reaches the ocean (e.g., the Colorado River in the southwest U.S.).[32]

Human impact on the biosphere is not limited to the land. Sixty percent of the human population lives within 100 km of an ocean coast, and humans consume 25% to 35% of the energy flow in coastal ocean waters. As of 1995, 22% of all ocean fisheries for human consumption were overexploited (resulting in population crashes of the targeted fish species), and another 44% were being exploited at their maximum sustainable level.[31] Overharvesting has put most of the world's whale species at risk of extinction.

Many coastal wetlands, mangrove forests, and coral reefs are destroyed or degraded by human activities. As much as 50% of worldwide mangrove forests have been transformed or destroyed.[31] In Indonesia, with the largest coral reef system in the world, 70% of the reefs have been severely degraded by dynamite fishing. Worldwide, 30% of all coral reefs have been destroyed by human activities, pollution, and coral bleaching that may be associated with global warming. Coastal water pollution has been linked to increased frequency of harmful algae blooms that cause extensive fish kills, and increased risk of shellfish poisoning for humans who eat seafood.[31]

The cumulative effects of all these human-caused changes to the Earth's land and oceans have increased the species extinction rate by 100 to 1,000 times over rates estimated for the period before human domination.[32]

The effects on personal health associated with worldwide loss of natural communities and species extinctions are highly variable from person to person. Pharmaceutical companies have found many substances produced by species in various natural communities to be useful sources of drugs to treat human illnesses. As the richness of species on Earth is depleted by extinction, we lose a wealth of genetic material that could be of great importance to human health. The loss of natural ecosystems also undermines the systems that function to make Earth a livable planet, contributing to such problems as global climate change, freshwater shortages, and increased frequency of destructive flooding.

Some have proposed that human evolution predisposes us to desire green spaces and diverse biological systems; this is called the *Biophilia hypothesis*.[34] That is, we are most happy when we are surrounded by natural beauty. Many have written about the human psychological benefits from natural communities. John Muir, a famous early environmentalist in the United States, wrote:

> Climb the mountains and get their good tidings. Nature's peace will flow into you as sunshine flows into trees. The winds will blow their own freshness into you, and the storms their energy, while cares drop off like autumn leaves.

Wallace Stegner wrote a passage that appears in the Wilderness Act passed by the U.S. Congress in 1964 to protect areas of intact ecosystems in the United States for the enjoyment of future generations:

> It was a lovely and terrible wilderness, such a wilderness as Christ and the prophets went out into; harshly and beautifully colored, broken and worn until its bones are exposed, its great sky without a smudge or a taint from Technocracy, and in hidden corners and pockets under its cliffs, the sudden poetry of springs. Save a piece of country like that intact, and it does not matter in the slightest that only a few people every year will go into it. That is precisely its value . . . We simply need that wild country available to us, even if we never do more than drive to its edge and look in. For it can be a means of reassuring ourselves of our sanity as creatures, a part of the geography of hope.

Both Muir and Stegner refer to the psychological benefits that humans derive simply from the knowledge

Recycling glass, paper, and metal can reduce land pollution and consumption of natural resources.

that natural communities and wildlife species still exist, as they always have, somewhere on our planet. For many, the loss of Earth's natural heritage would have profound adverse consequences for their emotional, psychological, and spiritual well-being. The thought of forever losing wilderness, coral reefs, rain forests, whales, pandas, tigers, and eagles can cause anger, frustration, depression, hopelessness, and despair.[35]

How can you or any one person exert any degree of personal control over such a great and complex threat to your physical, emotional, and spiritual health? Let's start with the little things: conserve energy, recycle and reuse what you can, limit your consumption of the world's resources to what you need, and join together with others of like mind to provide political and financial support to organizations that are working to solve these big problems (see the listing in the Star box below).

Another way you can reduce the negative environmental effects of your personal consumption of natural resources is to "buy green" when you can. In recent years,

Organizations Working to Address Environmental and Population Concerns

Population Issues

United Nations Family Planning Organization: **http://www.unfpa.org**

International Planned Parenthood Federation: **http://www.ippf.org**

The Population Institute: **http://www.populationinstitute.org**

Environmental Political Advocacy Groups

Sierra Club: **http://www.sierraclub.org**

Wilderness Society: **http://www.wilderness.org**

National Wildlife Federation: **http://www.nwf.org**

Natural Resources Defense Council: **http://www.nrdc.org**

Environmental Defense Fund: **http://www.environmentaldefense.org**

The League of Conservation Voters: **http://www.lcv.org**

Conservation of Natural Communities and Endangered Species

The Nature Conservancy: **http://nature.org**

World Wildlife Fund: **http://www.panda.org**

Source of Environmental Information

World Resources Institute: **http://www.worldwatch.org**

U.S. Environmental Protection Agency: **http://www.epa.gov**

environmental organizations have begun certification programs so that the consumer can identify which products are produced by "Earth-friendly" means (for more information, go to the website **http://www.newdream. org/buygreen/**). Examples of such products include sustainably harvested timber, shade-grown coffee, and organic food and cotton. Many "buy green" organizations also work to improve the economic conditions of small rural villages where the producers of their products live. These efforts at economic development are often associated with improved education opportunities that lead to reduced birth rates, slowing global human population growth that is the root cause for many environmental problems. For ideas on how to make environmentally sound choices in your life, see the Changing for the Better Box on page 503.

Taking Charge of Your Health

- Protect yourself from ultraviolet light. Always wear sunscreen, and make sure your sunglasses filter out UV rays.
- Have your home tested for radon, and install a radon reduction system if necessary.
- Install a water filtration device to remove contaminants from your drinking water.
- Keep your car in proper running condition to reduce the amount of noise and air pollution it produces.

- Reduce your personal impact on the environment by reducing your consumption of energy and recycling and reusing what you can, and using Earth-friendly products in your home.
- Take personal action on environmental issues using the suggestions outlined in the Changing for the Better box on page 503.

Summary

- Your environment contains a wide range of substances, living organisms, and forms of energy that may substantially impact one or more dimensions of your personal health.
- Environmental influences on personal health operate over a wide range of spatial scales, from the personal spaces of your home and workplace, to the common spaces of your community and region, to the global environment that supports all life on Earth.
- The most direct environmental health risks to your physical health are related to the presence of toxic substances or pathogenic organisms (pollutants) in the air and water of your personal and community environments.
- You can exert the greatest degree of control over your exposure to pollutants within the personal environment of your home and workplace. You can identify environmental health risks in your personal environment, and then eliminate or reduce these risks by changing your buying habits and eliminating pollutant sources.
- Air pollution in major urban areas can cause significant adverse health effects, especially for people who suffer from respiratory or cardiac disease.
- While you have no control over community air pollution, you can limit your exposure to these toxic substances by being aware of daily pollution levels and by restricting your outdoor activities when these levels are high.

- Much progress has been made in reducing community water pollution, but water in many rivers and lakes still contains chemicals and pathogens that can adversely affect your health.
- You should seek out information about any health advisories for wild foods you obtain from local rivers, and advisories regarding recreational use of those rivers.
- The U.S. Environmental Protection Agency monitors and regulates the quality of drinking water from municipal water suppliers, but it is up to you to ensure the safety of your drinking water if it comes from a private well.
- Improper disposal of toxic solid wastes in landfills designed for household waste is a major source of regional surface and groundwater pollution.
- You should never dispose of toxic household products (batteries, automotive fluids, pesticides, oil-based paint products) by simply putting them in the household trash or pouring them down a drain. Take them to specially designated toxic disposal locations.
- Loss of green space in your community and regional environment, associated with urban sprawl and unregulated land development can diminish your perceived quality of life, and reduce opportunities for exercise, which is important for maintaining good physical health.
- While you have limited personal control over the environment of your community and region, you can

still work to enhance your environment by joining others of like mind in groups that advocate environmental protection through the democratic political process.

- A rapidly expanding global human population, armed with increasingly more powerful technologies, is now degrading the global environment that sustains all life on Earth.
- At the current rate of human population growth, most scientists of the world warn of increased starvation and disease, decreased standards of living, and increased conflict over progressively decreasing supplies of natural resources.
- Human population growth can be substantially slowed by simply providing girls and women opportunities to become educated and gainfully employed, and access to contraception.
- Pollutants produced by humans are responsible for changes in the atmosphere that are altering climate patterns and allowing harmful solar radiation to reach the surface of the Earth.
- Changes in the global environment have potential to increase risks to human health, and to significantly harm many other species and natural communities.
- While individuals can do little to address global environmental problems, the solutions all start with individual choices about family size, resource consumption, and political candidates. The best path to a livable future for humankind is to do your part and have faith that others will do theirs.

Review Questions

1. What is radon, and what are the health risks associated with it? What actions can you take to minimize the health risks of radon?
2. Identify the sources and the potential health effects of the following common indoor air pollutants: carbon monoxide, volatile organic compounds, and biological pollutants such as mold, mildew, pollen, and pet dander. Describe actions you could take to minimize health risks from these pollutants.
3. What health risks are associated with lead and asbestos? What actions can you take to minimize these risks?
4. Describe actions you should take to safeguard drinking from a well on your own property.
5. What are the physical and emotional health effects of noise? What actions could you take to minimize the health risks of noise?
6. Tropospheric ozone and small particulate matter are community and regional air pollutants that have been linked to serious health risks. For each of these substances, describe the main human source(s), the effect(s) on human physical health, and what actions you could take to minimize your own risk of adverse health effects from these air pollutants.
7. What are "air toxics" and where do you think you are most likely to be exposed to these substances? What do you think you could do to minimize your personal health risk from air toxics?
8. What is "biological water pollution" and what is the main source of this pollution in your community's rivers, streams, and/or lakes? What are the health risks associated with biological water pollution? What can you do to minimize the risk to your personal health from this type of pollution?
9. Who is responsible for ensuring the safety of your drinking water if the source is a municipal water company? What can you do to minimize any health risks associated with your drinking water in this circumstance?
10. What is the main health risk associated with land pollution from solid waste landfills? What can you do to minimize your personal contribution to this type of pollution?
11. What is "green space," and why is it important to your personal health? What personal actions could you take to protect green space in your community or region?
12. What policies should the U.S. foreign aid agencies implement in poor underdeveloped countries to help them reduce their population growth rate? Explain how these policies would work toward this goal.
13. Global warming and stratospheric ozone depletion are large-scale changes in the global environment with uncertain, but potentially significant, health consequences. For each of these global changes, describe the cause(s) of environmental change, the potential health effects, and what might be done to minimize these effects.
14. Loss of natural habitats and species extinctions are major ecological problems, but do these phenomena represent any risk to *your* personal health? Your answer should reflect your own perceptions, and should provide some explanation for your assessment.
15. A well-known environmentalist slogan is, "Think globally, but act locally." Based on what you've learned in this chapter, describe how you think this slogan applies to your personal actions in response to environmental health risks.

References

1. U.S. Environmental Protection Agency. Healthy Buildings, Healthy People: A Vision for the 21st Century. 2003. **http://www.epa.gov/iaq/hbhp/index.html**

2. Consumer Product Safety Commission. Carbon Monoxide Questions and Answers. CPSC Document #466. 2003. **http://www.cpsc.gov/cpscpub/pubs/466.html**

3. U.S. Environmental Protection Agency. The Senseless Killer. 2003. **http://www.epa.gov/iaq/pubs/senseles.html**

4. U.S. Environmental Protection Agency. The Inside Story: A Guide to Indoor Air Quality. 1995. **http://www.epa.gov/iaq/pubs/insidest.html**

5. Thorn J, et al. Adult-Onset Asthma Linked to Mold and Tobacco Smoke Exposure. *Allergy* 56: 287–292, 2001.

6. U.S. Environmental Protection Agency. Sources of Indoor Air Pollution: Asbestos. 2003. **http://www.epa.gov/iaq/asbestos.html**

7. U.S. Environmental Protection Agency. Sources of Indoor Air Pollution: Biological Pollutants. 2003. **http://www.epa.gov/iaq/biologic.html**

8. National Safety Council. Radon. 2002. **http://www.nsc.org/ehc/radon.htm**

9. National Academy of Sciences. Biological Effects of Ionizing Radiation (BEIR) VI Report : "The Health Effects of Exposure to Indoor Radon." 1998. National Academy Press. **http://books.nap.edu/books/0309056454/html/**

10. National Academy of Science. Risk Assessment of Radon in Drinking Water. 1999. **http://www.nap.edu/books/0309062926/html/index.html**

11. U.S. Environmental Protection Agency. Sources of Indoor Air Pollution: Lead (Pb). 2003. **http://www.epa.gov/iaq/lead.html**

12. U.S. Department of Health and Human Services, Public Health Service, Agency for Toxic Substances and Disease Registry. Case Studies In Environmental Medicine: Lead Toxicity. 1995. **http://www.atsdr.cdc.gov/HEC/HSPH/caselead.html**

13. U.S. Environmental Protection Agency. Water on Tap: A Consumer's Guide to the Nation's Drinking Water. 2003. **http://www.epa.gov/safewater/wot/howsafe.html**

14. Townsend AR, et al. Human health effects of a changing global nitrogen cycle. *Frontiers in Ecology* 1: 240–246, 2003.

15. U.S. Environmental Protection Agency. Technical Factsheet on: Nitrate / Nitrite. 2002. **http://www.epa.gov/safewater/dwh/t-ioc/nitrates.html**

16. Gray LE, Ostby J. Effects of pesticides and toxic substances on behavioral and morphological reproductive development: endocrine versus no-endocrine mechanisms. *Toxicology and Industrial Health* 14: 159–184, 1998.

17. U.S. Environmental Protection Agency. Permeation and Leaching. 2003. **http://www.epa.gov/safewater/tcr/pdf/permleach.pdf**

18. Bell PA. Noise, pollution, and psychopathology. *In:* AMA Ghadirian and HE Lehmann (eds.): *Environment and Psychopathology.* Springer Publishing Co. New York, 1993.

19. U.S. Environmental Protection Agency. Draft Report on the Environment: Outdoor Air Quality. 2003. **http://www.epa.gov/indicators/roe/html/roeAirOut.htm**

20. Dockery DW and CA Pope III. Acute Respiratory Effects of Particulate Air Pollution. *Annual Review Public Health* 15, 107–132, 1994.

21. U.S. Environmental Protection Agency. Asthma Triggers—Related Topics—Ozone. 2003. **http://www.epa.gov/iaq/asthma/triggers/ozone.html**

22. McConnell R, et al. Asthma in exercising children exposed to ozone. *The Lancet* 359: 386–391, 2002.

23. U.S. Environmental Protection Agency. The National Air Toxics Assessment. 2002. **http://www.epa.gov/ttn/atw/nata**

24. U.S. Environmental Protection Agency. Drinking Water and Your Health, What You Need to Know, List of Drinking Water Contaminants & MCLs. 2003. **http://www.epa.gov/safewater/mcl.html#1**

25. U.S. Environmental Protection Agency. Municipal Solid Waste: Basic Facts. 2003. **http://www.epa.gov/epaoswer/non-hw/muncpl/facts.htm**

26. The Population Institute. **http://www.populationinstitute.org/**

27. Gasana J. Remember Rwanda? *World Watch* 15(5): 24–33, 2002.

28. Intergovernmental Panel on Climate Change. Climate Change 2001: Summary Report: Synthesis for Policy Makers. 2001. **http://www.ipcc.ch/pub/un/syreng/spm.pdf**

29. Petit JR, et al. Climate and atmospheric history of the past 420,000 years from the Vostok ice core, Antarctica. *Nature* 399: 429–436, 1999.

30. U.S. Environmental Protection Agency. The Science of Ozone Depletion. 2003. **http://www.epa.gov/docs/ozone/science/index.html**

31. Vitousek P, et al. Human domination of Earth's ecosystems. *Science* 277: 494–499, 1997.

32. World Resources Institute. 2003. **http://www.wri.org**

33. United Nations: Food and Agriculture Organization. **http://www.fao.org/desertification/default.asp?lang=en**

34. Wilson E. *Biophilia: The Human Bond with Other Species.* Harvard University Press, Cambridge, MA, 1984.

35. Gardner GT and Stern PC. *Environmental Problems and Human Behavior.* Allyn & Bacon, a Simon & Schuster Co. Needham Heights, MA, 1996.

As We Go to Press

Recent research reported in the journal *Environmental Science and Technology* reports that Americans are exposed to more cancer-causing air pollutants than is indicated by standard air quality assessments. Most air pollution data for the United States is collected at centrally located outdoor monitoring sites. However, most people spend over 90% of their time indoors. For this recent study, the investigators rigged 71 study subjects with lapel-mounted air filters that absorbed volatile organic compounds (VOCs). For 14 VOCs that are designated as "hazardous," the personal lapel-mounted sensors contained concentrations that were 3 to 60 times higher than samples taken at outdoor air quality monitors. Several of these VOCs are documented carcinogens. Environmental concentrations of many hazardous VOCs have decreased in recent years due to regulations developed under the Clean Air Act. Nonetheless, the results of this study indicated that even nonsmokers' personal exposure to airborne carcinogens is surprisingly high.

Fortunately, it is fairly easy to reduce your personal exposure to these hazardous substances. You should avoid cigarette smoke and air fresheners. You should hang recently dry-cleaned clothing in a well-ventilated area for a few hours. You should use cleaning agents and other household chemicals that contain VOCs only in well-ventilated spaces.

focus on

radiation from cell phones and electrical devices: environmental health hazard or not?

In 1992 a lawsuit filed in a Florida court alleged that radio frequency radiation (RFR) from cell phones caused the brain cancer and subsequent death of a woman. The concern and controversy about potential health effects of exposure to RFR has lasted long after this lawsuit was dismissed for lack of evidence. The potential problem with many cell phones is that the radio transmitter is placed next to the head, and millions of people are exposed to this radiation every day.

Scientific evidence for adverse health effects caused by RFR is limited. Some studies that exposed lab rats to constant, high levels of radio frequency radiation claim to have documented damage to DNA in brain cells that might later cause cancer. However, the amount of RFR to which these rats were exposed far exceeded the amount that a person would receive from normal use of a cell phone. Also, other animal studies found no cancer-related effects of exposure to RFR. Several large-scale epidemiological studies in a number of countries have compared the occurrence of various cancers of the brain and head between people who do and do not use cell phones. None of these studies found a link between exposure to cell phone RFR and cancer.

At the time of this writing, there is no scientifically credible evidence that using a cell phone poses a health risk beyond distracting you while driving.[1,2] However, cell phones have been in widespread use for only a relatively short period of time. There is no way to determine if long-term exposure to low levels of RFR

from a cell phone placed close to the head has cumulative effects that might pose a health risk.

If you are concerned about potential long-term health effects of RFR, and must use a cell phone for long periods of time, you might use a head set so that the transmitter in the phone can be placed away from your body. The intensity of RFR decreased rapidly over even very short distances to levels so low that it is very unlikely to be a health risk.

For information about potential health effects of radio frequency radiation sources in the workplace, go to the following website of the U.S. Dept. of Labor, Occupational Safety and Health Administration: **http://www.osha-slc. gov/SLTC/radiofrequencyradiation.**

Other kinds of non-ionizing radiation are a ubiquitous component of the environment of technologically advanced societies like that of the United States. Every electric wire and electronic device emits some form of non-ionizing radiation, including microwave, infrared, and ultraviolet radiation. Sources of non-ionizing radiation include microwave ovens, televisions, tanning lamps and black lights, home alarm systems, electric blankets, electric clothes dryers and ovens, and electricity transmission lines.

The health effects of various forms of non-ionizing radiation associated with modern electronic gadgets and electrical power lines are topics of some public controversy. A few studies have suggested that exposure to non-ionizing radiation or magnetic fields around electrical devices or power lines may slightly increase risk

for some cancers.[3,4] For example, one of these studies estimated that up to 8% of childhood leukemia cases in the U.S. were associated with living in proximity to power lines. However, the vast majority of studies of health effects of non-ionizing radiation have failed to find any increased risk of adverse health effects associated with household electronics or living in close proximity to high voltage power lines[5,6] (for a comprehensive review of the scientific literature, go to the website of J.E. Moulder, professor of radiation oncology at the Medical College of Wisconsin, **http://www.mcw.edu/gcrc/cop/ powerlines-cancer-FAQ/toc.html#C55).**

In a world where environmental health hazards are common, we must be careful to not blindly accept unsubstantiated claims regarding new hazards. However, we must also consider which is the lesser of two evils, to ban a product that is safe, or to allow a hazardous product on the market that causes damage to human health or natural systems. Sometimes governmental policies and regulations err on the side of caution, banning products even if there is only a hint of potential adverse effects. Sometimes dangerous products pass initial testing, only to cause devastating consequences when they are released into the environment. Just because a study fails to detect adverse effects of a new product does not mean that the product is safe. Finding the correct balance between caution and progress is difficult, both for governmental agencies and for individuals making choices in their own lives.

For Discussion . . .

How often do you use a cell phone? Do you worry about the effects of radio frequency radiation? What about other forms of non-ionizing radiation? Why or why not?

References

1. Foster KR. Are mobile phones safe? Institute of Electrical and Electronic Engineers (IEEE) Spectrum Online Volume 37, Number 8. 2000. **http://www.spectrum.ieee.org/publicfeature/aug00/prad.html**

2. U.S. Food and Drug Administration. *Cell Phone Facts: Consumer Information on Wireless Phones.* 2002.

3. Ahlbom A, Day N, et al: A pooled analysis of magnetic fields and childhood leukemia. *British Journal of Cancer* 83: 692–698, 2000.

4. UK Childhood Cancer Study Investigators. Childhood cancer and residential proximity to power lines. *Brit J Cancer* 83: 1573–1580, 2000.

5. Savitz DA, Loomis DP. Magnetic field exposure in relation to leukemia and brain cancer mortality among electric utility workers. *American Journal of Epidemiology* 141 (2): 123–128, 1995.

6. Greenland S, Sheppard AR, et al. A pooled analysis of magnetic fields, wirecodes, and childhood leukemia. *Epidemiology* 11: 624–634, 2000.

personal assessment

are you an environmentalist?

When asked, many people will say that they are an "environmentalist," including political leaders who are widely criticized for decisions perceived by others to be environmentally destructive. So what is an "environmentalist"? One definition of environmentalism is that it is an ideology that values and reveres Nature, and works to protect and preserve natural systems for both ethical reasons and because humankind depends on these systems for life. However, beyond this general statement environmentalists encompass a wide diversity of beliefs and practices. For some, their environmental beliefs are a form of religion, others function mainly in the political process, and some operate like terrorist groups who use violence to fight human economic development on behalf of Earth.[1] The wide diversity of beliefs and practices encompassed under "environmentalism" creates a situation where almost anyone could claim to be an environmentalist. Perhaps more useful criteria for determining if you are an environmentalist would be: (1) your awareness of how various human activities create environmental health hazards or degrade natural systems; (2) your willingness to consider your own role in creating environmental problems; and (3) your willingness to act in ways that reduce your personal risk from environmental hazards and your contribution to the causes of these hazards. These three criteria define a hierarchy of commitment to environmental protection. First you have to know a problem exists. Then you have to recognize your own part in creating that problem. The last, and most difficult, step is that you must be willing to reduce or eliminate your contribution to environmental problems. Your answers to the following questions will help you think about where you really stand on protecting the environment for yourself, your community, and all the rest of life on Earth.

Awareness of Environmental Problems

1. Have you ever read the water quality assessment provided by the supplier of your drinking water?
2. If your drinking water is from a well, do you know about potential sources of contamination (landfills or other waste disposal sites, large agricultural areas, confined feedlot livestock operations) in your watershed?
3. If your drinking water supply is from a well, do you know if your water contains potentially harmful contaminants?
4. Do you know whether or not your community wastewater treatment system occasionally dumps raw sewage into the local river during high rainfall events?
5. If you use a gas furnace or kerosene space heater, do you know whether or not these appliances are functioning properly so as to maximize energy efficiency and minimize risks from indoor air pollution?
6. Have you ever made a note of air pollution alerts or information about high ultraviolet radiation published in a local newspaper or presented on a local TV news program?
7. Have you ever searched for information on air, water, and land pollution in your community?
8. When you eat fish, are you aware of health advisories regarding contaminants in fish (e.g., mercury, PCBs) and recommendations that you limit the amount of the fish you consume?
9. When you purchase products, do you look at packaging materials for warnings that the product contains toxic chemicals?
10. When you listen to loud music, do you think about potential long-term damage to your hearing and the nuisance noise you create for your neighbors?
11. Do you know if your community (city, county, state) has a land-use management (zoning) plan?
12. When you see new economic developments (malls, superstores, warehouses, suburban housing developments) being constructed, do you wonder if wildlife habitat is being destroyed?
13. Do you know the proposed human causes of global warming and the potential consequences of this change in climate?
14. Do you know the causes and potential health effects of depletion of the stratospheric ozone layer?
15. Do you know the link between the wood you buy at a store like Menard's, Lowe's, and Home Depot and species extinctions?

Willingness to Consider Your Personal Environmental Impact

16. When you think about having a family of your own, do you worry about contributing to a rapidly growing human population that is responsible for widespread environmental degradation?
17. When you think about purchasing a vehicle, do you consider fuel efficiency more important than "image" sold by advertisers?
18. When you consider purchasing any product, do you consider the resources used, and pollution created, to produce that product?
19. When you purchase an electric appliance or a gas-powered device, do you consider energy efficiency?
20. When planning to build a new home, do you consider how your choices regarding location and amount of land could contribute to loss of green space and natural habitat?
21. When you use or dispose of household, yard, and automotive chemicals and fluids, do you consider that you may be contributing to local water pollution?
22. When you hear about global warming, do you recognize that your own use of electricity and gas-powered vehicles contributes to this problem?
23. Did you know that if you vent your home or automotive air conditioning system coolant while performing

do-it-yourself maintenance, you are contributing to the depletion of the stratospheric ozone layer?

24. When you purchase lumber, do you wonder if the wood you are buying was harvested using environmentally sound practices, or if critical wildlife habitats or wilderness was destroyed to produce the lumber?

25. Do you consider how your vote in public elections can affect government policies that impact the environment?

Willingness to Alter Your Lifestyle to Protect Yourself and the Environment

26. Would you limit the number of your own children to one or two so as to reduce your contribution to the problem of global human population explosion?

27. When you purchase a vehicle, is energy efficiency your main concern?

28. Would you use mass transit to travel from home to work, if it were available, to reduce your contribution to local air pollution and need for paving more land to expand highways?

29. When you buy a home, would you seek to minimize the distance from work and schools to reduce gas consumption, minimize air pollution, and reduce demand for construction of new roads?

30. When you buy a home, would you look for a smaller, energy-efficient home to minimize your contribution to natural resource exploitation and pollution associated with energy consumption?

31. When you buy lighting, do you buy energy-efficient lightbulbs (compact fluorescent and LED) that are initially more expensive, but more efficient and less expensive over the long term?

32. When furnishing your home, would you seek out water-efficient toilets, faucets, and shower heads that conserve freshwater and reduce demands on wastewater treatment systems?

33. Do you set the thermostat in your home to cooler temperatures in winter and warmer temperatures in summer to conserve energy?

34. Would you invest money and effort to better insulate your home so as to reduce energy needed for heating and cooling?

35. When buying food, would you be willing to pay more for organically grown foods that were produced without the use of pesticides and fertilizers that pollute the surrounding environment?

36. Would you buy locally grown foods to support farmers (and their green spaces) in your community and reduce energy spent on long-distance transport?

37. When purchasing wood products, would you buy more expensive wood that is certified to have been harvested using environmentally sound practices?

38. Would you be willing to have something less than the perfect lawn so that you avoid using fertilizers and pesticides that contaminate local waterways?

39. Would you limit your personal consumption of material goods to mainly those things you need, so as to reduce exploitation of natural resources?

40. When you dispose of household chemicals, automotive fluids, and spent batteries, do you make the extra effort to be sure they do not end up polluting the environment, like taking them to a Tox-Away Day location?

41. Do you make the effort to recycle paper, glass, plastic, and metals?

42. When you make purchases, do you look for products made from recycled materials (e.g., post-consumer recycled paper, "plastic wood," fleece clothing made from recycled plastic)?

43. Do you limit the noise that you produce (loud music, loud car or motorcycle engines, barking dogs) to reduce noise pollution in your neighborhood?

44. Do you contribute financial support to environmental groups that promote conservation and protection of natural resources through the legal and political systems?

45. When you consider candidates for public office, do you vote for the candidates who have strong records or position statements for environmental protection?

If the majority of your answers to questions 1 to 15 are "Yes," you are likely "environmentally aware." That is, you pay attention to news stories about environmental issues or have taken an environmental science course.

If most of your answers to questions 1 to 25 are "Yes," you are "environmentally conscious." That is, you are not only aware of the problems, but beginning to think about how these problems are related to your own lifestyle.

If the majority of your answers to questions 26 to 45 are "Yes," you are likely "environmentally active." That is, you are personally involved in efforts to address environmental problems through your own lifestyle choices and through the political process.

[1]Wikipedia (The Free Encyclopedia). **http://www.wikipedia.org/wiki/Environmentalism**

glossary

A

abortion induced premature termination of a pregnancy

absorption passage of nutrients or alcohol through the walls of the stomach or intestinal tract into the bloodstream

abuse any use of a legal or illegal drug that is detrimental to health

acquired immunity (AI) significant component of the immune system associated with the formation of antibodies and specialized blood cells that are capable of destroying pathogens

acupuncture insertion of fine needles into the body to alter electroenergy fields and cure disease

acute alcohol intoxication potentially fatal elevation of the blood alcohol concentration, often resulting from rapid consumption of large amounts of alcohol

acute rhinitis the common cold; the sudden onset of nasal inflammation

adaptive thermogenesis physiological response of the body to adjust its metabolic rate to the presence or absence of calories

additive effect the combined (but not exaggerated) effect produced by the concurrent use of two or more drugs

aerobic energy production body's production of energy when the respiratory and circulatory systems are able to process and transport a sufficient amount of oxygen to muscle cells

agent causal pathogen of a particular disease

air pollution refers to a wide variety of substances found in the atmosphere that can have adverse effects on human health, crop productivity, and natural communities

air toxics a class of 188 toxic air pollutants identified by the U.S. Environmental Protection Agency as known or suspected causes of cancer or other serious health effects

alarm stage the first stage of the stress response involving physiological, involuntary changes which are controlled by the hormonal and nervous system; the fight or flight response is activated in this stage

alcoholism primary chronic disease with genetic, psychosocial, and environmental factors influencing its development and manifestations

allopathy system of medical practice in which specific remedies (often pharmaceutical agents) are used to produce effects different from those produced by a disease or injury

alveoli thin, saclike terminal ends of the airways; the sites at which gases are exchanged between the blood and inhaled air

Alzheimer's disease gradual development of memory loss, confusion, and loss of reasoning; will eventually lead to total intellectual incapacitation, brain degeneration, and death

amino acids chief components of protein; synthesized by the body or obtained from dietary sources

amotivational syndrome behavioral pattern characterized by widespread apathy toward productive activities

anabolic steroids drugs that function like testosterone to produce increases in weight, strength, endurance, and aggressiveness

anaerobic energy production body's production of energy when needed amounts of oxygen are not readily available

anal intercourse a sexual act in which the erect penis is inserted into the rectum of a partner

androgyny the blending of both masculine and feminine characteristics

angina pectoris chest pain that results from impaired blood supply to the heart muscle

anorexia nervosa an eating disorder in which the individual weighs less than 85% of their expected weight, and has an intense fear of gaining weight; in females, menstruation ceases for at least 3 consecutive months. People with anorexia perceive themselves as overweight, even though they are underweight

anovulatory not ovulating

antagonistic effect effect produced when one drug nullifies (reduces, offsets) the effects of a second drug

antibodies chemical compounds produced by the immune system to destroy antigens and their toxins

arrhythmias irregularities of the heart's normal rhythm or beating pattern

artificially acquired immunity (AAI) type of acquired immunity resulting from the body's response to pathogens introduced into the body through immunizations

asbestos a term used to refer to a class of minerals that have a fibrous crystal structure

asphyxiation death resulting from lack of oxygen to the brain

atherosclerosis the buildup of plaque on the inner walls of arteries

attention deficit hyperactivity disorder (ADHD) inability to concentrate well on a specified task; often accompanied by above-normal physical movement; also called *hyperactivity*

autoimmune immune response against the cells of a person's own body

axon portion of a neuron that conducts electrical impulses to the dendrites of adjacent neurons; neurons typically have one axon

ayurveda traditional Indian medicine based on herbal remedies

B

balanced diet diet featuring food selections from each of the five food groups

ballistic stretching a "bouncing" form of stretching in which a muscle group is lengthened repetitively to produce multiple quick, forceful stretches

basic needs deficiency needs that are viewed as essential and fundamental, including physiological safety, belonging, and love and esteem needs

benign noncancerous; tumors that do not spread

beta blockers drugs that prevent overactivity of the heart, which results in angina pectoris

beta endorphins mood-enhancing, pain-reducing, opiate-like chemicals produced within a smoker's body in response to the presence of nicotine

bias and hate crimes criminal acts directed at a person or group solely because of a specific characteristic, such as race, religion, ethnic background, or other difference

binge eating disorder an eating disorder formerly referred to as compulsive over-eating disorder; binge eaters use food in the same way to cope as bulimics do, but do not engage in compensatory purging behavior

biological air pollutants living organisms or substances produced by living organisms that cause disease or allergic reactions, including bacteria, molds, mildew, viruses, dust mites, plant pollen, and animal dander, urine or feces

biological sexuality male and female aspects of sexuality

biological water pollutants disease-causing organisms that are found in water

biopsychological model a model that addresses how biological, psychological, and social factors interact and affect psychological health

bipolar disorder a mood disorder characterized by alternating episodes of depression and mania

birth control all of the procedures that can prevent the birth of a child

bisexual choosing members of both genders as one's sexual preference

blackout temporary state of amnesia experienced by a drinker; an inability to remember events that occur during a period of alcohol use

blood alcohol concentration (BAC) percentage of alcohol in a measured quantity of blood

BOD POD body composition system used to measure body fat through air displacement

body image our subjective perception of how our body appears

body mass index (BMI) numerical expression of body weight based on height and weight

bolus theory a theory of nicotine addiction based on the bolus (ball) of nicotine delivered to the brain with each inhalation of cigarette smoke

brand name specific name assigned to a patented drug or product by its manufacturer

bulimia nervosa an eating disorder in which individuals engage in episodes of binging, consuming unusually large amounts of food and feeling out of control, and engaging in some form of compensatory purging behavior to eliminate the food

C

calcium channel blockers drugs that prevent arterial spasms; used in the long-term management of angina pectoris

calendar method form of periodic abstinence in which the variable lengths of a woman's menstrual cycle are used to calculate her fertile period

calipers device to measure the thickness of a skinfold from which percent body fat can be calculated

calories units of heat (energy); specifically, 1 calorie equals the heat required to raise 1 kilogram of water $1°$ C

carbohydrates chemical compounds comprised of sugar or saccharide units; the body's primary source of energy

carbon monoxide a gaseous by-product of the incomplete combustion of natural gas, kerosene, heating oil, wood, coal, gasoline, and tobacco

carcinogens environmental agents that stimulate the development of cancerous changes within cells

cardiac muscle specialized muscle tissue that forms the middle (muscular) layer of the heart wall

cardiorespiratory endurance ability of the body to process and transport oxygen required by muscle cells so that these cells can continue to contract

cardiovascular pertaining to the heart (cardio) and blood vessels (vascular)

carjacking a crime that involves a thief's attempt to steal a car while the owner is behind the wheel; carjackings are usually random and unpredictable and often involve handguns

catabolism metabolic process of breaking down tissue for the purpose of converting it to energy

cerebrovascular occlusion blockage to arteries supplying blood to the cerebral cortex of the brain; resulting in a stroke

cervical cap small, thimble-shaped contraceptive device designed to fit over the cervix

cesarean delivery surgical removal of a fetus through the abdominal wall

chemical name name used to describe the molecular structure of a drug

chemoprevention the safe and effective use of dietary supplements in the prevention of illness and disease

child maltreatment the act or failure to act by a parent or caregiver, which results in abuse or neglect of a child or which places the child in imminent risk of serious harm

chiropractic manipulation of the vertebral column to relieve pressure and cure illness

chlamydia the most prevalent sexually transmitted disease; caused by a nongonococcal bacterium

cholesterol a primary form of fat found in the blood; lipid material manufactured within the body, as well as derived through dietary sources

chronic bronchitis persistent inflammation and infection of the smaller airways within the lungs

chronic fatigue syndrome (CFS) illness that causes severe exhaustion, fatigue, aches, and depression; mostly affects women in their thirties and forties

chronic stress a high level of physiological arousal for an extended period of time; it can also occur when an individual is not able to immediately react to a real or perceived threat

cilia small, hairlike structures that extend from cells that line the air passage

circadian rhythms The internal, biological clock that helps coordinate physiological processes to the 24-hour light/dark cycle

clinical depression a psychological disorder in which individuals experience a lack of motivation, decreased energy level, fatigue, social withdrawal, sleep disturbance, disturbance in appetite, diminished sex drive, feelings of worthlessness, and despair

codependence unhealthy relationship in which one person is addicted to alcohol or another drug and a person close to him or her is "addicted" to the alcoholic or drug user

cohabitation sharing of a residence by two unrelated, unmarried people; living together

coitus penile-vaginal intercourse

coitus interruptus (withdrawal) a contraceptive practice in which the erect penis is removed from the vagina before ejaculation

cold turkey immediate, total discontinuation of use of tobacco or other addictive substances

collateral circulation ability of nearby blood vessels to enlarge and carry additional blood around a blocked blood vessel

colonoscopy examination of the entire length of the colon, using a flexible fiberoptic scope to inspect the structure's lining

compliance willingness to follow the directions provided by another person

condom latex shield designed to cover the erect penis and retain semen on ejaculation

congestive heart failure inability of the heart to pump out all the blood that returns to it; can lead to dangerous fluid accumulation in veins, lungs, and kidneys

consumer fraud marketing of unreliable and ineffective services, products, or information under the guise of curing disease or improving health; quackery

contraception any procedure that prevents fertilization

contraceptive patch contraceptive skin patch containing estrogen and progestin; replaced each week for a three-week period

contraceptive ring thin, polymer contraceptive device containing estrogen and progestin; placed deep within the vagina for a three-week period

contraindications factors that make the use of a drug inappropriate or dangerous for a particular person

coronary arteries vessels that supply oxygenated blood and nutrients to heart muscle

coronary artery bypass surgery surgical procedure designed to improve blood flow to the heart by providing a new route for blood around points of blockage

corpus luteum cellular remnant of the graafian follicle after the release of an ovum

cross-tolerance transfer of tolerance from one drug to another within the same general category

cruciferous vegetables vegetables that have flowers with four leaves in the pattern of a cross

CT scan computed tomography scan; an x-ray procedure that is designed to visualize structures within the body that would not normally be seen through conventional x-ray procedures

cunnilingus oral stimulation of the vulva or clitoris

D

dehydration abnormal depletion of fluids from the body; severe dehydration can lead to death

dendrite portion of a neuron that receives electrical stimuli from adjacent neurons; neurons typically have several such branches or extensions

dependence general term that reflects the need to keep consuming a drug for psychological or physical reasons, or both

desertification a process that converts lands that historically supported grasslands, shrub lands, or dry forest to nonproductive desert

designated driver a person who abstains from or carefully limits alcohol use to drive others safely

desirable weight weight range deemed appropriate for people of a specific gender, age, and frame size

diaphragm soft rubber vaginal cup designed to cover the cervix

diastolic pressure blood pressure against blood vessel walls when the heart relaxes

dilation gradual expansion of an opening or passageway

dilation and curettage (D & C) surgical procedure in which the cervical canal is dilated to allow the uterine wall to be scraped

distillation the process of heating an alcohol solution and collecting its vapors into a more concentrated solution

distress stress that diminishes the quality of life; commonly associated with disease, illness, and maladaptation

drug synergism enhancement of a drug's effect as a result of the presence of additional drugs within the system

duration length of time one needs to exercise at the target heart rate to produce the training effect

E

ectopic pregnancy a pregnancy wherein the fertilized ovum implants at a site other than the uterus, typically in the fallopian tube

embolism potentially fatal situation in which a circulating blood clot lodges itself in a smaller vessel

emotional intelligence the ability to understand others and act wisely in human relations and measure how well you know your emotions, manage your emotions, motivate yourself, recognize emotions in others, and handle relationships

empower the ability to make choices and take responsibility for oneself

enabling in this case, the inadvertent support that some people provide to alcohol or drug abusers

enucleated egg an ovum with the nucleus removed

environment the physical conditions (temperature, humidity, light, presence of substances) and other living organisms that exist around your body

environmental tobacco smoke tobacco smoke that is diluted and stays within a common source of air

enzymes organic substances that control the rate of physiological reactions but are not themselves altered in the process

erection the engorgement of erectile tissue with blood; characteristic of the penis, clitoris, nipple, labia minora, and scrotum

ergogenic aids supplements that are taken to improve athletic performance

erotic dreams dreams whose content elicits a sexual response

estrogen ovarian hormone that initiates the development of the uterine wall

eustress stress that enhances the quality of life

exercise a subcategory of physical activity; it is planned, structured, repetitive, and purposive in the sense that an improvement or maintenance of physical fitness is an objective (Casperson, et al., 1985)

excitement stage initial arousal stage of the sexual response pattern

exhaustion stage the point at which the physical and psychological resources used to deal with stress have been consumed

F

false labor conditions that tend to resemble the start of true labor; may include irregular uterine contractions, pressure, and discomfort in the lower abdomen

FDA Schedule 1 list comprising drugs that hold a high potential for abuse but have no medical use

fecal coliform bacteria a category of bacteria that live within the intestines of warm-blooded animals. The presence of these bacteria is used as an indicator that water has been contaminated by feces

femininity behavioral expressions traditionally observed in females

fermentation chemical process whereby plant products are converted into alcohol by the action of yeast on carbohydrates

fertility ability to reproduce

fetal alcohol syndrome characteristic birth defects noted in the children of some women who consume alcohol during their pregnancies

fiber plant material that cannot be digested; found in cereal, fruits, and vegetables

fight-or-flight response the physiological response reaction to a stressor that prepares the body for confrontation or avoidance

flaccid nonerect; the state of erectile tissue when vasocongestion is not occurring

flexibility ability of joints to function through an intended range of motion

follicle-stimulating hormone (FSH) gonadotropic hormone required for initial development of ova (in the female) and sperm (in the male)

food additives chemical compounds that are intentionally or unintentionally added to our food supply that change some property of the food such as color or texture

food allergy a reaction in which the immune system attacks an otherwise harmless food or ingredient; allergic reactions can range from mildly unpleasant to life-threatening

food intolerance an adverse reaction to a specific food that does not involve the immune system; usually caused by an enzyme deficiency

foreplay activities, often involving touching and caressing, that prepare individuals for sexual intercourse

frequency number of times per week one should exercise to achieve a training effect

functional foods foods capable of contributing to the improvement/prevention of specific health problems

G

gait pattern of walking

gaseous phase portion of tobacco smoke containing carbon monoxide and many other physiologically active gaseous compounds

gateway drugs easily obtained legal or illegal drugs (alcohol, tobacco, marijuana) whose use may precede the use of less common illegal drugs

gender general term reflecting a biological basis of sexuality; the male gender or the female gender

gender adoption lengthy process of learning the behaviors that are traditional for one's gender

gender identification achievement of a personally satisfying interpretation of one's masculinity or feminity

gender identity recognition of one's gender

gender preference emotional and intellectual acceptance of one's gender

general adaptation syndrome (GAS) sequenced physiological response to the presence of a stressor; the alarm, resistance, and exhaustion stages of the stress response

generalized anxiety disorder (GAD) an anxiety disorder that involves experiencing intense and nonspecific anxiety for at least six months, in which the intensity and frequency of worry is excessive and out of proportion to the situation

genetic counseling medical counseling regarding the transmission and management of inherited conditions

genetic predisposition inherited tendency to develop a disease process if necessary environmental factors exist

gonads male or female sex glands; testes produce sperm and ovaries produce eggs

green space areas of land that are dominated by domesticated or natural vegeta-

tion, including rural farmland, city lawns and parks, and nature preserves

greenhouse gases a category of gases in the atmosphere that allow solar radiation to pass through the atmosphere to the Earth, but then trap the heat that is radiated from the Earth back toward space; greenhouse gases include water vapor, carbon dioxide, methane, nitrous oxide, and tropospheric ozone

H

hallucinogens psychoactive drugs capable of producing hallucinations (distortions of reality)

health claims statements attesting to a food's contribution to the improvement/prevention of specific health problems

health promotion movement in which knowledge, practices, and values are transmitted to people for their use in lengthening their lives, reducing the incidence of illness, and feeling better

healthy body weight body weight within a weight range appropriate for a person with an acceptable waist-to-hip ratio

herbalism an ancient form of healing in which herbal preparations are used to treat illness and disease

high-density lipoprotein (HDL) the type of lipoprotein that transports cholesterol from the bloodstream to the liver where it is eventually removed from the body; high levels of HDL are related to a reduction in heart disease

high-risk health behavior a behavioral pattern associated with a high risk of developing a chronic disease

holistic health broadest view of the composition of health; views health in terms of its physical, emotional, social, intellectual, spiritual, and occupational makeup

homeopathy the use of minute doses of herbs or minerals to stimulate healing

homicide the intentional killing of one person by another

hormone replacement therapy (HRT) medically administered estrogen and progestin to replace hormones lost at menopause

host negligence a legal term that reflects the failure of a host to provide reasonable care and safety for people visiting the host's residence or business

hot flashes temporary feelings of warmth experienced by women during and after menopause; caused by blood vessel dilation

human cloning the replication of a human being

human papillomavirus (HPV) sexually transmitted viruses, some of which are capable of causing precancerous changes in the cervix; causative agent for genital warts

hypercellular obesity form of obesity seen in individuals who possess an abnormally large number of fat cells

hyperglycemia elevated blood glucose levels; an important indicator of diabetes mellitus

hyperparathyroidism condition reflecting the overactive production of parathyroid hormone by the parathyroid glands

hypertonic saline solution salt solution with a concentration higher than that found in human fluids

hypoxia oxygen deprivation at the cellular level

I

immune system system of biochemical and cellular elements that protect the body from invading pathogens and foreign materials

immunizations laboratory-prepared pathogens that are introduced into the body for the purpose of stimulating the body's immune system

incest marriage or coitus (sexual intercourse) between closely related individuals

incubation stage time required for a pathogen to multiply significantly enough for signs and symptoms to appear

indoor air quality characteristics of air within homes, workplaces, and public buildings, including the presence and amount of oxygen, water vapor, and a wide range of substances that can have adverse effects on your health

infatuation a relatively temporary, intensely romantic attraction to another person

infertility inability of a male to impregnate or of a female to become pregnant

inhalants psychoactive drugs that enter the body through inhalation

inhibitions inner controls that prevent a person's engaging in certain types of behavior

insulin pancreatic hormone required by the body for the effective metabolism of glucose (blood sugar)

intensity level of effort one puts into an activity

interstitial cell stimulating hormone (ICSH) a gonadotropic hormone of the male required for the production of testosterone

intimacy any close, mutual verbal or nonverbal behavior within a relationship

intimate partner violence violence committed against a person by her or his current or former spouse, boyfriend, or girlfriend

intrauterine device (IUD) small plastic medicated or unmedicated device that when inserted in the uterus prevents continued pregnancy

ionizing radiation electromagnetic radiation that is capable of breaking chemical bonds, such as x-rays and gamma rays

isokinetic exercises muscular strength-training exercises that use machines to provide variable resistances throughout the full range of motion

isometric exercises muscular strength-training exercises that use a resistance so great that the resistance object cannot be moved

isotonic resistance exercises muscular strength-training exercises in which traditional barbells and dumbbells are used to provide variable resistances throughout the full range of motion

L

learned helplessness a theory of motivation explaining how individuals can learn to feel powerless, trapped, or defeated

learned optimism an attribution style, comprised of permanence, pervasiveness, and personalization; how people explain both positive and negative events in their lives, accounting for success and failure

lightening movement of fetus deeper into the pelvic cavity before the onset of the birth process

low-density lipoprotein (LDL) the type of lipoprotein that transports the largest amount of cholesterol in the bloodstream; high levels of LDL are related to heart disease

lumpectomy a surgical treatment for breast cancer in which a minimal amount of breast tissue is removed

luteinizing hormone (LH) female gonadotropic hormone required for fullest development and release of ova; ovulating hormone

Lyme disease systemic bacterial infection transmitted by deer ticks

M

mainstream smoke the smoke inhaled and then exhaled by a smoker

mania an extremely excitable state characterized by excessive energy, racing thoughts, impulsive and/or reckless behavior, irritability, and being prone to distraction

masculinity behavioral expressions traditionally observed in males

masturbation self-stimulation of the genitals

maximum contaminant level the highest concentration of a contaminant that is allowed in drinking water, as established and regulated by the U.S. Environmental Protection Agency

medical abortion an abortion caused by the use of prescribed drugs

medical power of attorney for health care a legal document that designates who will make health care decisions for people unable to do so for themselves

menarche time of a female's first menstrual cycle

menopause decline and eventual cessation of hormone production by the reproductive system

menstrual phase phase of the menstrual cycle during which the broken-down lining of the uterus (endometrium) is discharged from the body

metabolite breakdown product of a drug

metaneeds secondary concerns, such as spirituality, creativity, curiosity, beauty, philosophy, and justice, that can be addressed only after the basic needs are met

metastasis spread of cancerous cells from their site of origin to other areas of the body

misuse inappropriate use of legal drugs intended to be medications

monogamous paired relationship with one partner

mononuclear leukocytes large white blood cells that have only one nucleus

monounsaturated fats fats made of compounds in which one hydrogen-bonding position remains to be filled; semisolid at room temperature; derived primarily from peanut and olive oils

morbidity illness or disease

mortality death

MRI scan magnetic resonance imaging; an imaging procedure that uses a giant magnet to generate an image of body tissue

mucus clear, sticky material produced by specialized cells within the mucous membranes of the body; mucus traps much of the suspended particulate matter from tobacco smoke

multiorgasmic capacity potential to have several orgasms within a single period of sexual arousal

murmur an atypical heart sound that suggests a backwashing of blood into a chamber of the heart from which it has just left

muscular endurance the aspect of muscular fitness that deals with ability of a muscle or muscle group to repeatedly contract over a long period of time

muscular strength the aspect of physical fitness that deals with ability to contract skeletal muscles to a maximal level

myocardial infarction heart attack; the death of heart muscle as a result of a blockage in one of the coronary arteries

N

narcolepsy sleep-related disorder in which a person has a recurrent, overwhelming, and uncontrollable desire to sleep

narcotics psychoactive drugs derived from the oriental poppy plant; narcotics relieve pain and induce sleep

naturally acquired immunity (NAI) type of acquired immunity resulting from the body's response to naturally occurring pathogens

nature the innate factors that genetically determine personality traits

naturopathy a system of treatment that avoids drugs and surgery and emphasizes the use of natural agents to correct underlying imbalances

neuron nerve cell; the structural unit of the nervous system

nocturnal emission ejaculation that occurs during sleep; "wet dream"

nomogram graphic means of finding an unknown value

non-insulin-dependent (type 2) diabetes mellitus form of diabetes generally seen for the first time in people 35 years of age and older; adult-onset diabetes

non-ionizing radiation electromagnetic radiation that cannot break chemical bonds, but may excite electrons (ultraviolet radiation) or heat biological materials (infrared, radio frequency, and microwave radiation)

nonoxynol 9 a spermicide commonly used with contraceptive devices

nontraditional-age students administrative term used by colleges and universities for students who, for whatever reason, are pursuing undergraduate work at an age other than that associated with traditional college years (18–24)

norepinephrine adrenaline-like neurotransmitter produced within the nervous system

nurture the effect that the environment, people, and external factors have on personality

nutrients elements in foods that are required for the growth, repair, and regulation of body processes

O

obesity condition in which a person's body weight is 20% above desirable weight

obsessive-compulsive disorder an anxiety disorder characterized by obsessions—intrusive thoughts, images, or impulses causing a great deal of distress—and compulsions—repetitive behaviors aimed at reducing anxiety or stress that is associated with the obsessive thoughts

oncogenes genes that are believed to activate the development of cancer

oral contraceptive pill taken orally, composed of synthetic female hormones that prevent ovulation or implantation; "the pill"

orgasmic platform expanded outer third of the vagina that during the plateau phase of the sexual response grips the penis

orgasmic stage third stage of the sexual response pattern; the stage during which neuromuscular tension is released

orthodontics dental specialty that focuses on the proper alignment of the teeth

osteoarthritis arthritis that develops with age; largely caused by weight-bearing and deterioration of joints

osteopathy system of medical practice that combines allopathic principles with specific attention to postural mechanics of the body

osteoporosis the loss of calcium from the bone caused by the inability of the body to use dietary calcium; seen primarily in postmenopausal women

outercourse sexual activity that does not involve intercourse

overload principle principle whereby a person gradually increases the resistance load that must be moved or lifted

overweight condition in which body weight is 1%–19% above desirable weight

ovolactovegetarian diet diet that excludes the use of all meat but does allow the consumption of eggs and dairy products

ovulation the release of a mature egg from the ovary

oxidation in this case, the process that removes alcohol from the bloodstream

oxygen debt physical state that occurs when the body can no longer process and transport sufficient amounts of oxygen for continued muscle contraction

P

panic disorder an anxiety disorder characterized by panic attacks, in which individuals experience severe physical symptoms; these episodes can seemingly occur "out of the blue" or because of some trigger, and can last for a few minutes or for hours

pap test a cancer screening procedure in which cells are removed from the cervix and examined for precancerous changes

particulate phase portion of tobacco smoke composed of small suspended particles

passively acquired immunity (PAI) temporary immunity achieved by providing extrinsic antibodies to a person exposed to a particular pathogen

pathogen disease-causing agent

pelvic inflammatory disease (PID) acute or chronic infections of the peritoneum or lining of the abdominopelvic cavity; associated with a variety of symptoms and a potential cause of sterility

perfectionism a tendency to expect perfection in everything one does, with little tolerance for mistakes

periodic abstinence birth control methods that rely on a couple's avoidance of intercourse during the ovulatory phase of a woman's menstrual cycle; also called *fertility awareness* or *natural family planning*

periodontal disease destruction of soft tissue and bone that surround the teeth

peripheral artery disease (PAD) damage resulting from restricted blood flow to the extremities, especially the legs and feet

permanence one of three dimensions of an individual's attribution style, related to whether certain events are perceived as temporary or long-lasting

peritonitis inflammation of the peritoneum or lining of the abdominopelvic cavity

personalization another dimension of attribution style, related to whether an individual takes things personally or is more balanced in accepting responsibility for positive and negative events

pervasiveness another dimension of an individual's attribution style, related to whether events are perceived as specific to a situation or generalized

pesco-vegetarian diet a vegetarian diet that includes fish, dairy products, and eggs, along with plant foods

phenylpropanolamine (PPA) active chemical compound once found in most over-the-counter diet products

physical activity any bodily movement produced by skeletal muscles that results in energy expenditure (Casperson, et al., 1985)

physical fitness a set of attributes that people have or achieve that relates to the ability to perform physical activity (Casperson, et al., 1985)

placebo medications that contain no active ingredients

platonic close association between two people that does not include a sexual relationship

positive caloric balance caloric intake greater than caloric expenditure

post-abortion syndrome long-term negative psychological effects of abortion

postpartum period of time after the birth of a baby during which the uterus returns to its prepregnancy size

potentiated effect phenomenon whereby the use of one drug intensifies the effect of a second drug

preventive or prospective medicine physician-centered medical care in which areas of risk for chronic illnesses are identified so that they might be lowered

primary care health provider the physician who sees a patient on a regular basis, particularly for preventative health care

problem drinking alcohol use pattern in which a drinker's behavior creates personal difficulties or difficulties for other people

Prochaska's stages of change the six predictable stages—precontemplation, contemplation, preparation, action, maintenance, and termination—people go through in establishing new habits and patterns of behavior

procrastination a tendency to put off completing tasks until some later time, sometimes resulting in increased stress

procreation reproduction

prophylactic mastectomy elective (voluntary) removal of the breast or breasts to prevent the development of breast cancer

prophylactic oophorectomy surgical removal of the ovaries to prevent cancer in women at high risk of the disease

prostaglandins chemical substances that stimulate smooth muscle contractions

prostate-specific antigen (PSA) test a blood test used to identify prostate-specific antigen, an early indicator that the immune system has recognized and mounted a defense against prostate cancer

prosthodontics dental specialty that focuses on the construction and fitting of artificial appliances to replace missing teeth

proteins compounds composed of chains of amino acids; primary components of muscle and connective tissue

protooncogenes normal genes that hold the potential of becoming cancer-causing oncogenes

psychoactive drugs any substance capable of altering feelings, moods, or perceptions

psychological health a broadly based concept pertaining to cognitive functioning in conjunction with the way people express their emotions, cope with stress, adversity, and success, and adapt to changes in themselves and their environment

psychosocial sexuality masculine and feminine aspects of sexuality

puberty achievement of reproductive ability

pulmonary emphysema irreversible disease process of the lungs in which the alveoli are destroyed

pulmonary hypertension a serious form of high blood pressure that affects lung vessels

purging using vomiting, laxatives, diuretics, enemas, or other medications, or such means as excessive exercise to eliminate food

R

radio frequency radiation electromagnetic radiation with frequency in the range of 3 kilohertz to 300 megahertz, emitted by cell phones, radios, communications transmitters, and other electronic devices

radon a naturally occurring radioactive gas that is emitted during the decay of uranium in soil, rock, and water

reflexology massage applied to specific areas of the feet to treat illness and disease in other areas of the body

refractory errors abnormal patterns of light wave transmission through the structures of the eye

refractory phase that portion of the male's resolution stage during which sexual arousal cannot occur

regulatory genes genes within the cell that control cellular replication and specialization, DNA repair, and tumor suppression

relaxation response physiological state of opposition to the fight-or-flight response of the general adaptation syndrome

resistance stage the second stage of a response to a stressor, during which the body attempts to reestablish its equilibrium or internal balance

resolution stage fourth stage of the sexual response pattern; the return of the body to a preexcitement state

retinal hemorrhage uncontrolled bleeding from arteries within the eye's retina

rheumatic heart disease chronic damage to the heart (especially heart valves) resulting from a streptococcal infection within the heart; a complication associated with rheumatic fever

risk factor a biomedical index or behavioral pattern associated with chronic illness

S

salt sensitive descriptive of people whose bodies overreact to the presence of sodium by retaining fluid and thus increasing blood pressure

satiety state in which there is no longer a desire to eat; fullness

saturated fats dietary fats that influence the formation of cholesterol

schizophrenia one of the most severe mental disorders, characterized by profound distortions in one's thought processes, emotions, perceptions and behavior; symptoms may include hallucinations, delusions, disorganized thinking, and/or maintaining a rigid posture and not moving for hours

sclerotic changes thickening or hardening of tissues

self-actualization the highest level of psychological health at which one reaches his or her highest potential and values truth, beauty, goodness, spirituality, love, humor, and ingenuity

self-care movement trend toward individuals taking increased responsibility for prevention or management of certain health conditions

self-concept an individual's internal picture of him or herself; the way one sees oneself

self-esteem an individual's sense of pride, self-respect, value, and worth

self-fulfilling prophecy the tendency to inadvertently make something more likely to happen as a result of your own expectations and attitudes

semen secretion containing sperm and nutrients discharged from the male urethra at ejaculation

set point a genetically programmed range of body weight beyond which a person finds it difficult to gain or lose additional weight

sex flush reddish skin response that results from increasing sexual arousal

sex reassignment operation surgical procedure designed to remove the external genitalia and replace them with genitalia appropriate to the opposite gender

sexual fantasies fantasies with sexual themes; sexual daydreams or imaginary events

sexuality the quality of being sexual; can be viewed from many biological and psychosocial perspectives

sexually transmitted diseases (STDs) infectious diseases that are spread primarily through intimate sexual contact

shock profound collapse of many vital body functions; evident during acute alcohol intoxication and other serious health emergencies

sidestream smoke the smoke that comes from the burning end of a cigarette, pipe, or cigar

smegma cellular discharge that can accumulate beneath the clitoral hood and the foreskin of an uncircumcised penis

social phobia a phobia characterized by feelings of extreme dread and embarrassment in situations in which public speaking or social interaction is involved

sodomy generally refers to anal or oral sex; a legal term whose definition varies according to state law

solid waste pollutants that are in solid form, including non-hazardous household trash, industrial wastes, mining wastes, and sewage sludge from wastewater treatment plants

spermatogenesis process of sperm production

spermicides chemicals capable of killing sperm

stalking a crime involving an assailant's planned efforts to pursue an intended victim

static stretching the slow lengthening of a muscle group to an extended level of stretch followed by holding the extended position for 10–30 seconds

stem cells premature cells that have the potential to turn into any kind of cells

sterilization generally permanent birth control techniques that surgically disrupt the normal passage of ova or sperm

stimulants psychoactive drugs that stimulate the function of the central nervous system

stress the physiological and psychological state of disruption caused by the presence of an unanticipated, disruptive, or stimulating event

stress response the physiological and psychological responses to positive or negative events that are disruptive, unexpected, or stimulating

stressors factors or events, real or imagined, that elicit a state of stress

sudden cardiac death immediate death resulting from a sudden change in the rhythm of the heart

synapse location at which an electrical impulse from one neuron is transmitted to an adjacent neuron

synergistic drug effect heightened, exaggerated effect produced by the concurrent use of two or more drugs

systolic pressure blood pressure against blood vessel walls when the heart contracts

T

tar particulate phase of tobacco smoke with nicotine and water removed

target heart rate (THR) number of times per minute that the heart must contract to produce a training effect

test anxiety a form of performance anxiety that generates extreme feelings of distress in exam situations

therapeutic cloning the use of certain human replication techniques to reproduce body tissues and cells

thermic effect of food (TEF) refers to the amount of energy our bodies require for the digestion, absorption, and transportation of food

thorax the chest; portion of the torso above the diaphragm and within the rib cage

titration determining a particular level of a drug within the body

tolerance an acquired reaction to a drug; continued intake of the same dose has diminished results

toxic shock syndrome (TSS) potentially fatal condition resulting from the proliferation of certain bacteria in the vagina, whose toxins enter the blood circulation

trace elements minerals whose presence in the body occurs in very small amounts; micronutrient elements

transcervical balloon tuboplasty the use of inflatable balloon catheters to open blocked fallopian tubes; a procedure used for some women with fertility problems

transient ischemic attack (TIA) temporary spasm of a cerebral artery that produces symptoms similar to those of a minor stroke; often a forewarning of a true cerebrovascular accident

trimester three-month period of time; human pregnancies encompass three trimesters

tropospheric ozone ozone is comprised of three oxygen atoms that are bound into a single molecule; tropospheric ozone refers to this substance as it occurs in the lower layer of the atmosphere, close to the ground

tumor mass of cells; may be cancerous (malignant) or noncancerous (benign)

U

unintentional injuries injuries that occur without anyone's intending that harm be done

index

Food Guide Pyramid, 116
  heart disease prevention, 272
  home safety, 473–474
  maltreatment, 462, 463
  physical fitness, 81, 98, 269
  sexual abuse of, 468–469
Chippers, 241
Chiropractic, 436–437
Chlamydia, 350–351
Cholesterol, 111, 277–279
Cholesterol levels, 124, 275, 279
Chronic bronchitis, 252
Chronic conditions, 315–320, 325–326. *See also specific conditions*
Chronic fatigue syndrome, 329, 341
Chronic obstructive lung disease (COLD), 252
Chronic stress, 54–55
Cigar smoking, 239–240
Cigarette smoking. *See* Nicotine; Tobacco use
Cilia, 251, 369
Circadian rhythms, 66
Clinical breast examination, 300
Clinical depression, 35–36, 37
Clinical stage, of infection, 333
Clitoris, 370
Cloning, 415–416
Club drugs, 194
Cocaine, 189, 192–193
Codependence, 224
Coenzymes, 113
Cognitive self-talk, 69–70
Cohabitation, 384
Coinsurance, health insurance, 444
Coitus, 377, 379
Coitus interruptus, 398
Cold, common, 338–339
COLD (chronic obstructive lung disease), 252
Cold turkey, defined, 197
College students
  alcohol use, 211–213
  cigarette smoking, 237
  diversity of, 22–23
  minority students, 11–12, 22
  nontraditional-age, 11, 22
  students with disabilities, 12, 22
  traditional-age, 11, 22
Colonoscopy, 310
Colorectal cancer, 300, 309–310
Combination drug effects, 198
Combined pill, for birth control, 398, 406
Commercial weight reduction programs, 163–164
Commercials. *See* Advertising
Common cold, 338–339
Communication
  developing skills, 29
  with health care providers, 432
  nonverbal, 28–29
  for resolving conflict, 385
  and stress, 51
  with students with a disability, 53
  verbal, 28
Community environment, 484, 492–499
Community health promotion, 6–7
Companionate love, 383
Compatibility, in relationships, 383, 393

Complementary care practitioners, 436–438, 439
Compliance, 431
Compulsion, in addiction process, 185–186
Compulsive overeating, 170
Computer waste, 498
Condoms, 379, 398, 402–403
Conflict management, 29–30, 385
Confrontation, for drug dependence, 199
Congenital heart disease, 284–285
Congenital rubella syndrome (CRS), 285
Congestive heart failure, 285–286
Consultations, 435
Consumer advocacy groups, as health information source, 433
Consumer fraud, 450, 454–455
Consumerism assessment, 457
Contact inhibition, and cancer cells, 296
Contemplation stage, of change, 9
Contraception. *See also* Birth control
  versus birth control, 396–397
  defined, 396
  selecting method, 397, 399, 411, 427
Contraceptive patch, 398, 408–409
Contraceptive ring, 398, 408
Contraceptive sponge, 405
Contraceptives
  injectable, 398, 408
  oral, 254, 398, 406–408
"Contract for Life," 222
Contraindications, 407
Controlled fasting, 161, 163
Convalescence stage, of infection, 333
Cooldown phase, 92
Cord blood (stem) cells, 335–336
Corona, 370
Coronary arteries, 272
Coronary arteriography, 280
Coronary artery bypass surgery, 280
Coronary heart disease, 277–281
  diagnosis and coronary repair, 280–281
  emergency response to heart crises, 279–280
Corpus, 372
Corpus luteum, 373
Counseling, for depression, 35
Cowper's glands, 369
CPR (cardiopulmonary resuscitation), 280, 474
Crabs, 354
Crack cocaine, 193
Creatine, 97
Creativity, 42–44
Crime
  and alcohol use, 220–221, 230–231
  bias and hate crimes, 464, 466
  campus crime and alcohol use, 230
  illegal drug activity and homicide, 461
Crohn's disease, 316
Cross-tolerance, 189
Crosstraining, 97
Crosstraining shoes, 95–96
Crowning, during childbirth, 418
Cruciferous vegetables, 116
Crystal meth, 191
C-section, 419
CT scan, 283
Cultural factors, in obesity, 153
Cunnilingus, 379

Curette, 412
Cycle, menstrual, 372–373, 400
Cystitis, 355

D
Dancing, as aerobic exercise, 93–94
Date rape, 194, 467–468, 470
Death, causes of, 5, 10, 270, 271
Death rates, cancer, 297, 298, 312
Decline stage, of infection, 333
Deductibles, health insurance, 443
Dehydration, 114
Delirium tremens (DTs), 224
Delivery, 418. *See also* Childbirth
Dementia, 320
Dendrite, 184
Dengue, 359
Denial, 224–225
Dental dams, 379
Dentists, 439
Dependence, 188–189
Depo-Provera, 398, 408
Depressants, 190, 193–194, 203
Depression, 35–36, 37
Desertification, 501–502
Designated drivers, 209, 221–222
Designer drugs, 195
Desirable weight, 148
Developmental tasks, of young adulthood, 12–15
Dexfenfluramine, 164–165
Dextrose, 109
Diabetes mellitus
  and cardiovascular disease, 276
  insulin-dependent, 318–319
  non-insulin-dependent, 317–318, 319
Diaphragms, for birth control, 398, 403–404
Diastolic pressure, 281
Diet. *See also* Nutrition
  balanced, 115–116, 117, 118, 159
  and cancer prevention, 314
  and obesity, 154–155
  and weight management, 158, 159–161, 163–164
Dietary Guidelines for Americans, 131, 148
Dietary supplements, 126–128, 438
Dieting, and weight gain, 152–153
Dilation and curettage (D & C), 412
Dilation and evacuation (D & E), 412
Dionne quintuplets, 424
Diphtheria immunization, 337
Disabilities
  developmentally disabled athletes, 89
  students with, 12, 53
  violence against people with, 464
Disaccharides, 109
Disaster reactions, 70
Dissonance, and tobacco use, 245
Distillation, 213
Distress, 52–53
Diuresis, 318
Diversity
  Americans with Disabilities Act, 434
  bisexuals, 382
  college students, 22–23, 34
  developmentally disabled athletes, 89
  heart disease prevention, 272

urethra passageway through which urine leaves the urinary bladder

urethritis infection of the urethra

V

vasectomy surgical procedure in which the vasa deferentia are cut to prevent the passage of sperm from the testicles; the most common form of male sterilization

vegan vegetarian diet vegetarian diet that excludes the use of all animal products, including eggs and dairy products

virulent capable of causing disease

vitamins organic compounds that facilitate the action of enzymes

volatile organic compounds a wide variety of chemicals that contain carbon and readily evaporate into the air

W

wellness the promotion and achievement of optimal health, including physical, emotional, social, intellectual, spiritual, and occupational well-being

withdrawal illness uncomfortable, perhaps toxic response of the body as it attempts to maintain homeostasis in the absence of a drug; also called *abstinence syndrome*

Y

Yerkes-Dodson law a bell-shaped curve demonstrating that there is an optimal level of stress for peak performance. This law states that too little and too much stress are not helpful, while a moderate level of stress is positive and beneficial

Z

zero tolerance laws laws that severely restrict the right to drive for underage drinkers who have been convicted of driving under the influence of *any* alcohol

zoonosis the transmission of diseases from animals to humans

Credits

Chapter Two: p. 41 (Figure 2-1), based on "Hierarchy of Needs" from *Motivation and Personality,* 3rd ed. by Abraham H. Maslow. Revised by Robert Frager, et al., Harper & Row, Publishers, 1954, 1987; **p. 47 (Figure),** Data from Yankelovich Partners for Lutheran Brotherhood; **p. 49 (Personal Assessment),** From Study Guide and Personal Exploration for *Psychology applied to modern life; adjustment in the 80s,* by Wayne Weiten. Copyright © 1983 by Wadsworth, inc. Reprinted by permission of Brooks/Cole Publishing, Pacific Grove, CA 93950.

Chapter Three: p. 56 (Figure 3-3), Hebb, D.O. (1955). *Drive and the CNS (Conceptual Nervous System).* Psychological Review, 62 (4), 243–245; **p. 64 (Figure 3-5),** Data from the Wirthlin Report; **p. 93 (Personal Assessement),** Modified from Holmes TH, Rahe RH: The social adjustment rating scale, *Journal of Psychosomatic Research* 11:213218, 1967; **p. 77 (Personal Assessment),** Adapted with the permission of The Free Press, a Division of Simon and Schuster Adult Publishing Group, from *Never Good Enough: Freeing Yourself From The Chains of Perfectionism* by Monica Ramirez Basco, Ph.D. Copyright © 1999 by Monica Ramirez Basco. All rights reserved.

Chapter Four: p. 80 (Figure 4-1) Data from the Wirthlin Report; **pp. 92–93 (Star Box),** Copyright 1986, USA Today, excerpted with permission, art by Donald O'Connor; **p. 96, (Table 4-1),** Prentice, WE: *Fitness for college and life.* ed. 5; New York, 1997, McGraw Hill; **pp. 101–102 (Personal Assessment),** Data from the National Fitness Foundation.

Chapter Five: p. 118 (Table 5-2), Modified from Food and Nutrition Board, National Research Council: *Recommended dietary allowances,* ed. 10, Washington DC, 1989, National Academy of Sciences; **pp. 121–122 (Table 5-5),** US Department of Agriculture; **pp. 126–127 (Figure 5-4),** Data from US Food and Drug Administration and Wardlow G, Insel P: *Perspectives in Nutrition,* ed 3, St. Louis, 1986, Mosby.; **p. 133 (Figure 5-5),** US Department of Agriculture. **p. 141 (Personal Assessment)** From *Nutrition for a healthy life,* Courtesy of March Leeds.

Chapter Six: p. 148 (Table 6-1) Reprinted with permission of Metropolitan Life Insurance Company; **p. 149 (Table 6-2)** Based on data from Bannister EW, Brown SR: The relative energy requirements of physical activity. In HB Falls, editor: *Exercise physiology,* New York, 1968; **p. 184 (Figure 6-4),** Opinion Research Institue for *Simply Lite Foods;* **pp. 160–161 (Table 6-4),** Adapted from Guthrie H: Introductory nutrition, ed 7, St. Louis, 1989, Mosby.

Chapter Seven: p. 190 (Table 7-1), Modified from Muncie Star © 1987. Reprinted with permission. **p. 237 (Figure 7-2),** Source: American Management Association Survey; **p. 205 (Personal Assessment),** US Department of Education, A parent's guide to prevention.

Chapter Eight: p. 214 (Figure 8-2), Data from Core Institute: *2000 Statistics on alcohol and other drug use on American campuses,* Center for Alcohol and other Drug Studies, Student Health Programs, Southern Illinois University at Carbondale, 2000; **p. 216 (Figure 8-3),** Feldman, Understanding Psychology 5e, 2002, McGraw-Hill; **p. 218 (Figure 8-4),** From Wardlaw G: Perspectives in nutrition, ed 3, St. Louis, Mosby; **p. 224 (Changing for the Better),** Modified from brochure of the Indiana Alcohol Countermeasure Program; **p. 233 (Personal Assessment),** From *Are You Troubled by someone's drinking?* 1980, by Al-Anon Family Group Headquarters, Inc. Reprinted by permission of Al-Anon Family Group Headquarters, Inc.

Chapter Nine: p. 271 (Table 9-1), Data from *MMWR* 1999, 48(45): 1034–1039 and *MMWR* 2000, 49(SS-2):1-60; **p. 267 (Personal Assessment),** Reproduced with permission of the American Cancer Society.

Chapter Ten: p. 270 (Table 10-1) and **p. 271 (Figure 10-1),** Data from American Heart Association, *2001 Heart and stroke statistical update,* 2000, The Association; **p. 277 (Figure 10-3),** Reproduced with permission, © 1988, American Heart Association: Heart Facts; **p. 280 (Figure 10-4),** 1990 *Heart facts,* art by Donald O'Connor; **p. 291 (Personal Assessment),** From Howard E: *Health risks,* Tucson, 1985, Body Press.

Chapter Eleven: p. 296 (Figure 11-1), Data from National Cancer Institute: Horizons of cancer research, NIH Pub. No. 89-3011 © 1989; **pp. 300, 303, 309 (Changing for the Better),** American Cancer Society; **p. 313 (Changing for the Better),** Courtesy of the American Academy of Dermatology; **p. 327 (Personal Assessment),** American Cancer Society.

Chapter Twelve: p. 361 (Personal Assessment), Centers for Disease Control and Prevention, Atlanta.

Chapter Fourteen: p. 398 (Table 14-1), Adapted from Hatcher et al., *Contraceptive technology.* 17th rev. ed., 1998, Ardent Media, Inc; **p. 427 (Personal Assessment),** From Haas K, Haas A: Understanding sexuality, ed. 3, St. Louis, 1993, Mosby.

Chapter Fifteen: p. 435 (Changing for the Better), Source: Pell, AR: *Making the most of Medicare,* DCI Publishing, 1990, in insynch, Erie PA Spring 1994, Erie Insurance.

Chapter Sixteen: p. 463 (Figure 16-1), Courtesy of the National Committee to Prevent Child Abuse, Chicago, IL; **p. 470 (Changing for the Better),** From the American college Health Association; **p. 473 (Figure 16-2),** National Safety Council; **p. 475 (Changing for the Better),** Adapted from Pynoos J, Cohen E: *Creative ideas for a safe and livable home,* Washington DC, American Association of Retired Persons, 1992, and Van Tassel D: *Home safe home,* St. Louis, 1996, GenCare Health Systems.

Chapter Seventeen: p. 495 (Figure 17-2), Environmental Protection Agency.

Photo Credits

Chapter 1 p. 8, Ryan McVay/PhotoDisc/Getty Images; p. 14, Digital Vision; p. 16, Don Farrall/PhotoDisc/Getty Images

Chapter 2 p. 28, Buccina Studios/PhotoDisc/Getty Images; p. 34, Mel Curtis/PhotoDisc/Getty Images

Chapter 3 p. 61, PhotoLink/PhotoDisc/Getty Images; p. 62, Keith Brofsky/PhotoDisc/Getty Images; p. 66, Ryan McVay/PhotoDisc/Getty Images

Chapter 4 p. 84, Ryan McVay/Getty Images/PhotoDisc; p. 87, Ryan McVay/PhotoDisc/Getty Images; p. 92, Ryan McVay/PhotoDisc/Getty Images; p. 93, Ryan McVay/PhotoDisc/Getty Images; p. 96, Courtesy Stewart Halperin; p. 102, Ryan McVay/PhotoDisc/Getty Images; p. 105, Courtesy Stewart Halperin; p. 106, Courtesy Stewart Halperin

Chapter 5 p. 116, Ryan McVay/PhotoDisc/Getty Images; p. 125, © Royalty-Free/Corbis; p. 132, Ryan McVay/PhotoDisc/Getty Images

Chapter 6 p. 147, Suza Scalora/PhotoDisc/Getty Images; p. 150, © Custom Medical Stock Photo; p. 155, Ryan McVay/PhotoDisc/Getty Images; p. 166, Jack Star/PhotoLink/PhotoDisc/Getty Images

Chapter 7 p. 186, Image100; p. 191, PhotoDisc/Getty Images; p. 193, Jack Star/PhotoLink/PhotoDisc/Getty Images; p. 196, © The Cover Story/Corbis

Chapter 8 p. 211, Jim Arbogast/PhotoDisc/Getty Images; p. 212, SW Productions/PhotoDisc/Getty Images; p. 219T, © George Steinmetz; p. 219B, Courtesy Mothers Against Drunk Driving

Chapter 9 p. 241, Jack Star/PhotoLink/PhotoDisc/Getty Images; p. 245, © Royalty-Free/Corbis; p. 250, Courtesy Wayne Jackson; p. 253, © Photick/Superstock

Chapter 10 p. 271, Karl Weatherley/PhotoDisc/Getty Images; p. 275, Ryan McVay/PhotoDisc/Getty Images; p. 283, Keith Brofsky/PhotoDisc/Getty Images; p. 288, Ryan McVay/PhotoDisc/Getty Images

Chapter 11 p. 301, © Kevin Laubacher/Getty Images/Taxi; p. 312, From Thibodeau G., Patton, K. Anatomy and Physiology, 3/e, St. Louis, 1996. Mosby

Chapter 12 p. 338, Janis Christie/PhotoDisc/Getty Images; p. 352, © Phototake; p. 353, © Custom Medical Stock Photo

Chapter 13 p. 367, Digital Vision; p. 385, Buccina Studios/PhotoDisc/Getty Images; p. 389, Digital Vision

Chapter 14 p. 401, 402T, Courtesy Stewart Halperin; p. 402B, Linsley Photographics; p. 404, © Laura J.; p. Edwards; p. 405L, Laura J. Edwards; p. 405R, Courtesy Stewart Halperin; p. 406, Courtesy of Alza Corp.; p. 409, Courtesy Organon USA

Chapter 15 p. 434, Ryan McVay/PhotoDisc/Getty Images; p. 437, Anthony Saint James/PhotoDisc/Getty Images

Chapter 16 p. 470, Mitch Hrdlicka/PhotoDisc/Getty Images; p. 472, Ryan McVay/PhotoDisc/Getty Images; p. 474, Ryan McVay/PhotoDisc/Getty Images

Chapter 17 p. 490, Nick Koudis/Getty Images/PhotoDisc; p. 494, Kent Knudson/Getty Images/PhotoDisc; p. 501, Digital Vision; p. 502, Tomi/PhotoLink/Getty Images/PhotoDisc

Obsessive-compulsive disorder (OCD), 38, 39
Occupation, and cancer, 313–314
Older adults
    exercise, 92–93
    home safety, 473–474
    infectious disease, 337
    maltreatment, 462–463
    nutrition, 134
    prescription drug abuse, 203–204
    sexuality, 380
    sleep, 99
Olive oil, in Mediterranean Pyramid, 162
Oncogenes, 295
Online information. *See* Internet
Oogenesis, 372
Oophorectomy, prophylactic, 307
Opoids, 203
Opportunistic infections, 346
Optimism, 30–32
Optometrists, 440
Oral cancer, 255
Oral contraceptives, 254, 398, 406–408
Oral sex, 379
Organ donation, 449
Organic food labels, 124
Organizations
    consumer advocacy, 433
    environmental and population control, 503
    for responsible drinking, 222–223
Orgasm, 370
Orgasmic platform, 370
Orgasmic stage, of sexual response, 374, 376
Orlistat, 165
Orthodontics, 439
Osteoarthritis, 88
Osteopathy, 436
Osteoporosis, 87–88, 100
Outercourse, 396–397
Ovarian cancer, 306–307
Ovariectomy, 411
Ovaries, 372
Overload principle, 84–85
Over-the-counter (OTC) drugs, 447–448
Overweight, 146, 147, 154, 276. *See also* Obesity
Oviducts, 372, 373
Ovolactovegetarian diet, 132
Ovulation, 373
Oxidation rate, alcohol, 215
OxyContin, 197–198
Oxygen debt, 83

P
P53 gene, 295
Pancreatic cancer, 310
Panic disorder, 38, 39
Pap test, 300, 304, 305
Paracervical anesthetic, 411
ParaGard IUD, 398, 406
Parasitic worms, and infectious diseases, 331
Parenting, surrogate, 420
Partial-birth abortion, 413
Particulate matter, as air pollution source, 493–494
Particulate phase, of tobacco smoke, 246
Parties, and alcohol abuse, 221–222, 224
Part-time smokers, 241

Passionate love, 381, 383
Passive immunity, 335
Passive smoking, 255–257, 274
Passively acquired immunity, 334
Pasta, 107
Patellofemoral knee pain, 99
Pathogens, and infectious diseases, 330–331
Patient education, 21, 431
Patients' institutional rights, 442–443
PCP (phencyclidine), 195
Peak smokers, 242
Peckman, Jeff, 73
Pelvic inflammatory disease (PID), 351, 401, 406
Penis, 370
Pennebaker, James W., 58
Perfectionism, 63–64, 79
Pericarditis, 286
Periodic abstinence, as birth control method, 398, 399–401
Periodontal disease, and smokeless tobacco, 254
Peripheral artery disease, 286
Peritonitis, 351
Permanence, as attribution style dimension, 31
Personal environment, 484–492
Personal space, 29
Personalization, as attribution style dimension, 31–32
Pervasiveness, as attribution style dimension, 31
Pesco-vegetarian diet, 132
Pesticides, agricultural, 496
Pets, and stress management, 67
Phencyclidine (PCP), 195
Phenfen, 164
Phentermine, 164
Phenylpropanolamine, 164
Phlebitis, 286
Physical activity. *See also* Exercise
    and cardiovascular disease, 275
    defined, 82
    encouraging in children, 269
    and obesity, 155
Physical dependence, 188–189
Physical fitness, 81–106
    assessing, 105–106
    of children, 81, 98
    components, 83–87
    conditioning, 92
    cooldown, 92
    defined, 82
    program for, 88–92
    and sleep, 98–99
    warm-up, 92
Physical health, 16
Physical intervention, for weight management, 164–165
Physicians, 435, 436
Physiological dependence, 203
Physiological factors, in obesity, 151–152
Phytochemicals, 120, 123
Picovir, 339
Pipe smoking, 239–240
Placebo pills, 406
Placenta, 217, 418
Planned Parenthood Federation of America, 395–396, 420

Plaque, 277
Plasma cells, 335, 336
Plateau stage, of sexual response, 374, 375
Platelet adhesiveness, and nicotine, 249
Platonic cohabitation, 384
Pleconaril, 339
PMS (premenstrual syndrome), 373–374
Pneumococcal infection immunization, 337, 338
Pneumocystis carinii, 340
Pneumonia, 340
Podiatrists, 440
Point sources of pollution, 493, 495
Polio immunization, 337
Pollution
    air, 489, 492–495
    land, 496–497
    noise, 491–492
    nonpoint sources, 493, 495
    point sources, 493, 495
    water, 495–496
Polyps, 309
Polysaccharides, 109, 110
Population explosion, 499–500, 503
Portal of entry, and chain of infection, 332
Portal of exit, and chain of infection, 331–332
Portion control, 159, 175–177
Positive caloric balance, 146
Post-abortion syndrome, 413
Postovulation phase, of menstrual cycle, 373
Postpartum, defined, 418
Post-traumatic stress syndrome, 468
Posture, body, 29, 30
Potentiated effect, 198
Power line safety, 508
Precontemplation stage, of change, 9
Preemptive abortion, 411
Preferred provider organizations (PPOs), 445
Pregnancy, 414
    and alcohol use, 217–218, 219
    ectopic, 253, 408
    exercise during, 102–103
    signs of, 416
    and smoking, 253
    weight gain in, 152
Premeasured food plans, 161
Premenstrual syndrome (PMS), 373–374
Preovulation phase, of menstrual cycle, 373
Preparation stage, of change, 9
Prepuce, 370
Prescription drugs, 187, 203–204, 445, 446–447
President's Council on Physical Fitness and Sports, 105–106
Preventive medicine, 5–6, 435–436
Primary care health providers, 435
Prion, and infectious diseases, 331
Private hospitals, 441–442
Proactive approach to life, 32–33
Probiotics, 120, 123
Prochaska's Stages of Change, 9
Procrastination, 63
Procreation, 379
Prodromal stage, of infection, 333
Professional journals, as health information source, 3
Professional nurses, 440
Progestasert IUD, 406

health reference guide

Emotional Health

American Psychological Association
750 First Street, NE
Washington, DC 20002-4242
(202) 336-5500
www.apa.org

National Institute of Mental Health
Public Inquiries Branch
6001 Executive Boulevard
Room 8184 MSC 9663
Bethesda, MD 20892-9663
(301) 443-4513
www.nimh.nih.gov

National Mental Health Association
1021 Prince Street
Alexandra, VA 22314
(800) 969-NMHA
(703) 684-7722
(800) 433-5959 (TTY)
(416) 484-7750 (in Canada)
www.nmha.org

Fitness and Nutrition

American College of Sports Medicine
401 W. Michigan Street
Indianapolis, IN 46202-3233
(317) 637-9200
www.acsm.org

National Eating Disorders Association
603 Stewart St., Suite 803,
Seattle, WA 98101
(206) 382-3587
(800) 931-2237
www.nationaleatingdisorders.org

President's Council on Physical Fitness and Sports
Department W
200 Independence Ave., SW
Room 738-H
Washington, D.C. 20201-0004
(202) 690-9000
www.fitness.gov

Substance Abuse

Al-Anon Family Group Headquarters, Inc.
1600 Corporate Landing Parkway
Virginia Beach, VA 23454-5617
(757) 563-1600
www.al-anon.alateen.org

Alcoholics Anonymous
Grand Central Station
P.O. Box 459
New York, N.Y. 10163
(212) 870-3400
www.alcoholics-anonymous.org

Mothers Against Drunk Driving (MADD)
MADD National Office
511 E. John Carpenter Frwy. Suite 700
Irving, TX 75062
800-GET-MADD (438-6233)
www.madd.org/home

National Council on Alcoholism and Drug Dependence, Inc.
20 Exchange Place, Suite 2902
New York, NY 10005
800/NCA-CALL (24-hour referral)
www.ncadd.org

Remove Intoxicated Drivers (RID)
P.O. Box 520
Schenectady, NY 12301
(518) 393-HELP (4357)
www.rid-usa.org

Students Against Destructive Decisions (founded as Students Against Drunk Driving)
SADD National
P.O. Box 800
Marlborough, MA 01752
(877) SADD-INC
www.saddonline.com

Conditions and Diseases

American Social Health Association
P.O. Box 13827
Research Triangle Park, NC 27709
(919) 361-8400
www.ashastd.org

American Cancer Society
(800)-ACS-2345
www.cancer.org

American Diabetes Association
1701 North Beauregard Street
Alexandria, VA 22311
(800) DIABETES (342-2383)
www.diabetes.org

American Heart Association
7272 Greenville Avenue
Dallas, TX 75231
(800) AHA-USA-1 (242-8721)
www.americanheart.org

American Lung Association
61 Broadway, 6th Floor
New York, New York 10006
(800) LUNG-USA (586-4872)
www.lungusa.org

American Red Cross National Headquarters
2025 E Street, NW
Washington, DC 20006
(800) 435 7669
www.redcross.org

Asthma and Allergy Foundation of America (AAFA)
1233 20th Street, NW, Suite 402,
Washington, D.C. 20036
(800) 7-ASTHMA
www.aafa.org

Centers for Disease Control and Prevention
1600 Clifton Road
Atlanta, GA 30333
(800) 311-3435
www.cdc.gov

Juvenile Diabetes Research Foundation International
120 Wall Street
New York, NY 10005-4001
(800) 533-CURE (2873)
www.jdrf.org

Leukemia & Lymphoma Society
1311 Mamaroneck Ave.
White Plains, NY 10605
(800) 955-4572
www.leukemia-lymphoma.org

March of Dimes
1275 Mamaroneck Avenue
White Plains, NY 10605
www.marchofdimes.com

MedicAlert Foundation International
2323 Colorado Avenue
Turlock, CA 95382
(888) 633-4298
(209) 668-3333 from outside the U.S.
www.medicalert.org

National Headache Foundation
820 N. Orleans, Suite 217
Chicago, IL 60610
(888) NHF-5552
www.headaches.org

National Multiple Sclerosis Society
733 Third Avenue
New York, NY 10017
(800) Fight MS (344-4867)
www.nationalmssociety.org

**National Organization for
Rare Disorders**
55 Kenosia Avenue
PO Box 1968
Danbury, CT 06813-1968
(800) 999-6673 (voicemail only)
(203) 797-9590 (TDD Number)
www.rarediseases.org/

Project Inform
*Information, Advocacy, Inspiration for
People Living with HIV/AIDS*
205 13th Street, #2001
San Francisco, CA 94103
(800) 822-7422
(415) 558-9051 (in the San Francisco Bay
Area and internationally)
www.projinf.org

**Sickle Cell Disease Association of
America, Inc.**
200 Corporate Pointe, Suite 495
Culver City California 90230-8727
(800) 421-8453
www.sicklecelldisease.org

**Y-ME National Breast Cancer
Organization**
212 W. Van Buren, Suite 1000
Chicago, IL 60607-3908
(800) 221-2141
www.y-me.org

Sexuality, The Family, and Fertility Control

Childhelp USA® National Headquarters
15757 N. 78th Street
Scottsdale, Arizona 85260
(800) 4-A-CHILD (422-4453)
www.childhelpusa.org

National Abortion Federation – NAF
1755 Massachusetts Avenue
Suite 600
Washington, DC 20036
(877) 772-9100
www.prochoice.org

**National Center for Missing &
Exploited Children**
Charles B. Wang International Children's
Building
699 Prince Street
Alexandria, Virginia 22314-3175
(800) the-lost (843-5678)
www.ncmec.org

National Runaway Switchboard
3080 N. Lincoln Ave.
Chicago, IL 60657
(773) 880-9860
www.nrscrisisline.org

Prevent Child Abuse America
200 S. Michigan Avenue, 17th Floor
Chicago, IL 60604-2404
(312) 663-3520
www.preventchildabuse.org

Parents Anonymous Inc.
675 West Foothill Blvd., Suite 220
Claremont, CA 91711-3475
(909) 621-6184
www.parentsanonymous.org

Parents Without Partners, Inc.
1650 South Dixie Highway, Suite 510
Boca Raton, FL 33432
(561) 391-8833
www.parentswithoutpartners.org

**Planned Parenthood Federation
of America**
434 West 33rd St.
New York, NY 10001
(800) 230-PLAN
www.plannedparenthood.org

**Rape, Abuse & Incest National
Network (RAINN)**
635-B Pennsylvania Ave., SE
Washington, DC 20003
(800) 656-HOPE
www.rainn.org

Sudden Infant Death Syndrome Alliance
1314 Bedford Avenue, Suite 210
Baltimore, Maryland 21208
(800) 221-7437
www.sidsalliance.org

Consumer Safety

**National Highway Traffic Safety
Administration**
(888) DASH-2-DOT (327-4236)
http://www.nhtsa.dot.gov

**U.S. Consumer Product Safety
Commission**
4330 East-West Highway
Bethesda, Maryland 20814-4408
(800) 638-2772
(800) 638-8270 (TTY).
www.cpsc.gov

The Maturing Adult

Alzheimer's Association National Office
225 N. Michigan Ave., Fl. 17
Chicago, IL 60601
(800) 272-3900
www.alz.org

**American Association of Retired
People (AARP)**
601 E. Street NW
Washington, DC 20049
(888) OUR-AARP (687-2277)
www.aarp.org

Arthritis Consulting Services, Inc
2787 East Oakland Park Blvd.
Suite #204
Ft. Lauderdale, Florida 33306
(800) 327-3027
(954) 739-3202
www.stoparthritis.com

Partnership for Caring
1620 Eye Street NW, Suite 202,
Washington, DC 20006
(800) 989-9455
(202) 296-8071
www.partnershipforcaring.org

United Network for Organ Sharing
Post Office Box 2484
Richmond, Virginia 23218
(888) 894-6361
www.unos.org

NOTE: Check your local directory for
additional information on poison control,
suicide prevention, Social Security, and
for additional resources.